Practical Diabetes Care

Practical Diabetes Care

FOURTH EDITION

David Levy MD FRCP

Formerly Consultant Physician, Barts Health NHS Trust, Whipps Cross University Hospital, London
The London Diabetes Centre, Marylebone, London

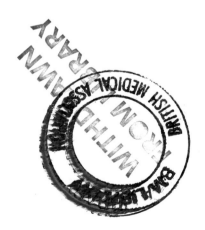

WILEY Blackwell

Registered Office(s)
John Wiley & Sons, Inc., 111 River Street, Hoboken, NJ 07030, USA
John Wiley & Sons Ltd, The Atrium, Southern Gate, Chichester, West Sussex, PO19 8SQ, UK

Editorial Office
9600 Garsington Road, Oxford, OX4 2DQ, UK
For details of our global editorial offices, customer services, and more information about Wiley products visit us at www.wiley.com.

Wiley also publishes its books in a variety of electronic formats and by print-on-demand. Some content that appears in standard print versions of this book may not be available in other formats.

Library of Congress Cataloging-in-Publication Data
Names: Levy, David, 1954– author.
Title: Practical diabetes care / by David Levy.
Description: Fourth edition. | Hoboken, NJ : Wiley, 2017. | Includes
    bibliographical references and index. |
Identifiers: LCCN 2017040598 (print) | LCCN 2017041148 (ebook) | ISBN
    9781119052234 (pdf) | ISBN 9781119052227 (epub) | ISBN 9781119052241 (pbk.)
Subjects: | MESH: Diabetes Mellitus–therapy | Diabetes Mellitus–diagnosis
Classification: LCC RC660 (ebook) | LCC RC660 (print) | NLM WK 815 | DDC
    616.4/62–dc23
LC record available at https://lccn.loc.gov/2017040598

Cover design: Wiley
Cover image: Courtesy of David Levy

Set in 8.5/10.5pt Frutiger by SPi Global, Pondicherry, India
Printed and bound in Malaysia by Vivar Printing Sdn Bhd

10 9 8 7 6 5 4 3 2 1

Contents

Acknowledgments

This book's peer reviewers have added clarity, focus and critical detail and have been astonishingly sweet and supportive. Without their clear advice I would have blundered up several, possibly many, more medical garden paths leading to cul-de-sacs all named Embarrassment Drive. I applaud their directionality and comradely scholarship.

My dear long-time friend and colleague Dr Tore Julsrud Berg (Oslo University Hospitals) reviewed Chapter 1 (Classification) and the two chapters on Type 1 diabetes (Chapters 7 and 8). Everything I have written over the years on Type 1 diabetes has been improved by his patience and encouragement. I can only aspire to his intense pragmatism combined with academic rigour (and to the wonderful modernist Oslo house meticulously treasured and preserved by Tore and his wife, Anne Valle).

Dr Edouard Mills, a specialist registrar in endocrinology who previously worked with me during his foundation training, meticulously and thoughtfully reviewed Chapter 2 (Diabetes emergencies) and Chapter 11 (Hypertension).

Dr Albert Mifsud gently chided and guided me about antibiotics in diabetic infections (Chapter 3) with the same patience my late colleague Dr Louise Neville had shown in earlier editions. I hope there are no remnants in the text of our intellectual fist-fights on the Whipps Cross wards (and many years ago at the Central Middlesex Hospital) – both part of the great outer circle of University Hospitals in London whose heyday of teaching, research and clinical care from the end of World War II up to the 1980s has been eclipsed by progressive resource starvation and massively increased clinical stresses over the past two decades.

Professor Miles Fisher, coiner of one of the great aphorisms of diabetes, reviewed Chapter 6 (Diabetes and the cardiovascular system) with the same speed and efficiency with which he no doubt traverses the glens of his native country by bike.

Helen Alston, specialist registrar in nephrology, brought me up to date on many renal secrets.

Carin Hume, a wonderfully practical dietician at London Medical who inhabits the real world of dietetics, even allowed me to pursue higher protein, lower carbohydrate diets in Chapter 8.

Professor Alan Sinclair, doyen of diabetes care in older people, forgave me the mere hemi-chapter I devoted to his critical subject (Chapter 14) and reminded me about the pervasive impact of frailty in older people with diabetes.

Dr Nicoletta Dozio and Dr Marina Scavini of the Diabetes Research Institute of San Raffaele Hospital in Milan helped with all the sections of the book relating to diabetes and pregnancy. Wonderful stays at Nicoletta's and Stefano's beautiful palazzo in Merate undoubtedly increased my retention rate of key facts in an area of diabetes practice that continues to be neglected by clinicians in primary and secondary care.

Professor Karim Meeran (Imperial Centre for Endocrinology) kindly provided me with access to the invaluable online manual of endocrine test protocols. He is happy to share the intranet link with all readers:

http://imperialendo.co.uk

Pretty well every paragraph of this book owes any breadth and new insight to Timo Pilgram, Senior Library Assistant at Whipps Cross University Hospital. Every reference I requested (and a lot of illustrations) pinged into my inbox in full text form within a few hours, sometimes minutes; but more important, dozens of references that I would never have found using my kindergarten skills in Boolean logic are here because of Timo's pure talents of modern librarianship, combined with curiosity and tenacity and seemingly unlimited manoeuvrability around the internet, shared by few clinicians. Imagination and new stories (as they now say everywhere) are possible only when these startling skills combust slightly after catalysis by the tiniest addition of serendipity. He deserves to be a co-author. More generally, librarianship in hospitals, just like libraries in the community, is inevitably an easy target of cost-cutting. Ensure, at least, that before they disappear from your own institution you understand their continuing centrality to the pursuit of modern medical thinking.

Most of the writing was done during 2016. My wife, Laura Liew, left me during the first nine months to gain a Grande Diplôme in cuisine and patisserie at the London Cordon Bleu School in Bloomsbury Square. Most days I could sit and write for twelve hours, by which time Laura had returned, usually exhausted, with a take-away box containing a French dish of staggering complexity and subtlety that had been the product of her industry and rigorous supervision and assessment by the teaching chefs. Practical Diabetes Care by day, lobster Thermidor for dinner: the haute cuisine recipe for extracting the best possible performance from an author. I thoroughly commend it.

Introduction

Excuses normally round off the preface, but I owe readers some up-front explanations: for a fourth edition that's at least three times weightier than the original of eighteen years ago, and one still penned by a single author. As to the first, maturity doesn't always bring concision and simplification (in music Brahms managed it, Schoenberg and Berg brought it to a state of crystalline perfection, but Wagner certainly didn't), and the relatively terse bulleted form (if not style) I managed in the dash to the millennium has yielded, through normal aging and a desire to try and write real sentences, to a more discursive approach. Recognizing the hazards to readers' patience, this new edition is riddled with Practice Points, which I hope are useful, in addition to the usual burden of devices (boxes, tables, figures etc.) that I suspect are the 21st century equivalent of the ornate Victorian section marker, and probably command a similar degree of attention.

A second problem, more substantive, is whether a single-author book has any meaning in the new world (let's set aside the equally important matters of books versus electronics, and textbooks versus monographs). In a tepid review of the last edition someone wondered (I paraphrase) how I had the brass neck to invade territory such as diet therapy in diabetes. But the reviewer made a minor category error in his understandable defence of a non-medical area, which I suspect he felt had been traduced by someone he considered a typical arrogant hospital doctor: his argument should have applied with at least equal force to the sections on cardiology, psychology and bits of pathophysiology for that matter. But of these other territorial meanderings there was no mention.

The conventional resolution is superficially simple: do multi-author, much as now everything is done multidisciplinary. There are wonderful multi-author books (as I write this, the *Textbook of Diabetes*, edited by Richard Holt and colleagues has reached its fifth edition, and from the same publisher the fourth edition of the wide-ranging *International Textbook of Diabetes*) and I have huge admiration for any editor brave enough to grapple with the stylistic lurchings and lumpy content that can gravitate to pet and hobby-horse topics of individual chapter authors. But probably through a combination of real and perceived pressures to comply the writing often homogenizes to standard passive academic prose, fuelled by the output of the meta-analysis industrial complex (of which more shortly) with a persistent risk of imbalance both within and between chapters, in addition to the risk of trying to update the non-updatable, when the best option, probably involving little more work, is to start from scratch.

I've gone for the easy options. First, I've restructured the contents and completely rewritten the book, strategies I hope have helped expunge old and less-relevant material. For example, I have now twinned diabetic eye disease with renal disease in the same chapter, and continued to de-emphasize the details of retinopathy, as the UK screening programme has – fortunately – taken over from individual doctors attempting to wield an ancient and non-illuminating ophthalmoscope in vaguely the right direction. Type 1 diabetes, now more commonly encountered in primary care, has a fully deserved greater prominence and there is a separate new chapter on technology, which of course is already out of date. More patients and even some practitioners are emphasizing the increasing evidence-base of non-pharmacological interventions in Type 2 diabetes, and

I have enjoyed elaborating the fascinating detail emerging in diet, weight loss and exercise. The chapter on the pharmacological treatment of Type 2 diabetes has also, despite my best efforts, expanded. This is not just because new agents have been introduced since the last edition in 2011 but we now have more evidence that helps us place classes of drugs more precisely than before. However, more than ever we must maintain a balanced approach to medication in relation to the wishes of patients and the burgeoning cost of new drugs, especially when used in combination. The trial portfolios that now accompany the launch of a new agent or insulin (some so self-important they have their own registered trademark) comprise bewildering numbers of individual studies, some of which explore minute gaps in therapeutic combinations that may not have occurred even to experienced practitioners. Superior brains might not make it to the end of the titles of some of the more rococo comparisons. Second, I have asked trusted colleagues to review some chapters and to deploy the electronic equivalent of the blue pencil. They deserve their more prominent place, and my thanks, in Acknowledgments rather than as another afterthought to the Introduction.

A fourth edition of any book should, above all, prompt general reflection, now a ubiquitous box-ticking requirement in appraisal and revalidation and therefore another thoroughly diminished component of our professional life. But let me explain one characteristic – increased true scepticism – that I hope the careful reader will detect throughout the book. During the first half of the first decade of the 2000s I was a strong advocate of the now largely discredited glitazone drugs. We'd already had a warning in the later 1990s: the first agent, troglitazone was a cause of fatal liver disease and in the United Kingdom was withdrawn within weeks of launch but it remained available elsewhere far too long. This terrible outcome, attributed to a pharmacologically gratuitous addition of a supposedly anti-oxidant vitamin moiety to the molecule, served to de-focus concerns about other, more widespread adverse effects, and when the two follow-on drugs, rosiglitazone and pioglitazone, were introduced in 1999, battle was joined: not in scrutinizing with greater ferocity their pros and cons but regrettably in a largely commercial feud around antiatherosclerotic actions and minutiae of differences in achieved lipid profiles, the aspirations of all of which disappeared in a puff of non-significances in clinical trial outcomes. At the same time we didn't yet have the results of the mega-trials of the middle and latter part of the decade and therefore hadn't properly understood the limited importance to patients of what were – and still are – relatively small changes in glucose levels in comparison with the clinical evidence of substantial weight gain, oedema and possible heart failure, and trial data of increased risk of fractures and anaemia. Statistical nit-picking still rumbles on over the possible increased risk of bladder malignancy with pioglitazone, at the same time as the drug itself is no longer prescribed.

In 2007, Nissen and Wolski published highly suggestive but contested meta-analyses raising further concerns, this time about increased cardiovascular risk associated with rosiglitazone; but groaning under an increasing burden of adverse effects the prescribing status of rosiglitazone was not changed until 2009. The combined belief system, that glycaemia is still of primary importance in the Type 2 syndrome, and that improvements in intermediate measures of atherosclerosis somehow meant something for patients, still hasn't been confined to its proper speculative place, and after a few years of relative calm, the potential antiatherosclerotic effects of the newest antihyperglycaemic agents are still eliciting hyper-excitable responses. As a result of all this activity, I hope you will detect a much more cautious and a properly critical approach to all drugs, including the seemingly interminable battle for supremacy over long-acting analogue insulins, which is tiresome after witnessing nearly two decades of angels and camels alike struggling for pole position at the extremities of small sharp structures, but clearly distracts from much more important and eminently fixable matters, especially in Type 1 diabetes, and has made the management of insulin-treated diabetes in the USA a nightmare for many patients because of cost. I am grateful for the thoughtful approach of Edwin Gale and John Yudkin, long-time techno- and pharma-cynics, for activating my own concerns. We're only a few years away from the centenary of the first use of insulin, and I don't think the heroic early clinicians would be much impressed with our persistent bickering over minute differences in nocturnal hypoglycaemia rates with long-acting analogues to try and convince ourselves and our patients that they are in any meaningful way better than NPH insulin. The more the arguments, the more it becomes clear that the superiority of a furiously defended insulin preparation is irrelevant compared with the way we work with patients to use insulin.

Two further concerns can probably be detected. First, the invasion of our medical lives by the increasingly raucous onslaught of systematic review and meta-analysis, which some commentators now believe is distorting research priorities. Evidence-based medicine, the broad principles of which we all subscribe to, is now within striking distance of being considered coterminous with systematic review and meta-analysis; that is, meta-analysis is moving to a privileged position as the highest form of evidence-based medicine. It is of course an important component of the evidence base, but in clinical diabetes our most reliable source should be the well-conducted clinical trial, published in a high quality peer-reviewed journal, preferably with all the supplementary data readily accessible, because for a variety of reasons much important information is relegated to supplementary data files. Forest plots, even more than woods, obscure the beautiful structure of individual trees.

Second, more important, is the balance between opinion and evidence. We are rapidly shifting, again in part under the baleful influence of meta-analysis, to declaring opinion unnecessary, and in its strong form, hazardous. In turn, this perverse view was based on the now largely derided 'experience' without which, so the medical educationalists tell us, we can practice the highest quality medicine, so long as we have access to a smartphone, guidelines and do competent handovers. But in this sense medicine remains, frustratingly, way behind the times. In other fields we have passed peak 'objectivity'; to take another musical analogy, the radical 'early music' movement of the 1970s and 1980s, which celebrated baroque music as inflexible machine-music translated directly from the dots on the unencumbered urtext page, has moved to a proper accommodation between textual accuracy and recognition that Kapellmeister Bach and his musicians were likely to be no less affected by the emotional impact of his miraculous music than twenty-first century listeners. I have, therefore, attempted here to present balanced information with an occasional personal view. Don't ignore the former (or preferably look for more and contradictory material) but at least consider the latter – and then discard it. There shouldn't be much difficulty in spotting the difference between the two.

Another tangential advantage of a single-author work is that I have been able to zig-zag my way through the manuscript right up to the time of submission, adding new information and references supplied by colleagues and friends. Chapter 1 is, therefore, as dated as, but no more than, Chapter 15. PMID numbers will help you track down papers that do not have consistent citations by entering the eight-digit number into the PubMed search box. I have deliberately included as many papers as possible that are available as free full text, with their associated seven-digit PMC (PubMed Central) identifiers. In trawling through hundreds of references I have been struck by the widely differing practices of quality journals; without naming individual publications I don't think are behaving very well – which I would have dearly loved to do – let me applaud at least the *New England Journal of Medicine*, which seems to maximize the availability of free full text articles, and without the mendacity of imposing a year's delay or, even more pernicious, making available a 'printer-friendly' version that isn't so friendly when your printer churns out 50% more paper because the article isn't properly formatted. These matters are far from trivial. They include the converse situation, pharma companies presumably paying for immediate full-text availability of research papers that support the use of their new agents, and also the startlingly perverse practice of issuing grand consensus statements, of which there are unstoppable torrents, with no free full text availability. Such practices distort the availability of research and scholarship and risk adding substantial bias to our views.

Though I know I tormented Pri Gibbons, my patient editor at Wiley Blackwell, by exceeding our original agreed word count at least twofold and delivering it at least two years late, writing it has been therapeutic for me, and I hope will be entertaining in places for readers. In this edition, originally commissioned by Oliver Walter, I have been guided by the principles and practices of Stephen Pinker, one of the finest modern scientific writers. He suggests at least three full re-writes of manuscripts and encouraged me in my first attempt to rigorously avoid the 'curse of knowledge' – the infuriating and anti-educational practice of 'experts' writing as if every reader has immediate command of as much information as the author, thereby obviating its primary educational purpose. Everyone considering writing non-fiction should first read his magical blend of serious linguistics and hilarious examples of grotesque misuse of English in *The Sense of Style* (Pinker, 2015). I didn't regret doing so. If there is any graceful writing in the book it's mostly due to Pinker's benign influence.

The previous edition drew warm comments from friends and colleagues, and someone even claimed that five years on they were still referring to it, which is heartening but also a bit scary. It was wonderful to see copies of translations of the third edition into, among other languages, Polish and Chinese. The latter reminded me that the widely-repeated and mostly self-serving fib of the 'diabetes epidemic' in the West is almost certainly true when applied to South East Asia, and though the literature is shockingly slender, I have tried to include discussion and references relevant to that critically important part of the world. In general I hope that this edition has slightly more international relevance than the technocratic focus of the previous three.

There are lots and lots of books on diabetes, and many have 'Care' somewhere in the title. The word was included in the title of the third edition at the 'request' of Wiley Blackwell, because a senior editorial team felt that 'Practical Diabetes' (as the first two editions were titled) couldn't exist (I disagree: nobody would object to a book called plain 'Practical Plumbing' or even – I think there are many already – 'Practical Philosophy'. There is a good popular journal in the United Kingom called 'Practical Diabetes' that hasn't felt the need for the obligatory 'care' designation). It doesn't matter: it's on the 'Practical' that I would like this book to be judged. But a book designed to help practising healthcare professionals can't just be a recipe book (nor, of course, can a good recipe book). Some of the chapter reviewers felt that the introductory stuff was a little heavy on background material and numbers, and they may be right. But if this book, like its predecessors, helps practitioners think about sleek minimalism in management, while suggesting an occasional evidence-based trick that might shorten the journey time for some patients, then I don't mind too much if readers omit some of the introductory bits.

BMA Library

BMA House, Tavistock Square, London WC1H 9JP

British Medical Association
BMA House
Tavistock Square
London
WC1H 9JP

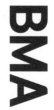

BMA

I'd love it if you could let me know about the balance from your viewpoint. But if you think it's pompous and doctor-ish, I'd like to be told as well. While a fifth edition recedes beyond some kind of event horizon, you never know.

David Levy
DavidLevyDM@gmail.com

Recommended reading

Pinker S (2015) *The Sense of Style: The Thinking Person's Guide to Writing in the 21st Century*. Penguin. ISBN: 978-0-241-95771-4.

Practical Diabetes Care is set in Frutiger, an elegant and clear Humanist sans-serif type-face designed in the mid-1970s by the Swiss typeface designer Adrian Frutiger (1928–2015). It is derived from a design first used in airport signs at Paris Charles de Gaulle in 1970–1. Together with Arial (1982) NHS Identity has adopted it as the only typeface permissible throughout the NHS, where it is used for all signage, and in its bold italic form, the NHS logotype itself.

Clinical trials and organizations: abbreviations and acronyms

Abbreviation/ acronym	Full title	Year of main trial publication	Notes
ACCOMPLISH	Avoiding Cardiovascular Events through Combination Therapy in Patients Living with Systolic Hypertension	2008	ACE-inhibitor + calcium channel blocker superior to ACE-inhibitor + thiazide for preventing CV events in high-risk hypertension.
ACCORD	Action to Control Cardiovascular Risk in Diabetes	2008	No advantage and possibly increased mortality in very tight glycaemic control (HbA$_{1c}$ 6.4% vs 7.5%) in Type 2. ACCORD BP study (2010): no micro/ macrovascular advantage in target SBP <120 vs 140 (slight benefit in progression of microalbuminuria). ACCORD LIPID (2010): no additional CV advantage of fenofibrate added to simvastatin.
ADA	American Diabetes Association	Founded 1940	
ADOPT	A Diabetes Outcome Progression Trial	2006	Durability of monotherapy in Type 2: rosiglitazone (withdrawn) > metformin > sulfonylurea.
ADVANCE	Action in Diabetes and Vascular Disease: Preterax And Modified-Release Controlled Evaluation	2008	No CV advantage with tight glycaemic control (HbA$_{1c}$ 6.3% vs 7.0%). Gliclazide was primary agent.
AIM-HIGH	Atherothrombosis Intervention in Metabolic Syndrome with Low HDL/High Triglycerides: Impact on Global Health Outcomes	2011	No CV advantage in adding niacin to statin (+ ezetimibe) in high-risk patients. A definitive study that effectively ended the clinical use of niacin in cardiovascular disease.

(Continued)

Abbreviation/ acronym	Full title	Year of main trial publication	Notes
ALLHAT	Antihypertensive and Lipid-Lowering Treatment to Prevent Heart Attack Trial	2002	A millennial blockbuster trial of initial monotherapy in hypertension. Amlodipine, chlortalidone and lisinopril had broadly similar CV outcomes. Doxazosin was discontinued because of lower efficacy.
ALTITUDE	Aliskiren Trial in Type 2 Diabetes Using Cardiorenal Endpoints	2012	Combination aliskiren (direct renin inhibitor) and angiotensin blockade did not reduce cardiac and renal endpoints, and increased the risk of hyperkalaemia and hypotension. Another study showing no benefit of dual angiotensin blockade.
ASCOT-BPLA	Anglo-Scandinavian Cardiac Outcomes Trial-Blood Pressure Lowering Arm	2005	β-blocker and bendroflumethiazide probably inferior in CV outcomes compared with amlodipine and perindopril. Modified-release doxazosin is effective for BP. The end of the era of β-blocker trials.
BASIL	Bypass versus Angioplasty in Severe Ischaemia of the Leg	2005	Initial angioplasty or bypass surgery in critical limb ischaemia have broadly similar outcomes, but surgery after failed angioplasty less successful than primary surgery – which still has a place.
CANVAS	Canagliflozin Cardiovascular Assessment Study	2017	Canagliflozin in high CV risk patients. 16% risk reduction in fatal cardiovascular events, non-fatal myocardial infarction or non-fatal stroke. Possible benefit on hard renal endpoints. Increased risk of toe amputations.
CARDS	Collaborative Atorvastatin Diabetes Study	2004	Major reductions in CV outcomes using atorvastatin 20 mg daily in Type 2 without overt vascular disease. Achieved LDL 2.0 mmol/l. Clear evidence for benefit of widespread statin treatment in Type 2.
CORAL	Cardiovascular Outcomes in Renal Atherosclerotic Lesions	2014	Renal artery stenting in systolic hypertension or CKD did not reduce cardiorenal endpoints compared with multimodal medical treatment.
DASH	Dietary Approaches to Stop Hypertension	1997	A pioneering study in lifestyle management of hypertension. Recommendations include: fruits, vegetables and low-fat dairy foods, and low total and saturated fat. In hypertensive people, mean systolic BP fall was 11 mm Hg.

Abbreviation/ acronym	Full title	Year of main trial publication	Notes
DIRECT	Dietary Intervention Randomized Controlled Trial	2008	In obesity weight loss was best maintained with a calorie-restricted Mediterranean diet or a non-calorie-restricted low-carbohydrate diet compared with a traditional low-fat restricted-calorie diet
DIRECT	Diabetic Retinopathy Candesartan Trials	2009	High-dose candesartan (32 mg daily) did not reduce progression of normo- to microalbuminuria in Type 1 or Type 2 diabetes. 'Prophylactic' angiotensin blockade does not prevent renal disease in normotension.
DCCT	Diabetes Control and Complications Trial	1993	Pivotal Type 1 trial. Risk of microvascular complications reduced by 50–75% after about 6 years of intensive control (HbA_{1c} 7%) compared with conventional control (HbA_{1c} 9%).
EASD	European Association for the Study of Diabetes	Founded 1965	
EDIC	Epidemiology of Diabetes Interventions and Complications	1994–	Continuing follow-up of the DCCT participants after randomization stopped. Continuing ('legacy') benefit of intensive control on microvascular complications, macrovascular events and all-cause mortality.
ELIXA	Evaluation of Lixisenatide in Acute Coronary Syndrome	2015	GLP-1-receptor analogue lixisenatide did not reduce event rates in Type 2 patients with recent acute coronary syndrome (see and compare LEADER).
EMPA-REG OUTCOME®	Empagliflozin, Cardiovascular Outcomes, and Mortality in Type 2 Diabetes	2015	Long-term trial of empagliflozin in Type 2 with advanced CV disease. Significant reduction in all-cause death, CV outcomes and heart failure admissions. No effect on stroke. Possibly the first clinical trial to have a registered trade-mark.
ESC	European Society of Cardiology	Founded 1950	
ESH	European Society of Hypertension	Founded 1989	
ETDRS	Early Treatment Diabetic Retinopathy Study		The Diabetic Retinopathy Study (1976) was the first to show that laser treatment preserved vision in proliferative retinopathy. Intervention at an earlier stage was not beneficial (ETDRS). The abbreviation remains as a widely-used scoring system for diabetic retinopathy.

(Continued)

Abbreviation/ acronym	Full title	Year of main trial publication	Notes
EURODIAB	EURODIAB IDDM Complications Study	1994	Epidemiological study of 3000 Type 1 (then 'IDDM') patients across Europe. A small embedded RCT (EUCLID) hinted that the ACE-inhibitor lisinopril may protect against development of retinopathy.
FIELD	Fenofibrate Intervention and Event Lowering in Diabetes	2005	The first of a series of important negative lipid trials, in this case the fibric acid drug fenofibrate, which did not reduce CV events except in the most insulin resistant group. Retinopathy and below-knee amputations were reduced.
FinnDiane	Finnish Diabetic Nephropathy study	2003–	Important longitudinal cohort study in Type 1 diabetes; main focus in diabetic renal disease, but many other topics covered, especially diet and activity.
FOURIER	Further Cardiovascular Outcomes Research with PCSK9 Inhibition in Subjects with Elevated Risk	2017	PCSK9 inhibitor evolocumab reduced CV events.
GISSI-HF	Gruppo Italiano per lo Studio della Streptochinasi nell'Infarto Miocardico – Heart Failure	2008	n-3 PUFA 1 g daily had small beneficial effect on death rate and hospital admissions in people with chronic heart failure (NYHA II-IV).
GISSI-Prevenzione	Gruppo Italiano per lo Studio della Streptochinasi nell'Infarto Miocardico – Prevenzione	1999	n-3 PUFA 1 g daily reduced CV death but not events in postmyocardial infarction patients. In this group moderate wine intake and advice on a Mediterranean diet were at least as effective as n-3 PUFA.
HPS	Heart Protection Study	2003	Simvastatin 40 mg daily for 5 years reduced major vascular events by about one-quarter in people with diabetes.
HPS2-THRIVE	Heart Protection Study 2–Treatment of HDL to Reduce the Incidence of Vascular Events	2014	Niacin did not reduce the risk of events in statin-treated people with established vascular disease and there was an increased risk of significant side effects. Another negative outcome trial for niacin therapy.
IDNT	Irbesartan Diabetic Nephropathy Trial	2001	Irbesartan and amlodipine were equally effective antihypertensive drugs in Type 2 nephropathy, but end-stage renal disease about one-quarter less likely with irbesartan treatment over 2½ years (see RENAAL).

Abbreviation/ acronym	Full title	Year of main trial publication	Notes
IDSA-IWGDF	Infectious Disease Society of America-International Working Group on the Diabetic Foot		USA guidelines on management of the diabetic foot.
IFCC	International Federation of Clinical Chemistry and Laboratory Medicine	1952	Body which introduced quantitative SI units (mmol/mol) for reporting of glycated haemoglobin measurements (full implementation in 2011 in UK; dual reporting with traditional DCCT % measurements continues in some countries).
IMPROVE-IT	Improved Reduction of Outcomes: Vytorin Efficacy International Trial	2015	Further risk reduction of 7% in CV endpoints when ezetimibe 10 mg daily was added to simvastatin 40 mg daily for 7 years in post-ACS patients. Mean achieved LDL 1.4 mmol/l, compared with 1.8 in simvastatin-treated patients.
JNC n	nth Report of the Joint National Committee on Prevention, Detection, Evaluation, and Treatment of High Blood pressure		Hypertension guidelines.
KDIGO	Kidney Disease: Improving Global Outcomes		Guidelines on managing renal disease issued by International Society of Nephrology. Novel heat map for risk stratification of renal disease using combined estimations of albuminuria and eGFR introduced in 2009.
LEADER	Liraglutide Effect and Action in Diabetes: Evaluation of Cardiovascular Outcome Results	2016	The GLP-1-receptor analogue liraglutide given for 4 years reduced some CV outcomes in Type 2 patients at high vascular risk.
LIFE	Losartan Intervention for Endpoint	2001	For the same antihypertensive effect losartan-based treatment reduced the risk of CV end-points more than atenolol.
Look AHEAD	Action for Health in Diabetes	2013	Ten years of intensive lifestyle intervention focusing on weight loss did not reduce CV events in Type 2 patients.
NHANES	National Health and Nutrition Examination Survey	Started early 1960s	Large-scale population-based health surveys in the USA.

(Continued)

Abbreviation/ acronym	Full title	Year of main trial publication	Notes
ONTARGET		2008	ACE-inhibitor + ARB reduced proteinuria more than ACE-inhibitor alone, but hard renal end-points more common with combined angiotensin blockade. Taken with results of ALTITUDE (q.v.): dual therapy of no benefit and consistently increased end-stage renal events and hyperkalaemia.
ORIGIN	Outcome Reduction with an Initial Glargine Intervention	2012	Insulin glargine given for 6 years in Type 2 diabetes and prediabetes did not reduce CV events compared with standard care. In a substudy n-3 PUFA 1 g daily did not reduce CV events. Insulin treatment does not carry cardiovascular benefits.
PATHWAY	Prevention and Treatment of Hypertension with Algorithm-based Therapy	2015 onwards	A series of studies in hypertension focusing particularly on the pathophysiology and management of resistant hypertension.
Pittsburgh EDC	Pittsburgh Epidemiology of Diabetes Complication Study	Study started 1986–1988, continuing	Important longitudinal study of childhood-onset Type 1 diabetes. Methods and results complement DCCT/EDIC.
PREDIMED	Prevención con Dieta Mediterránea	2013	Supplementing a traditional Mediterranean diet with 1 litre weekly of extra-virgin olive oil reduced the risk of CV events by 30% over 5 years. Some benefits were seen by supplementing with 30 g mixed nuts daily.
RENAAL	Reduction of Endpoints in NIDDM with the Angiotensin II Antagonist Losartan	2001	Losartan 50–100 mg daily for 3½ years reduced hard renal endpoints by 25% in Type 2 patients with established diabetic nephropathy. Similar to IDNT trial (q.v.) using irbesartan, and confirming prognostic benefit of angiotensin blockade in Type 2 nephropathy.
REGARDS	REasons for Geographic and Racial Differences in Stroke	Study started 2003–2007	Wide-ranging prospective study of risk factors for stroke in the USA.
ROADMAP	Randomized Olmesartan and Diabetes Microalbuminuria Prevention	2011	Olmesartan (ARB) reduced risk of progression to microalbuminuria in Type 2 with hypertension. (Increase in CV events.)
SEARCH	Search for Diabetes In Youth	2000–2020	USA national multicentre study of all types of diabetes in children and young adults.www. searchfordiabetes.org

Abbreviation/ acronym	Full title	Year of main trial publication	Notes
SHEP	Systolic Hypertension in the Elderly Program	1991	Placebo-controlled trial of chlortalidone in people over 60 with SBP >160 and DBP <90. 35% risk reduction in stroke, nearly 40% reduction in CV events.
SOS	Swedish Obese Subjects	2004	The largest prospective study of bariatric surgery vs medical treatment of obesity. CV events and mortality were reduced. There was a high rate of diabetes remission. Diabetes incidence was 80% lower after surgery.
Steno-2		2008	Multimodal management of risk factors in microalbuminuria reduced microvascular complications and CV outcomes (including mortality). After very long follow-up reduced CV events resulted in increased longevity.
STOP-NIDDM	Study to Prevent Non-Insulin-Dependent Diabetes Mellitus	2002	Acarbose reduced risk of progression of impaired glucose tolerance to Type 2. Also a hugely contested claim that acarbose reduced CV events (especially MI) and new-onset hypertension. A forgotten trial and a largely forgotten drug.
SUSTAIN-6	Trial to Evaluate Cardiovascular and Other Long-term Outcomes with Semaglutide in Subjects with Type 2 Diabetes	2016	Semaglutide in CV high-risk Type 2. CV death, and non-fatal MI and stroke were reduced.
SYMPLICITY HTN	Device name (SYMPLICITY)	2010 onwards	A series of studies of renal denervation in resistant hypertension. SYMPLICITY HTN-3 (2014), sham-procedure controlled, showed no significant effect on blood pressure control.
TNT	Treating to New Targets	2005	High-dose statin study. 20% risk reduction in CV events with high-dose atorvastatin (80 mg daily) compared with low dose (10 mg daily).
TREAT	Trial to Reduce Cardiovascular Events with Aranesp Therapy	2009	Definitive negative study of erythropoietin-stimulating agent (darbepoetin) in diabetic renal disease with anaemia. No reduction in mortality or CV events, and increased risk of stroke.

(Continued)

Abbreviation/ acronym	Full title	Year of main trial publication	Notes
UKPDS	United Kingdom Prospective Diabetes Study	1997	Truly iconic study in Type 2 diabetes. Glycaemic study: basket of microvascular complications reduced with HbA_{1c} 7.0% compared with 7.9%. Metformin reduced risk of myocardial infarction in obese people compared with diet therapy. Hypertension study: mortality, stroke, heart failure and microvascular complications reduced with tighter control. Glycaemia had some legacy effect.
VADT	Veterans Affairs Diabetes Trial	2009	Tight glycaemic control (HbA_{1c} 6.9% vs 8.4%) did not reduce the risk of CV events. Progression of albuminuria, but not retinopathy, was reduced.
VA-HIT	Veterans Affairs High Density Lipoprotein cholesterol Intervention Trial	1999	Fibric acid drug (gemfibrozil) reduced coronary events in men with low HDL levels (<1.0 mmol/l) and normal (for the time) LDL (<3.6 mmol/l). This positive trial stimulated widespread use of the fibric acid drugs until FIELD (q.v.).
VA NEPHRON-D	Veterans Affairs Nephropathy in Diabetes	2013	Dual angiotensin blockade in diabetic nephropathy (proteinuria and reduced eGFR). Losartan added to lisinopril (dual angiotensin blockade) did not reduce the risk of hard renal end points and significantly increased AKI and hyperkalaemia. Trial terminated early.

1 Classification, diagnosis and presentation

Key points

- The four major categories of diabetes are: Type 1, Type 2, gestational diabetes and other specific categories. The distinctions between Type 1 and Type 2 have been blurred latterly by clinically important syndromes, for example latent autoimmune diabetes of adults (LADA), which has some characteristics of Type 2, and Type 2 diabetes presenting with 'classical' Type 1 diabetic ketoacidosis ('Flatbush'-type diabetes)
- Diabetes is diagnosed with laboratory fasting plasma glucose ≥ 7.0 mmol/l, random glucose ≥ 11.1 mmol/l or $HbA_{1c} \geq 6.5\%$ (48 mmol/mol)
- The differential diagnosis is widest in adolescents and young adults. Tests for islet-related autoantibodies, for example, those to glutamic acid decarboxylase, are of help in this group
- There is still no worldwide agreement on the biochemical diagnosis of gestational diabetes, but fasting plasma glucose values between 5.6 and 6.9 mmol/l are proposed
- The diagnosis of diabetes out of pregnancy is now based solely on fasting glucose values and HbA_{1c}. The glucose tolerance test is obsolete in non-pregnant adults
- Cumulatively, uncommon causes account for a significant proportion of patients, especially pancreatic and monogenic diabetes

A PRACTICAL CLASSIFICATION OF DIABETES

The usual lists of types of diabetes, while comprehensive, are static and represent neither the frequency with which they are seen by general or even specialist practitioners, nor local differences in prevalence resulting from ethnicity and socioeconomic deprivation. So, for example, in the list of 'other specific types' of diabetes – a fascinating potpourri – the diabetes associated with a glucagonoma, seen perhaps a very few times in a lifetime by a specialist endocrinologist, is given the same apparent prominence as the much more common diabetes associated with pancreatic disease (mainly alcohol related). But before arriving at a practical discussion of some of the specific diabetes types – many of which must not be missed – we should consider the two major types, accounting for well over 90% of all cases: Type 1 and Type 2 diabetes.

In 1997, the American Diabetes Association proposed moving the classification towards one based on pathogenesis rather than treatment modality (even though the pathogenesis was not understood in full, either then or now). This resulted in, for example, a change in nomenclature from 'insulin-dependent diabetes' to 'Type 1 diabetes' (immune-mediated), and 'non-insulin-dependent' to 'Type 2 diabetes (insulin resistance with a variable contribution from insulin deficiency). Various other pathogenesis-based systems have been proposed, most recently one based on the centrality of β-cell stress,

Practical Diabetes Care, Fourth Edition. David Levy.
© 2018 John Wiley & Sons Ltd. Published 2018 by John Wiley & Sons Ltd.

dysfunction or loss through multiple pathways (Schwartz *et al.*, 2016). It is doubtful whether the clinician or patient will experience greater clarity from such complexity and for better or worse the current classification will remain.

TYPE 1 DIABETES

'Classical' Type 1 diabetes (**Table 1.1**) is relatively uncommon and occurs in about one in 300 of a northern, white population, usually in children and pre-adolescents, though it can occur at any age (including the elderly). Its multiple previous names are – importantly – now obsolete. These include:

- Insulin-dependent diabetes
- Juvenile-onset diabetes
- IDDM (insulin-dependent diabetes mellitus). There has been a recent tendency to start using this term again, probably because in speech it is a euphonious abbreviation, in the same way as 'NIDDM' is for Type 2 diabetes. In practice it is coterminous with Type 1 diabetes, but 'IDDM' was dropped because not all patients with autoimmune diabetes require insulin treatment from the start, especially those with later-onset diabetes. The hazard is that 'IDDM' can become a cover-all term that includes insulin-treated Type 2 patients, thus dangerously de-emphasizing the continued need for insulin treatment without interruption in people with true Type 1 diabetes
- Ketosis-prone diabetes, ketosis being the simple but reliable clinical phenotype of insulin deficiency; but the spectrum of ketosis-prone diabetes is now wider than classical Type 1 diabetes

Epidemiology; Type 1 diabetes in China

The epidemiology of Type 1 diabetes is fascinating, and mostly unexplained. It has a greater than 300-fold difference worldwide between countries of low incidence (e.g. China, Venezuela) and high incidence (e.g. Finland, much of northern Europe and Sardinia). Even within Europe the difference is tenfold, but there is a consistent difference between north (high incidence) and south (low), and west (high) and east (low). Very little is known about Type 1 diabetes in areas of low incidence but large populations, where the total burden may be high, but in Zhejiang, a rapidly developing province in south-east China, there has been a rapid increase in the under-fives (noted in many other countries too), and the mean age at diagnosis in children and adolescents fell by 1.6 years to 13 years over a short period between 2007 and 2013 (Wu *et al.*, 2016). The phenotype of Type 1 diabetes in China is not well described but a large registry of Han Chinese from Guangdong (formerly Canton in South China, bordering Hong Kong and Macau) between 2000 and 2011 paints a striking picture (Yang *et al.*, 2016):

- Older onset than in Europe: median age 28 years (compared with 14 in Germany, 9 in the USA), though with the same slight excess in males (54%)
- Patients are very slim (median body mass index (BMI) 20); 30% were underweight (BMI <20)
- There is a high prevalence of diabetic ketoacidosis at onset (50%), typical of countries where the incidence of Type 1 diabetes is low
- A significant proportion of patients had microvascular complications (retinopathy 8%, nephropathy 20%), implying a slow onset

Table 1.1 Phenotypic features of Type 1 diabetes.

Classical phenotypic characteristic	Modifiers	Importance for practitioners
White	Ethnicity and migration	In the UK, the incidence of Type 1 diabetes is probably almost as high in South Asian and African Caribbean people who have immigrated as in those of European heritage, but the overall prevalence is lower. Non-white ethnic groups at high risk of Type 1 diabetes include North Africans and Kuwaitis. White ethnic groups increasingly represented in the UK include the ex-Communist countries of Eastern Europe and the Baltic states (Estonia, Latvia and Lithuania). Increasing distance eastwards and towards the equator is associated with a much reduced risk, so African people, South Americans and those from South-East Asia (especially China and Japan), have a very low risk of Type 1 diabetes – though there is always a small background risk which may be rapidly increasing (see below).
Onset in childhood and pre-adolescence	Age and secular trends	In high-risk countries, e.g. Scandinavia, peak incidence is at 10 years in girls, 13 in boys. After 16, the incidence falls rapidly and, thereafter, slowly over the next 20 years, at which point it merges into latent autoimmune diabetes of adults (LADA). The incidence in the under 5s is increasing more rapidly than in older age groups, but absolute numbers in this age group are still low.
Onset	Age	Onset is acute with short preceding hyperglycaemia; with increasing age the clinical onset tends to be slower as the immunological assault on the β-cells weakens.
Lean body phenotype	Trends in obesity	Children are usually slim even before any weight loss that occurs before diagnosis. Older patients with antibody-positive diabetes (Type 1 diabetes or LADA) tend to be slightly overweight (e.g. mean BMI 26–27), less so than Type 2 patients (e.g. BMI 29–31), but it is not possible to make a presumptive diagnosis on body phenotype unless the patient is strictly of normal weight.
Ketosis	Age	Immunological attack on the β cells is most virulent in younger children; ketosis is a reliable indicator of insulin deficiency and, therefore, of presumed Type 1 diabetes. Beta-cell reserve is higher in older people developing Type 1 diabetes and ketosis may be intermittent or not apparent.
Microvascular complications		Microvascular complications, especially retinopathy and neuropathy, are almost never present at the time of diagnosis.
Family history		Powerful genetic factors are at play and nearly all patients will be HLA-DR3 and DR4 positive; but they do not affect the phenotype. Only about 5% of Type 1 patients have a positive family history in first-degree relatives (compare the variable but much higher rate in Type 2).

> **Practice point**
>
> Younger people developing Type 1 diabetes are usually thin despite the increase in population levels of obesity.

Awareness of Type 1 diabetes is increasing in the general population and in parents of those diagnosed. Where there have been specific education programmes to further increase awareness, fewer children present in diabetic ketoacidosis.

The diagnostic problem may be most difficult at onset, especially in adolescents (see later) and older people, but management not based on a proper diagnosis can be problematic later in life, especially as most Type 1 diabetics can now be expected to live as long as non-diabetic people. Recognizing long-standing Type 1 diabetes in older people is the major difficulty (see **Chapter 14**). Typically, when insulin-treated patients move to a different part of the country or abroad, they can carry with them an array of obsolete diagnostic labels. The hazard – real – is that they will be reallocated on account of their age alone to 'insulin-treated Type 2 diabetes'. The hazards of this should not need pointing out, but it is a common scenario.

> **Practice point**
>
> Older insulin-treated people may have either Type 1 or Type 2 diabetes. This important distinction is blurred by the old label 'IDDM'. If there is any doubt, especially in the emergency situation, regard insulin-treated older people with long-standing diabetes as being Type 1 and fully dependent on insulin.

Further clinical pointers to Type 1 diabetes
- Duration of insulin treatment: if continuous and started when the patient was under 30 years old, then Type 1 diabetes is highly likely
- A non-overweight, white person of any age treated with insulin alone should be considered to have Type 1 diabetes. Many patients now live without significant complications for 50 years or more (they are likely to be in their 60s and 70s). They often need only tiny doses of insulin (e.g. <20 units/day) but are fully insulin-requiring and will develop ketosis if insulin is withdrawn
- Continuing the treatment theme: someone on full insulin treatment (a regimen that covers night-time and meal times, without non-insulin agents) is very likely to have Type 1 diabetes (**Chapter 7**). Some Type 1 patients take metformin as well, either because they are overweight, with some degree of insulin resistance, or because they have polycystic ovarian syndrome, but these cases are unusual (**Chapter 7**)

AUTOIMMUNE ASSOCIATIONS OF TYPE 1 DIABETES

There is a wide array of autoimmune conditions linked more or less strongly (and some speculatively because of their rarity) to Type 1 diabetes (**Box 1.1**). They pose a significant diagnostic problem because of their subtle symptoms and gradual onset, and there is a hazard that non-specific symptoms will be attributed to some aspect of the underlying diabetes.

> **Box 1.1** Autoimmune conditions associated with Type 1 diabetes.
>
> **Established organ-specific conditions**
> - Autoimmune thyroid disease, especially Hashimoto's thyroiditis; Graves' hyperthyroidism much less common (~1% prevalence)
> - Coeliac disease (clinical prevalence 1–8%, autoantibody positivity 8–14%)
> - Addison's disease (clinical prevalence 0.5%)
> - Pernicious anaemia (clinical prevalence 2–4%, much higher rates of positive parietal cell antibodies, 10–15% in children, 15–25% adults)
>
> **Possible associations**
> *Organ-specific*
> - Primary ovarian failure
> - Autoimmune hepatitis
> - Primary biliary cirrhosis
> - Renal tubular acidosis
> - Vitiligo
> - Hypophysitis
> - Myasthenia gravis
> - Multiple sclerosis (speculative)
> - Idiopathic thrombocytopenic purpura (speculative)
>
> *Non-organ-specific*
> - Juvenile rheumatoid arthritis
> - Rheumatoid arthritis
> - Sjögren's syndrome
> - Systemic lupus erythematosus

Could there be an emerging associated autoimmune problem? is an important question always to bear in mind, regardless of the duration of Type 1 diabetes. The commonest are autoimmune thyroid disease, coeliac and Addison's disease. Up to 80% of patients will be hypothyroid at 20 years; this very high prevalence warrants annual thyroid function testing.

TYPE 2 DIABETES

Because Type 2 diabetes is at least 10 times more common than Type 1, there is a tendency for clinicians to default to Type 2 when considering a diagnosis, especially in older and overweight or obese people. From the safety point of view, the tendency should be more to question whether any patient could have autoimmune diabetes. In adults, the need to alter our focus is seen increasingly commonly in the 'Flatbush' form of Type 2 diabetes that frequently presents with diabetic ketoacidosis, where the biochemical picture is indistinguishable from that of classical Type 1 diabetes-associated ketoacidosis. But in most cases there is little or no diagnostic difficulty (**Table 1.2**).

The over-representation of non-white ethnic groups in surveys of people with Type 2 diabetes is as striking as the over-representation of white people with Type 1. The importance of ethnicity as a risk factor for Type 2 diabetes cannot be overstated; data from the United Kingdom are shown in **Figure 1.1**.

Table 1.2 Diagnosing Type 2 diabetes in adults.

Classical phenotypic characteristic	Modifiers	Significance/Importance for practitioners
Ethnic minority (South Asian and African Caribbean in the UK)	Immigration Increasing prevalence of obesity	In the UK the prevalence of Type 2 diabetes in South Asians is twice that of white people (14% vs 7%). That of African-Caribbeans is intermediate, about 10%.
Onset in middle age	Increasing obesity in youth	In the UK, Type 2 diabetes is diagnosed 6–7 years earlier in South Asian and African-Caribbean people than in white people. Mean age of onset ~59 years (52 in South Asians and African-Caribbeans); compare the much younger age at onset in the USA in all ethnicities (mean ~45 years). Despite the increase in population obesity, Type 2 diabetes in adolescence is very uncommon in the UK, even in ethnic minority youth (Chapter 14)
Centrally obese phenotype	Increasing obesity	Visceral fat is critical; ectopic fat may have organ-specific effects (Chapter 13).
Absent ketosis	Factors increasing insulin resistance and decreasing β cell function, e.g. intercurrent infection or glucocorticoid use	If there is significant ketonuria, then treat as if insulin-deficient; absent ketonuria is characteristic of Type 2 and LADA
Microvascular complications		If present, then very likely Type 2 diabetes (characteristic long asymptomatic prodrome with significant hyperglycaemia and associated metabolic syndrome abnormalities). However, micro- and macrovascular complications are much less common in ethnic minorities at diagnosis.
Family history		Powerful. Risk is increased threefold if there is one parent with Type 2 diabetes, sevenfold if both, and fivefold if at least one sibling has diabetes. Overall prevalence of Type 2 diabetes: ~14% of people with family history (compared with 3% with no family history; USA data, Annis *et al.*, 2005).

Source: Winkley *et al.*, 2013 (UK ethnicity data). Reproduced with permission of Springer.

Latent autoimmune diabetes of adults (LADA): a valuable epidemiological concept, but of limited value in immediate clinical decision-making

This is a variable but increasingly common form of autoimmune diabetes, up to three times more prevalent than Type 1 diabetes, and therefore much more common than childhood-onset Type 1 diabetes. It is similar to other organ-specific autoimmune conditions, as it can occur throughout later life, and was first described in the

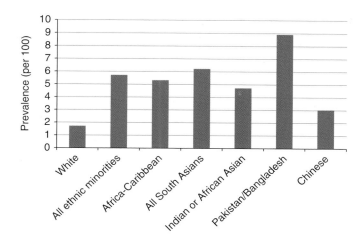

Figure 1.1 Prevalence of Type 2 diabetes in the United Kingdom by ethnicity (age- and sex-standardized). *Source*: Holman *et al.*, 2011. Reproduced with permission of John Wiley and Sons.

mid-1970s, around the same time as the discovery of islet-cell antibodies. Its formal definition comprises:

- patients aged 30–70 years
- presence of diabetes-associated autoantibodies
- insulin treatment that did not start before six months after diagnosis.

It is only the last criterion, the arbitrary time frame within which insulin is started, that distinguishes LADA from Type 1 diabetes in older people. It is a retrospective diagnosis and does not help in the immediate characterization and management of newly-presenting patients, where clinical features and the presence of ketones indicate the need to start insulin treatment.

In the UK CARDS study, 7% of 'Type 2' patients were positive for GAD antibodies at recruitment, and by the end of the study, with a mean known duration of diabetes ~12 years, more than one-half were still not using insulin. Importantly, they were no more likely to have vascular complications compared with the insulin treated group (Hawa *et al.*, 2014). Its variable presentation and progress is due to at least five contributing domains (**Figure 1.2**).

In the Action LADA programme, Hawa *et al.* (2013) studied over 6000 adult patients across Europe. Findings are summarised in **Table 1.3**. Even in retrospective group comparisons there are few phenotypic differences between adult-onset Type 1 and LADA, the most striking of which is age (mean 42 years for Type 1 diabetes, 50 for LADA), and higher BMI (29 vs 26). The gender ratio is the same (50:50), as is systolic blood pressure and the lipid profile. However, the clinical profile is highly modified by the specific study. For example, in the ADOPT study of patients clinically diagnosed with Type 2 diabetes the LADA group, comprising 4% of the study population, had the same mean age as the Type 2 patients (57 years), but because this was a study in European and American subjects, BMI was overall higher (31-32) than in Action LADA (Zinman *et al.* 2004).

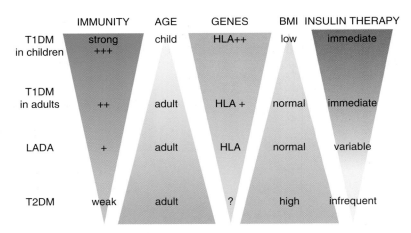

Figure 1.2 The spectrum of autoimmune diabetes. Five important continuously variable domains interact to produce the broadening modes of presentation of autoimmune diabetes. *Source*: Leslie *et al.*, 2008. Reproduced with permission of John Wiley and Sons.

Table 1.3 Characteristics of LADA in Europe.

Mean age at diagnosis	52 years
Males	59%
Ethnicity	Caucasian 85%, Middle East 4.5%, Asian 2.5%, African 1.2%, other ethnicities 7.2%
Autoantibodies	Overall GADA positivity 91% Other single autoantibody prevalences: IA-2A 5.0%, ZnT8A 2.3% (very low) Two or more autoantibodies: 24.1%

Source: Hawa *et al.,* 2013. Reproduced with permission of American Diabetes Association.

Clinical diagnosis of autoimmune diabetes in older people

For clinical purposes, therefore, we need to adopt a basket of characteristics in order to diagnose autoimmune diabetes in older individuals presenting with hyperglycaemia:

- age >30 years
- subacute symptoms, duration usually under six months, for example, typical osmotic symptoms, unintentional weight loss, but not infections or blurred vision
- minor degree of weight loss
- lack of family history of diabetes
- presence of family or personal history of other autoimmune conditions
- in Europe, normal weight or overweight, rather than obese
- intermittent or 1+ or less ketonuria (analyse urine for ketones at every visit).

Clinicians will not receive a routine anti-GAD antibody (GADA) result from the laboratory for several weeks. GADA positivity confirms the diagnosis but 10% are GADA negative. Other diabetes-related autoantibodies (anti-IA-2A and ZnT8A) are not routinely available, and in any case much less frequently positive in later-onset compared with childhood-onset diabetes. If there is no ketonuria and blood glucose levels are modest (e.g. around 15 mmol/l), start a trial of antidiabetic medication (metformin + secretagogue, either a sulfonylurea or repaglinide). The place of the DPP-4 inhibitors is not known in this clinical situation; they are weak secretagogues compared with a sulfonylurea (see **Chapter 10**). One of the major clinical features of LADA patients with poor β-cell reserve is a weak or absent response to non-insulin agents. If blood glucose levels are still in double figures about two weeks after starting a sulfonylurea, then this constitutes primary sulfonylurea failure and insulin treatment is needed. Because these patients are not especially insulin resistant, metformin mono-therapy is unwise because the response may be minimal. Clinicians alerted to autoim-munity by requesting GADA tests that turn out to be positive tend to suggest earlier insulin treatment, though in many cases it is not needed: GADA positivity implies an autoimmune process affecting the islets, but not necessarily severe enough to cause insulin deficiency of a degree that mandates insulin treatment. Fasting insulin and C-peptide measurements have not been studied prospectively (see below for the clinical place of these tests).

Practice point

If clinicians learn that 'Type 2' patients are GAD antibody positive (about 1 in 20), they are more likely to suggest early insulin treatment, which may not be necessary. Observe carefully for signs of oral agent failure (poor glycaemic response to standard drugs, weight loss, intermittent ketonuria).

The emerging role of C-peptide measurements: valuable to confirm or revise the need for insulin treatment in patients previously started on insulin treatment

C-peptide and insulin are secreted in equimolar concentrations from β-cells, so measur-ing C-peptide is potentially valuable in assessing endogenous insulin secretion in people taking insulin. There is broad agreement that a random non-fasting blood C-peptide measurement <0.2 nmol/l indicates absolute insulin deficiency. Assays are reliable and standardized and C-peptide is more stable than previously thought, up to six hours in serum gel or plain sample tube and up to 24 hours in whole blood collected in EDTA. A stimulated C-peptide measurement, commonly used in academic studies and clinical trials, is not necessary. Samples should be taken >90 minutes after a meal, and when blood glucose is >8 mmol/l. It is unreliable in the presence of hypoglycaemia (blood glu-cose <4 mmol/l). Finally, it must be interpreted with caution in the early stages (up to year 3) of diabetes. During a honeymoon period of Type 1 diabetes, C-peptide levels are likely to be high, and they can be transiently low in newly-diagnosed Type 2 diabetes that is accompanied by severe hyperglycaemia.

However, it still has value, not so much in formal diagnosis but in the common and difficult clinical situations where it is difficult to distinguish between Type 1, Type 2 and monogenic (MODY) diabetes in a patient taking insulin. In short, in certain common clinical circumstances it will answer the important therapeutic question: does this patient continue to need insulin? (**Table 1.4**) (Jones and Hattersley, 2013). Importantly, it is inde-pendent of the simple clinical characteristics (age, ethnicity, degree of obesity) that – as the data on LADA show – are increasingly unreliable in diagnosis. C-peptide measure-ments may also be of use as a simple biomarker of response to drugs, for example GLP-1 receptor agonists (see **Chapter 10**).

Practice point

Consider using a random blood C-peptide measurement to determine whether or not an insulin-taking patient with an unclear diagnosis some years before is truly insulin deficient. A value <0.2 nmol/l suggests severe insulin deficiency and the need to continue insulin treatment.

Table **1.4** Clinical situations in which C-peptide measurement may help clinical decision making in insulin-taking patients.

Clinical situation	C-peptide measurement (non-fasting 'random' blood measurement (nmol/l) or home postmeal urinary C-peptide-creatinine ratio (nmol/nmol)
Absolute insulin deficiency, i.e. Type 1 diabetes	<0.2
Likely Type 1 diabetes/inability to achieve glycaemic control with non-insulin therapies	<0.6
Suggests Type 2 or MODY in a patient with presumed Type 1 diabetes diagnosed >3–5 years previously	>0.2
Consider MODY/Type 2 diabetes in young person at diagnosis	>1

Source: Jones and Hattersley, 2013. Reproduced with permission of John Wiley & Sons.

ADOLESCENTS AND YOUNG PEOPLE

The differential diagnosis of diabetes is widest during adolescence and young adulthood, and while the typical acute onset of Type 1 diabetes is still the commonest presentation, the SEARCH study in the USA found that over 40% of cases were *not* Type 1 diabetes (Hamman *et al.*, 2014):

- Type 1 diabetes and obesity (16% of cases)
- typical Type 1 diabetes (55%)
- typical Type 2 diabetes (26%)
- no autoimmunity or insulin resistance (10%):
  - monogenic diabetes (8%) – HNF-1α, glucokinase, HNF-4α
- secondary diabetes (uncommon in youth)
- other genetic types.

Formal diagnosis is critical in this group, and urgent specialist referral is needed.

TYPE 2 DIABETES PRESENTING WITH DIABETIC KETOACIDOSIS ('FLATBUSH' DIABETES)

This is a now common but still perplexing presentation of Type 2 diabetes, first described in Africa in the 1960s and 1970s, but characterized in the 1990s in obese African-American men in their 30s living in the Flatbush area of Brooklyn, hence its informal name (Banerji *et al.*, 1994). It presents with diabetic ketoacidosis, sometimes severe and indistinguishable from the ketoacidosis of Type 1 diabetes. However it is autoantibody negative and the acute insulin deficiency that precipitates ketoacidosis – and requires insulin treatment in the early stages – remits, often permanently. Patients often need insulin only for a short time (average 3½ months), and they are prone to hypoglycaemia even on low doses of insulin shortly after discharge from hospital. Complete remission, defined as good glycaemic control on diet alone, occurs in 30–40% of cases, even if there is no weight loss. Relapse into diabetic ketoacidosis occurs but is uncommon. There are no long-term follow-up studies, which would be difficult because so many patients need no medication at all and are likely to be lost to follow-up. This presentation of Type 2 diabetes is becoming more common in the United Kingdom and practitioners in areas with ethnic minority patients will regularly encounter it. It is now a common presentation in African-American youth in the USA (it was described in 1987 in a group of Florida children, average age 13, but because they had a strong family history of diabetes presenting in a similar way, it was originally thought to be a form of MODY). There is also an isolated case report of a patient in India.

Practice point

'Flatbush' Type 2 diabetes in obese African or African-Americans frequently presents acutely as ketoacidosis, indistinguishable from the ketoacidosis of Type1. Discharge patients on insulin, but they need frequent follow-up, as most will not need insulin beyond a few months.

TYPE 2 DIABETES IN CHILDREN AND ADOLESCENTS

Although Type 1 diabetes is still by far the commonest form of diabetes in USA youth, the SEARCH study in people under 20 found that 15% of diabetes cases in the white population were Type 2, increasing to 45% in Hispanics and 60% in African-Americans. Sixty percent were girls (Writing Group for the SEARCH Group, 2007). In the UK Type 2 diabetes in young people is very uncommon, around one-twentieth the incidence in the USA, and was not even described until 2002. Some of the difference in incidence is due to a higher proportion of ethnic minorities in the USA, and by population obesity levels, but there is likely to be ascertainment bias, as patients in late adolescence may not be captured by paediatric data collection. Many will be in the asymptomatic prodromal phase, whose duration is unknown, but, as in adults, likely to be several years.

Diabetes diagnosed on oral glucose tolerance test was found in only ~1% of obese white children over 12 years of age in Germany, and a similar proportion in overweight or obese 10–17 year olds in Michigan. Given the prevalence of obesity around 20%, Type 2 diabetes is undiagnosed in the majority of young people. In ethnic minority populations, systematic examination for axillary acanthosis nigricans, the classical cutaneous marker of insulin resistance, when added to elevated BMI and a positive family history, reliably identifies people at high risk; this straightforward clinical approach has been used in screening programmes in the USA (Lee *et al.*, 2013; see **Chapter 5**). To the list of risk factors should probably be added antipsychotic medication, which carries a two- to threefold increased risk of Type 2 diabetes that emerges soon after starting treatment, though the absolute risk still remains very low (Galling *et al.*, 2016).

In primary care, there is a good case for opportunistic screening, especially of overweight or obese children with one or more parents with Type 2 diabetes, using HbA_{1c} rather than fasting glucose measurements (as recommended by the American Diabetes Association guidelines). However, we must not get too obsessed with glucose levels: elevated systolic blood pressure is the most prevalent treatable abnormality associated with insulin resistance in this age group.

Practice point

Type 2 diabetes in adolescence is uncommon in Europe, but be alert for it in young obese ethnic minority people with a positive family history, especially if there is axillary acanthosis nigricans.

OTHER SPECIFIC TYPES OF DIABETES

Fulminant diabetes

This is a fascinating form of antibody-negative diabetes (i.e. classified as Type 1B in contrast to the much more common antibody-positive form, Type 1A). It was first described in 2000. Most cases occur in South East Asian countries, especially Japan (where 5000–7000 cases have been reported), South Korea, the Philippines and Thailand, where autoimmune Type 1 diabetes is uncommon (Imagawa and Hanafusa, 2011). A handful of cases have occurred in Caucasians in France.

The phenotype is variable. Most cases occur in the third and fourth decades, and individuals are not usually notably thin. The onset is abrupt and the duration of symptoms usually less than a week before presentation. A viral precipitant is likely. Gastrointestinal symptoms are prominent and can result in a sometimes hazardous delay in diagnosis. Pancreatic enzymes are often elevated, suggesting exocrine involvement in the inflammatory process. Patients present in severe diabetic ketoacidosis (pH <7.1), often with blunted consciousness, and there is a significant mortality. Strikingly, the HbA_{1C} at onset is nearly normal, around 6% (42), confirming the hyperacute onset. Any autoimmunity is feeble, and although certain HLA types are emerging, they are different from those of Type 1A diabetes. There are very few long-term studies, but in a nine-year follow-up in Japan, in spite of better glycaemic control than patients with acute-onset Type 1 diabetes and no difference in the prevalence of microalbuminuria, impaired renal function (eGFR <60 ml/min) was about twice as common (Takahashi et al., 2017). Other striking differences from Type 1A diabetes are likely to emerge in future.

Monogenic diabetes

The several forms of monogenic diabetes comprise only 1–2% of all cases of diabetes but they are mechanistically fascinating and clinically challenging, as they often present as only mildly atypical forms of Type 1 and Type 2 diabetes. Misra and Hattersley (2017) list features that should alert the clinician to monogenic diabetes:

- atypical presentations of Type 1 or Type 2 diabetes; they may coexist by chance with either of the major forms
- autosomal dominant family history (or maternal inheritance in the mitochondrial disorders)
- diagnosis within the first six months of life (possible mutations of the Kir6.2 and SUR1 subunits of the potassium channel of the pancreatic β cell)
- unusual clinical features, for example sensorineural deafness, acanthosis nigricans in the absence of obesity, partial lipodystrophy (muscular, thin limbs associated with elevated triglycerides and insulin resistance).

The most common phenotype is that of maturity-onset diabetes of the young (MODY), broadly divided into glucokinase and transcription factor types, both showing autosomal dominant inheritance.

syndrome (cortisol), phaeochromocytomas (catecholamines, especially noradrenaline) and glucagonoma. Several studies have uncovered excess cortisol in up to 10% of people with poorly-controlled Type 2 diabetes. The significance of these findings is disputed but vigilance is needed, as the gross textbook phenotype of Cushing's is just that, and many patients will not present with striae, buffalo humps or osteoporotic fractures. More promising therapeutically is the relatively recent discovery of the complexity of intracellular cortisol metabolism and its importance in obesity and Type 2 diabetes. For example, the enzyme 11β-hydroxysteroid dehydrogenase 1 (11β-HSD1), present in adipose tissue and the liver, generates intracellular cortisol from cortisone and is a potent stimulator of adipogenesis, giving rise to the colourful concept of 'Cushing's disease of the omentum'. A few years ago there was intense pharmacological interest in the blood glucose-lowering effects of selective blockers of this pathway. In Phase 2 clinical studies HbA_{1c} levels fell by ~0.5%, associated with some weight reduction and improvement in lipid profiles (Rosenstock et al., 2010), and another agent improved fatty liver in non-diabetic subjects. The development of this potentially valuable group of drugs for Type 2 diabetes has stalled recently. Protocols for the laboratory diagnosis of endocrine disorders associated with hypertension are outlined in **Chapter 11**.

Practice point

Among the long list of rare endocrine disorders associated with Type 2 diabetes, very few will present with hyperglycaemia. There is much interest in cortisol overproduction in adipose tissue and the liver that may contribute to Type 2 diabetes and the metabolic syndrome, but nothing yet of therapeutic value.

New-onset diabetes after transplantation (NODAT)
This is a common and important multifactorial form of diabetes. It is not clear whether it is a distinct form of diabetes or, more likely, a form of Type 2 diabetes accelerated by multiple factors caused by transplantation (Sharif and Cohney, 2016). It shares features of both insulin resistance and β-cell failure. Drugs, especially the calcineurin inhibitors (ciclosporin and tacrolimus) contribute; sirolimus is under suspicion. Ascertainment is difficult. Most patients do not have standardized formal diabetes assessments before transplantation; in both end-stage renal and liver diseases, many patients have complex states of dysglycaemia before transplantation. But transplantation is undoubtedly an added risk: a year after renal transplantation, 10–20% have diabetes on a glucose tolerance test, compared with only about 5% of non-transplanted patients. It carries a poor prognosis for organ and patient survival and cardiovascular events, with up to threefold increased risks. All vascular risk factors must be rigorously managed and joint management with the transplant team would be wise, though not always achieved in the real world. There are no documented major interactions between modern antirejection drugs and non-insulin agents for the treatment of glycaemia but it is always wise to check before prescribing; compromise of a transplanted organ is always more important than modest short-term hyperglycaemia.

Practice point

New-onset diabetes after transplantation is common. Always additionally check HbA_{1c} in transplant patients when requesting routine laboratory tests.

PREGNANCY AND GESTATIONAL DIABETES MELLITUS

Hyperglycaemia of some degree occurs in about 1 in 6 pregnancies worldwide, of which one-sixth are probably newly-diagnosed diabetes, mostly Type 2, and the remainder gestational diabetes mellitus (GDM).

GDM is hyperglycaemia that does not meet the criteria for frank diabetes with onset or first recognition during pregnancy. The diagnosis is independent of treatment modality and GDM must be distinguished from pregnancy in patients with pre-existing Type 1 or 2 diabetes, and the uncommon cases of Type 1 or Type 2 diabetes newly diagnosed during pregnancy. Risk factors for GDM are shown in **Box 1.2**. Type 2 diabetes is increasing in women of childbearing age, especially in ethnic minority groups, but is still relatively uncommon. The importance of prepregnancy counselling in patients with known diabetes is widely recognized but systematic implementation is elusive and, even in Type 1 diabetes, around 30% of pregnancies in the United Kingdom are unplanned, and up to 50% are unplanned in the USA (see **Chapter 14**). Curiously, prepregnancy counselling in Type 1 diabetes is less effective than in Type 2 (Dozio, 2016).

If developing the criteria for the laboratory diagnosis of diabetes itself has been troublesome, the difficulties pale into insignificance beside the tortured disagreements that still haunt the quantitative definition of GDM. To both outsiders and patients this must seem incomprehensible; after all, GDM was first identified in the mid-1960s. However, there are recommendations that are likely to come into widespread use in some high-resource health systems (**Box 1.3**) (Hod *et al.*, 2015)**.** About 50% of pregnant women have one or more risk factors for GDM and this very high prevalence has encouraged the consensus that all women should be tested. Although morbidity lies on a continuum of glucose levels, with no obvious inflection points, GDM carries risks for the mother (caesarean deliveries, birth trauma, hypertensive disorders of pregnancy, including pre-eclampsia, and of course, Type 2 diabetes), and for the foetus and offspring (macrosomia, shoulder dystocia and other birth injuries, respiratory distress, hypoglycaemia, polycythaemia and hyperbilirubinaemia; in the longer term, increased risk of obesity, metabolic syndrome, dysglycaemia and diabetes). In 2010, the International Association of the Diabetes and Pregnancy Study Groups (IADPSG) proposed universal screening with a 75-g oral glucose tolerance test (OGTT) between 24 and 28 weeks, or at any other time during pregnancy. Despite widespread support, there is still concern about

---

Box 1.2 Risk factors for GDM.

- Ethnicity (in the UK South Asian – especially India, Pakistan or Bangladesh; Black Caribbean; Middle East)
- Older age
- High parity
- Overweight and obesity; short stature
- Excessive weight gain in the index pregnancy
- Polycystic ovarian syndrome
- History of diabetes in first-degree relatives
- History of poor pregnancy outcomes (macrosomia, foetal loss)
- Pre-eclampsia
- Multiple pregnancy

Source: Hod *et al.*, 2015. Reproduced with permission of John Wiley & Sons.

Box 1.3 Pregnancy and diabetes.

Protocol in high-resource settings
- Screen for diabetes in pregnancy at booking/first trimester, using fasting or random plasma glucose or HbA$_{1c}$
- If negative, perform 75-g 2-h oral glucose tolerance test at 24–28 weeks

Diagnosis of overt diabetes in pregnancy:
- FPG ≥7.0 mmol/l (126 mg/dl), ± 2-h value on oral glucose tolerance test ≥11.1 mmol/l (200 mg/dl) *or*
- Random plasma glucose ≥11.1 mmol/l (200 mg/dl), associated with signs and symptoms of diabetes
- HbA$_{1c}$ ≥6.5% (48) (ADA recommendation)

Diagnosis of GDM
These criteria are considered appropriate for different ethnicities, with perhaps the exception of Chinese people. One or more of:
- FPG 5.1–6.9 mmol/l (92–125 mg/dl)
- 1-h post 65-g oral glucose load ≥10 mmol/l (180)
- 2-h post 65-g oral glucose load 8.5–11.0 (153–199)

Elevated random plasma glucose in early pregnancy (at booking); value of ≥7.5 mmol/l is better than maternal age or BMI in predicting GDM (Meek *et al.*, 2016).

Source: Hod et al., 2015. Reproduced with permission of John Wiley & Sons.

the poor clinical predictive value of these criteria, while at the same time increasing the risk of overdiagnosis and overtreatment. We are left with a plethora of protocols in use in different countries and in individual institutions. Critically, the historical two-stage diagnostic process established for many years in the USA is still recommended, and this will be the major barrier to wider acceptance of the IADPSG cut-offs.

DIAGNOSIS OF DIABETES IN NON-PREGNANT ADULTS (BOX 1.4)

The oral glucose tolerance test is obsolete for diagnosing diabetes in the non-pregnant adult, and although its proposed demise was well-signalled for years, it is still frequently requested. Laboratory fasting venous plasma glucose or whole blood HbA$_{1c}$ are the only accepted measurements, though measurements using laboratory-standard point-of-care devices (e.g. HemoCue) are acceptable. Measurement of HbA$_{1c}$ is now so reliable that a DCCT- or IFCC-traceable HbA$_{1c}$ of 6.5% (48) or above can and where available should be used to diagnose diabetes. The epidemiological evidence for the cut-point of 6.5% is the same as that for fasting plasma glucose values: the prevalence of definite retinopathy diagnostic of diabetes (moderate non-proliferative or worse) is vanishingly small at lower values. There is voluminous data indicating that cardiovascular disease risk begins to climb from a much lower baseline within the non-diabetic range, but this is a continuous spectrum, so diagnostic criteria cannot be established. The use of diagnostic HbA$_{1c}$ values has rapidly increased in well-resourced countries, and was adopted by the WHO in 2011.

Practice point

In the absence of symptoms, fasting plasma glucose ≥7.0 mmol/l or random HbA$_{1c}$ ≥6.5% (48) is diagnostic of diabetes. No further tests are required.

Practice point

The oral glucose tolerance test is troublesome, time- consuming and expensive; it is obsolete apart from its important place in obstetric practice.

Box 1.4 Diagnosis of diabetes.

- HbA_{1c} ≥6.5% (48 mmol/mol) *or*
- Fasting plasma glucose ≥7.0 mmol/l (126 mg/dl)
- Random plasma glucose ≥11.1 mmol/l (200 mg/dl) in the presence of symptoms (this is a highly abnormal value, but like all diagnostic measurements, must be measured in a laboratory and not with home blood glucose testing devices)
- The oral glucose tolerance test is no longer used for diagnosis except in obstetric practice
- Where the initial result is close to the diagnostic value, a repeat measurement is recommended. If two tests have been initially done, and one is above the cut-point, then this should be the one to be repeated
- The simplicity of these tests compared with the OGTT means that they are simple to repeat in practice. Diagnostic HbA_{1c} is especially valuable in:
  - ○ Hospitalized patients where intercurrent illness usually increases insulin resistance resulting in transiently high glucose levels but a strictly normal HbA_{1c} ('stress hyperglycaemia')
  - ○ Patients who have deliberately lost weight when they recognize symptoms, and who then present with normal fasting glucose values.

PREDIABETES

A term as fraught and difficult as the 'metabolic syndrome' (of which it is a component; see **Chapter 13**); in both instances, furious debates about the diagnostic criteria have dominated the discussion rather than their clinical significance. The world cannot even agree a cut-point value for 'prediabetes', let alone accurately guide prognosis for progression to diabetes, variously estimated at 4–9% annually (diagnostic glucose criteria are shown in **Box 1.5**). Nevertheless, we can at least be grateful that the oral glucose tolerance test-defined 'impaired glucose tolerance' (and its contorted partner 'impaired glucose tolerance' with 'impaired fasting glucose') has now disappeared. A huge proportion of the population of the USA has prediabetes on either fasting glucose levels or HbA_{1c} – one-third of those over 20, and one-half of those over 65 (Bansal, 2015). Nevertheless, for an individual it is a valuable portal to the recognition of the cluster of insulin-resistance characteristics that might predispose to premature cardiovascular disease, and may well be associated with significant health problems of more pressing

Box 1.5 Biochemical definitions of prediabetes.

World Health Organization (WHO)
Fasting plasma glucose 6.1–6.9 mmol/l (110–125 mg/dl)

American Diabetes Association
Fasting plasma glucose 5.6–6.9 mmol/l (100–125 mg/dl) *or*
HbA_{1c} 5.7–6.4% (39–46 mmol/mol)

concern, especially hypertension, non-alcoholic fatty liver disease and obstructive sleep apnoea. The place for glucose-lowering pharmacotherapy is limited to metformin in some people (see **Chapter 9**) and structured educational support to begin and maintain meaningful weight loss and exercise levels remains the most effective intervention to reduce the risk of progression to diabetes.

It is also unhelpful to regard these biochemical states as static. For example, using continuous glucose monitoring techniques in people with definitely normal glucose status (low fasting glucose and strictly normal HbA_{1c}), three-quarters spent a median 30 minutes in each 24-hour period at glucose levels >7.8 mmol/l (140 mg/dl) and 7% had a peak glucose level diagnostic of diabetes (>11.1 mmol/l, 200 mg/dl) (Borg et al., 2010). Degrees of glucose tolerance are bound to change with changes in weight and exercise over a longer time-frame; these will, in part, account for advanced diabetic complications that are seen in some patients at the time of formal diagnosis. Careful consideration of overall cardiovascular risk factors and informed, focused discussion is the right approach.

Practice point

Prediabetes, defined as fasting glucose 5.6 (or 6.1) mmol/l to 6.9 mmol/l is best considered an indicator of other 'metabolic syndrome' characteristics, rather than a glucose value that exceeds an arbitrary level and therefore warrants 'treatment'.

References

Annis AM, Caulder MS, Cook ML, Duquette D. Family history, diabetes, and other demographic and risk factors among participants of the National Health and Nutrition Examination Survey 1999–2002. *Prev Chronic Dis* 2005;2:A19 [PMID: 15888230] PMC1327713.

Banerji MA, Chaiken RL, Huey H et al. GAD antibody negative NIDDM in adult black subjects with diabetic ketoacidosis and increased frequency of human leukocyte antigen DR3 and DR4. *Flatbush diabetes. Diabetes* 1994;43:741–5 [PMID: 8194658].

Bansal N. Prediabetes diagnosis and treatment: a review. *World J Diabetes* 2015;6:296–303 [PMID: 25789110] PMC4360422.

Borg K, Kuenen JC, Carstensen B et al. Real-life glycaemic profiles in non-diabetic individuals with low fasting glucose and normal HbA1c: the A1C-Derived Average Glucose (ADAG) study, *Diabetologia* 2010;53:1608–11 [PMID:20396998] PMC2892065.

Dozio N. Pregnancy planning in Type 1 diabetes, in Levy D: *Type 1 Diabetes*, 2nd edn (Oxford Diabetes Library). Oxford: Oxford University Press, 2016, pp.189–203.

Galling B, Roldán A, Nielsen RE et al. Type 2 diabetes mellitus in youth exposed to antipsychotics: a systematic review and meta-analysis. *JAMA Psychiatry* 2016;73:247–59 [PMID: 26792761].

Hamman RF, Bell RA, Dabelea D. SEARCH for Diabetes in Youth Study Group. The SEARCH for Diabetes in Youth study: rationale, findings, and future directions. *Diabetes Care* 2014;37:3336–44 [PMID: 25414389] PMC4237981.

Hawa MI, Kolb H, Schloot N et al. Action LADA Consortium. Adult-onset autoimmune diabetes in Europe is prevalent with a broad clinical phenotype: Action LADA 7. *Diabetes Care* 2013;36:908–13 [PMID: 23248199] PMC3609504.

Hawa MI, Buchan AP, Ola T et al. LADA and CARDS: a prospective study of clinical outcome in established adult-onset autoimmune diabetes. *Diabetes Care* 2014;37: 1643–9 [PMID: 24722498].

Hod M, Kapur A, Sacks DA et al. The International Federation of Gynecology and Obstetrics (FIGO) Initiative on gestation diabetes mellitus: a pragmatic guide for diagnosis, management, and care. *Int J Gynaecol Obstet* 2015;131 Suppl 3:S173–211 [PMID: 26433807].

Holman N, Forouhi NG, Goyder E, Wild SH. The Association of Public Health Observatories (APHO) Diabetes Prevalence Model: estimates of total diabetes prevalence for England, 2010–2030. *Diabet Med* 2011;27:575–82 [PMID: 21480968].

Imagawa A, Hanafusa T. Fulminant type 1 diabetes – an important subtype in East Asia. *Diabetes Metab Res Rev* 2011;27:959–64 [PMID: 22069293].

Jones AG, Hattersley AT. The clinical utility of C-peptide measurement in the care of patients with diabetes. *Diabetic Med* 2013:30:803–17 [PMID: 23413806] Free full text.

Lee JM, Gebremariam A, Woolford SJ et al. A risk score for identifying overweight adolescents with dysglycemia in primary care settings. *J Pediatr Endocrinol Metab* 2013;26:477–88 [PMID: 23435184] PMC3837697.

Leslie RD, Kolb H, Schloot NC et al. Diabetes classification: grey zones, sound and smoke: Action LADA 1. *Diabetes Metab Res Rev* 2008;24:511–9 [PMID: 18615859].

Levy D. Acute pancreatitis, in Levy D: *The Hands-on Guide to Diabetes Care in Hospital*. Chichester: John Wiley & Sons Ltd, 2016, pp. 62–65.

Lu Y, Rodriguez LA, Malgerud L et al. New-onset type 2 diabetes, elevated HbA1c, anti-diabetic medications, and risk of pancreatic cancer. *Br J Cancer* 2015;113:1607–14 [PMID: 26575601] PMC4705881.

Ma RC, Chan JC. Type 2 diabetes in East Asians: similarities and differences with populations in Europe and the United States. *Ann N Y Acad Sci* 2013;1281:64–91 [PMID: 23551121] PMC3708105.

Meek CL, Murphy HR, Simmons D. Random plasma glucose in early pregnancy is a better predictor of gestational diabetes diagnosis than maternal obesity. *Diabetologia* 2016;59:445–52 [PMID: 26589686] PMC442503.

Misra S, Hattersley AT. Monogenic causes of diabetes, in (eds) Holt RI et al.: *Textbook of Diabetes*, 5th edn. Chichester: John Wiley & Sons Ltd, 2017, pp. 243–261.

Nyamdorj R, Pitkäniemi J, Tuomilehto J et al. DECODA and DECODE Study Groups. Ethnic comparison of the association of undiagnosed diabetes with obesity. *Int J Obes (Lond)* 2010;34:332–9 [PMID: 19884891].

Onandy GM, Stolfi A. Insulin and oral agents for managing cystic fibrosis-related diabetes. *Cochrane Database Syst Rev* 2016;4:CD004730 [PMID: 27087121].

Pedersen SB, Langsted A, Nordestgaard BG. Nonfasting mild-to-moderate hypertriglyceridemia and risk of acute pancreatitis. *JAMA Intern Med* 2016;176:1834–1842 [PMID: 27820614].

Rosentock J, Banarer S, Fonseca V et al. INCB13739-202 Principal Investigators. The 11-beta-hydroxysteroid dehydrogenase type 1 inhibitor INCB13739 improves hyperglycemia in patients with type 2 diabetes inadequately controlled by metformin monotherapy. *Diabetes Care* 2010;33:1516–22 [PMID: 20413513] PMC2890352.

Schwartz SS, Epstein S, Corkey BE et al. The time is right for a new classification system for diabetes: rationale and implications of the β-cell-centric classification schema. *Diabetes Care* 2016;39:179–86 [PMID: 26798148] PMC5317235.

Sharif A, Cohney S. Post-transplantation diabetes – state of the art. *Lancet Diabetes Endocrinol* 2016;4:337–49 [PMID: 26632096].

Shivaprasad C, Pulikkal AA, Kumar KM. Pacncreatic exocrine insufficiency in type 1 and type 2 diabetics of Indian origin. *Pancreatology* 2015;15:616–9 [PMID: 26549275].

Takahashi N, Tsujimoto T, Chujo D, Kajio H. High risk of renal dysfunction in patients with fulminant type 1 diabetes. *J Diabetes Investig* 2017 [Epub ahead of print]. [PMID: 28267278].

Winkley K, Thomas SM, Sivaprasad S et al. The clinical characteristics at diagnosis of type 2 diabetes in a multi-ethnic population: the South London Diabetes cohort (SOUL-D). *Diabetologia* 2013;56:1272–81 [PMID: 23494447].

Writing Group for the SEARCH for Diabetes in Youth Study Group, Dabelea D, Bell RA, D'Agostino RB Jr et al. Incidence of diabetes in youth in the United States. *JAMA* 2007;297;2716–24 [PMID: 17595272] Free full text.

Wu HB, Zhong JM, Hu RY et al. Rapidly rising incidence of Type 1 diabetes in children and adolescents aged 0–19 years in Zhejiang, China, 2007 to 2013. *Diabet Med* 2016;33:1339–46 [PMID: 26499360].

Yang W, Liu J, Shan Z *et al.* Acarbose compared with metformin as initial therapy in patients with newly diagnosed type 2 diabetes: an open-label, non-inferiority randomised trial. *Lancet Diabetes Endocrinol* 2014;2:46–55 [PMID: 24622668].

Yang D, Deng H, Luo G *et al.* Demographic and clinical characteristics of patients with type 1 diabetes mellitus: a multicenter registry study in Guangdong, China. *J Diabetes* 2016;8:847–853 [PMID: 26663759].

Zinman B, Kahn SE, Haffner SM *et al.* ADOPT Study Group. Phenotypic characteristics of GAD antibody-positive recently diagnosed patients with type 2 diabetes in North America and Europe. *Diabetes* 2004;53:3193–200 [PMID: 15561950] Free full text.

2 Diabetes emergencies

Key points

- Moderately severe hyperglycaemia in an otherwise well patient with known diabetes (e.g. blood glucose up to 25 mmol/l) rarely requires hospital admission, but a full medical and laboratory assessment is always needed
- Modest hyperglycaemia, for example blood glucose 15–20 mmol/l in an unwell patient or one with significant ketosis may be a medical emergency
- In diabetic ketoacidosis, fixed-dose intravenous soluble insulin (e.g. 6 units/h) will rapidly correct ketosis; insulin at a lower dose should be started in the hyperosmolar hyperglycaemic state only after rehydration is well under way
- Hypoglycaemia is recognized as a major threat in both Type 1 and 2 diabetes; the morbidity and mortality from severe hypoglycaemia is much higher than from hyperglycaemia
- Always try to find a reason for an episode of severe hypoglycaemia
- People with diabetic foot infections, usually from a neuropathic foot ulcer, often need admission to intercept rapid progression. If discharged, make a water-tight follow up appointment with the specialist foot service or multidisciplinary foot team

INTRODUCTION: ABSOLUTE BLOOD GLUCOSE LEVELS ARE A POOR GUIDE TO MEDICAL SEVERITY

The relationship between the blood glucose level and the hazard it poses to a patient is weak. This is because in Type 1 diabetes the problem is insulin deficiency and consequent ketosis and acidosis, and this can occur at almost normal blood glucose levels. In Type 2 diabetes, the threat is a hyperosmolar state, usually in an older person with comorbidity and impaired renal function. Any patient with a blood glucose level in the mid-20s or above requires a very careful but focused examination, but in the majority of cases urgent referral to hospital and an unnecessary admission can be avoided. Type 1 patients become rapidly very sick as a result of ketosis and acidosis, and they will nearly always present directly to the emergency services. In addition, many will be acutely aware of symptoms and the circumstances under which they have become unwell. Type 2 patients with an impending hyperosmolar state usually have a much longer history and are also very sick at presentation. Unfortunately, their immediate carers and medical attendants are not always aware of symptoms, especially if patients already have some degree of cognitive impairment or pre-existing major mental illness. The early part of this chapter, therefore, is directed towards establishing an overall picture of the at-risk patient, especially those with Type 2 diabetes.

Practical Diabetes Care, Fourth Edition. David Levy.
© 2018 John Wiley & Sons Ltd. Published 2018 by John Wiley & Sons Ltd.

Practice point

In the acute setting, absolute blood glucose levels are less important than ketosis in Type 1 diabetes and hyperosmolarity in Type 2.

The management of hyperglycaemic emergencies is summarized in sound guidance documents, adherence to which very likely improves outcomes (see **Further reading**). But the evidence on which they are founded is old in the case of Type 1 diabetes and very slim in Type 2 diabetes. Now that we have empirically established management strategies, further clinical trials are exceedingly difficult to devise. Particularly troublesome is the lack of literature on the hyperosmolar state; not only its management (which actually would be amenable to clinical trial) but even simple registries of clinical characteristics of patients. Because Type 2 diabetes is so pleomorphic, presentations vary according to the ethnicity of the local population (for example 'Flatbush' Type 2 diabetes presenting as ketoacidosis), but there are other characteristics that may have changed over time, as the presentations of Type 1 diabetes themselves have changed (see **Chapter 1**).

ACUTE HYPERGLYCAEMIA PRESENTING TO PRIMARY CARE TEAMS

Every patient initially needs a measurement of capillary blood glucose and urinary ketones, or where available capillary ketones. Patients fall into several groups.

Patients with no previous history of diabetes presenting with hyperglycaemia out of hospital for the first time (Table 2.1)

Always consult previous biochemistry where it is available. Values, while not at levels diagnostic of diabetes, may still have been (in retrospect) abnormal, even though they are unlikely to have been flagged up as abnormal on an automated laboratory report. So although diabetes is defined as fasting glucose ≥7.0 mmol/l, a value of 6.0 mmol/l a year or two ago was clearly abnormal, especially in a young person, and hints at a diagnosis of Type 2 diabetes or latent autoimmune diabetes of adults (LADA). Do not ignore random measurements either:for example, 8 or 9 mmol/l is probably abnormal, though not diagnostic (≥11.1 mmol/l).

Newly-presenting Type 2 diabetes

The majority of patients fall into this group. The Whitehall II Study shows clearly the trajectory of glycaemia before the onset of Type 2 diabetes (**Figure 2.1**), slowly climbing from a fasting value around 5.5 mmol/l 12–14 years before diagnosis with a much more rapid increase in the two years preceding diagnosis. This is associated with a sharp decrease in β-cell function over the same 2-year period (Tabák *et al.*, 2009).

Practice point

Fasting and random glucose levels rise very steeply in the two years before diagnosis. Fasting glucose values ~6.0–6.5 mmol/l, while not diagnostic of diabetes, are formally 'prediabetic' and warrant follow-up, though there is no agreement on how it should be done.

Type 2 diabetes occasionally presents as a hyperglycaemic hyperosmolar state, but not nearly as frequently as Type 1 presents with diabetic ketoacidosis. Hyperosmolarity is often associated with blunted consciousness, so a final security check would be a laboratory glucose measurement together with creatinine (urea) and electrolytes.

Table 2.1 The newly hyperglycaemic patient.

Clinical scenario	Consider diagnosis	Immediate investigations	Decision
Younger, non-obese, white <30 years (minimal family history)	Assume Type 1. Remember that young people from Eastern Europe are also at high risk of Type 1 diabetes*	CBG Urinary/capillary ketones	Rapid direct referral (same day) to local secondary care team
White, non-obese, 30–40 years (minimal family history)	Suspect Type 1 (LADA?)	CBG Urinary/capillary ketones	If CBG <20 mmol/l, and ketones negative,** start treatment as Type 2 (include sulfonylurea) and urgent referral
Ethnic minority and/or obese >30 years (positive family history)	Likely Type 2	CBG Urinary/capillary ketones If any hint of impaired mental state, urgent creatinine + electrolytes to exclude hyperosmolarity	If ketones negative, start treatment as Type 2 (metformin + sulfonylurea)
Special group at risk of DKA: obese African/African-Caribbean males ('Flatbush'-type diabetes)	Probably Type 2, but likely to be acutely insulin-deficient with full-blown DKA	CBG Urinary/capillary ketones	Positive ketones, ask to attend emergency department. If negative, start medication for Type 2 diabetes

CBG = capillary blood glucose; DKA = diabetic ketoacidosis; LADA = latent autoimmune diabetes of adults.
*Eastern Europe (Baltic states – Latvia, Estonia, Lithuania – and Poland, Romania, Bulgaria, Czech Republic and Hungary). The incidence of Type 1 diabetes in these countries is lower than the United Kingdom but there is a large young working population, so newly-presenting Type 1 diabetes is fairly common.
**Capillary blood ketone measurements which detect the dominant ionized ketone body, β-hydroxybutyric acid, and urine dipstick for ketones are equally sensitive in detecting diabetic ketoacidosis, but the blood measurement is more specific (e.g. nearly 80% compared with 35%), therefore more valuable in excluding DKA (Arora et al., 2011).

If patients are otherwise well and free of ketosis, they should start medication to relieve symptomatic hyperglycaemia while awaiting the appropriate education programme. The jury is still out on the question of whether lifelong metformin is needed in these patients (see **Chapter 10** for a more detailed discussion). The long-term vascular benefits of metformin have probably been overstated, but its undoubted safety and very low risk of hypoglycaemia make it a secure choice in patients of all ages (it is safe in pregnancy) and occupations. Start with non-modified release metformin 500 mg twice daily; if there are osmotic symptoms, these require additional short-term sulfonylurea treatment, for example gliclazide 40 mg twice daily (this will require concise education about hypoglycaemia, especially in the middle of the morning/before lunch). Frequent reviews with the benefit of an early dietetic review should allow most patients to revert

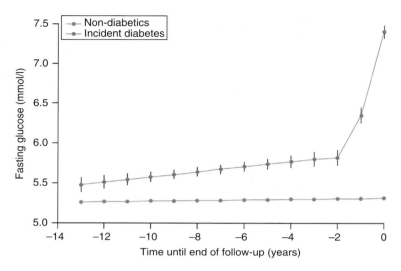

Figure 2.1 In civil servants who developed diabetes, fasting glucose levels rise gradually but imperceptibly for at least 10 years before increasing rapidly into the diabetic range in the two years before diagnosis. *Source*: Tabák *et al.*, 2009. Reproduced with permission of Elsevier.

to metformin only, or in some determined patients diet alone, once glucose levels are optimum. There is general agreement on target HbA_{1c} <7.0–7.5% (53–58), though guidelines are more coy on fasting glucose targets (the American Diabetes Association suggests 4.5–7.0 mmol/l; see **Chapter 10**). Aim to minimize the dose of sulfonylurea and, preferably, with intensive input into non-pharmacological approaches, to discontinue it completely; up-titration of metformin to 2 g/day is a better pharmacological option.

Known diabetes patients presenting with unusually high glucose but without an obvious precipitant (Table 2.2)

Table 2.2 High glucose levels in patients with known diabetes.

Clinical scenario	Consider diagnosis	Immediate investigations	Decision
Type 1	Poorly-controlled or ketotic Ketotic (insulin omitted?)	CBG Urinary/capillary ketones Review historical HbA_{1c} measurements if available	If insulin omission, reinforce regular insulin injection, or ensure new prescription is issued. Urgent direct referral to local secondary care team. If ketosis (urinary ketones ≥1+), rapid same-day referral – but ensure insulin is not omitted in the meantime
Type 2	Poorly-controlled	CBG Urinary/capillary ketones Review medication. Has there been new oral steroid treatment or antipsychotic medication?	If urinary ketones negative, reinforce regular diabetes medication. If steroids responsible, increase or start sulfonylurea, and consider daytime insulin

Recently-diagnosed patients with Type 2 diabetes who have been started on treatment but are still hyperglycaemic

Many patients, even those presenting with marked hyperglycaemia, are started on metformin alone. Even with initial stringent diet restrictions, this may not be sufficient to settle hyperglycaemia over the first few days and patients understandably become anxious if blood glucose values are still in double figures. The only rapidly-effective medication under these circumstances is a sulfonylurea, which should begin to act within 24 hours. Review the patient via telephone in 48 hours. If blood glucose levels are still in double figures, this *may* be non-obvious Type 1 or LADA. However, blood glucose levels at presentation of Type 2 diabetes reflect the degree of β-cell depletion, so patients already severely hyperglycaemic when diagnosed are likely to need insulin sooner rather than later.

ACUTE HYPERGLYCAEMIA PRESENTING TO SECONDARY CARE TEAMS (ESPECIALLY EMERGENCY DEPARTMENTS) (Levy, 2016)

A different spectrum of hyperglycaemia patients presents to the emergency department. They also need careful, though not necessarily prolonged, evaluation.

Known type 1 patients

A much higher proportion of Type 1 patients will come to the emergency department than to primary care teams; many are well used to random glucose levels in the high teens and low 20s especially after meals and if they have also omitted a mealtime dose of insulin (**Figure 2.2**). If they present to the emergency department they are likely to have an additional problem:

- Early diabetic ketoacidosis (DKA) (many will recognize its onset).
- Omitting insulin because they have run out of insulin supplies.

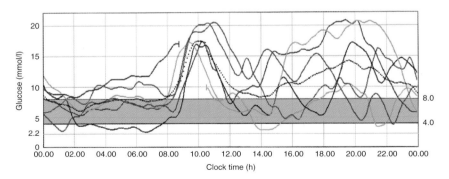

Figure 2.2 Real-life glucose levels in a Type 1 patient, measured continuously over six days (this patient was using an insulin pump, though with poor glucose levels). There is a long hypoglycaemic episode one night and highly unstable levels during the day with frequent peak values between 15 and 20 mmol/l. Note the consistent rapid rise after breakfast, a combination of the dawn phenomenon, possibly exacerbated by high-carbohydrate breakfast cereals.

- The increasing number of patients using insulin pumps (**Chapter 8**) often have 24-hour access to diabetes specialist nurses; they are usually very well-motivated and if they attend an emergency department they are likely to be unwell. Pump malfunction leading to ketosis and diabetic ketoacidosis is very unusual with modern devices (see **Chapter 8**). Ketosis and early ketoacidosis is managed in the same way as a patient using multiple dose insulin, with fluids and variable rate intravenous insulin infusion ('insulin drip').

> **Practice point**
>
> Type 1 patients who come to the emergency department with high blood glucose levels need careful assessment, preferably by the specialist diabetes team.

Assessment

- Get a capillary blood ketone measurement on all Type 1 patients in the emergency department.
- If >1.5 mmol/l, the patient should be admitted.
- Check venous blood gases for pH and bicarbonate: if pH <7.3 and bicarbonate <17 mmol/l, respectively, this is diabetic ketoacidosis: admit.
- Infection: viral upper respiratory illnesses and gastroenteritis predominate, but look out for less common bacterial infections (skin, foot).
- If venous blood gases are normal, then this is poorly-controlled Type 1 diabetes with some degree of insulin deficiency. It may be early ketoacidosis. Admit, initially for 4–6 hours of intravenous insulin (variable rate intravenous insulin infusion/'insulin drip') and rehydration. Admit if ketosis does not completely resolve.
- Ask the diabetes team to see the patient straight away. Diabetes specialist nurses are likely to know individually many of the Type 1 patients attending a hospital clinic There is a small number of patients, usually young females, with recurrent ketoacidosis (DKA-prone 'brittle diabetes'). They will be known to the diabetes team, and may also be well known to the emergency department. They always need admission.

> **Practice point**
>
> Capillary ketone measurements of β-hydroxybutyrate are more specific for diabetic ketoacidosis than urine dipsticks and are, therefore, more reliable in excluding ketoacidosis. Patients can be more accurately triaged.

Type 2 diabetes

There are four groups of patients frequently encountered in emergency departments:

1. Patients with known Type 2 diabetes, often self-presenting because of osmotic symptoms or high self-measured blood glucose levels.
2. Newly-diagnosed Type 2 diabetes patients, usually referred in by their primary care team because of 'high' blood glucose levels, or possible ketosis on urinalysis in the primary care clinic.
3. Hyperosmolar hyperglycaemic state (HHS; see later).
4. Black African or African-Caribbean patients with 'Flatbush'-type diabetes and diabetic ketoacidosis.

The role of the emergency physician is to exclude the last two groups with incipient or actual hyperosmolar state (HHS), DKA or mixed DKA/HHS, and once this has been done to suggest appropriate medication changes.

Mandatory tests in all patients:

- Capillary blood glucose.
- Urinary ketones, or preferably capillary blood ketones.
- Creatinine and electrolytes to calculate osmolarity: $(2 \times [Na] + [glucose] + [urea])$. Hyperosmolarity >320 mOsmol/kg; severe hyperosmolarity >340.

HHS is nearly always associated with blood glucose levels >30 mmol/l, sometimes much higher. To avoid errors in interpretation of capillary glucose levels and missing the diagnosis of HHS, clinicians must be familiar with the equipment used for capillary glucose measurement in their department. Many units have a networked system, such as the FreeStyle Precision Pro, which reads up to a maximum of 500 mg/dl (27.7 or 27.8 mmol/l). At glucose levels higher than this the 'greater than' (>) sign is displayed but, critically, it may not be transcribed into the clinical notes, so '27.7' may mislead clinicians into thinking their patient may not have very severe hyperglycaemia. Values of 27.7 or 27.8 should prompt another sample for a laboratory venous glucose measurement (**Figure 2.3**).

Known Type 2 diabetes

This is a very common presentation, usually with asymptomatic 'high' blood glucose levels. Although the glucose numbers may be high, unless there is an associated medical condition requiring admission (often an infection), these cases can be managed by close liaison between the emergency department and the patient's primary care team. In some instances, they have been told about arbitrary 'threshold' values for glucose that pose a risk. The highest values are seen in patients taking insulin, especially a multiple-dose insulin regimen, which is often inefficient in managing hyperglycaemia, particularly in obese patients (see **Chapter 10**). Its presence itself often indicates poor overall control.

In otherwise uncomplicated Type 2 patients, increase medication, but in the emergency setting limit it to metformin and sulfonylureas. No other drugs will have a sufficiently rapid effect. Possibilities:

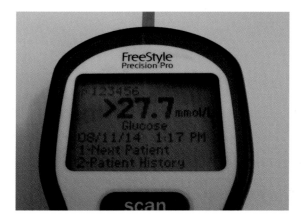

Figure 2.3 Hospital-based glucose meter (FreeStyle), showing the maximum measurable level (27.7 mmol/l = 500 mg/dl). If the '>' sign is omitted in transcription, very severe hyperglycaemia can be missed.

- Ensure the patient is adhering to their medication and that they have adequate supplies.
- Increase metformin to the maximum effective dose, that is 2 g daily (1 g bd), but this manoeuvre will be slow to reduce severe hyperglycaemia, so temporarily add a sulfonylurea.
- If the patient is taking metformin only, then add the most widely used sulfonylurea in the United Kingdom, gliclazide 40 mg bd. Instruct the patient about hypoglycaemia, characteristically maximum 3–4 hours after the dose.
- If the patient is already taking gliclazide, increase to the maximum effective dose, 80 mg bd.
- If the patient is already taking maximum metformin + maximum effective sulfonylurea, only insulin has any chance of acting quickly enough, but it is difficult to start insulin treatment in the emergency department. If the diabetes team is on-site, ask them to see the patient. Otherwise, instruct the patient in a simple zero sugar, low carbohydrate diet in the short term, and emphasize adherence.

If there has been a genuine and major deterioration in overall glycaemic control, make robust arrangements for an assessment with the intention of an insulin start (most likely basal overnight insulin). Where insulin starts are done varies from area to area, and if you are uncertain whether the patient's general practice team is confident with insulin, ensure the referral goes to the secondary care team. They will know local arrangements and how to activate them quickly. Patients must not be lost in the bureaucracy (a general aim, of course, but especially important where urgent insulin treatment is needed).

Newly-diagnosed Type 2 diabetes

A common presentation to emergency departments. Some patients present with typical osmotic symptoms. The referring primary care practitioner and the patient are often very anxious about 'high' blood glucose levels. There is usually no diagnostic problem but bear in mind the possibility of early 'Flatbush' diabetes with ketosis in black patients. You need to be able to give the patient a rapid and, concise introduction to Type 2 diabetes in addition to starting medication.

> **Practice point**
>
> Patients newly presenting with Type 2 diabetes rarely need admission, but always measure capillary ketones to exclude DKA, and if patients are unwell, check electrolytes to exclude hyperosmolarity (>320 mOsmol/kg).

Diet

As above – firm instructions to stop not only all sugar, which patients may already be doing, but non-diet soft drinks, biscuits and cakes, and soft sweet fruit. In addition, suggest a severe reduction in carbohydrate intake (bread, pasta, rice, potatoes, crisps, chips) pending the patient meeting a dietician. If the patient is already self-testing, there is no need to further intensify the testing regime, and, with firm reassurance, try and persuade anxious people testing too often to reduce the frequency. At this most receptive time, it is worthwhile reminding the patient that weight loss and dietary control will reduce the need for medication (see **Chapter 9**) and (a lurking fear for many patients) if it is maintained, probably reduce the need for insulin treatment.

Medication

If patients are symptomatic, and have not already been started on medication, prescribe a sulfonylurea (gliclazide 40 mg bd) in addition to metformin 500 mg bd (if eGFR is

>30 ml/min). Mention hypoglycaemia, which is a risk when compliance with your recommended simple dietary regimen is adopted (which it will be).

Communication

Ensure that a concise summary gets to the patient's primary care team. Electronic communication is more secure.

DIABETIC KETOACIDOSIS (DKA)

The era of high mortality from DKA is thankfully long over. Mortality in the modern era is very low, even in patients admitted to ICU (1% in a study from New Zealand and Australia) (Venkatesh *et al.*, 2015). However, a high proportion of cases of DKA now occur in Type 2 patients – 27% in the same study – and because of age, higher comorbidity and the poor prognosis associated with hyperosmolarity, renal impairment and dehydration, mortality in this group was much higher, 2.4%.

While in-hospital mortality is now very low, mortality was 9% in the year following an episode of severe DKA in a study from Edmonton, Canada, and 35% were readmitted. The reasons for this poor longer term outlook are complex and related to the factors that may have precipitated the episode, including poor adherence to insulin and medical appointments, and underlying psychosocial problems (Azevedo *et al.*, 2014). In children and young people cerebral oedema remains a serious complication of the treatment of DKA and has long-term neuropsychological sequelae; severe DKA itself without cerebral oedema is associated with changes on brain MRI scans and functional impairment, especially of memory, which persists for six months after the acute episode (Cameron *et al.*, 2014). Even in resource-rich countries, 20–40% of new Type 1 patients present in DKA, and several countries have successfully used intensive educational programmes to reduce this rate. DKA at presentation of Type 1 is strongly associated with long-term poor control. In one study under-18 s in Colorado with severe DKA tracked consistently at a mean HbA_{1c} 1.3% higher than those without DKA, and those with mild or moderate DKA nearly 1% higher (Duca *et al.*, 2017). It is not known whether early interception with an educational programme can help ameliorate this poor prognostic indicator.

DKA basics

DKA is a state of insulin deficiency, causing ketosis and acidosis. It is associated with hyperglycaemia but often not of a dramatic degree. The clinical severity of DKA, including the degree of depressed sensorium, is related to the severity of metabolic acidosis, not to the level of hyperglycaemia. However, to fulfil the formal definition all the following are needed:

- hyperglycaemia ('officially' [USA] BG >14 mmol/l)
- ketosis (urinary ketones ≥2+ (>3.9 mmol/l), capillary ketones usually >4 mmol/l)
- acidosis (venous pH <7.3)
- venous bicarbonate ≤17 mmol/l.

Hyperglycaemia with up to moderate ketonuria used to be a very common scenario in poorly-controlled Type 1 diabetes but it is now unusual. Early compensated DKA is occasionally seen, with low bicarbonate but normal pH through buffering of ketoacids by bicarbonate. Recall there are other causes of metabolic acidosis and ketosis and, as discussed above, various states of diabetes that do not amount to full-blown diagnosis. Because the management of DKA is intensive and protocolized it is important to make a secure diagnosis and to bear in mind unusual features even after treatment has started (**Figure 2.4**).

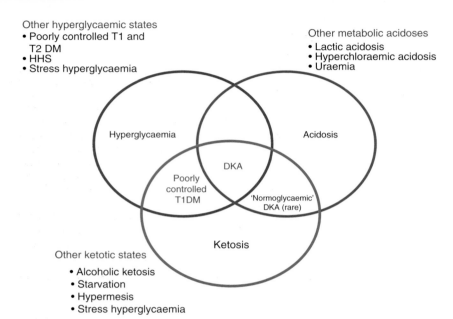

Other hyperglycaemic states
- Poorly controlled T1 and T2 DM
- HHS
- Stress hyperglycaemia

Other metabolic acidoses
- Lactic acidosis
- Hyperchloraemic acidosis
- Uraemia

Hyperglycaemia

Acidosis

DKA

Poorly controlled T1DM

'Normoglycaemic' DKA (rare)

Ketosis

Other ketotic states
- Alcoholic ketosis
- Starvation
- Hypermesis
- Stress hyperglycaemia

Figure 2.4 The differential diagnosis of DKA, including the spectrum of poorly-controlled diabetes that does not fulfil formal biochemical criteria of DKA. Source: Adapted from Fisher and Kitabchi, 1983. Reproduced with permission of Oxford University Press.

Causes
- Infection (30–40% of cases), predominantly gastrointestinal.
- Omitting insulin (15–30%):
  - not observing the sick-day rule to continue insulin treatment uninterrupted, even when ill and not eating
  - running out of insulin supplies
  - in young people, partying in association with a combination of alcohol, substances, vomiting and omitting overnight insulin.
- Drugs, especially cocaine.
- 'Brittle diabetes': recurrent DKA, usually in young women, with unstable diabetes.
- Patients, again often young women who have disordered eating (see **Chapter 15**) and frequently omit insulin in order to lose weight.
- Gastroparesis.
- *Immune-checkpoint inhibitors*, monoclonal antibodies increasingly used in cancer treatment (especially melanoma, non-small cell lung cancer and renal cancer). Agents include the PD-1 inhibitors nivolumab and pembrolizumab, the PD-L1 inhibitor atezolizumab, and the CTLA-4 inhibitor ipilimubab. Endocrine side-effects are common, especially hypophysitis causing hypopituitarism, adrenalitis precipitating acute Addison's disease, and thyroiditis (Torino *et al.*, 2016). From 2015, there were sporadic reports of acute-onset DKA, amounting to fulminant diabetes in one case reported from Japan. Autoimmune markers are absent. High vigilance is needed in these patients who are often already ill, and where symptoms may be masked and not easily recognized.

DKA in Type 2 diabetes

There are three important groups:

- 'Flatbush'-type diabetes (see **Chapter 1**).
- DKA caused by SGLT2 inhibitors ('flozins'). Rare, but relatively normoglycaemic DKA is recognized with this group of drugs used in combination with insulin or other agents in Type 2 diabetes (see **Chapter 10**). Multiple mechanisms may be responsible (Taylor *et al.*, 2015). They are effective glucose-lowering drugs and, in insulin-treated patients, insulin can often be reduced to doses that may not be sufficient to suppress lipolysis and ketosis. In addition, they may reduce renal excretion of ketoacids and increase glucagon secretion from pancreatic α-cells. The clinical concern is that because the drugs act primarily by increasing renal glycosuria, patients may be relatively normoglycaemic (this occurs in other states, for example, malnutrition or, classically but fortunately now extremely rarely, in pregnancy); this is another reminder that severity of DKA relates to the degree of acidosis and not hyperglycaemia.
- Type 2 patients with acute illnesses and those taking high dose steroids increasingly present either with DKA or mixed DKA and hyperosmolarity. Hyperglycaemic emergencies are no respecters of even the most sophisticated classifications of diabetes.

Indicators of severity

Simple clinical and biochemical indicators will direct the urgency and intensity of treatment (**Table 2.3**).

Table 2.3 Indicators of severity in DKA. In some countries all patients with DKA are managed on ICU. Patients with mild (pH 7.25–7.30) or moderately severe (pH 7.00–7.24) acidosis can be managed in an acute admissions unit or specialist ward, but not on a general medical (or surgical) ward. Clinically unwell or sick patients require an ICU outreach team referral.

Feature	Significance	Action
Clinical		
Shock		Urgent ICU referral
Kussmaul respiration	Severe metabolic acidosis (pH <7.0)	ICU assessment
Impaired conscious level	Severe metabolic derangement; cerebral oedema, especially in young patients, other intracranial diagnosis	Brain CT scan; ICU assessment
Abdominal pain	Severe metabolic acidosis	Surgical assessment and serum amylase
Laboratory		
Osmolarity >320	Possible mixed DKA/HHS	ICU referral
pH <7.0	May be resistant to treatment	
Leucocytosis >25	Probable infection	Temperature may be normal or low; full infection screen
Elevated amylase	Correlates with pH and osmolarity	If associated with abdominal pain, get abdominal CT scan for acute pancreatitis

Outline of management

For detailed guidance, see the Joint British Diabetes Societies guideline (**Further reading**).

Contact your hospital diabetes inpatient team as soon as you know that a patient with likely DKA is in the emergency department.

Immediate investigations

- Capillary glucose and ketones; if glucose >27.7 mmol/l, request formal laboratory glucose.
- Cr + electrolytes, FBC, CRP.
- Venous blood gases (VBG).
- In sick patients or acute kidney injury: lactate, creatine kinase, amylase, phosphate, troponin.

Acute management – up to four hours

- Monitoring: hourly blood glucose and capillary ketones, hourly VBG.
- *Fluid:* use 0.9% sodium chloride. PlasmaLyte 148 or Hartmann's would be preferable (because their sodium concentration is 140 mmol/l compared with 154 mmol/l), but these solutions contain only 5 mmol/l potassium chloride, which is inadequate.

   Duration of each litre of 0.9% NaCl:

   Initially 1 hr, then 2 hours, 2, 4, 4 and 6–8 hours

   Use potassium chloride 40 mmol/l once serum potassium is known (potassium measurements from venous blood gas printouts are accurate enough for this purpose). Although there is a significant fluid deficit to make up (5–8 litres is usually quoted) and most DKA patients are young and without cardiovascular comorbidity, truly 'aggressive' fluid infusion regimens, for example infusing 4–6 litres in the first few hours risks fluid overload and cerebral oedema in teenagers. Shock is very unusual in DKA and usually means another process, for example sepsis. Involve the ICU team immediately.
- *Intravenous bicarbonate is of no value and should not be given.* Senior ICU staff, who see metabolic acidosis almost daily, may opt to use sodium bicarbonate in very severe or resistant acidosis, but usually only as a holding measure before starting definitive treatment, for example haemofiltration.
- *Insulin. Fixed-dose soluble (or fast-acting analogue) insulin given intravenously via syringe pump at 6 units/h.* Most hospitals use this as it works efficiently to suppress ketosis and is unlikely to result in prescribing or administration errors. Some guidelines suggest a weight-based dose, that is 0.1 units/kg/h, but it has not been shown to be clinically superior, there are practical difficulties in weighing people in the emergency setting (and the accuracy of estimated weights of patients, especially when they are supine, has not yet been subjected to a rigorous study).

Practice point

Ensure that the patient receives the usual dose of their normal subcutaneous long-acting insulin at the appropriate time.

The current sound recommendation is to continue insulin infusion at 6 units/h to ensure ketosis is continually suppressed, but to supplement the rehydrating fluids with 10% glucose infused at 100 ml/h once blood glucose is <14 mmol/l, in order to prevent hypoglycaemia. This fixed-dose regimen further reduces the risk of insulin administration errors. Therefore, use a triple infusion regimen (all infusions can be given through the same cannula):

- rehydrating fluids
- intravenous insulin at 6 units/h
- 10% glucose at 125 ml/h (500 ml 4-hourly).

Practice point

Intravenous insulin suppresses ketosis. Continue to give it at 6 units/h until ketosis has fully resolved.

By 4 hours, venous pH should be rising steadily, and blood glucose and capillary ketones falling. In particular if the pH is not responding to fluids, get the ICU team to review (and consider co-existing problems, for example sepsis, acute pancreatitis, other intra-abdominal pathology).

Management from 4–12 hours

- Start triple intravenous infusion as necessary.
- Ensure electrolytes are checked at 8 hours.
- Hypernatraemia, commonly seen in HHS, is uncommon in DKA, unless too much sodium chloride has been infused too rapidly.
- Hypokalaemia, often in the range 3.0–3.5 mmol/l, is common and potentially hazardous. Vigorously replace potassium chloride.

Eating and drinking

Uncomplicated DKA is now managed proficiently and patients are often well enough to be eating and drinking within 12 hours of admission. When capillary ketones are less than 1.0 mmol/l, discontinue intravenous insulin and the patient can start their usual insulin. (In the general ward setting where capillary glucose monitoring may not be regular do not discontinue intravenous insulin late in the day; plan to do so early the following morning.) If the patient is drinking normally, and electrolytes are normal, fluids can be discontinued as well. But ketosis can be slow to resolve in some patients, in which case intravenous insulin and the 10% glucose infusion should be continued until capillary ketones are negative, even if the patient is eating and drinking. Conversely, patients admitted with an underlying gastrointestinal problem, usually vomiting, may not be eating once ketosis has resolved. Use a variable rate intravenous insulin infusion with 5% glucose until patients are eating.

The introduction of capillary ketone measurements has significantly reduced the length of stay in cases of DKA. This is because intravenous insulin was previously continued until urinary ketones were negative. However, while a major urinary ketone, acetoacetate, does not contribute to systemic acidosis, it persists long after the major ketone, β-hydroxybutyric acid, which is detected by the quantitative blood strips, has disappeared from the circulation.

Practice point

Urinary ketones persist after plasma β-hydroxybutyrate has disappeared. Using capillary rather than urine ketone measurements can shorten length of stay.

Planning for discharge

Ensure the inpatient diabetes team has reviewed the patient. If the team is not available, communicate with them securely and ensure the patient also has their contact details. Patients should be reviewed by the team within a few days of discharge. Get a brief senior review before discharge.

The insulin regimen on discharge

Reinforce, in writing if necessary, the insulin regimen (brand of insulin, dosage). In known Type 1 patients (the majority of admissions) do not change the insulin regimen unless it is immediately apparent that it has been responsible for the admission (unlikely, compared with poor adherence to that regimen). Do not empirically change brands of insulin if the patient is using preparations you are unfamiliar with. Differences in minutiae of action of insulin between competing brands are never responsible for admission with DKA and any changes of insulin must be considered very carefully in discussion with the patient (see **Chapter 7**). Changes must never be made if a patient is not admitted to their usual hospital on the basis that they do not use the current preferred insulin of the admitting hospital (or the pharmacy does not stock the patient's usual brand).

Ensure patients have sufficient insulin to immediately reinstate their usual regimen on discharge. Insulin in a locked house to which they have no access or which is a train ride away is not of much use. Issue an emergency prescription if necessary (remember to prescribe needles for injection). Ward-based pharmacists are an invaluable resource, but may not be accessible at weekends.

Practice point

Do not suggest substantive changes to insulin brands or regimens to someone admitted with DKA. Reinforce adherence to the current regimen and discuss changes in the clinic setting.

In newly-diagnosed Type 1 patients it is traditional to add up the previous 24 hours' intravenous insulin requirements and divide the total by the number of insulin injections. The statistical correlation between intravenous and subcutaneous insulin requirements is weak, especially when they have been given the 10% glucose/6 units/h insulin regimen. In addition, newly-diagnosed patients may be entering partial remission ('honeymoon') and insulin requirements may rapidly fall. A starting dose based on weight (e.g. 0.5 units/kg/day, divided up approximately 40% as basal insulin, 60% meal-time insulin) is safer. If an experienced diabetologist is available, tap into their experience.

Write a concise discharge summary that focuses on the underlying cause of the episode and future management, and not on the details of how long it took for the pH to normalize or whether there was a transient problem with serum phosphate levels.

HYPEROSMOLAR HYPERGLYCAEMIC STATE (HHS), PREVIOUSLY CALLED 'HONK' (HYPEROSMOLAR NONKETOTIC [STATE])

For detailed guidance, see guidelines from the Joint British Diabetes Societies and the 2015 update (Further reading).

HHS is often much more challenging to treat than DKA. It occurs in Type 2 patients and about 50% of cases are new presentations – compared with 20–40% of Type 1 patients presenting in DKA. Drugs are frequent culprits, notably recent high dose glucocorticoids for any reason, but particularly in cancer patients. General concerns in this hazardous condition include:

- Older patients with cardiovascular comorbidities.
- A high mortality quoted at about 10–20%, which has not changed over the past 20 years, though this seems much higher than the experience of most physicians. Regardless, it still carries substantial morbidity and mortality (Umpierrez and Korytkowski, 2016).
- Frequent pre-existing renal impairment and, very commonly, acute kidney injury on admission.
- Variable presentation, often with non-specific symptoms, for example increasing drowsiness, reluctance to eat and drink, especially hazardous in a warm spell.
- A less acute prodromal phase than DKA, usually several days or a week.
- Severe biochemical derangements and much more severe hyperglycaemia than in DKA.
- An even less convincing evidence base for its physiology or treatment than DKA (HHS/HONK was barely recognized before the 1970s). It is widely stated to be due to a partial insulin deficiency state, where insulin secretion is sufficient to suppress ketosis but not to stimulate peripheral glucose uptake; as in DKA, excess counterregulatory hormones exacerbate the hyperglycaemia through glycogenolysis and other mechanisms.
- 'Aggressive' fluid replacement and insulin treatment are even more hazardous than in the management of DKA. Gentle correction of severely deranged biochemistry with very frequent clinical and laboratory monitoring is needed in this situation.

Practice point

The hyperosmolar hyperglycaemic state is more difficult to manage than diabetic ketoacidosis and has greater morbidity and mortality, especially in the elderly. Most patients will benefit from intensive care team advice.

There is no formal definition, other than the mandatory hyperosmolarity, but key features are:

- *Hyperosmolarity* (>320 mOsmol/kg); severe hyperosmolarity >340 mOsmol/kg. The most widely used definition of osmolarity is $2 \times [Na^+] + [urea] + [glucose]$. The potassium term is too small to make any clinical difference.
- *Hyperglycaemia*, with glucose levels frequently >30 mmol/l, and sometimes much higher. The severe hyperglycaemia (and profound dehydration) contribute to a high thromboembolic risk.
- *Acidosis* and *ketosis* are not usually present. If there is acidosis, it is likely to be caused by existing chronic kidney disease, metformin (lactic acidosis) or sepsis, sometimes in combination.
- *Hypernatraemia* and risk of osmotic demyelination.

A particularly hazardous 'package' of adverse features is described, comprising:

- Serum creatinine >300 μmol/l.
- Osmolarity >340 mOsmol/kg.
- Low Glasgow Coma Scale score, for example 6 or lower.
- Oliguria.
- Acidosis.

Patients with most of these features need immediate ICU care.

Outline of management

Immediate investigations

Venous blood gases (specifically note lactate level), biochemistry, full blood count and C-reactive protein; always include a laboratory glucose measurement because they can be spectacularly high (occasionally >100 mmol/l). A simultaneous blood glucose will also allow calculation of true sodium concentration, which is genuinely depressed in severe hyperglycaemia because of osmotic shifts but when corrected may reveal severe hyper-natraemia. Calculate using the following formula:

$$\text{True}\left[Na^+\right]=\text{laboratory}\left[Na^+\right]+\left[\text{glucose}\,(mmol\,/\,l)\,/\,4\right]$$

and continue to do this calculation with repeat biochemical tests.

Sick patients will warrant, in addition:

- Troponin, creatine kinase (especially if patients have been found at home on the floor), magnesium and amylase.
- They are often elderly, so carry out a full screen for sepsis (always remember to look at the feet and pressure areas for ulceration).

Immediate management

Once initial biochemistry is through, liaise with the ICU team (it will be involved sooner if the patient arrives shocked). Patients are more likely to need ICU care than those with DKA.

Fluid replacement

Start fluid replacement with 0.9% sodium chloride, 1 litre over one hour. Many patients will be hyperkalaemic as a result of acute kidney injury and previous treatment with angiotensin blocking drugs. The potassium concentration derived from venous blood gas printouts is reliable in the acute phase. Thereafter, a suggested regimen for duration of each litre of 0.9% sodium chloride is:

> (1 hour), then 2 hours, 4, 4, 6, 6, 8 hours

But this will need to be adjusted in the light of biochemistry and the clinical state of the patient. Avoid massive initial infusions of rehydrating fluid without careful discussion with the ICU team. There is a case for cautious use of hypotonic fluids if there is hypernatrae-mia after correction for glucose (e.g. serum sodium >150 mmol/l). Appropriate fluids could be sodium chloride 0.45% or PlasmaLyte 148, but this is a senior decision and must be meticulously monitored with frequent laboratory tests.

Insulin

There is no need to start immediate insulin treatment. Non-insulin mediated glucose disposal (i.e. renal) will cause blood glucose levels to fall with rehydration, and rapid osmotic shifts induced by insulin from the vasculature into the extracellular fluid may precipitate cardiovascular collapse; similar reasoning is behind the concerns over osmotic shifts in the central nervous system resulting in central pontine myelinolysis, though clini-cally both outcomes are fortunately extremely uncommon. Many guidelines suggest delaying intravenous insulin treatment for 1–2 hours, some advocate delaying it for up to 12 hours, and there are suggestions that insulin may barely be needed at all. However, there is often very severe hyperglycaemia and, because patients may not be monitored in the same high-dependency area throughout this period, there is a risk that no insulin will be given over a long period.

Because there is no ketosis to suppress, the DKA regimen of fixed dose insulin at 6 units/h is too high, as the blood glucose level is likely to fall precipitously, with possible associated rapid changes in serum sodium concentration. The Joint British Diabetes Societies recommend a fixed-dose intravenous insulin regimen, as in diabetic ketoacidosis, but at a lower dose (e.g. 0.05 units/kg body weight/h). This will, in many cases, result in only slightly lower doses than in DKA management, but clinically it may be too high to establish a slow and steady fall in glucose levels, and there are the same concerns here as in DKA surrounding estimation of body weight in the emergency setting. It is probably wise to start with a lower fixed dose, for example 2 units/h, with hourly laboratory or capillary glucose measurements. On the basis of the rate of fall, alter the insulin infusion rate as necessary; initially increase only by 1 unit/h, to maintain a slow and steady fall in glucose levels if possible (e.g. ~3 mmol/h). This requires continual vigilance, and regular communication with senior clinicians with wide experience of managing this very tricky metabolic state.

Once blood glucose levels fall to 10–14 mmol/l, maintain the same low dose insulin to maintain the blood glucose level. Alternatively, start a standard variable rate intravenous insulin infusion if blood glucose levels are unstable, or if the patient has started eating. Because they are often much sicker than DKA patients, they may not be eating for several days.

Anticoagulation

All patients will receive standard prophylaxis against venous thromboembolism. Hyperosmolarity is strongly associated with venous and arterial thrombosis (cerebrovascular, peripheral vascular and intra-abdominal), and this risk may persist for weeks after discharge. If admission osmolarity is >330 mOsmol/kg, consider full-dose anticoagulation and continue it for perhaps a month after discharge.

> **Practice point**
>
> Consider perhaps a month of venous thromboembolism prophylaxis after discharge in patients admitted with severe hyperosmolarity, especially the elderly and those with known vascular disease.

Diabetes management after resolution of HHS

Patients with the hyperosmolar state usually need a longer admission than DKA patients, which gives the admitting and diabetes teams time to consider the best options for diabetes treatment. Ensure there is a recent HbA$_{1c}$ measurement to help the discussion. Not infrequently, HHS was precipitated by omission of medication or insulin in the week or two before admission, which may not be apparent from the initial history. There are evident problems intensifying a regimen that was not being taken in the first place. Explore the reasons.

Patients previously treated with insulin

Many Type 2 patients will require intensification of insulin treatment, for example increasing basal overnight insulin, moving from basal overnight insulin to basal-plus or perhaps twice-daily biphasic insulin, or occasionally from twice-daily to multiple dose insulin (though – see **Chapter 10** – there is often no benefit from this). Intensification is particularly important if the patient is in poor overall control or there has been progressive weight loss indicating insulin deficiency. Non-insulin agents can be reinstated in addition but persistent poor renal function (eGFR <30 ml/min) will be a contraindication to metformin in many patients.

Patients previously treated with non-insulin agents

Discuss with the diabetes team. If HHS was precipitated by omitting diabetes medication, then they can be reinstated with careful follow up and discussion about adherence, but discuss an insulin start with patients who:

- Had ketosis with hyperosmolarity, that is a mixed HHS/DKA picture.
- Have had a gradual deterioration in control over the past few years, often patients with long-standing diabetes who may have gradually lost weight and may not be obese.
- Are in very poor control, for example, HbA$_{1c}$ >9% (75) on maximum non-insulin agents and good medication compliance.
- Were started on steroids that precipitated the HHS.
- There has been poor compliance with medication before admission and where once-daily insulin can be reliably given by carers, relatives or community nurses.

Newly-presenting patients with clear-cut Type 2 diabetes

Eventually many patients will be well controlled on diet alone, or diet with metformin. However, metformin acts slowly and many will have poor renal function (i.e. eGFR <30 ml/min) that precludes any metformin treatment. Here, the best option is short-term treatment with a sulfonylurea. Start gliclazide 40 mg bd, or if a once-daily drug is preferable, low dose glimepiride, for example 1 mg daily with breakfast, or modified-release gliclazide 30 mg.

HYPOGLYCAEMIA

Acute, severe hypoglycaemia is equally frequent in Type 1 and insulin-treated Type 2 patients. The detailed criteria for thresholds for hypoglycaemia issued by various bodies are not important in the emergency setting but patients presenting to hospital will generally have blood glucose levels of 3.0 mmol/l or less, at which level cognition is likely to be impaired, though perhaps not obviously so. However, symptoms are not always clear-cut and are affected by, among many other things, circumstances (alcohol, drugs), duration of diabetes and previous experience of hypoglycaemia.

Once the immediate emergency has been resolved, wherever possible try and find an explanation. Many events are explained by the usual causes: insulin taken in the wrong dose, at the wrong time, with insufficient food, with excess alcohol or exercise, or a combination of these factors. Recurrent hypoglycaemia at a stereotyped time of day or circumstance requires some sleuthing but is usually due to too much insulin (including 'stacking' resulting from the combined effects of two or more insulin injections). Severe hypoglycaemic events cluster in Type 1 patients: one episode of severe hypoglycaemia can generate a degree of hypoglycaemia unawareness and further events. It should be remembered that the primary cause of death in Type 1 patients under 40 years is an acute complication, especially hypoglycaemia. This includes the terrible 'dead in bed syndrome', where a previously well Type 1 patient is found in an undisturbed bed, and which accounts for 5% of all deaths in long-term follow-up of childhood-onset diabetes (Gagnum et al., 2017).

Practice point

In many countries severe hypoglycaemia has fallen progressively in the face of overall improved glycaemic control in Type 1 patients, but it is still a notable cause of death in otherwise well young people.

Only the severest hypoglycaemic events will be managed in the emergency department. Paramedics are superb at managing it out of hospital and, once treated and recovered, many patients decline the offer of a review in hospital, especially as many events happen at night. This means they are less likely to have education or adjustment of medication. If a patient with hypoglycaemia presents to the emergency department, the event should be considered unusual and hazardous to the patient, and should be followed up. While there are no studies that report the long-term outcomes for patients presenting to emergency departments with hypoglycaemia, there is a strong association (causality not proven, it should be noted) between a single severe hypoglycaemic episode while a hospital inpatient (blood glucose <2.2 mmol/l) and increased mortality over the following year (Turchin *et al.*, 2009). The outlook should be assumed to be poor for patients treated for hypoglycaemia in the emergency department and while, at the very least, detailed discharge instructions should be given, in a large series one in two patients had none documented (Rowe *et al.*, 2015).

Practice point

Ensure all patients with severe hypoglycaemia have a clear management plan in a discharge summary and can implement the needed changes or reductions in medication or insulin.

Consider unusual presentations:

- Seizure (remember that idiopathic epilepsy is ~3 times more common in people with Type 1 diabetes; Dafoulas *et al.*, 2017).
- Hemiparesis.
- Aggressive behaviour, sometimes to people in authority.
- 'He's been drinking, doctor'.
- Acute back pain (opisthotonos or rarely crush fracture of thoracic vertebra caused by fitting).

Consider unusual causes:

- Overdosage of insulin or sulfonylurea. Bear in mind factitious or accidental sulfonylurea overdosage. Many sulfonylureas can be measured in plasma and factitious insulin overdose in non-diabetic individuals can be diagnosed through a combination of high serum insulin and low C-peptide levels (reflecting suppression of endogenous insulin secretion by hypoglycaemia).
- New-onset endocrine disorders, especially Addison's disease, which is strongly associated with Type 1 diabetes (see **Chapter 1**), and hypopituitarism. The onset is often insidious, with increasing frequency of hypoglycaemia despite decreasing insulin doses.
- Impaired absorption: gastroenteritis, coeliac disease.
- Impaired gastric emptying: gastroparesis (see **Chapter 5**).

- Pregnancy-related causes: early pregnancy (decreased insulin requirements at 8–12 weeks combined possibly with nausea/hyperemesis), failure to decrease insulin post-partum, breastfeeding.

Sulfonylurea-induced hypoglycaemia (also see Chapter 10)

Around 3% of patients taking a sulfonylurea report a severe hypoglycaemic reaction in the previous year, and 2% coma and hospitalization (Schloot *et al.*, 2016). Hypoglycaemia caused by a sulfonylurea occurs in patients with significant comorbidity (advanced age, long-standing diabetes, macrovascular disease and impaired renal function). Because there is a high risk of recurrent hypoglycaemia (around one-third of patients) they should generally be admitted; average length of stay is three days and there is a small but definite in-hospital mortality rate of around 1% (Braatvedt *et al.*, 2014). Very severe cases with recurrent hypoglycaemia (in both adults and children) respond well to treatment with subcutaneous octreotide (Glatstein *et al.*, 2012). Discontinue the sulfonylurea; because they show a weak dose-response relationship, simply reducing the dose and then discharging the patient is not secure management. Patients require careful follow-up.

Non-diabetic hypoglycaemia seems to be more common these days. If blood glucose <2.5 mmol/l, always try to take blood for C-peptide and insulin levels; this may be a critical opportunity to make a clear diagnosis.

Management

Blood glucose levels are likely to be high after emergency treatment out of hospital. Track the sequence by reading the ambulance/paramedic records, which are usually meticulous. Treating any rebound hyperglycaemia with a variable rate insulin infusion (VRIII, 'sliding scale', insulin drip) is illogical and may be dangerous if the reason for the hypoglycaemic episode was a long-acting insulin or sulfonylurea.

Treatment

Glucagon. Give 1 mg intramuscularly using the standard kit. It increases hepatic glycogen-olysis, so works more slowly than intravenous glucose. Use it freely if there is likely to be a delay in establishing intravenous access. It is less effective in malnourished people, in liver disease and sulfonylurea-induced hypoglycaemia, where intravenous glucose is needed. Intranasal glucagon is effective and safe, and will be valuable when introduced.

Intravenous glucose. 20% is now given rather than 50% because it is less injurious to vein walls if it extravasates. Give 20% glucose, 100 ml over five minutes. In sulfonylurea-induced hypoglycaemia follow the 20% glucose with a 10% glucose infusion at 100 ml/h.

Follow-up

- Get as full a history as possible. Ask the diabetes team to see the patient.
- Give substantial carbohydrate: 2–3 slices of bread, or several biscuits.
- Monitor capillary glucose every 30 minutes until in the range 7–10 mmol/l.
- If the patient is due a meal shortly after an episode of severe hypoglycaemia, ensure that some of an intended dose of insulin, for example 30%, is given.

When to admit

- Patients with sulfonylurea-induced hypoglycaemia, which is likely to be prolonged and severe (short-acting agents, such as tolbutamide, are no longer used).
- Where it is not clear when long-acting or mixed insulin was last taken, or how long the patient had been unconscious before the hypoglycaemia was detected.

- If there is residual neurological deficit or prolonged coma after treatment, get an urgent brain CT (which was required in about 1 in 7 people in a large study from Canada; Rowe *et al.*, 2015); people with diabetes and hypoglycaemia may also have cerebral infarction or haemorrhage, head injury, cerebral oedema or co-existing poisoning with alcohol or drugs.
- Patients living on their own who cannot be closely supervised over the next 24 hours. The clustering of episodes of severe hypoglycaemia in Type 1 diabetes has already been mentioned.
- Recurrent hypoglycaemia after apparent initial successful treatment (liver disease, overdose with long-acting insulin or sulfonylurea, intentional or otherwise).

> **Practice point**
>
> Severe hypoglycaemia is always a significant medical event. Never treat and discharge without an agreed follow-up plan that involves the diabetes team.

Driving

Requiring treatment for severe hypoglycaemia in an emergency department is considered a significant medical event. The UK rules on driving and hypoglycaemia, considerably tightened in 2011, are simple. A group 1 (car) licence holder is permitted only one episode of severe hypoglycaemia in a 12-month period; group 2 holders (vocational – lorries, buses) must not have any severe hypoglycaemia. Inform the patient that if the current episode exceeds the limit for their particular licence, they are obliged to inform the DVLA. Recognize the seriousness of possible consequences, especially for vocational drivers. This is another reason for the patient to be seen promptly by the diabetes team.

THE DIABETIC FOOT (SEE CHAPTER 3)

Lower limb amputations in people with diabetes are thankfully less common now. However, as a result of better conservative management, chronic foot ulceration may be more frequent. Regardless, it is a very common emergency presentation in both primary and secondary care. The key principle is that antibiotics, while important in the management of acute diabetic foot ulceration with infection, are by themselves inadequate. Most ulcers are neuropathic and not vascular, and offloading with meticulous wound care is the key to resolution. Since the mean age of patients presenting with diabetic foot ulceration is around 60 years, this is an older population, with 40% or more living on their own. They are unlikely to be properly managed if they are sent home. In primary care, a rapid referral to the multidisciplinary diabetes team or the specialist podiatrists should be made where possible; patients who arrive in the emergency department with infected foot ulceration should be discharged home only if there is a small and minimally infected ulcer, for example surrounded by <2 cm cellulitis. Even then, infection can progress rapidly in an insensitive foot.

If the patient is discharged from the emergency department, ensure:

- There is a secure referral to the relevant podiatry team.
- Remind the patient to return if the infection worsens (though this is often a counsel of perfection in people with diminished pain sensation). Ideally the patient or a carer should inspect the foot (and the inside of footwear for objects) every day.

- Issue a prescription for antibiotics that can be immediately filled, for example co-amoxiclav 625 i tds for a week; ciprofloxacin 500 mg bd or clindamycin 300 mg tds in penicillin-sensitive individuals.

References

Arora S, Henderson SO, Long T, Menchine M. Diagnostic accuracy of point-of-care testing for diabetic ketoacidosis at emergency-department triage: β-hydroxybutyrate versus the urine dipstick. *Diabetes Care* 2011;34:852–4 [PMID: 21307381] PMC3064039.

Azevedo LC, Choi H, Simmonds K et al. Incidence and long-term outcomes of critically ill adult patients with moderate-to-severe diabetic ketoacidosis: retrospective matched cohort study. *J Crit Care* 2014;29:971–7 [PMID: 25220529].

Braatvedt GD, Sykes AJ, Panossian Z, McNeill D. The clinical course of patients with type 2 diabetes presenting to the hospital with sulfonylurea-induced hypoglycaemia. *Diabetes Technol Ther* 2014;16:661–6 [PMID: 25010949].

Cameron FJ, Scratch SE, Nadebaum C et al. DKA Brain Injury Study Group. Neurological consequences of diabetic ketoacidosis at initial presentation of type 1 diabetes in a prospective cohort study of children. *Diabetes Care* 2014;37:1554–62 [PMID: 24855156] PMC4179516.

Dafoulas GE, Toulis KA, Mccorry D et al. Type 1 diabetes mellitus and risk of incidence epilepsy: a population-based open-cohort study. *Diabetologia* 2017;60:258–61 [PMID: 27796422].

Duca LM, Wang B, Rewers M, Rewers A. Diabetic ketoacidosis at diagnosis of type 1 diabetes predicts poor long-term glycemic control. *Diabetes Care* 2017;40:1249–55 [PMID: 28667128].

Fisher JN, Kitabchi AE. A randomized study of phosphate therapy in the treatment of diabetic ketoacidosis. *J Clin Endocrinol Metab* 1983;57:177–80 [PMID: 6406531].

Gagnum V, Stene LC, Jenssen TG et al. Causes of death in childhood-onset Type 1 diabetes: long-term follow-up. *Diabet Med* 2017;34:56–63 [PMID: 26996105].

Glatstein M, Scolnik D, Bentur Y. Octreotide for the treatment of sulfonylurea poisoning. *Clin Toxicol (Phila)* 2012;50:795–804 [PMID: 23046209].

Levy D. The Hands-on Guide to Diabetes Care in Hospital. Chichester: John Wiley & Sons Ltd, 2016, pp. 26–31.

Rowe BH, Singh M, Villa-Roel C et al. Acute management and outcomes of patients with diabetes mellitus presenting to Canadian emergency departments with hypoglycaemia. *Can J Diabetes* 2015; 39 Suppl 4:9–18 [PMID: 26541486].

Schloot NC, Haupt A, Schütt M et al. Risk of severe hypoglycaemia in sulfonylurea-treated patients from diabetes centres in Germany/Austria: how big is the problem? Which patients are at risk? *Diabetes Metab Res Rev* 2016;32:316–24 [PMID: 26409039].

Tabák AG, Jokela M, Akbaraly TN et al. Trajectories of glycaemia, insulin sensitivity, and insulin secretion before diagnosis of type 2 diabetes: an analysis from the Whitehall II study. *Lancet* 2009;373:2215–21 [PMID: 19515410] PMC2726723.

Taylor SI, Blau JE, Rother KJ. SGLT2 inhibitors may predispose to ketoacidosis. *J Clin Endocrinol Metab* 2015;100:2849–52 [PMID: 26086329] PMC4525004.

Torino F, Corsello SM, Salvatori R. Endocrinological side-effects of immune checkpoint inhibitors. *Curr Opin Oncol* 2016;28:278–87 [PMID: 27136136].

Turchin A, Matheny ME, Shubina M et al. Hypoglycemia and clinical outcomes in patients with diabetes hospitalized in the general ward. *Diabetes Care* 2009;32:1153–7 [PMID:19564471] Free full-text.

Umpierrez G, Korytkowski M. Diabetic emergencies – ketoacidosis, hyperglycaemia hyperosmolar state and hypoglycaemia. *Nat Rev Endocrinol* 2016;12:222–32 [PMID: 26893262].

Venkatesh B, Pilcher D, Prins J et al. Incidence and outcome of adults with diabetic ketoacidosis admitted to ICUs in Australia and New Zealand. *Crit Care* 2015;19:451 [PMID: 26715333] PMC4699354.

Further reading

Management of DKA

Joint British Diabetes Societies for Inpatient Care Guideline. The management of diabetic ketoacidosis in adults (revised September 2013). www.diabetologists-abcd.org.uk/JBDS/JBDS.htm; last accessed 3 August 2017.

Management of HHS

Joint British Diabetes Societies for Inpatient Care Guideline. Management of the hyperosmolar hyperglycaemic state (HHS) in adults with diabetes (August 2012). www.diabetologists-abcd.org.uk/JBDS/JBDS.htm; last accessed 3 August 2017.

Scott AR; Joint British Diabetes Societies (JBDS) for Inpatient Care; JBDS hyperosmolar hyperglycaemic guidelines group. Management of hyperosmolar hyperglycaemic state in adults with diabetes. *Diabet Med* 2015;32:714–24 [PMID: 25980647].

General inpatient management including diabetes emergencies

Levy D. The Hands-on Guide to Diabetes Care in Hospital. Chichester: John Wiley & Sons Ltd, 2016.

App for iPhone and iPad

Levy D, Cubitt A. *Diabetes in Practice*, 2012.

3 Infections and the diabetic foot

Key points

- Bacterial infections are a persistent threat to people with diabetes
- There is a higher risk of medium- and long-term complications. They often need more intensive treatment than in non-diabetic individuals and require careful follow-up
- Infections related to neuropathic foot ulcers require intensive antibiotic treatment but also need meticulous wound care and pressure offloading
- Staphylococcal infections are particularly prevalent
- Postoperative infections are more common. Although the evidence for tight glycaemic control reducing infection rates is not convincing, try to maintain perioperative blood glucose levels at the fairly stringent general in-hospital levels currently recommended, that is <10 mmol/l
- Ensure immunizations are up to date in everyone with diabetes

INTRODUCTION

Infection is an ever-present risk for people with diabetes and encompasses a spectrum from fulminating life-threatening episodes, for example necrotising fasciitis, to low-level chronic inflammatory conditions, such as periodontal disease. Infection must be uppermost in the mind of the practitioner whenever a diabetic patient presents with non-specific symptoms. High blood glucose levels predispose to some acute infections, especially postoperative, but multiple other, glucose-independent mechanisms seem to be involved, such as the low-level inflammatory state of Type 2 diabetes. Micro- and macrovascular disease, neuropathy and subtly abnormal immunology, the latter particularly in Type 1 diabetes, may contribute. Epidemiological studies abound, as do numerous case reports of unusual infections caused by unusual organisms. Most studies are unlikely to be sufficiently detailed to highlight increased risks of important infections, except, for example, the well-known links between poorly-controlled diabetes and staphylococcal and candidal infections. Relatively uncommon comorbidities, for example Type 2 diabetes and hepatitis C, are mechanistically fascinating but therapeutic innovations resulting from these observations are generally uninspiring. Historical links, for example between diabetes and tuberculosis, are re-emerging and potentially concerning. The evidence base for treating even very common and life-threatening infections, foot infections, is distressingly weak, in spite of heroic efforts spanning decades (Uçkay et al., 2015).

Practical Diabetes Care, Fourth Edition. David Levy.
© 2018 John Wiley & Sons Ltd. Published 2018 by John Wiley & Sons Ltd.

TYPES OF INFECTIONS

- *Common infections* in people without diabetes are also common in people with diabetes. Whether people with well-controlled diabetes have overall an increased risk of chest and urinary tract infections is still not known, but complicated infections are more frequent.
- *Common infections occurring in unusual sites*, especially staphylococcal infections. Never overlook the staph.
- *Unusual infections occurring in unusual sites*. Textbooks repeat the dyad of rare infections nearly always linked with poorly controlled diabetes: rhinocerebral mucormycosis and 'malignant' otitis externa. More common, though equally destructive and potentially fatal, is necrotising fasciitis and its variants (see later).
- *Occult infections presenting with non-localizing features*. Abrupt worsening of glucose control or pyrexia of unknown origin are major challenges. New imaging techniques are useful in these diagnostically difficult cases, for example fluorodeoxyglucose positron emission tomography (FDG-PET). Other, more generally available radiological techniques, especially MRI scanning, are valuable, but only if properly informed by clinical insight and not requested blindly or routinely.

METHICILLIN-RESISTANT *STAPHYLOCOCCUS AUREUS* AND *CLOSTRIDIUM DIFFICILE* INFECTIONS

Methicillin-resistant *Staphylococcus aureus* (MRSA)

Type 2 diabetes is not itself a risk factor for asymptomatic carriage of either sensitive or methicillin-resistant staphylococcus and the high rates reported in single-centre studies are usually in patients with multiple hospitalizations. About 40% of both diabetic and non-diabetic patients carry *S. aureus* in the nose or axilla, but only 1% of community diabetes patients carry MRSA (Hart *et al.*, 2015). Nasal MRSA colonization and MRSA foot infection are not closely linked, but a nose swab negative for MRSA has been reported to reliably exclude MRSA infection in the foot (Lavery *et al.*, 2014). Prevalence data from individual reports must be interpreted with care because multiple factors will affect the rates of infection and detection, including overall changes in MRSA carriage in local populations in relation to national and local prescribing policies and to the near-universal screening of hospitalized patients.

MRSA in foot ulcers is associated with osteomyelitis, previous antibiotic use or hospitalization, long-duration and larger ulcers, and MRSA infections requiring hospital admission are, not surprisingly, associated with higher antibiotic use and longer stay. Nasal MRSA carriage increases the risk of wound infection or dehiscence after lower-extremity amputation. The most serious outcome of MRSA infection, bloodstream infection, is especially common in males, and about 25% of cases occur in people with diabetes. However, MRSA bloodstream infection does not seem to carry a higher mortality in people with diabetes, even though they are older than non-diabetic patients; this may be because very high mortality is associated with an unknown primary infection, while more cases in diabetes are related to evident soft tissue infections, frequently of the foot (Kaasch *et al.*, 2014).

Practice point

Staphylococcus aureus poses a continual threat to people with diabetes. Local factors determine the additional hazard posed by MRSA.

Clostridium difficile

C. difficile infection is not associated with diabetes itself. The majority occur in hospital and, since antibiotic usage is likely to be longer and more intensive in diabetic inpatients, hospitalized people with diabetes might be more at risk, but there is no evidence for this – even of asymptomatic carriage in people with foot ulcers. There is, however, some intriguing and rather more convincing preliminary data that metformin, by altering gut microbiota, may reduce the incidence of *C. difficile* stool positivity. Heart failure, however, may be a risk factor in people with diabetes, and proton pump inhibitor treatment is a clear risk factor, something to bear in mind when reviewing medication in diabetic foot patients (McCreight *et al.*, 2016).

Antibiotic restrictions

The very high incidence of *C. difficile* infections in the mid-2000s led to more restrictive hospital policies for prescribing antibiotics that were particularly associated with infection, that is fluoroquinolones, carbapenems, second, third and fourth generation cephalosporins and penicillin combinations (e.g. amoxicillin/clavulanic acid), in favour of narrower-spectrum agents, including gentamicin, vancomycin and other penicillins (e.g. ampicillin). Clindamycin is an interesting and important agent that was historically associated with an up to threefold increased risk of antibiotic-associated diarrhoea, though this seems to have changed dramatically and it is almost unheard of now. It is considered a broad-spectrum antibiotic, though it has no Gram-negative activity, and it is not recommended in guidelines that restrict the use of, among others, the so-called '4C' antibiotics (cephalosporins, co-amoxiclav, clindamycin and ciprofloxacin). It is, however, widely used and is valuable in penicillin-hypersensitive or allergic patients.

CHEST INFECTIONS

Symptoms of chest infection are less marked in people with diabetes; they notice less cough, sputum and pleuritic chest pain, and the onset of the infection may be less acute. Invasive pneumococcal infection is more common in people with diabetes and although the risk has decreased since the millennium, there is still a nearly fourfold increased risk (similar to that of people with asthma; Weyckyer *et al.*, 2016), which is higher in the under-60s and even higher in smokers. While recognizing that the pneumococcal vaccine is less effective in people with diabetes, these poor outcomes reinforce the need for widespread pneumococcal immunization. Diabetes is also a risk factor for community-acquired pneumonia, with an excess risk of up to 40% compared with the non-diabetic population. In one survey from a USA hospital, about 20% of patients admitted with community-acquired pneumonia had diabetes; patients with complications had a higher mortality. Long duration, poor glycaemic control and younger age (e.g. under 40) are emerging risk factors, but young Type 1 patients in good glycaemic control (HbA$_{1c}$ <7%, 53) still run much higher risks of pneumonia, with an associated standardized mortality rate of 5–6 (Magliano *et al.*, 2015), possibly reflecting deficient innate immunity.

Practice point

Pneumococcal pneumonia is a risk to all people with diabetes, including Type 1 and younger Type 2 patients. Immunization is important.

Respiratory infections with specific organisms are also more common in diabetes, for example:

- *Staphylococcus aureus.*
- *Mycobacterium tuberculosis.* Tuberculosis and diabetes have long been associated. In the 1930s and 1940s, nearly three-quarters of Type 1 patients under 20 had evidence of tuberculosis. The link is re-emerging, predominantly in countries where tuberculosis is endemic, with a usually-quoted threefold increased risk in people with diabetes. Tuberculosis in people with diabetes may be more extensive, more difficult to treat and have a worse outcome. The rapid increase in Type 2 diabetes in developing countries is an alarming potential public health problem itself, without the additional burden of another chronic disease and its management. The relationship is bidirectional. A large database survey in the United Kingdom found only a modestly increased relative risk (30%) of tuberculosis among people with diabetes (Pealing *et al.*, 2015); in the USA Hispanic individuals (but not white or black patients) hospitalized for tuberculosis had a 70% increased risk of diabetes. There is an alert that advanced renal impairment (G4 or 5) may add to this risk. In the United Kingdom there are no current recommendations for tuberculosis screening of high risk groups, but clinicians need to be aware of a link that many think is only of historical interest.
- Gram-negative organisms, especially *Klebsiella pneumoniae*, and associated empyema.

INFECTIONS AFTER SURGERY

There are countless retrospective and case-control studies of both preoperative glycaemic control and perioperative glycaemic control, most of them in patients undergoing coronary artery bypass grafting (CABG). None have given definitive answers, because none are prospective or approach adequate sample size. Poor preoperative glycaemia (e.g. HbA_{1c} >8.5%, 69 mmol/mol, or admission glucose >9.2 mmol/l, 166 mg/dl) is associated with increased risk of major superficial and deep infections, including mediastinitis, thoracotomy site, septicaemia and vein harvest site. Non-modifiable factors, especially renal impairment and obesity (BMI >30) are at least as important in all surgery, so the cumulative risk in many Type 2 patients may be high. Several retrospective studies have indicated that a preoperative HbA_{1c} >8% (64) is significantly associated with wound infections in general and orthopaedic surgery (Hwang *et al.*, 2015).

A randomized trial of tight versus less-tight glycaemic control in CABG showed no benefit in a basket of postoperative complications, but the numbers studied and the separation of mean glucose levels between the two groups (7.3 vs 8.6 mmol/l) were small. The same trial also compared diabetic with non-diabetic patients and again raised the thorny issue of tight glucose control in non-diabetic subjects; non-diabetic subjects maintained at the lower level had a significantly lower complication rate than those at the higher level (Umpierrez *et al.*, 2015).

Practice point

Preoperative HbA_{1c} ≥8.5% (69) carries an increased risk of major infective complications but no trials have established a practical target range for optimal perioperative glycaemic in general surgery.

Bilateral internal mammary artery grafts and associated ischaemia contribute to the most feared complication of CABG, chronic sternal wound infections, and there is good randomized control trial data that perioperative continuous intravenous insulin (UK: 'sliding scale', VRIII), resulting in mean glucose level ~7 mmol/l, compared with bolus subcutaneous insulin (USA: 'sliding scale'), resulting in mean 11 mmol/l, significantly reduces this risk. This is encouragingly practical in the real world (Ogawa *et al.*, 2016). If blood glucose levels can be reduced further without hypoglycaemia, additional benefits seem to emerge. In a proof-of-concept study from Japan using an artificial pancreas in surgical ICU patients routinely given parenteral nutrition, near-normoglycaemia (4.4–6.1 mmol/l) more than halved the rate of surgical site infections compared with higher levels (7.7–10.0 mmol/l), though preoperative glycaemic control in the sub-group with diabetes was already superb (mean HbA_{1c} was non-diabetic at 5.6% (38); Okabayashi *et al.*, 2014).

Negative-pressure dressings and, possibly, hyperbaric oxygen therapy may be of value in these uncommon but severe infections. Diabetes does not seem to be a risk factor for infections of pacemakers or cardioverter-defibrillators.

Orthopaedic surgery

All orthopaedic procedures that have been studied (including hip, knee, ankle and shoulder) are associated with an increased risk of postoperative complications in people with diabetes, including surgical site, urinary tract and lower respiratory infections. Most seriously, patients with diabetes more frequently need revision surgery for deep infection after hip replacement surgery, and peri-prosthetic joint infection is 3–4 times more common. Spinal anaesthesia in hip arthroplasty reduces immediate postoperative hyperglycaemia in both diabetic and non-diabetic people and, although scaling up this trial to show meaningful outcome benefit would be formidable, it may be a consideration in individual patients in persistently poor glycaemic control (Gottschalk *et al.*, 2014).

SOFT TISSUE INFECTIONS

Cellulitis

A spreading infection of the epidermis, dermis and subcutaneous fat, at least twice as common in diabetes. Cellulitis, usually of the lower leg, but occasionally spreading to the thigh, is often recurrent and serious enough to warrant repeated hospital admissions; it frequently occurs in patients with foot ulcers. If the patient does not have a foot ulcer, the microbiology of cellulitis is the same as in non-diabetic individuals, that is predominantly β-haemolytic streptococci, with an uncertain but quite high prevalence of *Staphylococcus aureus*. Antibiotics active against Gram-negative organisms are often given but they are not needed if there is no diabetic foot ulcer. Anaerobic organisms are not involved and do not need to be covered in mild-to-moderate infections. Fissuring and maceration between the toes is a common factor behind recurrent infection; always examine the feet, even if they are not clinically involved. Assiduously clearing up a localized infection while neglecting an evident risk factor for recurrence is unwise.

Practice point

In patients admitted with cellulitis, address general foot care and hygiene, especially fungal infection between the toes, as well as managing the acute infection.

Even straightforward cellulitis in diabetic patients can be difficult to treat. Blistering is prominent; culture of fluid from an unbroken blister is usually recommended, but only when there are additional complications, for example ischaemia or associated ulceration. Unless demarcated and involving a small area, patients should be admitted for at least 24–48 hours of intravenous antibiotics. Early conversion to oral antibiotics is strongly encouraged but should be guided only by definite signs of clinical improvement and not by protocol or pressure on beds. Where there is a large volume of infected tissue, especially if accompanied by ischaemia or marked oedema, 2–4 weeks treatment is often needed. Reducing oedema is very important to ensure antibiotics can get to the infected tissue and minimize the risk of further skin breaks. Loop diuretics are valuable. Bed rest is critical and can be achieved in the usual home environment only in the imaginations of those attempting to reduce the length of inpatient admissions. Extensive desquamation during recovery is characteristic of streptococcal infection.

Practice point

When cellulitis occurs with a foot ulcer or lower limb ischaemia, the patient needs admission to start intravenous antibiotics and ensure maximum bed rest and foot elevation.

Treatment

Mild cellulitis: oral antibiotics – minimum seven days
- Co-amoxiclav 625 i tds.
- Clindamycin 300–450 mg qds in penicillin-hypersensitive patients.
- Flucloxacillin 500 mg qds is usually recommended, with clarithromycin as an alternative in penicillin-hypersensitive patients; adherence to a four-times-daily regimen may not be good.

Trimethoprim-sulfamethoxazole is widely used in the USA, and in uncomplicated cellulitis with or without abscess (surgically treated if necessary) is as effective and safe as clindamycin. These regimens are indicative only, and if the patient is not admitted they still need follow-up in an ambulatory care setting, from where they can be rapidly admitted if there is deterioration or no improvement.

Moderate-to-severe cellulitis: intravenous antibiotics for at least five days followed by 2–4 weeks of oral therapy
- Benzylpenicillin and flucloxacillin 1 g each qds (but remember the high demands of this regimen on nursing staff).
- Clindamycin 300–450 mg qds (and in penicillin hypersensitivity).
- Vancomycin 1 g bd in MRSA or suspected MRSA, or penicillin-hypersensitive.
- Co-amoxiclav 1.2 g tds.
- *Systemically unwell patients* who have had previous antibiotic treatment, possibly oral agents which have not been effective:
  ○ Ceftazidime 1–2 g tds until more specific advice and possibly culture results are available.
  ○ Alternatives: ceftriaxone or cefotaxime.
  ○ Daptomycin and linezolid are probably more effective than vancomycin, but local protocols for the use of these drugs and their availability for emergency use are likely to vary; seek microbiology advice.

Necrotizing fasciitis

A fulminating gangrene of the subcutaneous tissue caused by rapidly spreading micro-vascular thrombosis affecting subcutaneous fat, dermis, muscle and deep fascia. Between 25 and 60% of cases occur in people with diabetes. Other associated factors include obesity, cancer, chronic kidney disease, heart failure, alcoholism, immunosup-pression and peripheral vascular disease (van Stigt *et al.*, 2016). Trauma, sometimes trivial and frequently overlooked, precipitates many cases but abdominal surgery is sometimes the cause. It usually occurs in the limbs but any area of the skin can be affected, especially the head and neck, where it is usually of dental origin. Mortality is still very high, 25% or more, from overwhelming sepsis and multi-organ failure. Awareness of this dreadful condition is much greater now but it is still very difficult to diagnose in its early stages, especially as laboratory indicators, other than perhaps an elevated C-reactive protein, may be initially normal; it is also, thankfully, still a very rare condition. Because of its deep and not cutaneous origin, local tenderness may be unimpressive. However, it rapidly progresses to skin blistering and irregular dusky blue and black patches. It is a surgical emergency requiring intensive medical support. Urgent and widespread surgical intervention, often requiring amputation, can be lifesaving. Think of necrotizing fasciitis in any diabetic patient with severe cellulitis. Confirm with urgent imaging: ultrasound and CT will demonstrate gas formation and its extent (**Figure 3.1**). The use of scoring systems for assessing severity are of little help when the overwhelming priorities are making the diagnosis and ensuring immediate surgical and intensive care support.

> **Practice point**
>
> Always consider the possibility of necrotising fasciitis in diabetic patients with severe cellulitis.

The Infectious Diseases Society of America highlights five important clinical features of necrotizing fasciitis (Stevens *et al.*, 2014):

1. Failure to respond to initial antibiotic therapy.
2. Systemic toxicity, often associated with delirium.
3. Beyond the area of apparent skin involvement subcutaneous tissues feel hard and wooden.
4. Bullous lesions (characteristically containing 'dishwater'-like fluid, not pus.)
5. Skin necrosis or ecchymoses.

Microbiology

- Monomicrobial: predominantly group A β-haemolytic streptococcus (especially *S. pyogenes*; Type 2 necrotizing fasciitis, usually involving the limbs).
- *Fournier's gangrene* is a specific form of polymicrobial (Type 1) necrotizing fasciitis involv-ing the perineum, genitalia and perianal area. Bacteria frequently identified include *S. aureus*, *E. coli* and anaerobes (clostridia, *Bacteroides* or anaerobic streptococci).
- Community-acquired MRSA-associated necrotizing fasciitis is increasingly described, usually associated with other underlying medical conditions including diabetes.
- *Vibrio vulnificus*, found in warm coastal waters of the southern hemisphere and in its seafood, is increasingly implicated, as are other Gram-negative organisms (Type 3 necrotizing fasciitis).

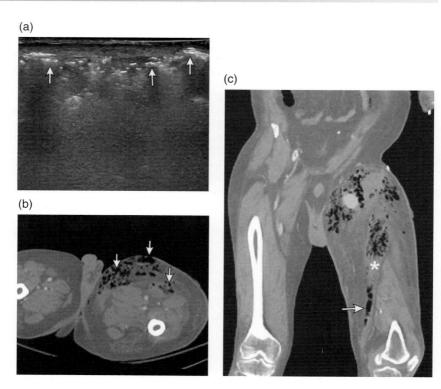

Figure 3.1 Radiology of necrotising fasciitis. (a) Ultrasound image of the left groin showing multiple pockets of soft tissue gas (arrows). This establishes the diagnosis and confirms an emergency, but urgent CT is needed to demonstrate its full extent. (b) Corresponding axial CT scan confirming multiple soft tissue gas pockets. (c) Coronal reformatted CT image of the left thigh. Gas pockets extend from the groin to the upper knee. Gas is seen in the sartorius muscle (asterisk) that extends into its insertion (arrow). *Source*: Reproduced with permission of Dr Sergei Kuzmich, Barts Health, Whipps Cross University Hospital.

Management

Obtain immediate senior surgical and intensive care advice, closely followed by microbiology. High dose benzylpenicillin (e.g. >14 g/day) and clindamycin (900 mg tds) are usually recommended for streptococcal infection, and a carbapenem (e.g. imipenem, meropenem) or piperacillin/tazobactam for suspected Fournier's gangrene. Hyperbaric oxygen may reduce tissue loss and reduce mortality, but is rarely available quickly enough, and there is no systematic evidence for benefit. We will await meaningful clinical trials a very long time.

DIABETIC FOOT INFECTIONS

These are nearly always related to foot ulcers and remain the commonest reason for hospital admission and for lower limb amputation. Peripheral arterial disease is definitely diminishing as a contributory cause of ulceration and infection, allowing neuropathic foot ulceration to dominate even more; chronicity and recurrent infection with resistant organisms, predominantly MRSA and extended-spectrum β-lactamase-producing Gram-negative rods (e.g. *E. coli, K. pneumoniae*), not *S. aureus*, are now the major burden of isolates from foot ulcers in individuals living in the United Kingdom, India, Africa and the Middle East. (MRSA prevalence may also be very low in other areas compared with northern populations, so locality and therefore local guidelines are critically important.)

Mild infections (IDSA-IWGDF classification: <2 cm cellulitis around the ulcer, infection limited to skin and subcutaneous tissue) can be managed in the ambulatory setting, but a fully-functioning diabetes foot team and frequent follow-up is required. The aim of treatment is not so much to heal the ulcer, which is a longer-term goal, but to rapidly deal with infection and its consequences, especially abscesses and osteomyelitis. Always consider the patient's wider environment when assessing whether or not to admit. Patients who are socially isolated (very common) or living in poor housing conditions with the possibility of poor hygienic surroundings should be admitted, even if the infection is judged to be mild; infections are much less likely to clear under these circumstances and relieving pressure on the ulcer and foot is much more effective in the inpatient setting. Antibiotics alone are not sufficient.

Practice point

Antibiotics are necessary for foot infections associated with ulcers, but wound care and pressure relief are critical for rapid resolution and reducing recurrent infections. Always request a plain radiograph of the affected foot.

General management points

- Inform and involve the diabetic foot team as soon as possible, especially if the patient is admitted via the acute surgeons.
- Always remove dressings and clothing from feet and examine them carefully, especially looking for evidence of abscess (specialist podiatrists are adept at detecting them).
- Symptoms are less dramatic in patients with advanced neuropathy and patients are unlikely to have significant pain (consider what symptoms you would have with a deep infected ulcer that might be eroding underlying bone). Some patients mention a non-specific and not very well localized discomfort that would not elicit much of a response from a clinician were it were not associated with a penetrating ulcer.
- *Initial radiology*. Infections can spread and osteomyelitis can develop very quickly. Always request a plain radiograph of the foot, even if the last one is recent. MRI is helpful for diagnosing and localizing collections of pus, but there is now a tendency to request an MRI in a majority of patients, sometimes even before the plain radiograph has been done. There are several reasons for avoiding the MRI reflex. The most important is that there must be a good clinical reason; in addition, there is likely to be a delay in getting the scan, during which time clinical reasoning may be put on hold and treatment delayed. Finally, patients often have old lesions of the foot, amputations and other surgical interventions, and scans can be very difficult to interpret (**Box 3.1**). Plain radiographs may not show convincing changes of osteomyelitis for several weeks (see below), but that is no reason not to get cheap serial studies.
- Deep cultures of ulcers are recommended, but they are of little value in most infections. Microbiological results will not be forthcoming for several days and the significance of many organisms (including MRSA) is dubious.

Box 3.1 Indications for MRI of the diabetic foot.

- If you suspect deep infection – abscess, necrotizing fasciitis (but delay in getting the investigation must never delay urgent surgical intervention).
- As an aid in diagnosing Charcot neuroarthropathy (see main text).
- To detect the presence of osteomyelitis and then evaluate its extent when plain radiography is equivocal or even negative.
- Clinical mid-foot and metatarsal fractures that are not clearly seen on plain radiography, but which present predominantly with foot swelling, bruising or new deformity – or a bone was heard to crack. Minor trauma can cause multiple fractures in people with insensitive feet.

Antibiotic therapy

Antibiotics should cover the most likely pathogenic organisms, that is *S. aureus*, streptococci and *Enterobacteriaceae*. Perhaps surprisingly, there is no definitive evidence to support the use of any specific antibiotic or combinations of antibiotics and local guidelines are still the mainstays of decision making. Bacteriostatic agents do not seem to be less effective than bactericidal agents and pharmacokinetic considerations apparently do not mandate the use of intravenous over oral administration. The key consideration is oral bioavailability, which favours agents such as clindamycin, ciprofloxacin, rifampicin, co-trimoxazole and linezolid, but not the frequently-prescribed flucloxacillin and definitely not penicillin V (phenoxymethylpenicillin). In acute infections arising from chronic ulcers, the initial combination of parenteral benzylpenicillin and flucloxacillin is not optimum because of resistance and the presence of Gram-negative organisms. Consider:

- Co-amoxiclav 1.2 g iv qds.
- Ceftriaxone 1 g daily, up to 2–4 g daily in severe or likely mixed infections, and in penicillin-hypersensitive patients.
- Piperacillin-tazobactam or meropenem in likely mixed infections (these will probably cover *Psudomonas* spp).

But the primary resource is local guidance and local microbiology team, which should be part of the multidisciplinary foot team (Levy, 2016).

Anaerobes

Anti-anaerobic antibiotics (e.g. metronidazole) are often prescribed in people with foot ulcer-related infection, but anaerobes may simply be colonizers in ischaemic and necrotic tissue rather than organisms that worsen outcomes. Initial empirical antibiotic therapy has limited effectiveness against most anaerobes and wound debridement and surgery are the primary treatments for necrosis and abscesses (Charles *et al.*, 2015).

Dressings

Simple dressings are as effective as foam, hydrocolloid or alginate dressings. Clean the wound with saline-soaked gauze, cover with povidone-iodine dressing (if there is no iodine allergy) and wrap with non-adhesive foam dressing, then a light layer of conforming bandage, using minimal adhesive tape and as little as possible in contact with the skin. The scalpel of the specialist podiatrist is a powerful implement when used to debride wounds and remove adherent exudate to expose granulating tissue; no 'advanced' dressing has a remotely similar efficacy. Where there is extensive wound exudate without crusting, sterile larval treatment ('maggot therapy') can be dramatically effective, especially where there is MRSA infection (Bowling *et al.*, 2007). We may even shortly be able to use transgenic maggots that secrete a human growth factor, a potentially dramatic blend of traditional medicine and science fiction (Linger *et al.*, 2016).

Comprehensive management of the diabetic foot

While dealing with infection is often the most pressing immediate concern, other aspects of management are critical in ensuring optimum healing. Their importance increases once the acute infection has settled and, in most cases, the patients will then be under outpatient care, when they are even more important.

Pressure relief

Relieving pressure on the ulcer is a mainstay of management and maintaining mobility rather than the unachievable bed rest of former times is universally recommended. Where available, total contact casting is usually preferred, though there was no difference in the time to healing, about seven weeks, when contact casting was compared with a removable boot, for example of the Aircast type widely used in the United Kingdom (Lavery *et al.*, 2015).

Total contact casting has a long history. It must be done by trained professionals who understand that the methods, aims and precautions differ from those used in fracture management. It is generally safe and effective but complications occur, especially new heel ulcers, mostly in the second week of treatment. Most resolve but even in expert centres around 1% were associated with a partial foot amputation (Owings *et al.*, 2016). It is not known whether removable boots have the same risks; though they are removed at bedtime, pressure-induced damage to neuropathic skin can occur very rapidly and repeatedly taking the cast on and off may pose some risk. However, on balance, the expert application of a removable boot by a specialist podiatrist with frequent wound care and review is probably preferable in many care settings.

Practice point

Excessive, abnormal pressures always contribute to neuropathic foot ulceration, which will not heal without pressure relief. Removable boots of the Aircast type are probably as effective as formal total contact casting.

Management of peripheral vascular disease

Peripheral vascular disease has a different distribution in diabetic patients:

- There is relative sparing of the aorto-iliac segments.
- Femoral disease is common. Localized calcified plaque is frequent in the common femoral artery and often extends into the superficial and profunda femoris arteries.
- Disease in the arteries below the knee is characteristic but foot (pedal) vessels are often patent.

Clinical assessment of the peripheral vasculature is important but often difficult for the non-specialist. It is important to take care in assessing the presence or absence of all four foot pulses. In people with foot ulceration, absent foot pulses predict that nearly half will not heal. In addition, there is a strong general association between absent foot pulses and all future macrovascular events. In the ADVANCE study there was a strong gradient of increasing risk with increasing numbers of impalpable pulses (Mohammedi *et al.*, 2016).

Simple measurements are valuable: an ankle pressure <80 mm Hg or toe pressure <50 mm Hg is associated with high risk of amputation. Ankle brachial pressure index (ABPI) is also simple to measure. Values outside the normal range (0.9–1.3) strongly indicate peripheral arterial disease but raised ankle pressure caused by calcification or incompressibility of the calf vessels is common. Simply elevating the limb will stop foot blood flow in those with low perfusion pressures. Low transcutaneous oxygen measurements in the skin of the foot (<50 mm Hg) are also associated with poor wound healing (Albayati and Shearman, 2013). Duplex ultrasound will indicate the extent of disease and degree of stenosis, and help plan intervention. CT angiography is widely performed, though vascular calcification can degrade the image quality and the vasculature of the foot is often not well seen (important if planning distal bypass surgery). Details apart, patients must not be planned for any lower limb amputation without a full vascular assessment. This should not need stating.

The management of patients with advanced limb ischaemia ('severe' and 'critical' are widely used terms that do not have agreed definitions) is still not established and the results of the single controlled trial (BASIL), which compared initial strategies of either angioplasty or bypass surgery, are still picked over (see the critique by Conte, 2010). Over 40% of the patients in this large study had diabetes. Broadly, there was no difference in overall survival and amputation-free survival. Among the post hoc analysis findings, two are clinically relevant: (i) prosthetic grafts perform poorly compared with vein grafts and (ii) patients who needed surgery after angioplasty did less well than the primary surgical group. The alternative procedures must therefore be considered together and angioplasty should not be assumed always to be the best primary intervention.

Practice point

In the BASIL 1 trial, surgery after failed angioplasty had a lower success rate than primary surgery. Consider all interventional options.

A more general consideration is that after intervention mortality is usually due to ischaemia elsewhere or comorbidities and not to the peripheral vascular disease. Since the BASIL I trial, countless endovascular techniques and devices (e.g. stents of various types, atherectomy) have been introduced, nearly all without evidence of benefit. Standard radiological interventions can be dramatically successful, at least in the short term, and when meticulously performed by experts (**Figure 3.2**).

Adjunctive treatments for non-healing ulcers

Specialized dressings

Specialized and new wound dressings are not regulated in the same way as pharmaceutical products. Many are designed to liquefy or absorb exudate; all have their advocates, some of the medical evangelical variety, but 'spin' in research reports is frequent and 70% of papers without statistically significant primary outcomes (many not even stated) made misleading statements about their effects (Lockyer et al., 2013). The best option is often physical debridement of adherent fibrinous exudate, followed by simple dressings carefully applied (**Figure 3.3**).

(a)   (b)   (c)

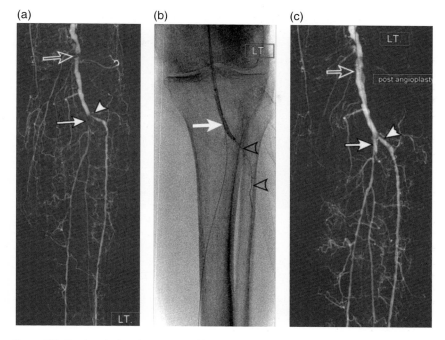

Figure 3.2 Distal angioplasty in a 68-year-old man with Type 2 diabetes and a non-healing foot ulcer. (a) Pre-angioplasty angiogram shows stenosis of the popliteal artery (non-filled arrow), origin of the anterior tibial artery (arrowhead) and tibioperoneal trunk (arrow). (b) Traversing the stenotic segments with a wire (non-filled arrowheads) and dilating with balloons (arrows). (c) Post-angioplasty angiogram shows improved flow through previously stenosed segments. *Source*: Reproduced with permission of Dr Sandeep Pathak and Dr Sergei Kuzmich, Whipps Cross University Hospital.

Growth factors

Of considerable theoretical and biological interest, several growth factors have been introduced for the treatment of ulcers not responding to standard management. Some, including the best-known, platelet-derived growth factor (becaplermin), are prepared by recombinant technology, but there are many others. They are usually applied topically as part of a comprehensive wound-management programme. Trials have been inadequately powered and many suffer systematic errors (bias). All are very expensive.

Skin grafts and tissue-engineered skin

Tissue-engineered skin products are another appealing high-tech group. When trial results were pooled, grafts and engineered products together increased the chance of an ulcer healing and there were fewer amputations in the experimental group, but discriminating differential benefit between the different engineered products is not possible. Long-term effectiveness has not been demonstrated and cost effectiveness, again with very expensive procedures and products, is not known (Santema *et al.*, 2016). Human amniotic dressings and, inevitably, stem cell therapy, are currently of research interest in biotechnology circles.

(a)

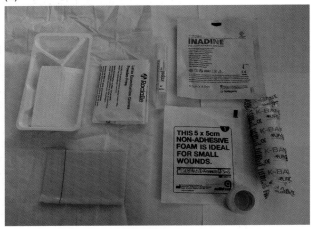

(b)   (c)

(d)   (e)

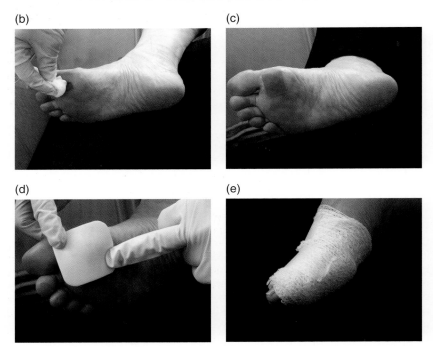

Figure 3.3 A simple dressing technique for diabetic foot ulcers. This should take less than 10 minutes. (a) Use a standard dressing pack and aseptic technique. In addition: iodine dressing (top right), non-adhesive foam dressing (e.g. Allevyn), adhesive tape and K band bandage. (b) Use saline-soaked dressing to thoroughly clean the wound. (c) Cut the iodine dressing to a size just sufficient to cover the wound. If the patient is sensitive to iodine, use a simple non-adhesive dry dressing. (d) Cover with a non-adhesive foam dressing cut to size if necessary (do not use tape). (e) Cover lightly but firmly with the conforming bandage, using only sufficient to hold the dressings in place. Use minimal adhesive tape and do not attach it to skin, as it can damage delicate neuropathic skin. *Source*: Levy, 2016. Reproduced with permission of John Wiley and Sons.

Hyperbaric oxygen treatment

Systemic hyperbaric oxygen is widely used in the USA and Europe for diabetic foot ulcers. There are sound biological reasons why hyperbaric oxygen might promote wound healing through improved oxidative killing of bacteria and systematic reviews have supported improved wound healing and reduced amputation rates. However, a definitive randomized trial using sham treatment (air breathing) in the control group showed no reduction in the risk of amputation or improvement in wound healing at three months (Fedorko et al., 2016). As well as being a good example of the limitations of systematic reviews and meta-analyses in the face of a single meticulously-designed controlled trial, the study should dampen any residual enthusiasm for this appealing treatment, though further trials seem to be in progress. While occasionally used in patients with refractory osteomyelitis, there is – unfortunately – no trial evidence to support its use.

> **Practice point**
>
> Hyperbaric oxygen therapy is of no value in the management of non-healing diabetic foot ulcers.

Negative-pressure wound therapy, widely used in general surgery, can be helpful in individual cases of foot ulceration,but is best used for large ulcers and large soft-tissue deficits, especially after partial foot amputations. However, it has never been subjected to a randomized trial, though the benefits reported in a German multicentre trial started in 2011 were considered insufficient to warrant reimbursement for the treatment (Seidel et al., 2014).

CHARCOT NEUROARTHROPATHY

Charcot neuroarthropathy is a serious and still poorly understood destructive arthropathy affecting bones, joints and soft tissues of the foot and ankle; it is associated with fractures and dislocations, and strongly linked to long diabetes duration accompanied by advanced sensory and autonomic neuropathy. Ultimately, the process causes deformity that compromises function, markedly changes loading patterns in the foot and can cause foot ulceration in sites not typical for usual neuropathic ulcers (that is other than the plantar surface under the first and fifth metatarsal heads) (**Figure 3.4**). It occurs only in patients with advanced sensory and autonomic neuropathy and, while characteristic of long-standing Type 1 diabetes with associated microvascular complications, it occurs in Type 2 patients. The classical site of the Charcot process is the midfoot, where fracture-dislocations of the tarso-metatarsal joints (Lisfranc) eventually result in deformity – the so-called rocker-bottom foot – and which can lead to ulceration caused by displaced mid-foot bones (**Figure 3.4**; La Fontaine et al., 2016). About 50% of patients can identify an episode of trauma – though not always major – that seems to set off a massive inflammatory reaction, resulting in the typical presentation of painless swelling, associated with increased blood flow to the foot, a markedly warm foot to the touch, and which may also lead to the characteristic rapid progression of patchy osteopenia of the mid-foot bones. Some patients describe a poorly-localized dull ache.

Delay in making the diagnosis in a largely insensitive foot is common and understandable but it is a rapidly progressing condition; even when the diagnosis is not clear, follow-up, with plain radiographs every week or two in the first instance, is important. Even then, 'silent' stress bone injuries may be difficult to spot, though MRI can do so more reliably. The Charcot foot should always be considered in patients with subacute

(a)

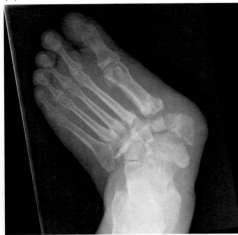

(b)

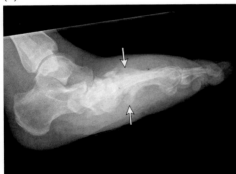

(c)

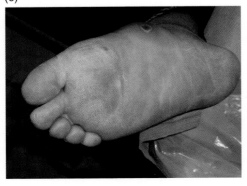

Figure 3.4 Advanced Charcot neuroarthropathy. (a) and (b) Anteroposterior and lateral radiographs of the foot of a male 72-year-old Type 2 patient about six months after the earliest radiological changes were detected. By this stage there is significant foot deformity with severe dislocation of all the tarsometatarsal joints, progressive destruction of the tarsometatarsal and intermetatarsal joints and heterotopic new bone formation (arrows). (c) Typical appearance of a 'Charcot foot': flattened arches and medial displacement of the navicular with secondary ulceration from footwear. 35-year male with 15 years' Type 1 diabetes. He twisted his ankle, but continued to walk on it for two weeks because he had no pain. *Source*: Radiographs reproduced with permission of Dr Sergei Kuzmich, Whipps Cross University Hospital.

unilateral foot swelling who have had no previous foot ulceration. The differential diagnoses include cellulitis, osteomyelitis, deep vein thrombosis and gout; primary osteomyelitis in an intact foot would be unusual, but once there is ulceration, secondary infection is a concern (**Figure 3.4c**). In the absence of ulceration, the presence of bone marrow oedema on MRI hints strongly at a Charcot process.

Practice point

Painless warm foot swelling without ulceration in a patient with advanced diabetic complications should be managed as an early Charcot process.

Management

Initial management is to immobilize the foot as soon as the process has been diagnosed – or better, as soon as there is reasonable clinical suspicion. As in the ulcerated foot, total contact casting is preferred, but a prefabricated walking cast, for example Aircast, is a good start, and in a UK survey was associated with more rapid resolution, though this is a long-term condition and patients and their team need to be aware that a year of treatment is likely (Game et al., 2012). The evident osteopenia of the mid-foot bones led to a vogue for treatment with antiresorptive treatment with bisphosphonates. They may help reduce symptoms more quickly, and certainly simple biochemical markers of bone turnover settle, but treatment probably has little impact on meaningful outcomes (Petrova and Edmonds, 2017). (However, it is a good opportunity to think about bone health in the patient and supplement with vitamin D where needed; in addition, in thin Type 1 patients with long-standing diabetes, and especially if there are eating disorders, consider bone densitometry; see **Chapter 5**.) Custom orthotic footwear is needed once the acute episode is over but these highly threatened patients require careful long-term follow-up.

Surgical intervention at a relatively early stage is becoming more popular, but requires discussion with and advice from surgeons with a major specialist interest in the area. The aims of surgery are to stabilize the foot and to reduce prominent pressure points and the risk of ulceration. Simple interventions, such as Achilles tendon lengthening with excision of bony prominences, can be valuable; some patients require extensive reconstruction with arthrodesis. Do not neglect likely associated complications, especially diabetic kidney disease.

OSTEOMYELITIS

Presentation and imaging

Osteomyelitis is a dominant theme in the chronicity of diabetic foot ulceration and a major contributor to the need for very long term antibiotic treatment with its attendant risks. Even when an ulcer is clinically not infected, around 15% will have osteomyelitis; this proportion rises to two-thirds in hospitalized patients. In most cases, osteomyelitis arises from breaks in the skin, usually a chronic plantar ulcer, but the portal of entrance may appear trivial by the time the patient presents. This is particularly common in osteomyelitis of the toes, where small puncture wounds in the flexures and tips of the toes can heal up after infection has entered. It is, therefore, clinically difficult to exclude osteomyelitis, but an ulcer larger than 2 cm^2 together with a positive 'probe-to-bone' test using a blunt metal probe should provoke a particularly diligent search for osteomyelitis, as it is likely to be present (Lam *et al.*, 2016). Where there is a classical neuropathic ulcer overlying the first or fifth metatarsal heads, protective fibrofatty pads are usually thin and osteomyelitis should be assumed.

Consider Charcot neuroarthropathy if there is radiological suspicion of osteomyelitis, especially of the mid-foot bones, but without clinical ulceration. A painless, red, warm and swollen 'sausage toe'– the dusky swelling is probably due to local ischaemia – is usually associated with osteomyelitis. Changes on plain radiography are notoriously difficult to interpret in the early stages but they can rapidly progress (**Figure 3.5**). While MRI can be helpful, the appearances of osteomyelitis are difficult to distinguish from those of Charcot neuroarthropathy (and the two can co-exist) and careful sequential plain radiography can be helpful.

Practice point

A 'sausage toe' usually harbours osteomyelitis. The distal discolouration of the toe is probably due to septic thrombosis and not to peripheral vascular disease.

Microbiology

The causative organism is usually *S. aureus*, sensitive or otherwise. There may be associated pyogenic streptococci and even coliforms, which would not be surprising in the common scenario of osteomyelitis with a contiguous chronic foot ulcer, but the prime

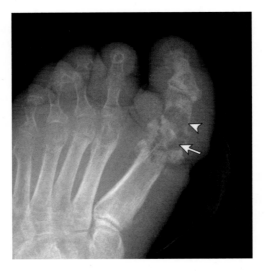

Figure 3.5 Advanced osteomyelitis of the great toe. There are extensive changes in the proximal phalanx (arrowhead) and head of the first metatarsal (arrow), with marked soft tissue swelling. The state of the skin and subcutaneous tissues will often determine whether the patient should have early surgery, which must always be especially carefully considered when the great toe is affected, because of its profound importance on mobility and gait. Infection can spread proximally very rapidly. *Source*: Reproduced with permission of Dr Sergei Kuzmich, Whipps Cross University Hospital.

target for antimicrobial treatment is the staphylococcus. Bone biopsy is often proposed where, for example, there has been no response to long-term empirical antibiotic treatment, but the practical difficulties of obtaining biopsies outside the specialist or research setting are formidable. In any case, there is good agreement between microbiology of deep wound swabs and culture of bone biopsy.

Antibiotic treatment

Unequivocal, extensive proximal osteomyelitis of the foot, fortunately uncommon, has a poor outlook. In a study of USA veterans a quarter of patients needed some form of surgery and 10% came to leg amputation (Barshes et al., 2016). However, the much more common situation of forefoot osteomyelitis – usually of the phalanges – is now usually successfully managed medically with long courses of bone-penetrating antibiotics, preferably oral. There is reasonable clinical trial evidence for this approach using single courses as short as six weeks with no evidence that longer courses increase cure rates (Tone et al., 2015). There is no need for surgery in the first place: antibiotics give the same healing rate over the same period, but a significant proportion (perhaps around 20%) will need surgery after failure of antibiotic treatment (Lázaro-Martinez et al., 2014).

The range of antibiotics used with apparent success is very wide and dogmatism is not warranted; even the ability of individual agents to penetrate bone is not related to their clinical effects on infection. However, do not underestimate the difficulty of adherence to such a long course of treatment, nor the real-life problems of patients obtaining continuous supplies of antibiotics. Most studies have used quinolones (e.g. ciprofloxacin 500 mg bd or levofloxacin 500 mg daily), with a reported cure rate of 60–80%. They are well-tolerated in ambulatory practice and the once-, or at most, twice-daily dosing is probably an advantage in ensuring adherence over long periods. Warn patients to stop antibiotics immediately without reference to a healthcare professional if they develop diarrhoea.

- Adjunctive rifampicin (600–900 mg daily) seems to decrease relapse rates and fusidic acid 500 mg bd or tds has a long history of effective use. These agents must not be used in isolation, and microbiology support is needed in recommending them.
- Clindamycin (150–300 mg qds) is appropriate but the multiple daily dosing is troublesome.
- Trimethoprim-sulfamethoxazole (co-trimoxazole) has a strong evidence base and is widely used in the USA, but as in soft-tissue infections, not in the United Kingdom.

Practice point

Six weeks of quinolone antibiotics or clindamycin will successfully treat distal osteomyelitis in around three-quarters of patients. Adding rifampicin or fusidic acid may increase the cure rate.

Haematogenous spread of *Staphylococcus aureus* from osteomyelitis

Haematogenous spread of staphylococcus is well recognized. Levels of alertness need to be high: the spine, especially the intervertebral discs, seems to be particularly vulnerable but extra-skeletal spread is described (to, among others, the endocardium, pericardium, pacemakers and implantable defibrillators) (Dherange et al., 2015), and even to the eye, causing endophthalmitis (Shenoy et al., 2016). Acute onset of skeletal pain in patients with current or even apparently successfully treated osteomyelitis requires repeated blood culture, radiological investigation and continued follow-up. Relapses are described decades after the initial infection, reflecting the ability of staphylococci to remain viable but not replicating while evading host defences. Importantly, make sure that surgeons are aware of active infection and ulceration, especially of the feet when planning even anatomically remote surgery. This will often be cataract surgery, but any open ophthalmological procedure should be postponed if possible while active infection is present.

Practice point

Where possible, defer eye surgery in people with any diabetic foot infection.

URINARY TRACT INFECTIONS

Any doubts about the relationship between poor glycaemic control and infections previously discussed must be set aside when considering urinary tract infections (UTI). They are around twice as frequent in diabetic patients, especially those in poor glycaemic control, compared with non-diabetic people, and are prone to being bilateral and involving the upper tracts, yet are less frequently accompanied by typical symptoms. The healthcare implications are significant: nearly 13% of women with diabetes and 4% of men develop a urinary tract infection in any year (Nitzan et al., 2015). Fungal infections, usually due to candida, are more frequent. Healthcare and urinary catheter-related infections are more common and resistant pathogens more likely, for example:

- extended-spectrum beta-lactamase and carbapenem-resistant *Enterobacteriaceae*
- fluoroquinolone-resistant uropathogens
- vancomycin-resistant *Enterococci*.

Asymptomatic bacteriuria in Type 2 patients is about three times as prevalent compared with control subjects. The prevalence further increases with longer duration but not with worse glycaemic control. In addition to urinary infections, males are also more prone to acute and chronic prostatic infections, including infections after transrectal biopsy.

Practice point

All diabetic patients with urinary tract infections need intensive treatment and investigation.

There is a traditional array of explanations for the higher risk of urinary infections. Strangely, the seemingly evident role of glycosuria was debated for a long time, but the definitely increased risk associated with SGLT2 inhibitors, which substantially increase glycosuria, should modify the epidemiological view, though so far these agents do not seem to be associated with an increased risk of pyelonephritis (see later and **Chapter 10**). Neuropathy affecting the lower tract, resulting in small but significant postmicturition residual urine, contributes to the increased overall risk.

Asymptomatic bacteriuria

Asymptomatic bacteriuria is common in older women with diabetes. Opinion has wavered over whether it should be treated, as there was a hint that it might predict a higher risk of developing symptomatic urinary infections, but a randomized trial did not find any difference between antibiotic- and placebo-treated groups in the rate of symptomatic urinary infection, hospitalization or pyelonephritis (Nicolle *et al.*, 2006), and a careful natural history study found that asymptomatic bacteriuria was benign from the point of view of renal function, frequently recurred and was often ineradicable. Pregnancy, therefore, remains the only circumstance where asymptomatic bacteriuria must be treated.

Practice point

Do not treat asymptomatic bacteriuria except in pregnancy.

Management of symptomatic urinary tract infections (Table 3.1)

Treat bacterial cystitis for a full five days. Pyelonephritis is treated as in non-diabetic people but bacteraemia is 3–4 times more likely, so blood culture is mandatory. Outpatient management with oral antibiotics is sometimes recommended but, because of the likelihood of bacteraemia, unpredictable response to treatment and further complications, especially perinephric abscess, these patients should be initially managed in hospital. For the same reason, even if community intravenous antibiotics are logistically possible in your locality, an initial brief admission is wise. Emphysematous pyelonephritis, usually caused by *E. coli* that for poorly-understood reasons tend to become gas forming, is rare but very serious; fortunately, intensive medical treatment is now usually successful, replacing the urgent nephrectomy of the past (**Figure 3.6**).

Infections in patients with chronic kidney disease

The markedly increased risk of infection in dialysis patients is evident in everyday hospital practice. The spectrum includes infections specific to the process of dialysis and also the high prevalence of foot ulceration. In the FinnDiane study in Type 1 diabetes, the risk of hospitalization with infection increased with the degree of renal disease (e.g. twofold relative risk in macroalbuminuric patients, 11-fold in dialysis patients, and sevenfold in renal transplant patients) (Simonsen *et al.*, 2015).

Genito-urinary infections in patients taking SGLT2 inhibitor drugs (see Chapter 10)

The SGLT2 inhibitors (flozins) are now widely used. The resulting glycosuria is heavy and persistent as long as the medication is taken. Genital fungal infections occur in about 5% of patients with a three- to fivefold increased risk compared with placebo. In a meta-analysis of randomized trials, urinary tract infections were found to be higher with dapagliflozin (Li *et al.*, 2016) and canagliflozin (Qiu *et al.*, 2017), so they are clearly a class effect of these drugs.

Practice point

Urinary tract infections are more common in patients treated with SGLT2 inhibitors. They should not be used in people with recurrent urinary infection.

ABDOMINAL INFECTIONS

Abdominal infections remain a persistent trap. The commonest infection, peritonitis in patients on peritoneal dialysis, is intercepted through rigorous protocols in renal units but symptoms caused by sporadic infections may be attenuated by reduced visceral abdominal sensitivity, well documented in patients with advanced autonomic neuropathy.

Table 3.1 Management of urinary tract infections in people with diabetes.

Infection	Clinical features	Diagnostic procedures	Microbiology	Suggested treatment	Comments
Cystitis	Frequency, dysuria, suprapubic pain	Urine culture USS KUB to exclude upper tract involvement	E. coli, Proteus spp.	Nitrofurantoin 50mg qds or trimethoprim 200mg bd for 5 days Quinolones, β-lactams	Less common organisms: Klebsiella spp., group B streptococci, enterococci, Pseudomonas
Pyelonephritis	Fever, loin pain	Urine and blood culture USS KUB	E coli, Proteus spp.	Gentamicin followed by co-amoxiclav 1.2 g every 8 hrs In the very sick: ceftazidime 0.5–1 g every 12 hrs or ceftriaxone 1–2 g once daily or piperacillin-tazobactam 4.5 g every 12 hours Total duration of treatment at least 14 days	Potential bilateral involvement. Oral outpatient treatment is sometimes recommended, but risk of poor response and progression
Emphysematous pyelonephritis	Fever, loin pain, poor response to initial antibiotics	Plain KUB film, ultrasound, CT scan	E coli, other Gram-negative bacilli (e.g. Klebsiella, Proteus). Occasionally anaerobes Treatment as for pyelonephritis	As above. Close microbiology liaison	Medical treatment nearly always successful, but always involve urology team urgently. Percutaneous drainage, hyperbaric oxygen may be of value, nephrectomy very rarely needed
Perinephric abscess	Fever, loin pain, poor response to antibiotics (fever persisting for >4days after start of antibiotics)	USS KUB, CT scan	E coli, other Gram-negative bacilli, S. aureus from haematogenous spread	As above. Close microbiology liaison	Urgent urological advice over surgical drainage
Papillary necrosis	Fever, loin and abdominal pain	USS KUB, CT urogram			
Fungal infection	Any of symptoms above can occur, depending on site of infection	Difficult to diagnose, and to distinguish from urine colonization; urine culture	Candida spp	Oral fluconazole (close liaison with microbiology)	

USS KUB: Ultrasound scan kidney, ureter, bladder

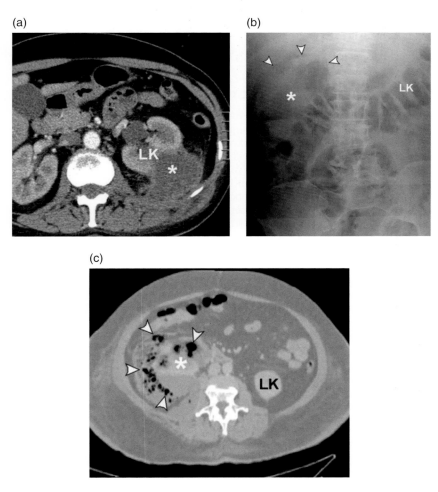

Figure 3.6 Renal abscess and emphysematous pyelonephritis: complicated renal tract infections characteristic of diabetes. (a) Enhanced axial CT scan showing left renal abscess (asterisk) consisting of a thick-walled fluid collection with peripheral enhancement. (b) and (c) Emphysematous pyelonephritis. (b) Plain abdominal radiograph shows free gas (arrowheads) around the right kidney (asterisk) and outlining it. (c) Corresponding axial CT image confirming pockets of gas (arrowheads) in and around the right kidney (asterisk). Normal left kidney.
Source: Dr Sergei Kuzmich, Whipps Cross University Hospital.

In a pyrexia of unknown origin always scrutinize the abdomen. Consider, in addition to the common conditions (acute cholecystitis, diverticular disease):

- emphysematous cholecystitis
- gynaecological infections
- bacterial hepatic abscess (usually *Klebsiella* spp. though relatively uncommon in the United Kingdom)

- psoas abscess (see later)
- | retroperitoneal abscess.

CT, or in diagnostically resistant cases PET-CT, will help. Remember the high radiation doses of these investigations.

MUSCULOSKELETAL INFECTIONS

Much more varied in their presentation than even abdominal infections, musculoskeletal infections in people with diabetes can remain undiagnosed for a long time, even though pain is as prominent as in non-diabetic subjects; the key problem is their distribution, which is wide, and their co-existence with other symptomatic but less threatening musculoskeletal problems, especially spinal. *Staphylococcus aureus* is the usual culprit and seems to have a particular predilection for the spine, causing vertebral osteomyelitis (though the streptococcus and pneumococcus are occasional causes). Local spread is common, resulting in paraspinal abscesses. As in the foot, high levels of suspicion should be maintained and new-onset spinal pain, especially in people with current or historical foot ulcers, needs careful investigation, backed up by targeted imaging discussed in detail with radiologists. Other related conditions include:

- *Septic arthritis* (including the sternoclavicular joint).
- *Epidural abscess.*
- *Discitis*, sometimes associated with vertebral osteomyelitis, increasingly frequent in patients on chronic haemodialysis, and presenting with insidious back pain. Infections can be bacterial or fungal.
- *Iliopsoas abscess* (classically presenting with fever, flank pain and limitation of hip movements, with a positive psoas sign – worsening pain on hip flexion). Frequent secondary causes include vertebral osteomyelitis and discitis, genitourinary infections, and less commonly bowel infections and trauma.
- *Pyomyositis*, which usually involves the quadriceps. Though not infective, diabetic muscle infarction (diabetic myonecrosis) can present in the same way. It usually occurs in poorly controlled diabetes with established microvascular complications, especially renal.

VIRAL INFECTIONS AND IMMUNIZATIONS

Hepatitis C (HCV)

For a long time hepatitis C has been known to be associated with insulin resistance, and hepatitis C is linked to a higher risk of Type 2 diabetes. The research literature is large, more because of the importance of the mechanisms than present management options. There is speculation aplenty, for example that the virus has inhibitory effects on insulin signalling pathways. In some studies, insulin resistance characteristics were associated with a worse clinical outcome of hepatitis C infection; of potential importance, improved lifestyle and metformin treatment, presumably by improving insulin resistance, have been linked with better sustained viral remission. The relationships between insulin resistance, Type 2 diabetes and the new direct-acting antiviral drugs are not known.

Immunizations

Type 1 diabetes

In addition to the childhood vaccines, Type 1 patients should be encouraged to have pneumococcal immunization and the annual seasonal influenza vaccine. In the United Kingdom, students in school year 13 and first-time university students are now offered the meningitis ACWY vaccine. In the USA, hepatitis B immunization is recommended for all people with diabetes under 60.

Type 2 diabetes

Herpes zoster infections are more common in people with Type 2 diabetes, but not in Type 1. The risk increases with age and is three- to fourfold higher in the over 65s. Postherpetic neuralgia may be more common in people with diabetes. Currently varicella zoster vaccine is offered to those aged 70 in the United Kingdom. Pneumococcal and seasonal flu immunizations are important; population attainment with flu jabs is especially impressive in the United Kingdom (73% of people aged 65 and over; OECD, 2016).

PERIODONTAL DISEASE AND DENTAL HEALTH

Dental health must not be neglected in diabetes, as it is strongly associated with periodontitis, a chronic inflammatory condition caused by bacterial colonization and which results in destruction of tissues between the tooth surface and gingiva, and connective tissue attaching the tooth. Alveolar bone loss eventually leads to tooth loss. There is great interest in the reciprocal interaction between the intense local inflammatory response seen in advanced periodontitis and the pro-inflammatory state of Type 2 and, to a much lesser extent, Type 1 diabetes. Although dental decay is probably not more prevalent in Type 1 individuals than in non-diabetic people, there are various abnormalities, for example lower salivary flow, that may contribute to the significantly higher gingival index seen in Type 1 patients that is independent of glycaemic control. Smoking, another major risk factor for periodontal disease, adds to the oral burden.

Quantifying periodontal disease is the major methodological sticking point in clinical studies but the clinically relevant question – does glycaemic control improve if significant periodontal disease is treated? – has a tentative answer, at least in Type 2 diabetes, where HbA_{1c} reduction is modest (~0.3%) but possibly meaningful (Simpson et al., 2015). There are no studies reported in Type 1 diabetes. While patients with diabetes already have a formidable list of self-care matters to attend to, it is worthwhile reminding them of the significance of regular dental examinations. There is recurrent epidemiological evidence for a weak link between periodontal disease and coronary artery atherosclerosis (Stewart and West, 2016), but there are no adequately powered trials, and clinicians would do well to remember that it was not very long ago that macrolide antibiotic-sensitive infectious agents were widely thought (and hoped) to be responsible for coronary artery disease, another of the many neat inflammatory hypotheses now consigned to the archives.

References

Albayati MA, Shearman CP. Peripheral arterial disease and bypass surgery in the diabetic lower limb. Med Clin North Am 2013;97:821–34 [PMID: 23992894].

Barshes NR, Mindru C, Ashong C et al. Treatment failure and leg amputation among patients with foot osteomyelitis. Int J Low Extrem Wounds 2016;15:303–12 [PMID: 27581112].

Bowling FL, Salgami EV, Boulton AJ. Larval therapy: a novel treatment in eliminating methicillin-resistant Staphylococcus aureus from diabetic foot ulcers. Diabetes Care 2007;30:370–1 [PMID: 17259512].

Charles PG, Uçkay I, Kressmann B et al. The role of anaerobes in diabetic foot infections. Anaerobe 2015;34:8–13 [PMID: 25841893].

Conte MS. Bypass versus Angioplasty in Severe Ischaemia of the Leg (BASIL) and the (hoped for) dawn of evidence-based treatment for advanced limb ischemia. Vasc Surg 2010;51:69S–75S [PMID: 20435263] Free full-text.

Dherange PA, Patel S, Enakpene E, Suryanarayana P. From bone to heart: a case of MRSA osteomyelitis with haematogenous spread to the pericardium. *BMJ Case Rep* 2015 Dec 7;2015 [PMID: 26643184].

Fedorko L, Bowen JM, Jones W *et al.* Hyperbaric oxygen therapy does not reduce indications for amputations in patients with diabetes with nonhealing ulcers of the lower limb: a prospective, double-blind, randomized controlled clinical trial. *Diabetes Care* 2016;39:392–9 [PMID: 26740639].

Game FL, Catlow R, Jones GR *et al.* Audit of acute Charcot's disease in the UK: the CDUK study. *Diabetologia* 2012;55:32–5 [PMID: 22065087].

Gottschalk A, Rink B, Smektala R *et al.* Spinal anesthesia protects against perioperative hyperglycemia in patients undergoing hip arthroplasty. *J Clin Anesth* 2014;26:455–60 [PMID: 25200644].

Hart J, Hamilton EJ, Makepeace A *et al.* Prevalence, risk factors and sequelae of Staphylococcus aureus carriage in diabetes: the Freemantle Diabetes Study Phase II. *J Diabetes Complications* 2015;29:1092–7 [PMID: 26243688].

Hwang JS, Kim SJ, Bamne AB *et al.* Do glycemic markers predict occurrence of complications after total knee arthroplasty in patients with diabetes? *Cin Orthop Relat Res* 2015;473:1726–31 [PMID: 25404402] PMC4385343.

Kaasch AJ, Barlow G, Edgeworth JD *et al.* Staphylococcus aureus bloodstream infection: a pooled analysis of five prospective, observational studies. *J Infect* 2014;68:242–51 [PMID: 24247070] PMC4136490.

La Fontaine J Lavery L, Jude E. Current concepts of Charcot foot in diabetic patients. *Foot (Edinb)* 2016;26:7–14 [PMID: 26802944].

Lam K, van Asten SA, Nguyen T *et al.* Diagnostic accuracy of probe to bone to detect osteomyelitis in the diabetic foot: a systematic survey. *Clin Infect Dis* 2016;63:944–8 [PMID: 27369321].

Lavery LA, Fontaine JL, Bhavan K *et al.* Risk factors for methicillin-resistant *Staphylococcus aureus* in diabetic foot infections. *Diabet Foot Ankle* 2014;5 [PMID: 24765246] Free full-text.

Lavery LA, Higgins KR, La Fontaine J *et al.* Randomised clinical trial to compare total contact casts, healing sandals and a shear-reducing removable boot to heal diabetic foot ulcers. *Int Wound J* 2015;12:710–5 [PMID: 24618113].

Lázaro-Martinez JL, Aragón-Sánchez J, Garcia-Morales E. Antibiotics versus conservative surgery for treating diabetic foot osteomyelitis: a randomizes comparative trial. *Diabetes Care* 2014;37:789–95 [PMID: 24130347].

Levy D. Infections in diabetes, in Levy D: *The Hands-on Guide to Diabetes Care in Hospital.* Chichester: John Wiley & Sons Ltd, 2016, pp. 66–84.

Li D, Wang T, Shen S *et al.* Urinary tract and genital infections in patients with type 2 diabetes treated with sodium-glucose co-transporter 2 inhibitors: a meta-analysis of randomized controlled trials. *Diabetes Obes Metab* 2017;19:348–55 [PMID: 27862830].

Linger RJ, Belikoff EJ, Yan Y *et al.* Towards next generation maggot debridement therapy: transgenic Lucilla sericata larvae that produce and secrete a human growth factor. *BMC Biotechnol* 2016;16:30 [PMID: 27006073] PMC4804476.

Lockyer S, Hodgson R, Durnville JC, Cullum N. 'Spin' in wound care research: the reporting and interpretation of randomized controlled trials with statistically non-significant primary outcome results or unspecified primary outcomes. *Trials* 2013;14:371 [PMID: 24195770] PMC3832286.

Magliano DJ, Harding JL, Cohen K *et al.* Excess risk of dying from infectious causes in those with type 1 and type 2 diabetes. *Diabetes Care* 2015;38:1274–80 [PMID: 26070592].

McCreight LJ, Bailey CJ, Pearson ER. Metformin and the gastrointestinal tract. *Diabetologia* 2016;59:426–35 [PMID: 26780750] PMC4742508.

Mohammedi K, Woodward M, Zoungas S *et al.* ADVANCE Collaborative Group. Absence of peripheral pulses and risk of major vascular outcomes in patients with type 2 diabetes. *Diabetes Care* 2016;39:2270–2277 [PMID: 27679583].

Nicolle LE, Shanel GG, Harding GK. Microbiological outcomes in women with diabetes and untreated asymptomatic bacteriuria. *World J Urol* 2006;24:61–65 [PMID:16389540].

Nitzan O, Elias M, Chazan B, Saliba W. Urinary tract infections in patients with type 2 diabetes mellitus: review of prevalence, diagnosis, and management. *Diabetes Metab Syndr Obes* 2015;8:129–36 [PMID: 25759592] PMC 4346284.

OECD. *Health at a Glance: Europe 2016. State of Health in the EU Cycle*, p. 147. http://www.oecd.org/els/health-systems/health-at-a-glance-europe-23056088.htm; last accessed 5 August 2017.

Ogawa S, Okawa Y, Sawada K *et al*. Continuous postoperative insulin infusion reduces deep sternal wound infection in patients with diabetes undergoing coronary artery bypass grafting using bilateral internal mammary artery grafts: a propensity-matched analysis. *Eur J Cardiothorac Surgery* 2016; 49:420–6 [PMID: 25825261].

Okabayashi T, Shima Y, Sumiyoshi T *et al*. Intensive versus intermediate glucose control in surgical intensive care unit patients. *Diabetes Care* 2014; 37: 1516–24 [PMID: 24623024].

Owings TM, Nicolosi N, Suba JM, Botek G. Evaluating iatrogenic complications of the total-contact cast. An 8-year retrospective review at Cleveland Clinic. *J Am Podiatr Med Assoc* 2016;106:1–6 [PMID: 26895354].

Pealing L, Wing K, Mathur R *et al*. Risk of tuberculosis in patients with diabetes: population based cohort study using the UK Clinical Practice Research Datalink. *BMC Med* 2015;13:135 [PMID: 26048371] PMC4470065.

Petrova NL, Edmonds ME. Conservative and pharmacologic treatments for the diabetic Charcot foot. *Clin Podiatr Med Surg* 2017;34:15–24 [PMID: 27865311].

Qui R, Balis D, Xie J *et al*. Longer-term safety and tolerability of canagliflozin in patients with type 2 diabetes: a pooled analysis. *Curr Med Res Opin* 2017;33:553–62 [PMID: 27977934].

Santema TB, Poyck PP, Ubbink DT. Skin grafting and tissue replacement for treating foot ulcers in people with diabetes. *Cochrane Database Syst Rev* 2016; 11:2 [PMID: 26866804].

Seidel D, Matthes T, Lefering R *et al*. Negative pressure wound therapy versus standard wound care in chronic diabetic foot wounds: study protocol for a randomized controlled trial. *Trials* 2014;15:344 [PMID: 25158846] PMC4156638.

Shenoy SB, Thotakura M, Kamath Y, Bekur R. Endogenous ophthalmitis in patients with MRSA septicaemia: a case series and review of literature. *Ocul Immunol Inflamm* 2016;24:515–20 [PMID: 26222985].

Simonsen JR, Harjutsalo V, Järvinen A *et al*. FinnDiane Study Group. Bacterial infections in patients with type 1 diabetes: a 14-year follow-up study. *BMJ Open Diabetes Res* 2015;3:e000067 [PMID: 25767718] PMC4352693.

Simpson TC, Weldon JC, Worthington HV *et al*. Treatment of periodontal disease for glycaemic control in people with diabetes mellitus. *Cochrane Database Syst Rev* 2015;6:CD004714 [PMID: 26545069].

Stevens DL, Bisno AL, Chambers HF *et al*. Infectious Diseases Society of America. Practice guidelines for the diagnosis and management of skin and soft tissue infections: 2014 update by the Infectious Diseases Society of America. *Clin Infect Dis* 2014;59:e10–52 [PMID: 23973422].

Stewart R, West M. Increasing evidence for an association between periodontitis and cardiovascular disease. *Circulation* 2016;133:549–51 [PMID: 2672522].

van Stigt SF, de Vries J, Bijker JB *et al*. Review of 58 patients with necrotizing fasciitis in the Netherlands. *World J Emerg Surg* 2016;11:21 [PMID: 27239222] PMC4884415.

Tone A, Nguyen S, Devemy F *et al*. Six-week versus twelve-week antibiotic therapy for nonsurgically treated diabetic foot osteomyelitis: a multicentre open-label controlled randomized trial. *Diabetes Care* 2015;38:302–7 [PMID: 25414157].

Uçkay I, Aragón-Sánchez J, Lew D, Lipsky BA. Diabetic foot infections: what have we learned in the last 30 years? *Int J Infect Dis* 2015;40:81–91 [PMID: 26460089] Free full-text.

Umpierrez G, Cardona S, Pasquel F *et al*. Randomized controlled trial of intensive versus conservative glucose control in patients undergoing coronary artery bypass graft surgery: GLUCO-CABG Trial. *Diabetes Care* 2015;38:1665–72 [PMID: 26180108] PMC 4542267.

Weycker D, Farkouh RA, Strutton DR *et al*. Rates and costs of invasive pneumococcal disease and pneumonia with underlying medical conditions. *BMC Health Serv Res* 2016;16:182 [PMID: 27177430] PMC4867996.

Guidelines

Lipsky BA, Berendt AR, Cornia PB *et al*. 2012 Infectious Diseases Society of America clinical practice guideline for the diagnosis and treatment of diabetic foot infections. *J Am Podiatr Med Assoc* 2013;103:2–7 [PMID: 23328846].

NICE. Diabetic foot problems: prevention and management (August 2015). nice.org.uk/guidance/ng19; last accessed 5 August 2017.

Stevens DL, Bisno AL, Chambers HF *et al*. Infectious Diseases Society of America. Practice guidelines for the diagnosis and management of skin and soft tissue infections: 2014 update by the Infectious Diseases Society of America. *Clin Infect Dis* 2014;59:e10–52 [PMID: 23973422].

4 Eyes and kidneys

Key points

Eyes

- The incidence of sight-threatening retinopathy fell after the introduction of retinal screening programmes – but it still occurs
- In Type 1 diabetes, any degree of diabetic retinopathy indicates long-term poor glycaemic control
- In Type 2 diabetes the presence of retinopathy should provoke a careful review of glycaemia, blood pressure and lipids: multiple factors are involved, not just hyperglycaemia
- Maculopathy is common in both Type 1 and Type 2 diabetes. The treatment is intravitreal injection with anti-VEGF drugs

Kidneys

- Cardiovascular and renal risk should be assessed using measures of both eGFR and albuminuria, preferably with the KDIGO 'heat chart'
- 'Microalbuminuria' = moderately increased albuminuria; 'macroalbuminuria' = severely increased albuminuria
- In Type 1 diabetes, the primary approach to patients with moderately increased albuminuria is to improve glycaemic control, preferably to HbA_{1c} levels ~7.5% (53) or lower
- In Type 2 diabetes a portfolio of active intervention, emphasizing blood pressure control and LDL lowering, reduces meaningful renal endpoints and reduces other major complications, including cardiovascular events
- Use maximum long-term ACE-inhibitor treatment in all patients with albuminuria in A2 or A3 categories. ACE-inhibitors may have cardiac benefits not shared by angiotensin receptor blockers
- Renal transplantation is preferable to dialysis
- Drug interactions, often serious, are much more common in patients with CKD; patients need frequent and careful medication reviews

INTRODUCTION

Many practitioners will now only be tangentially involved with diabetic retinopathy because the responsibility for its management is now shared largely between the local screening service and hospital ophthalmologists. Even in secondary care few doctors are confident in direct ophthalmoscopy. However, diabetic retinopathy is only one problem that affects the eyes of people with diabetes, which is associated with raised intraocular pressure and chronic open-angle glaucoma, too. Retinal venous and arterial occlusions are also more common. Age-related macular degeneration has some pathogenic features

Practical Diabetes Care, Fourth Edition. David Levy.
© 2018 John Wiley & Sons Ltd. Published 2018 by John Wiley & Sons Ltd.

in common with diabetic maculopathy and both are now successfully treated with anti-vascular endothelial growth factor (anti-VEGF) agents.

Practice point

Patients with diabetes need comprehensive ocular health checks as well as photographic screening for retinopathy.

Sight-threatening retinopathy is happily much less common in both Type 1 and Type 2 diabetes than it used to be. For example, in the large but possibly not representative T1D Exchange Clinic Registry of American Type 1 patients under 21, none had been given treatment for retinopathy (Beauchamp *et al.*, 2016), but any degree of retinopathy more than minimal background signifies poor – often very poor – long-term glucose control, and is a marker for generalized vascular disease. The latter may not be appreciated either by the routine retinal screening service or the secondary care ophthalmology teams reporting or acting on the photographs. The highest risk group is people with renal impairment, and about 10% of this group has sight-threatening retinopathy, mostly pre-proliferative and proliferative (Pugliese *et al.*, 2012). Effective interventions will depend on the severity of retinopathy and the type of diabetes. Glycaemia is by far the most important factor driving retinopathy in Type 1 diabetes; any degree of sustained retinopathy should trigger interventions to help improve glucose control and keep it improved. However, in Type 2 diabetes glycaemia is only one of several factors involved in retinopathy, especially the typical lesions of maculopathy, and not surprisingly multi-modal intervention is needed.

In contrast with retinopathy, primary care practitioners are very closely involved in diabetic renal disease. Routine screening is solely their responsibility. Early renal disease and associated hypertension in Type 2 diabetes need detailed intervention, and because of the continuing high prevalence of more advanced renal disease they are expected to manage patients with estimated glomerular filtration rate (eGFR) as low as 30 ml/min. Recognition and referral are key tasks in patients with retinopathy but diagnosis and often complex management are needed in diabetic kidney disease.

DIABETIC RETINOPATHY

Screening programmes

Local retinal screening programmes started soon after mobile camera technology became available in the 1980s. By 2008 all patients in the United Kingdom were being systematically screened. Many countries with national health services were in the forefront of developing screening programmes, some national (e.g. the UK countries, Iceland, Czech Republic), others regional (e.g. Denmark, Hungary). The impact of these costly programmes was not investigated prospectively and, although there is a convincing association between screening and a reduction in severe retinopathy and significant visual loss, there is also evidence that outcomes were improving in the two decades or more before screening was widely available (Wong *et al.*, 2009). Nevertheless, the Finnish programme was associated with a near-90% reduction in visual impairment over only five years and it is most unlikely that improvement in risk factors could have had such a rapid impact. Sight-threatening retinopathy has fallen in both Type 1 and Type 2 diabetes, but whether to an equal extent is not possible to establish without comprehensive prospective studies.

In the Welsh screening programme all degrees of retinopathy were more prevalent in Type 1 diabetes (sight-threatening retinopathy four times more common) but the overall burden of retinopathy is much greater in Type 2 (Thomas et al., 2015). One canard that can fortunately finally be put to rest: diabetic retinopathy is no longer the commonest cause of blindness in the 16–64 year age group in England and Wales. In 2009–2010, and for the first time in fifty years, it was overtaken by blindness due to inherited retinal conditions (Liew et al., 2014).

> **Practice point**
>
> Diabetic retinopathy is no longer the commonest cause of blindness in people of working age.

Coverage by the UK screening service is good; for example, in an area of South London that is not especially deprived, only 1.5% of the eligible population had not been screened in the past 18 months. Reasons for not attending were a mix of patient-related factors (other commitments, anxiety and misinformation about screening) and system-level factors (practical problems such as errors in addresses) (Strutton et al., 2016). The concern is that severe retinopathy may be unduly highly concentrated within this very small group and go undetected.

> **Practice point**
>
> Screening for retinopathy is in large part responsible for a significant fall in the incidence of sight-threatening retinopathy.

Early worsening of retinopathy with tight glycaemic control

This interesting phenomenon was first described in the 1980s in important early studies of tight glycaemic control in Type 1 diabetes and later confirmed in the large Diabetes Control and Complications Trial (DCCT) cohort. Progression of retinopathy to the point of proliferation and multiple cotton-wool spots occurred most frequently in subjects with high baseline HbA_{1c}, where the fall in HbA_{1c} after starting intensification was >2%, and where there was already significant background retinopathy. It was common, occurring in 13% of intensively treated DCCT subjects during the first year, but the majority of cases were asymptomatic and only detected on retinal photography. In the long term, the risk of progression of retinopathy was much lower with tight glycaemic control, and perhaps the natural history has changed since the DCCT, with a lower prevalence of significant retinopathy overall, as general levels of glycaemia improve, resulting in fewer patients encountering massive falls in HbA_{1c}. Nonetheless transient worsening should be borne in mind in the management of patients during preconception and early pregnancy, and in patients starting pump treatment, where rapid changes in HbA_{1c} can occur. It has not been described after pancreas transplantation, perhaps because many of these patients have advanced 'burnt-out' laser-treated retinopathy. Limited data in Type 2 patients after bariatric surgery, which usually results in immediate and profound reduction in glucose levels, is reassuring in showing no major differences in progression of retinopathy between surgical patients and patients in a medical obesity programme (Miras et al., 2015). However, the proportion of patients with any retinopathy in these studies is low and marked deterioration is described in those with background diabetic retinopathy or worse; they all need careful ophthalmological follow-up. A prominent concern, the possible exacerbation of maculopathy, especially ischaemic, needs detailed prospective follow-up using optical coherence tomography (OCT).

Practice point

When HbA_{1c} rapidly improves by 2% or more ensure that retinal screening is intensified, especially in people with Type 1.

Retinopathy in Type 1 diabetes

Proliferative retinopathy is often thought to occur only in Type 1 diabetes, and maculopathy restricted to Type 2, but screening programmes have uncovered a more mixed picture. For example, in the Welsh screening survey from 2005–2009, maculopathy was the presentation in 4.2% of Type 1 patients but in only 1.4% of Type 2 patients. However, proliferative retinopathy is still the characteristic endpoint of retinopathy in Type 1 diabetes.

Earlier stages of diabetic retinopathy are classified as non-proliferative diabetic retinopathy (NPDR). Microaneurysms (dot haemorrhages) and larger blot haemorrhages first occur at the posterior pole. Flitting microaneurysms due to capillary occlusions are also common—they may reflect disturbed haemodynamics caused by fluctuating blood glucose levels. Persistent minor background retinopathy causes no visual disturbance but increased numbers of microaneurysms predict a higher risk of proliferative diabetic retinopathy (PDR) and maculopathy (Rasmussen *et al.*, 2015). Glycaemic control dominates the prognosis. For example, in the DCCT NPDR progressed in only 5.5% of patients who had a mean HbA_{1c} of 6% (42), while 20% progressed at 8% (64) (DCCT, 1993). NPDR is also associated with a higher risk of other microvascular complications, especially microalbuminuria, and not surprisingly there is a hint of a higher risk of macrovascular events.

Medical treatment of background retinopathy

Only intensification of glycaemic control, whatever the HbA_{1c} level, and smoking cessation are of proven value in helping retinopathy resolve. Non-insulin treatments are much less important. In the RASS study (Harindhanavudhi *et al.*, 2011) an ACE-inhibitor (enalapril 20 mg daily) or angiotensin receptor blocker (ARB) (losartan 50 mg daily) reduced progression of retinopathy, especially in those with worse control (HbA_{1c} >7.5%, 58). However, angiotensin blockade is at best of borderline benefit, as shown by the DIRECT-Protect 1 study (Chaturvedi *et al.*, 2008), in which candesartan 32 mg taken daily for five years did not improve mild- to- moderate background retinopathy. Angiotensin blockade is of no value in primary prevention and should only be used if there are other indications, for example microalbuminuria or hypertension. Likewise, aspirin and statins beyond their usual indications are of no help.

Practice point

Even minor degrees of persistent retinopathy in Type 1 patients indicate poor glycaemic control requiring intensive medical and educational input. Angiotensin blocking drugs, aspirin and statins are of no additional benefit.

Preprolifcrative retinopathy

The term preproliferative retinopathy does not appear in the widely used ETDRS retin-opathy grading scheme and the formal diagnosis (and the very difficult decision if and when to apply laser treatment) is firmly in the hands of ophthalmologists. The term 'moderately severe non-proliferative retinopathy' is synonymous in practice with the pre-proliferative state. It comprises multiple blot haemorrhages, venous beading or redupli-cation and prominent intraretinal microvascular abnormalities (IRMAs). Multiple cotton wool spots (previously known as soft exudates) are characteristic of these advanced stages but they often occur in smaller numbers in less severe retinopathy, so they are not considered diagnostic. Preproliferative retinopathy is likely to be associated with microal-buminuria or proteinuria, subclinical coronary artery disease and certainly with severe long-standing hyperglycaemia. It requires careful joint management between ophthal-mologists and the diabetes team, but this liaison may be less likely now that diabetic retinopathy is often considered separate from the metabolic state that caused it. In addi-tion, because glycaemic control is usually poor, adherence likewise, ophthalmologists seeing these patients should ensure that they are given the opportunity to get back into the diabetes system, which they may have left a good number of years ago. Laser treat-ment does not help. Management is glycaemic improvement and smoking cessation, with obsessive follow-up from diabetes and eye teams.

Practice point

Preproliferative/severe non-proliferative retinopathy denotes high risk for progression to prolif-eration, but laser treatment at this stage does not help: radical improvement in glycaemia and smoking cessation are the correct treatments.

An important trial found that even intensive diabetes assessments and education delivered in the clinic by the ophthalmology team did not improve glycaemia or other markers (body mass index, blood pressure and diabetes self-management practices) (Aiello et al., 2015). Given this outcome, electronically-generated exhortations to improve glycaemic control, routinely included in retinal screening reports to patients, are likely to be futile and of only gestural value.

Practice point

Do your best to ensure that patients with severe degrees of retinopathy are re-integrated into the specialist diabetes network, and do not remain predominantly under the care of ophthalmologists.

DCCT/EDIC: long-term ocular outcomes

Very long-term legacy effects are now emerging in the follow-up of the DCCT cohort, EDIC (Epidemiology of Diabetes Interventions and Complications). The benefits of tight glycaemic control over the randomized phase, lasting seven years, have been docu-mented over an increasing time span, even though HbA_{1c} in the two cohorts converged around 8% (64) shortly after the end of the randomized trial. For example, after a median 23 years follow-up, there was still a 40–50% risk reduction in the need for ocular surgery (mostly for advanced diabetic eye disease) in the previously intensively treated group.

Other surgical interventions that were significantly reduced included cataract, vitrectomy and glaucoma-related operations (DCCT/EDIC, 2015). Non-surgical interventions (for example photocoagulation, anti-VEGF treatment) also continued at a lower cumulative rate but, because of substantial risk reduction in the previous conventionally treated group, the annual incidence is now approximately the same in both groups.

Maculopathy

Maculopathy is retinopathy at or near the fovea and is potentially sight-threatening. Although characteristic of Type 2 diabetes, it is not limited to it. Its prevalence is nearly three times higher than in Type 2, but the total burden is naturally much greater in Type 2. This is of little concern to the individual patient, Type 1 or 2, threatened with visual loss. Although there is no glycaemic 'threshold' for its development in Type 1, the mean HbA_{1c} in patients progressing to laser treatment for macular oedema was ~8.8% (73). The need for treatment was associated with a change (in either direction) of 0.5% HbA_{1c} and also with changes in blood pressure, highlighting again the need for careful retinal monitoring if there are major and rapid changes in glycaemia (Sander et al., 2013).

> **Practice point**
>
> Although there is no specific 'threshold' for development of high-risk retinopathy in Type 1 diabetes, HbA_{1c} consistently about 9% (75) or higher is emerging as a concerning level.

Proliferative retinopathy

In the Diabetic Retinopathy Study of 40 years ago laser photocoagulation halved the risk of severe visual impairment, and this benefit in proliferative retinopathy has been replicated in other studies. However, functional outcomes were not followed in the long term. Fortunately proliferative retinopathy is uncommon, though a UK teaching hospital clinic reported about ten new cases a year, strongly associated with high levels of social deprivation (Lane et al., 2015). These are likely to be people who have not engaged with diabetes services.

New vessels develop at the disc (NVD), where they are more likely to bleed than new vessels elsewhere (NVE) in the retina. The standard approach is scatter laser treatment (around 2000 burns) delivered in two short sessions of 10–15 minutes. It is usually well tolerated, though some patients get severe discomfort and pain. Intravitreal anti-VEGF treatment with ranibizumab had some advantages over panretinal phocotoagulation in one study (e.g. improved work productivity and driving outcomes) but most other outcomes were the same (Beaulieu et al., 2016).

Advanced diabetic eye disease and visual loss

Proliferative retinopathy causes visual loss through an intense fibrovascular response to retinal ischaemia and preretinal haemorrhage. Early intervention with increasingly sophisticated techniques of vitreoretinal surgery has improved the visual prognosis.

In the Europe-wide EURODIAB study reporting in the mid-1990s, severe visual impairment (visual acuity ≤6/60 in the better eye) occurred in 2.3% of Type 1 patients. In Arhus, Denmark the prevalence in 2003 was much lower, 0.6%; two-thirds of cases were due to proliferative retinopathy (Jeppesen and Beck, 2004). This low figure is probably representative of countries with advanced healthcare. Despite these encouraging recent data, patients are still fearful, and their concerns are rarely articulated to healthcare professionals.

Retinopathy in Type 2 diabetes

The natural history of retinopathy in Type 2 diabetes is different from that in Type 1, but although proliferative retinopathy in Type 1 is not encountered within ten years of diagnosis, sensitive screening tests used in the DCCT detected some degree of retinopathy in the majority of patients after five years. Given the long prediagnosis presence of intermittent hyperglycaemia and other abnormalities in Type 2 diabetes, retinopathy at presentation would be expected in some patients. In the newly-diagnosed patients enrolled in the United Kingdom Prospective Diabetes Study (UKPDS), 20% had microaneurysms or more advanced retinopathy in both eyes, and this proportion does not seem to have changed: in a contemporary study from Wales, 17% of newly-diagnosed patients had retinopathy. The presence of retinopathy was associated with various indicators of reduced β-cell function rather than of insulin resistance, reaffirming the contribution of both fasting and postprandial hyperglycaemia in the development of early retinopathy (Roy Chowdhury et al., 2016), and higher C-peptide levels at baseline in the VADT study of older Type 2 patients was linked to lower risk of retinopathy and of slower progression.

Practice point

In Type 2 diabetes hyperglycaemia is only one factor driving retinopathy. Hypertension and lipids are important as well.

Maculopathy

Maculopathy is a common form of sight-threatening retinopathy and, although its incidence is lower in Type 2 (see above), prevalence is much greater. It was detected in 10% of the VADT cohort, two to three times more frequently in Hispanic and African-American people, and was associated with diastolic hypertension and an increased risk of amputation (Emanuele et al., 2009), although several studies have not found an association with coronary artery disease. The pathological lesion causing visual loss is macular oedema, but it can be reliably detected only with optical coherence tomography (OCT), now routinely used in ophthalmology clinics, though interested optometrists are increasingly using it in private community clinics. It cannot be diagnosed on photographic retinal screening and surrogate measures are used to infer its presence. A subtle sign is pallor surrounding microaneurysms near the macula. More evident are waxy yellow exudates seen in exudative maculopathy, classically in a circular (circinate) formation. Other forms include focal maculopathy, diffuse maculopathy, ischaemic maculopathy caused by capillary closure and indicated by a pale macula with large blot haemorrhages, cotton-wool spots and cystoid maculopathy. Fluorescein angiography is still used for accurate diagnosis of ischaemic maculopathy.

Practice point

Maculopathy in Type 2 diabetes is a marker of significant more generalized vascular disease.

Multiple mechanisms have been proposed, of which the most relevant to treatment is VEGF-induced vascular permeability. Poor glycaemic control is frequent, but maculopathy, particularly ischaemic maculopathy, is a complication that persists for a long time, and some patients eventually have near-normal HbA_{1c} levels (this may be the ocular equivalent of the 'burnt-out' phenomenon seen in patients with advanced renal disease; see later). The epidemiology of visual loss in Type 2 diabetes reflects the age of the patients. In Denmark in 2003, registered blindness was two-and-a-half-times more frequent than in Type 1 patients, but age-related macular degeneration, proliferative diabetic retinopathy and maculopathy each comprised about 20% of the total (Jeppesen and Bek, 2004). However the continuing overall trends are encouraging: in Scotland in the decade between 2000 and 2009, blindness incidence in people with diabetes fell by nearly 11% each year.

Treatment: laser and intravitreal anti-VEGF agents

Laser treatment was first used in the mid-1980s and focal laser (grid laser for diffuse macular oedema) became established as standard intervention. However, it was never convincingly shown to reduce visual impairment and, although it is still used, it has been largely superseded by intravitreal anti-VEGF drugs which improve vision at all levels of baseline visual loss. In the Diabetic Retinopathy Clinical Research Network trial (2015) patients were randomized to three anti-VEGF compounds (bevacizumab – Avastin; ranibizumab – Lucentis; and aflibercept – Eylea) for one year. All were effective where visual loss was mild; aflibercept improved vision more than the others when visual loss was more severe and this effect persisted up to two years. Optimal treatment is intensive. Patients received a median nine injections (range 8–11) in the first year and most patients had additional laser treatment. Intravitreal steroids are still used in patients with chronic macular oedema that has not responded to other treatments. They may be as effective as anti-VEGF treatments in improving vision but visual loss from steroid-induced cataract is a common complication, as is raised intraocular pressure.

Practice point

Intensive intravitreal anti-VEGF therapy is the only treatment that preserves vision in maculopathy. Supplementary focal or grid laser is often used.

Other medical treatments

Tight blood pressure control in the UKPDS reduced the need for laser treatment of maculopathy, but at lower baseline blood pressure levels the ACCORD study found that there was no effect. Fortunately in these high-risk patients there is already a watertight case for good hypertension control (see **Chapter 11**). There are case reports of exudative maculopathy responding to intensive lipid lowering, but these patients at high cardiovascular risk should already be taking this treatment. The FIELD study (Keech et al., 2005) in Type 2 patents was persuasive that fenofibrate reduced the need for laser treatment. The prodigious ACCORD eye study found that fenofibrate in combination with a statin reduced progression of retinopathy, but only in patients with microaneurysms or mild NPDR. In practice it is difficult to recommend a lipid-modifying agent for a non-lipid related condition, moreover in a small subset of that condition, and also one that in the same study did not reduce cardiovascular events; nevertheless, in Australia fenofibrate has a licence for use in retinopathy. An encouraging substudy within the PREDIMED diet study (see **Chapter 9**) found that Type 2 patients who reported a daily intake of omega-3 fatty acids of at least 500 mg had a 50% reduced risk of developing adjudicated sight-threatening diabetic retinopathy over six years. This intake is easily achievable in practice by eating two or more portions of oily fish every week (Sala-Vila et al., 2016).

Practice point

Good blood pressure control and generous omega-3 fatty acid intake from fish reduce the risk of retinopathy in Type 2 diabetes.

Other eye complications related to diabetes

Cataract

Cataract occurs earlier and progresses faster in people with diabetes than in the non-diabetic population. In Type 1 patients it occurs about 20 years earlier than in non-diabetic people, and by 25 years duration one in three have cataract; it is therefore a common problem in people in their 30s and 40s.

Cataract obscures retinopathy and retinopathy incidence increases after surgery. Surgery for cataract is more difficult and visual outcomes are not as good. Complications include posterior capsule opacification, pseudophakic macular oedema (more common in patients with retinopathy), retinal detachment and endophthalmitis. Simvastatin with ezetimibe used in combination in a trial investigating its effects on aortic stenosis did not have any beneficial effects on the aortic valve but reduced the risk of developing cataract by nearly 50% in those with the largest fall in LDL (Bang *et al.*, 2015).

Diabetes eventually emerges in meta-analyses as a risk factor for glaucoma, but the association is probably only with Type 2 and not Type 1. Uveitis, in spite of its autoimmune connotations, is much more common in Type 2 than Type 1 diabetes.

Practice point

Cataracts can be visually significant for Type 1 patients in their 30s and 40s.

Retinal vascular occlusions

Occlusions of the retinal artery (and its branches) are common and, as in non-diabetic people, the risk increases with cumulative intensity of atherosclerotic risk factors. Retinal vein occlusions are also associated with diabetes and the metabolic syndrome; smoking is a risk factor for both arterial and venous occlusion. Patients usually present to emergency eye teams with acute visual symptoms.

Retinal artery occlusions

Central and branch retinal artery occlusions are often caused by microemboli from atherosclerotic plaques and calcific cardiac valves. The retina may at first look normal but it is usually whitened and opacified (segmental in the case of a branch occlusion).The cherry-red spot is characteristic. Investigate with a carotid Doppler study and echocardiogram. Intensive cardiovascular risk intervention (including formal smoking cessation advice) is needed. There are no specific ophthalmological interventions.

Retinal vein occlusions

Retinal vein occlusion is more common than arterial; again, both central and branch forms occur. Hypertension is a major risk factor but ocular hypertension and glaucoma are local risk factors. The 'tomato splash' retinal appearance is dramatic and characteristic and the widespread haemorrhages are sometimes mistaken for advanced retinopathy. Arterial risk management is primary but, if there have been previous venous thromboembolic events, investigate for a prothrombotic cause. Vascular leakage leads to retinal oedema, often treated with intravitreal anti-VEGF drugs that are licensed for this indication and for which there is evidence from small trials. A large study found that whether or not there was ischaemia aspirin did not improve visual outcomes and it should be withheld (Hayreh *et al.*, 2011).

> **Practice point**
>
> Optimize all cardiovascular risk factors in patients who have had a retinal artery or vein occlusion. Withhold aspirin in patients with vein occlusions.

Nonarteritic anterior ischaemic optic neuropathy
This is discussed in **Chapter 5**.

DIABETIC RENAL DISEASE

Like most other aspects of diabetes, especially Type 2, diabetic renal disease usually attracts the same cliches, including the ubiquitous 'epidemic' and 'unaffordable'. While the situation in many regions, especially Africa, the Middle East and South East Asia, is undoubtedly troubling in prospect, in other countries with advanced healthcare economies the incidence of end-stage renal disease (ESRD) in Type 1 diabetes has certainly fallen, in some countries to very low levels, and there is encouraging data from other countries that ESRD in Type 2 diabetes may have peaked. The increasing prevalence of Type 2 diabetes will undoubtedly strain health resources but the Steno-2 study (see later) confirmed that relatively modest but sustained interventions in glycaemia and cardiovascular risk factors could disproportionately benefit all important outcomes in patients with early established renal disease. Unfortunately there is no evidence to help us decide whether vigorous interventions in large proportions of the Type 2 population with the earliest indicators of renal disease – that is, low levels of microalbuminuria – will be of benefit in reducing meaningful outcomes many years hence.

Nomenclature
In addition to the relatively recent significant change to thinking of renal function in terms of estimated glomerular filtration rate (eGFR) and not serum creatinine levels, there have been more recent changes that add the dimension of albuminuria to eGFR category in a valuable attempt to encourage a more nuanced feel to severity, as both eGFR and albuminuria independently predict cardiovascular and renal outcomes (**Figure 4.1**). The overall consequence is that chronic kidney disease (CKD) has now returned to being a clinical diagnosis rather than one based on a single measurement with rigid cut points; this is an especially welcome introduction that combats the sclerosis of guidelines dictated by cut-points.

Microalbuminuria and macroalbuminuria
'Microalbuminuria' was first described in the 1970s by Professor Harry Keen (1925– 2013) and his colleagues working at Guy's Hospital, London. The term was convenient but somewhat imprecise in implying a distinct molecular form of albumin, rather than the intended 'very small amounts' – compare macroprolactin in endocrinology, for example – and KDIGO (Kidney Disease: Improving Global Outcomes) proposes that the term 'microalbuminuria' should be replaced by 'moderately increased' albuminuria and

				Presistent albuminuria categories Description and range		
Prognosis of CKD by GFR and Albuminuria Categories: KDIGO 2012				**A1**	**A2**	**A3**
				Normal to mildly increased	Moderately increased	Severely increased
				<30 mg/g <3 mg/mmol	30–300 mg/g 3–30 mg/mmol	>300 mg/g >30 mg/mmol
GFR categories (ml/min/ 1.73 m²) description and range	G1	Normal or high	≥90			
	G2	Mildly decreased	60–89			
	G3a	Mildly to moderately decreased	45–59			
	G3b	Moderately to severely decreased	30–44			
	G4	Severely decreased	15–29			
	G5	Kidney failure	<15			

Green: low risk (if no other markers of kidney disease, no CKD); Yellow: moderately increased risk; Orange: high risk; Red, very high risk.

Figure 4.1 Chronic kidney disease 'heat map'. Renal disease is more fully characterized as a global risk incorporating both eGFR (G1–G5 categories) and albuminuria (A1–A3 categories): each independently predict cardiovascular and renal outcomes. *Source*: Kidney Disease: Improving Global Outcomes (see *Further reading*). Reproduced with kind permission from KDIGO.

'macroalbuminuria' by 'severely increased' albuminuria. Although cut-points are still defined, using the new terms will help promote the concept that there is a continuity of risk (**Figure 4.2**). There are, however, considerable practical difficulties in real-life implementation. 'Microalbuminuria' is a term originally coined by diabetologists and it is not going to disappear soon from their lexicon. In addition, there is a large body of invaluable clinical trial data that used old nomenclature and also measurements and techniques that are no longer used (for example, 24-hour and timed – usually overnight – urine collections, each with their associated reference ranges). Although there is a statistical correlation between all the measurements of urinary albumin, these are often not helpful when attempting to make therapeutic decisions in the individual. The situation is not dissimilar to the move from the DCCT to IFCC reporting measurements for HbA_{1c} and plurality, while ensuring as much harmonization as possible at the same time as carefully defining terms, is the best approach.

Practice point

Encourage the use of 'moderately increased albuminuria' in place of the older and less accurate 'microalbuminuria', and 'severely increased albuminuria' in place of 'macroalbuminuria'.

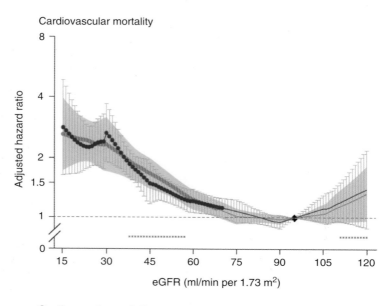

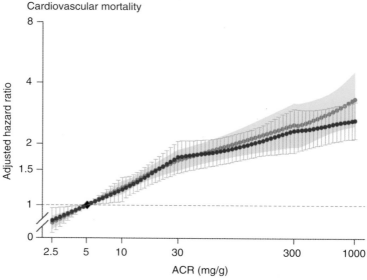

Figure 4.2 Cardiovascular mortality and renal function in a meta-analysis of people with diabetes (red points) and without (blue points), showing continuous changes with eGFR and albumin creatinine ratio (ACR). The reference points (adjusted hazard ratio = 1) are 95 ml/min for eGFR and ACR 5 (mg/g) – ~0.5 mg/mmol. The unexpected finding is that for a given eGFR and degree of albuminuria, cardiovascular mortality is similar in diabetic and non-diabetic patients: it is the renal disease itself that confers the increased risk. However, the increased risk of renal disease in diabetes confers the much greater individual risk and burden of disease in the population. *Source:* Fox *et al.*, 2012. Reproduced with permission of Elsevier.

It has been known for a long time, but still not sufficiently appreciated, that diabetic renal disease in both Type 1 and 2 diabetes is associated more with cardiovascular disease than end-stage renal disease (ESRD), as a competing risk. It is not oversimplifying, merely confirming, the outcomes of the Steno-2 study, to state that obsessive attention to cardiovascular risk factors will (so long as maximum angiotensin blockade is included in the therapeutic regimen) reduce all-cause mortality (mostly cardiovascular) in patients with renal disease. However, once moderately severe diabetic kidney disease occurs, ethnicity modifies these risks. For example, in the TREAT study of an erythropoietin-stimulating agent, in which diabetic patients of all ethnicities had standardized intensive care over 2½ years follow-up, black patients had a 50% increased risk of progressing to ESRD, while myocardial infarction and coronary revascularisation were about 40% lower (this advantage did not extend to strokes, which occurred at a similar rate). The increased burden of ESRD was not explained by conventional risk factors and should heighten our awareness of risk factors in the long prodromal period before severely increased albuminuria and impaired renal function occur (Lewis *et al.*, 2015).

Renal disease in Type 1 diabetes
The classical picture is a long period of normoalbuminuria and normal blood pressure in a patient with poorly-controlled diabetes, followed by progressing albuminuria and absent nocturnal dipping on ambulatory blood pressure monitoring, succeeded by a phase of accelerating proteinuria, sometimes in the nephrotic range, relentlessly falling eGFR and ending in ESRD in the third or fourth decade after diagnosis, with an associated terrible risk of cardiovascular disease and mortality (**Figure 4.3**). This picture is

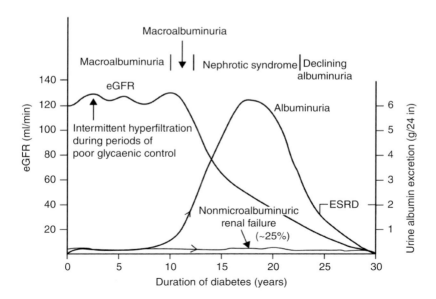

Figure 4.3 The characteristic course of renal disease in Type 1 diabetes. One of the main aims of long-term tight glycaemic control is to radically alter this pattern, with a view to indefinitely postponing the high mortality conferred by moderately and severely increased albuminuria. The trajectory of albuminuria is not seen in about 25% of patients, who do not develop moderately elevated albuminuria, yet progress to ESRD.

fortunately now much less common in many countries with advanced healthcare systems. For example, in Swedish patients diagnosed with Type 1 diabetes between 1977 and 1985, fewer than 1% developed ESRD; in the same country the age at which renal replacement therapy started increased from 53 to 56 years over the period 1995–2010, while the number of patients requiring replacement therapy fell (Toppe et al., 2014). Dialysis rates across Europe stabilized during the 1990s in spite of the increase in prevalence of Type 1 diabetes and overall improved survival.

Bear in mind the following points, which have emerged from careful long-term studies in defined populations of Type 1 patients:

- *Progressive renal impairment with no past or current evidence of significant proteinuria*. In Type 2 diabetes, some of these cases will be accounted for by non-diabetic non-proteinuric renal disease, for example hypertensive or renovascular disease. However, these are unlikely in Type 1 diabetes, where, nevertheless, about one in four patients with eGFR <60 ml/min have never had evidence of significant proteinuria (Molitch et al., 2010). That they have diabetic renal disease is clear, as biopsies show characteristic diabetic features of at least similar severity to those seen in proteinuric patients. This large subgroup adds further value to the heat-map approach.
- *The high rate of spontaneous remission of microalbuminuria/moderately elevated albuminuria (and even proteinuria) in Type 1 diabetes*. The reasons are unknown. Importantly, there is lack of convincing evidence for the benefits of angiotensin blockade treatment in patients with early microalbuminuria. Frequent observation is usually the best approach (see later).
- Finally, when albuminuria is present it remains a very powerful predictor of overall mortality. Recent reports of long-term studies in Type 1 diabetes (for example the Pittsburgh Epidemiology of Diabetes Complications and the FinnDiane Study) now ascribe nearly all the excess mortality in Type 1 diabetes to the presence of renal disease; in its absence, life expectancy is the same as that of the non-diabetic population (Orchard et al., 2010).

Practice point

Low-level albuminuria frequently goes away spontaneously in Type 1 patients. Do not rush to angiotensin blockade treatment in normotensive individuals.

Renal disease in Type 2 diabetes

Because Type 2 diabetes presents at such a variety of times through its natural history, the course of renal disease is highly variable. In addition, common co-existing conditions – obesity and hypertension – make renal disease in Type 2 diabetes a heterogeneous and complex condition to diagnose and manage. Unlike Type 1 where patients never have diabetes-related albuminuria at diagnosis, around 10% of Type 2 patients have microalbuminuria at diagnosis and a very small proportion overt proteinuria. A systematic survey of patients in the USA with known Type 2 diabetes found that 9% had eGFR <45 ml/min, that is G3b or worse; this rose to 19% in those aged 65 and over (Bailey et al., 2014). There was significantly elevated urinary albumin excretion (>30 mg/g, >3 mg/mmol) in 32% overall and nearly 40% in older people. Although in the UKPDS only about 2% of Type 2 patients progressed from macroalbuminuria to significant renal impairment or renal replacement therapy each year, this represents a large number of patients. Type 2 diabetes is still the commonest reason for renal replacement therapy and around 50% of dialysis patients have diabetes as an underlying or probably underlying cause. It is also becoming a major problem in the developing world; for example in China in 2010, the prevalence of diabetes overtook glomerulonephritis as the commonest reason for hospitalization with CKD, and the gap widened progressively over the next five years (Zhang *et al.*, 2016).

Non-diabetic nephropathies and the impact of obesity

While established diabetic renal disease has a simple clinical definition (hypertension, stick-positive proteinuria [macroalbuminuria/severely increased albuminuria] and impaired renal function in someone with diabetes), there is continuing concern that the breadth of the definition may allow patients with non-diabetic renal disease, perhaps treatable with more specific therapies, to slip through the net. Standard serological tests (e.g. ANF, ANCA, urine and blood tests for myeloma, and complement levels) are still often requested, though they are weak predictors of findings on renal biopsy, and are of little value where there are no specific clinical indicators of non-diabetic renal disease.

The value of the ultimate test, renal biopsy, is still debated and several groups continue to urge its wider use. In a survey of a large number of current renal biopsies in the USA, nearly a quarter of the specimens were taken from people with diabetes (Sharma *et al.*, 2013). Admittedly, as a group the patients had unequivocal features of advanced renal disease, with mean serum creatinine 220 μmol/l and nephrotic-range proteinuria (median 4.3 g/day). Of these, on biopsy a third each had features of diabetic nephropathy alone, non-diabetic renal disease alone and a combination, so that nearly 60% of renal biopsies showed some non-diabetic features. Non-diabetic renal conditions most often seen in diabetic renal biopsy include IgA nephropathy, focal segmental glomerulosclerosis (FSGS) and membranous glomerulonephritis, though features of 'acute tubular necrosis' were common and seen in nearly 30%. Reduced renal reserve and a susceptibility to intrarenal haemodynamic instability under the influence of angiotensin-blocking agents might be responsible. Although specifically treatable non-diabetic kidney diseases were uncovered, no clinical follow-up was reported, so it is not known whether they actually received treatment additional to standard management. From this and other studies, renal biopsy might be indicated in some of the following situations:

- Sudden development of nephrotic-range proteinuria
- Short duration of otherwise uncomplicated Type 1 diabetes, at a stage when diabetic nephropathy would be unusual
- A shorter duration of Type 2 diabetes e.g. around 5 years, with sub-nephrotic range proteinuria
- Non-resolving acute kidney injury.

There is growing awareness of the contribution of obesity to renal disease, characterized on biopsy by a specific form of focal segmental glomerulosclerosis. It is rare in otherwise uncomplicated obesity; other insults, probably operating through changes in intraglomerular pressures, are needed. While not quite a disease entity in search of a specific treatment, the literature on pathophysiology considerably outweighs that on useful therapy. Until there are reliable biomarkers for this currently histologically-defined condition, and whether obesity surgery therefore has an impact on it, it will remain of interest. Biopsy data in well characterized Type 2 patients is sparse, but normoalbuminuric patients show much less marked typical diabetes changes – atherosclerosis and hypertension are probably significant contributing factors (Ekinci *et al.*, 2013).

Practice point

Non-diabetic renal disease may occur quite frequently in people with Type 2 diabetes but rarely warrants biopsy unless there are highly atypical clinical features, for example, documented recent onset of heavy proteinuria.

Renal function: estimated glomerular filtration rate (eGFR)

Reporting renal function as eGFR using the MDRD (Modification of Diet in Renal Disease) equation is now firmly established as the single definitive measure. Alternative equations, for example the Chronic Kidney Disease Epidemiology Collaboration (CKD-EPI), have been proposed but its increased accuracy at higher GFR levels may not extend to people with diabetes. However, the generalist needs to recognize that modest reductions in eGFR alone should not be used to diagnose 'chronic kidney disease', which is a major diagnosis and which has many implications for the individual patient. The use of eGFR measurements has had very little impact on meaningful changes in practice and outcomes (Akbari et al., 2015). The limitations of eGFR reporting need emphasizing (**Box 4.1**).

eGFR categories (G1–G5)

The five eGFR categories are now well established and carry an independent risk of cardiovascular disease (**Table 4.1**).

Recently, cystatin C (one of several candidate low molecular weight serum proteins) has been promoted as a more reliable indicator of renal function than serum creatinine. Its place in routine practice is contested, because it has not been shown to change outcomes, even though it may estimate risk more accurately. Situations where cystatin C measurements might be more accurate in acute management as opposed to predicting long-term complications are not agreed, but cystatin C is less affected by muscle mass than serum creatinine and might be valuable in patients with impaired renal function undergoing weight-loss surgery. USA guidelines (KDIGO) also propose using cystatin C-derived eGFR for diagnosis in people with $eGFR_{creatinine}$ 45–59 without other markers of kidney damage.

Box 4.1 The effects of eGFR reporting.

Measurement accuracy

Limited accuracy (for example, in up to one-fifth of patients with eGFR <60 ml/min, the true GFR value is adrift by >30% of the reported estimate).

Clinical implications

- eGFR is frequently deranged by physiological stress, including acute illness, changes in hydration state and medications. Great caution is needed in hospitalised patients
- No clinically meaningful improvements in outcomes have been reported with the use of eGFR reporting
- In Canada eGFR reporting resulted in increased prescribing of angiotensin blockade treatment in CKD patients over 65 years of age. It is not known whether this change also occurred in people with diabetes
- There has been a slight reduction in the proportion of late referrals to nephrology services, but no convincing evidence that patients with eGFR <30 ml/min have been increasingly referred
- Women and elderly people were referred in substantially increased numbers
- Appropriate referrals increased, though so did inappropriate referrals.

Source: Akbari et al., 2015. Reproduced with permission of Elsevier.

Table 4.1 Categories of eGFR and diabetes.

GFR category	Value (ml/min/1.73 m²)	Description	Cardiovascular risk (odds ratio, univariate, non-diabetic subjects)	Comments
G1	≥90	Normal or high	1.0	Only normal if no other evidence of renal disease. Possibility of elevated eGFR during periods of hyperfiltration (poor glycaemic control), though this probably does not increased the risk of developing mildly-elevated albuminuria. Annual screening for: eGFR, ACR, serum potassium.
G2	60–89	Mildly decreased	1.1	Risk of cardiovascular disease greater than that of requiring renal replacement therapy
G3a	45–59	Mildly to moderately decreased	1.5	Use metformin with increasing caution, as the eGFR falls within these categories, and adjust doses of
G3b	30–44	Moderately to severely decreased	2.2	other diabetes and non-diabetes drugs (see Chapter 10). Increasing risk of anaemia and bone disease (check blood count, B12, folate, ferritin and bone screen including parathyroid hormone levels at least annually). Ensure patients are vitamin D replete (multiple current guidelines – ask for advice if uncertain). Specialist referral or advice where there is a suspicion of non-diabetic renal disease and for management planning. Risk of mortality from cardiovascular disease at this advanced stage is still greater than that from ESRD.
G4	15–29	Severely decreased	14	Refer to nephrologist.
G5	<15	Kidney failure	10 to >50	

ACR: albumin creatinine ratio; ESRD: end-stage renal disease.

Albuminuria

Persistent albuminuria categories (KDIGO) **(Table 4.2)**

In health, albumin creatinine ratio (ACR) is <1 mg/mmol. The threshold of 3, that is at least a threefold increase, is therefore thought to reliably indicate abnormality. There has been a lot of work deriving gender-specific measurements, resulting in slightly higher ACR measurements in males than females because of their higher levels of creatinine

Table 4.2 Categories of persistent albuminuria.

Albuminuria category	Description	ACR (mg/mmol)	PCR (mg/mmol)	Reagent stick result
A1	Normal to mildly increased	<3	<15	−ve to trace
A2	Moderately increased	3–30	15–50	Trace to 1+
A3	Severely increased	>30	>50	1+ or greater
[A4]	Nephrotic-range proteinuria	>220		

PCR: protein creatinine ratio; the A4 category is proposed

excretion, but given the variability of the measurement, current guidelines no longer make a gender distinction.

Practice point

Full characterization of renal disease in diabetes now requires recording both the eGFR category (1–5) and the albuminuria category (1–3).

Technical aspects of measuring albuminuria

It is now standard to measure only albumin. Albuminuria is especially prognostic in diabetes, as well as hypertension. In every way it is preferable than measuring total protein, though in non-diabetic conditions, for example monoclonal gammopathies, it may have specific advantages. Laboratory measurements are generally preferred, though automated reading of urine dipsticks, now widely used in hospital practice, reduces inter-operator variability. While only semi-quantitative, they are of diagnostic value. For example, nearly one-half of all patients with 1+ or greater stick test result had a laboratory ACR measurement >3. Fully quantitative point of care tests (e.g. DCA 2000+, Siemens) similar to those for HbA_{1c} give rapid results and have high performance measures.

Practice point

1+ or greater stick-positive albumin predicts ACR >3 mmol/mol, that is moderately increased albuminuria/microalbuminuria.

Early morning urine (first pass) measurements are valuable, as they correlate well with 24-hour measurements and have relatively low intra-individual variability. However, random samples are acceptable.

Intra-individual variation in albumin excretion is substantially reduced when expressed as the familiar ACR, rather than albumin concentration (mg/l), though concentrations are routinely reported in laboratory outputs. Timed urine measurements (24 hour or timed overnight specimens), routine not very long ago, are now obsolete.

Factors affecting urinary ACR

- Strenuous exercise in normal individuals can increase ACR to 6–8 mg/mmol but it returns to normal within 24 hours.
- Symptomatic urinary tract infection. Asymptomatic infections or bacteriuria do not cause albuminuria.

- Menstrual blood contamination.
- Upright posture (orthostatic proteinuria) – hence in part the lower variability of ACR measured in early morning urine specimens.
- Fever, systemic infection.
- Pre-analytical problems: urine samples are stable for a week at 4 °C and for much longer at −70 °C; at −20 °C there can be albumin loss.

Confirmation of albuminuria

The current recommendation is to confirm an elevated ACR (≥3 mg/mmol) with two further samples over the next two months. Albuminuria is confirmed if one or both of the samples are positive. This complicated procedure needs to be put into context. For example, it is extremely important in a young Type 1 person with borderline elevated ACR on the first sample – given the high rate of spontaneous regression of albuminuria, we would not want to commit someone, especially if normotensive, to treatment with angiotensin-blocking agents without definitive confirmation. On the other hand, an initial sample with ACR measurement in the moderately or severely increased range, especially in a Type 2 patient, may not justify further measurements of ACR.

Management of diabetic renal disease

'Renoprotection' with angiotensin blocking agents

The near-ubiquitous use of angiotensin blocking agents, ACE inhibitors and angiotensin receptor blockers (ARBs) in hypertension and their profound effects on proteinuria have led to the widespread view that they may be useful in preventing renal disease even in the absence of hypertension and albuminuria. There is strikingly little evidence for this.

Type 1

Two important long-term studies showed that angiotensin blockade in normotensive normoalbuminuric patients does not reduce the risk of progression to microalbuminuria. Drugs used were high-dose candesartan, 32 mg daily in the DIRECT study (Bilous et al., 2009), and enalapril 20 mg daily and losartan 100 mg daily in the RASS study (Mauer et al., 2009). In the RASS study, neither albumin excretion rate nor glomerular histology on renal biopsies showed any changes after treatment, but progression to microalbuminuria was slightly more common after losartan compared with placebo or enalapril. While this was not seen with candesartan in DIRECT, it is further indirect evidence that first-line angiotensin blockade in Type 1 patients should be with an ACE-inhibitor and not an ARB.

Type 2

The benefits of angiotensin blockade in preventing progression from normoalbuminuria to microalbuminuria in Type 2 patients are not clear. The risk of progressing from normoalbuminuria to microalbuminuria in the BENEDICT study was reduced by 50% after five years of treatment with the ACE inhibitor trandolapril, but this is not surprising in a definitely hypertensive population. Candesartan 32 mg daily did not have the same effect either in normotensive patients (mean blood pressure 123/75 mm Hg) or in those with relatively well-controlled hypertension (140/80) in the DIRECT-Renal study. The largest study, ROADMAP, used olmesartan 40 mg daily for three years in patients with mild hypertension (mean baseline blood pressure 137/80 mm Hg). There was about a 20% risk reduction in progression to microalbuminuria, but fatal cardiovascular events were increased in the olmesartan group (Haller et al., 2011).

Practice point

'Renoprotection' with angiotensin blockade in patients with normal ACR and blood pressure does not have an evidence base in either Type 1 or Type 2 diabetes.

Management of moderately increased ACR (microalbuminuria, 3–30 mg/mmol, A2)

Welcome though the proposed changes are to the nomenclature, the long-standing partition into normo-, micro- and macroalbuminuria (nephropathy) was long used in clinical trials, with microalbuminuria defined as ACR 3-30, and macroalbuminuria >30 mg/mmol. Actually, many used the then 'gold standard' 24 hour urinary albumin measurement and the DCCT used a slightly higher threshold to define microalbuminuria than was conventional (40 mg/24 hours for the DCCT, 30 mg/24 hours generally). The inevitable confusion and difficulty of translating the results of different studies can be used productively to manage patients, especially Type 1 patients, more clinically, and less obsessively according to cut-points.

Type 1 diabetes

The usual presentation of albuminuria in Type 1 patients is an elevated ACR on a routine annual screening test in a young person with ten or more years of poor glycaemic control, for example HbA_{1c} ~9% (75), but with strictly normal blood pressure, normal eGFR and no dyslipidaemia – in other words isolated albuminuria (though there may be minor retinopathy). The tendency, reinforced by guidelines, mostly from Type 2 diabetes, would be to promptly start treatment with an ACE inhibitor, accompanied by a lipid-lowering agent. The temptation to do this should be resisted in an evidence-based way.

First, albuminuria up to the moderately elevated range, especially if in the lower part of the range, frequently spontaneously regresses. This was documented in the DCCT, where ~80% of young people with albuminuria as high as 360 mg/24 hours ('macroalbuminuria') regressed, interestingly whether or not treated with an ACE inhibitor. Regression was most likely if HbA_{1c} was <8.0% (64), systolic blood pressure <115 mm Hg and total cholesterol <5.1 mmol/l (though the use of lipid-lowering treatment in this age group has no evidence) (Salardi et al., 2011).

Second, the primary treatment of an elevated ACR, which is a microvascular complication, is to improve glycaemic control. Young Type 1 patients who developed microalbuminuria had a mean HbA_{1c} >8.2% (66) in the average 10 years since diagnosis (Perrin et al., 2010). Improving glycaemia is the priority, though patients in the same study also had systolic hypertension (see later). Glycaemic improvement needs detailed and focused input from the diabetes specialist team, initially to help the patient manage problems with their existing insulin regimen and possibly to consider insulin pump treatment, if the patient is not already using it. It needs emphasizing to these sometimes demotivated patients that this is a reversible, not just a treatable, complication.

Practice point

Primary management of isolated mildly elevated albuminuria/microalbuminuria in Type 1 patients with normal blood pressure (<120/80 mm Hg) is with rigorous diabetes team input with the aim of reducing HbA_{1c}.

Hypertension

Patients with persistent albuminuria will usually be hypertensive. In young people (Perrin et al., 2010) ambulatory blood pressure profiles were clearly abnormal, with daytime mean systolic pressure >130 mm Hg, and nighttime average >120. Here the use of angiotensin blocking agents – for the hypertension – is important.

Investigations

Further investigations are unnecessary, unless there has been a recent change in albuminuria from A1 to A2 or A3. Routine ultrasound scan of the kidney and urinary tract is normal. There may be large kidneys, characteristically associated with poor glycaemic control. Previously there was concern that large kidneys were linked to acceleration of renal disease, but it is an epiphenomenon and not causal.

Management

Studies in the 1990s showed that ACE inhibitor treatment was of value in delaying progression of albuminuria. Its value is currently less clear-cut and more recent studies have not been able to show a link between duration of treatment and likelihood of progression (Ficociello et al., 2007). The conclusion is that glycaemia needs improving over the long term (mean HbA_{1c} in this study was >9.5% [80]) – combined with consistent ACE inhibitor treatment.

How should ACE inhibitor treatment be managed in patients planning pregnancy or who become pregnant? Angiotensin blocking agents are clearly hazardous to the foetus when taken during the second and third trimesters but in the DIRECT studies, so long as candesartan (the ARB used in this suite of trials) was not taken beyond eight weeks, there was no increase in foetal morbidity or congenital malformations. Women planning pregnancy who need angiotensin blockade for albuminuria should, therefore, not discontinue it and treatment should not be withheld merely because patients are of childbearing age (Porta et al., 2011). Intensive education is needed.

Practice point

Angiotensin blocking agents are toxic to the foetus during the second and third trimesters, but seem safe up to eight weeks of pregnancy. Discontinue them as soon as pregnancy is confirmed.

Type 2 diabetes – Steno-2

There is no area of diabetes practice where the benefits of multimodal treatment are greater than in Type 2 patients with moderately-increased albuminuria. The important Steno-2 study (Gaede et al., 2008) randomized Type 2 patients with established microalbuminuria (median 78 mg/24 hours) – and therefore at higher cardiovascular risk – to intensive or less intensive treatment over nearly eight years. Achieved levels and targets proposed in the protocol for the intensive group are shown in **Box 4.2**. There were clinically meaningful lower risks of retinopathy, nephropathy and autonomic (but not somatic) neuropathy, and cardiovascular events were reduced by about 50%.

At the end of the randomization phase, patients were followed observationally for a further 5½ years. The legacy effect of the more intensive input was associated with:

- nearly 50% reduction in the risk of cardiovascular death and events
- only one person progressing to ESRD, compared with six in the less-intensive group (statistically significant)
- nearly 60% reduction in the need for laser therapy.

> **Box 4.2** Steno-2 trial. Achieved levels of risk factors in patients with moderately elevated albuminuria. Protocol targets in parentheses.
>
> - BP 140/74 mm Hg (<130/75)
> - HbA$_{1c}$ 7.7%, 61 (<6.5%, 48)
> - Total cholesterol 3.8 mmol/l (<4.5–4.9)
> - Total triglycerides 1.1 mmol/l (<1.3)
> - Full dose ACE inhibitor or ARB treatment
> - Aspirin in patients with known cardiovascular disease
> - Smoking cessation.

After 21 years follow-up a median eight years of life were gained, largely due to freedom from cardiovascular events (Gæde *et al.*, 2016). This is an astonishing vindication of multimodal secondary treatment.

> **Practice point**
>
> Type 2 patients with moderately increased albuminuria gain significant life-years (due to prevention of cardiovascular events) from moderate multimodal intervention (glycaemia, angiotensin blockade, blood pressure control, statin and aspirin).

Glycaemia

These are remarkable findings, but even more so given the modest glycaemia achieved (mean HbA$_{1c}$ 7.7%, 61). The ACCORD study confirmed that moderate rather than low HbA$_{1c}$ levels should be targeted in people with renal impairment. In the main study (see **Chapter 10**), intensive glycaemic control (achieved mean HbA$_{1c}$ 6.4% (46)) was associated with an increased risk of cardiovascular and all-cause mortality compared with the less-tight control group (achieved mean HbA$_{1c}$ 7.5%, 58). In patients with CKD 1–3 (patients with more advanced renal impairment were excluded from the trial) the results are even clearer (Papademetriou *et al.*, 2015). In intensively-treated patients:

- All-cause mortality was increased by 30%, cardiovascular mortality by 40% (not associated with baseline use of metformin or thiazolidinediones).
- Mortality increased within six months of randomization, by which time glycaemic separation between the two groups was already at the levels maintained throughout the rest of the trial.
- Hypoglycaemia rates were twice as high, severe hypoglycaemia requiring assistance three times higher.

As in the main study, the trial can offer no explanation for these findings. The modest renal benefits of tight glycaemic control seen in the ACCORD study (for example 10% risk reduction for developing microalbuminuria) will in practice be limited to a small group of patients with no CKD and at low risk of hypoglycaemia. In most patients any slight benefit is likely to be considerably outweighed by the risks of increased cardiovascular events and severe hypoglycaemia.

> **Practice point**
>
> In Type 2 patients with any degree of CKD, avoid very low HbA$_{1c}$ levels, for example 6.4% (46) or lower: values around 7% (53 mmol/l) are likely to be safe.

Angiotensin blockade

In the most informative clinical trial, full-dose irbesartan (300 mg daily) reduced by about 70% the risk of progressing to severely-elevated albuminuria (macroalbuminuria) in patients with similar levels of albuminuria to those in Steno-2 (Parving *et al.*, 2001). Lower-dose irbesartan (150 mg daily) was less effective and despite similar blood pressure levels the placebo group had the highest risk of progression. There was no difference in the rate of fall of GFR in a comparative study of the ARB telmisartan 40–80 mg daily and enalapril 10–20 mg daily, so either class of angiotensin blocker could be used in this clinical group; however, patients should still be given an initial trial of an ACE inhibitor, given the suggestive evidence of a cardiovascular benefit over ARB agents.

Although ascribing benefits to one factor or another in a multi-interventional trial is hazardous, using the UKPDS approximations, the authors of Steno-2 judged that lipid and blood pressure control were more important than glycaemia, a view supported by later trials (see **Chapter 10**).

> **Practice point**
>
> In patients with moderately increased albuminuria (microalbuminuria) blood pressure control (e.g. <140/75 mm Hg) and cholesterol control (e.g. <4.0 mmol/l) are probably more important in reducing cardiovascular and renal outcomes than intensive glycaemic control.

Management of severely increased albuminuria (macroalbuminuria, >30 mg/mmol, A3)

The new classification removes the need for the use of the older term 'diabetic nephropathy', which was a clinical syndrome consisting of:

- severely increased albuminuria
- hypertension
- progressive deterioration in renal function.

Admittedly this syndrome is largely captured in the lower right quadrant of the heat map, but the older term does include the notion of progression, together with the likely presence of hypertension, which is usually severe and often resistant (see **Chapter 11**). It also encompasses the common nephrotic syndrome (see later) that predicts rapid progression of renal impairment.

Management

Patients with diabetic renal disease are increasingly managed in an intensive clinic environment with both renal and diabetes physicians and their associated specialist nursing teams. A randomized trial in a mixed population of Type 1 and Type 2 patients with eGFR category G3b or worse found that those with G4 (15–29 ml/min) had a lower risk of progression to dialysis and a lower risk of cardiovascular events when seen in a specialist clinic every 1–3 months for up to six years compared with usual care (Chen *et al.*, 2015), but there was no benefit in patients with eGFR category G3b or better (data on glycaemia was not quoted). This reinforces the UK NICE guidance not to refer patients with lesser degrees of renal impairment (but G3b still requires intensive treatment in primary or secondary care – see below).

All patients should have a renal tract ultrasound scan. In Type 2 diabetic patients, typically middle-aged or older, other renal tract pathologies are important:

- Normal renal length is about 11 cm and correlates weakly with height and body mass index. Mean renal length is about 10 cm in South Asian and oriental subjects. Importantly, even in advanced diabetic renal disease, the kidneys are not especially small (~10 cm), compared with the typically shrunken kidneys (~8 cm) of advanced chronic non-diabetic renal disease. Although adult polycystic kidney disease is not associated with diabetes, it may coexist.
- Obstruction (stones, tumour, prostatic enlargement, papilla).
- Discrepancy in kidney size: if marked, that is >1 cm, it suggests renal artery stenosis.
- Bladder size and residual volume (there should be none): neuropathic bladder.

Glycaemia

Multimodal intervention here is mandatory and there are no prospective randomized trials that have studied glycaemia itself. Glucose control should be as good as possible but there are inevitably limited resources available for even these complex patients, and efforts should be made not to devote disproportionate time to attempts to improve glycaemia while blood pressure, lipids and management of the very high vascular risk are relatively neglected; optimum glycaemia is difficult to attain without increasing the risk of hypoglycaemia, and most patients have been in poor control for many years. This should not mean ignoring glycaemia: on current limited evidence HbA_{1c} >9% (75) carries a poor prognosis, so values <8% (64) could be a realistic goal. Prescribe glucose-lowering medication with careful regard to dose reductions in renal impairment (see **Chapter 10**).

Practice point

In patients with severely increased albuminuria, aim for HbA_{1c} <8% (64).

Angiotensin blockade

The prototype ACE inhibitor drug captopril was established in 1993 as treatment that could delay the progression of renal failure to a greater extent than equivalent blood pressure reduction using non-angiotensin blockade treatment. However, these patients are often severely hypertensive and angiotensin blockade is likely to be only one of several antihypertensive medications needed.

There can now be no head-to-head studies of ACE inhibitor treatment compared with ARBs but, wherever possible, use the established recommended ACE inhibitor treatment first, and change to an ARB only if there are adverse effects – predominantly cough. Accepting the poor blood pressure dose–response relationship for most ACE inhibitors (see **Chapter 11**), maximum tolerated doses should always be used. Examples include:

- Lisinopril 40 mg daily (this dose, higher than the standard one, has been shown, at least in Type 1 patients, to be meaningfully more effective in reducing proteinuria: Schjoedt *et al.*, 2009)

- Ramipril 10 mg daily
- Perindopril 8 mg daily
- Enalapril 20-40 mg daily.

Angiotensin blockade in patients with severely-increased albuminuria and decreased eGFR

This is a very important group of patients at high risk of cardiovascular disease and rapid progression to end-stage renal disease. However, major trials have shown that at least the renal endpoints can be meaningfully deferred. Two trials, both using then novel ARBs were reported in 2001: IDNT (irbesartan 300 mg daily) and RENAAL (losartan 100 mg daily). Patients were in the highest risk categories, with moderate renal impairment (serum creatinine 150–170 μmol/l) and heavy proteinuria (ACR 140 mg/mmol). An average of three or four antihypertensive agents was needed to achieve relatively modest blood pressure levels (around 140/75 mm Hg, target <135/85). The risk of reaching the hard renal endpoints was reduced by about 25%. Very importantly, in the IDNT trial, a separate group was treated primarily with amlodipine. Achieved blood pressure was the same as in the irbesartan-treated group but the renal benefits were no greater than in the placebo group. Amlodipine is therefore an effective antihypertensive agent but does not reduce proteinuria. The IDNT trial also showed a clear relationship between the degree of albuminuria above 1 g per 24 hours and the rate of decline in renal function: about one-third of patients with nephrotic-range proteinuria (see later) reached a significant renal end point within three years (Atkins et al., 2005).

Practice point

The highest-risk patients, with severely increased albuminuria and elevated serum creatinine, require maximum angiotensin blockade to reduce hard renal endpoints. In Type 2 patients either losartan 100 mg daily or irbesartan 300 mg daily have trial-based evidence for their use. Renal outcomes dominate in this group.

These were predominantly renal trials, with no particular efforts to address cardiovascular risk factors or glycaemia (mean baseline HbA_{1c} was 8.5% (69)). Lipids were very poorly controlled by current standards (mean cholesterol 5.8 mmo/l, LDL 3.7 mmol/l). Even so, in a combined analysis of the IDNT and RENAAL trials, ESRD occurred in nearly 20% of the patients; this was 2.5 times more frequent than cardiovascular death and 1.5 times more frequent than all-cause mortality. The very poor renal prognosis in this threatened group must still be borne in mind (Packham et al., 2012).

Dual ACE inhibitor and ARB treatment

It has long been assumed that more complete angiotensin blockade with combination treatment using an ACE inhibitor and an ARB would have renal benefits additional to those resulting from the use of one agent only; several small early studies hinted that this may be the case. Trials in heart failure based on the same notion did not show uniform benefit but there were no signals of harm. Dual therapy therefore came to be widely used in proteinuric renal patients and even in resistant hypertension. However, a portfolio of troubling adverse effects, with no benefits in formal renal outcomes, emerged in trials in non-diabetic renal disease reporting from the mid-2000s onwards, for example the ONTARGET (2008) and ALTITUDE (2012) trials. Adverse renal endpoints – dialysis, doubling of serum creatinine and death – were increased in both these large trials.

Finally, in Type 2 diabetes, VA NEPHRON-D trialled a combination of lisinopril (up to 40 mg daily) and losartan (up to 100 mg daily) against losartan alone (Fried *et al.*, 2013). As in the RENAAL and IDNT trials most patients had advanced renal disease: mean eGFR was 54 ml/min, approximately one-third each in eGFR categories G3b, G3a and G1/G2, and severely increased albuminuria (A3, median ACR 85 mg/mmol). The trial was stopped early. This was due to a combination of lack of benefit (the decline in renal function was not slowed by dual therapy and there were no differences in renal or mortality outcomes) and a spectrum of serious adverse effects similar to that seen in the non-diabetic studies, especially a higher risk of acute kidney injury and hyperkalaemia (serum potassium >6 mmol/l). Cumulative four-year mortality was 20%, confirmation in a modern study of the historically poor prognosis of advanced kidney disease (there was a similar mortality in the RENAAL study recruiting in the late 1990s, though patients in that study had more advanced disease, with heavier proteinuria and lower eGFR).

Practice point

Dual ACE inhibitor and ARB treatment confers no renal benefit and can be harmful. Avoid the combination.

It might be imagined that given this consistent pattern of non-benefit and harm, there would be no reason to start or continue dual therapy in contemporary practice. Some authors have contended that the VA NEPHRON-D trial should not have been terminated prematurely and continue to propose the use of combination treatment in carefully-monitored patients. This is difficult to justify given the consistent and adverse outcomes in several trials of different clinical groups, and the failure to prospectively identify any specific groups who definitively benefited. There can be no reason to start or continue dual angiotensin blockade treatment in any routine setting.

Blood pressure target

The discussion about blood pressure targets in diabetes is especially vigorous (see **Chapter 11**). KDIGO recommends ≤130/≤80 mm Hg. Values should be <140/90, but systolic pressure should not be lower than 120 mm Hg, a level that in the ACCORD study was associated with higher risks of ESRD, while conferring no cardiovascular benefits, apart from the expected reduction in stroke risk. Even these levels are often difficult to achieve, given the combination of stiff arteries, nocturnal hypertension with a non-dipping pattern on ambulatory blood pressure monitoring and, most troublesome of all, postural hypotension in a small proportion of patients. Home blood pressure monitoring is extremely valuable and need not be burdensome. Duplicate measurements morning and evening on three or more days was prognostic in the important FinnDiane study in Finnish Type 1 patients (Niranen *et al.*, 2011).

SPECIAL SITUATIONS

Nephrotic-range proteinuria

The heavy albuminuria of the nephrotic syndrome (>220 mg/mmol) is probably more common than is thought. This may be partly due to laboratory methods, which often do not measure and report ACR values in this range, resulting in this important diagnosis being missed. In the IDNT study more than 40% of the participants had nephrotic syndrome. The other, traditional, components of the syndrome are still relevant. When they are present, serum albumin <35 g/l, cholesterol >6.7 mmol/l or statin use, and peripheral oedema or use of loop diuretic, together they increase the risk of doubling of proteinuria by a further threefold (Stoycheff et al. 2009). In the IDNT study doubling of proteinuria above 1 g/day was associated with a doubling of the risk of a hard renal endpoint. The clinical hazard is highlighted by the heat map: renal risk is still very high even when baseline eGFR is normal (**Figure 4.1**). Although maximum angiotensin blockade does not guarantee success in reducing proteinuria, if it falls by >50% in the first year of treatment the rate of renal progression is halved.

'Burnt-out' diabetes

A graphic term that is pathologically imprecise, yet conveys a set of important clinical messages. 'Burnt-out' diabetes describes a state of near-normoglycaemia common in patients with G4 and G5 categories of eGFR (<30 ml/min), though it can exist in elderly patients without renal impairment (see **Chapter 14**). For example, two-thirds of dialysis patients have HbA_{1c} <7.0% (53), and one-third <6.0% (42). Factors contributing to this state include:

- prescribed medications
- decreased renal insulin degradation and clearance
- declining renal gluconeogenesis
- decreased food intake, loss of lean body mass and fat (sometimes dramatic, though patients may still be overweight) (Park et al., 2012).

As we have seen, there is no benefit and possibly considerable harm in tight glycaemic control in this group, as patients are often hypoglycaemia unaware. Blood glucose medication needs frequent review and usually dose reduction, focusing primarily on insulin and sulfonylureas. Although diabetes teams are much more vigilant these days about metformin dosing in renal impairment, patients often have many medications and metformin has a tendency to persist in prescriptions after it should have been reduced in dose or withdrawn (see **Chapter 10**).

Practice point

Patients with established renal disease often have low HbA_{1c} measurements (e.g. <7.0%, 53). This often means they are taking too much diabetic medication/insulin: review and adjust frequently.

Renal artery stenosis

The diagnosis and management of atherosclerotic renal artery stenosis was previously a major concern when it was thought to be an important contributor to the progression of CKD, though it was recognized that treatment did not improve blood pressure control. Usually asymptomatic, though often associated with atherosclerosis elsewhere, and therefore common in Type 2 diabetes, it was often investigated after finding unequal kidney size on ultrasound; however, it can present acutely with 'flash' pulmonary oedema relating to renin–angiotensin–aldosterone pathway activation. Revascularisation was widely performed. Randomized studies in the mid-2000s (e.g. CORAL) found that revascularization did not improve renal or cardiovascular outcomes or reduce death rates. In a regrettable but by no means unique state of so-called 'stagnating equipoise', the trials are now being pored over for alleged bias, with the usual hope that we can now identify specific groups of patients who will benefit from intervention using the new biology of speculative biomarkers and cellular technology. Inevitably, more robust studies are called for (Sag *et al.*, 2016).

While invasive treatment remains in its uncertain state, identification of atherosclerotic renal artery disease is still of practical importance. It identifies a group at especially high vascular risk and patients would benefit from non-invasive cardiac testing, a carotid Doppler scan and careful examination for peripheral vascular disease (arterial bruits in particular). Although renal function may deteriorate markedly after starting angiotensin blocking treatment (see **Chapter 11**), it is uncommon even in this group and, most importantly, angiotensin blockade is particularly beneficial and may even reduce mortality (Hackam *et al.*, 2007). The minor risks highlight – yet again – the need for frequent monitoring of renal function after starting angiotensin blocking treatment.

Practice point

Invasive treatments for atherosclerotic renal artery disease are no longer performed but patients are at high vascular risk and benefit from angiotensin blocking treatment.

Management of patients with eGFR G3b (<45 ml/min) or worse

Patients with moderately or severely decreased eGFR are commonly seen in both primary and secondary care. G3b is the CKD stage where guidelines recommend considering a secondary care referral, but in most cases patients will have much of their care delivered in the community. The comments below are elaborated from the guidelines of Bilo *et al.* (2015).

Glycaemia

Apart from meta-analysis there are no single trials that can guide practice. However, the results of ACCORD (which included patients with Stage 3 CKD) must be taken seriously and HbA_{1c} <7.5% (58) should be assessed critically in the individual, especially with regard to hypoglycaemia. Lower values are probably harmful.

Angiotensin blockade

Most patients will have been taking an angiotensin blocker before they develop G3b. While angiotensin blockade does not improve cardiovascular outcomes, the IDNT and RENAAL trials (see earlier) showed renal benefit. However, hypotension is common in this group and, if necessary, non-angiotensin blocking drugs should be withdrawn first. Hyperkalaemia usually precludes angiotensin blockade much earlier in the course of diabetic renal disease, so hyperkalaemia is not usually a concern at this stage.

Lipid lowering

Nearly all patients will be taking a statin, unless they are wholly intolerant of them, by the time they reach G3b. LDL lowering has no effect on progression to renal endpoints and probably does not reduce stroke risk. Question patients carefully about musculoskeletal symptoms, especially if they are taking high doses of statins, though there is little trial evidence that adverse effects with statins in CKD patients are more frequent. All patients in G3b and G4 should be taking maximum recommended statin doses (**Box 4.3**), but several studies have found there is no cardiovascular or renal benefit in starting statins once patients have ESRD or are on renal replacement therapy. Ezetimibe monotherapy is safe in CKD, but efficacy has been shown only in combination with statin

Box 4.3 Maximum recommended doses of statins when eGFR <45 ml/min.

- Atorvastatin 20 mg
- Rosuvastatin 10 mg
- Simvastatin/ezetimibe 20/10 mg
- Pravastatin 40 mg
- Simvastatin 40 mg

(*Source*: Wanner et al., 2014. Reproduced with permission of Elsevier.)

treatment. There is no evidence that LDL targets should be different in CKD patients, or that statins of different potencies should be used.

All patients will probably be taking aspirin. However, patients with CKD G5 (eGFR <15 ml/min) are at increased bleeding risk and aspirin is of uncertain benefit in this group.

Diet

Patients benefit from specialized dietary advice. Overweight patients need especially careful advice in view of the risk of non-fat loss and malnutrition. The benefits and practicalities of implementing a traditional 'low protein' diet for patients with advanced diabetic kidney disease are still discussed at length. A lower protein intake, for example 0.8 g protein/kg/day, may slow eGFR fall, and higher intakes, for example 1.2 g/kg/day, are not recommended. Patients should not adopt the informally widely recommended high protein diets. Salt intake should be less than 2.0–2.3 g/day and patients should be encouraged to avoid processed food and fast food.

Ischaemic heart disease

Highly prevalent in these patients with multiple risk factors but usually without symptoms – except for heart failure. In patients without CKD all non-invasive tests give inconsistent results (see **Chapter 6**); they are even less reliable in CKD patients. Given these limitations we need to recognize that ischaemic heart disease is the commonest cause of death in these patients, so simple tests – resting ECG, echocardiography and myocardial perfusion scanning – should be requested more often than they are. The slightest hint of symptoms, which may only be mild shortness of breath, should prompt investigation. All patients have pretransplantation coronary angiography and carotid Doppler scans.

Renal bone disease

Nephrologists have moved from actively treating renal bone disease to a state of much greater uncertainty, as it is not clear what levels of serum phosphate or parathyroid hormone should be targeted. There is, therefore, more uncertainty about the use of phosphate binders, which in any case are not the province of the generalist or diabetologist. More relevant to the generalist, the place and dose of vitamin D supplements and vitamin D analogues is not known either and, in particular, there are no data on vitamin D supplements and meaningful renal outcomes. In a response to the KDIGO recommendations, Canadian nephrologists suggested that in patients with eGFR >30 ml/min (i.e. nearly all patients managed in primary care and secondary care diabetologists) routine supplementation with 800–1000 IU/day is all that is needed. In patients with eGFR <30, doses up to ~4000 IU/day are suggested, but treatment is not mandatory (Moist et al., 2013).

> **Practice point**
>
> Consider routine vitamin D supplementation (800–1000 IU/day) in all patients with eGFR >30 ml/min if they are not already taking it.

Anaemia

The typical normochromic anaemia of erythropoietin deficiency occurs at a higher eGFR than in non-diabetic renal disease; at G3 about 20% have a haemoglobin <11 g/dl. Include a full blood count in routine tests in patients with eGFR <30 ml/min. Early clinical studies hinted that generous haemoglobin values (e.g. 13 g/dl) were associated with improved renal outcomes and held out the hope of decreased cardiovascular outcomes. These resulted in the widespread use of erythropoietin-stimulating agents (ESA), especially recombinant human erythropoietin. The definitive study in Type 2 patients, TREAT (Pfeffer *et al.*, 2009) used another recombinant ESA, darbepoeitin, in patients with eGFR ~30 ml/min, and anaemia (mean haemoglobin concentration 10.6 g/dl), again randomized to higher haemoglobin (mean achieved 12.6 g/dl) and lower (10.6). Overall cardiovascular events were not increased at the higher haemoglobin concentration, but stroke risk was doubled, and venous and arterial thromboembolic events, and reported hypertension, increased; there was no discernible impact on measures of quality of life.

Co-existing iron deficiency is common and correcting it is important to optimize the benefit of any ESA treatment. This is particularly important in view of the lower recommended haemoglobin level. Oral and intravenous iron are equally effective but intravenous iron is a simple single treatment, and better tolerated with a possibly better effect on quality of life measures than oral. Intravenous iron is widely used by nephrology teams but diabetes teams and general practitioners should be more aware of its value. Having corrected iron (and where necessary B12 and folate) deficiency, if patients are still anaemic then ask the nephrology team to help out.

Monitoring glycaemia in patients with advanced renal impairment

This is methodologically and scientifically a fraught area. ESAs increase the number of younger red cells, which will be less exposed to glycaemia, resulting in factitiously lower HbA_{1c} measurements. On the other hand HbA_{1c} is higher in people with iron deficiency and iron deficiency anaemia (English *et al.*, 2015). The effect of uraemia itself is also variable, so although HbA_{1c} measurements are unreliable in advanced renal impairment, it is not easy to determine whether they under- or overestimate true HbA_{1c} measurements in individuals – and it may vary with circumstances. Avoiding hypoglycaemia in patients with advanced CKD is critically important, so systematic and meaningful overestimates of HbA_{1c} would be clinically the most important to identify.

Glycated albumin and fructosamine have often been advocated as more reliable measures of glycaemic control in renal failure. Neither has much evidence supporting their use. On balance, judicious use of home blood glucose monitoring is the most reliable method and diagnostic continuous glucose monitoring if there is a high suspicion of hypoglycaemia and hypoglycaemia unawareness. Patients are often symptomatic and burdened with multiple medical matters, so suggest minimal testing, taking into account likely times of hypoglycaemia. Moderate levels of glycaemia are appropriate. A reasonable HbA_{1c} range in these patients is considered to be 7.5–8.0% (58–64); the approximate associated glucose levels (derived from the ADAG study) would be 8–10 mmol/l (Wei *et al.*, 2014).

Peripheral vascular disease and peripheral neuropathy

The toll of foot lesions in patients with advanced diabetic kidney disease remains high but there is no evidence that routine screening for peripheral vascular disease or neuropathy (which is nearly always present in these patients) is of value. Palpation of foot pulses is still the most reliable reassurance that there is no significant peripheral arterial disease; because of stiff arteries Doppler testing is unreliable and difficult in the many patients with peripheral oedema, which itself has multiple contributory causes (stasis, venous disease, heart failure and low albumin states). The best safeguard in this highly threatened population is repeated education of patients and carers about rapid and frequent foot checks, and extreme vigilance by clinicians. Patients are often admitted to hospital with infected foot ulcers and pregangrenous lesions. Involve the hospital diabetes foot team at an early stage.

End-stage renal disease (ESRD)

A complex area, with little formal guidance. Even the timing of dialysis is not agreed, though nephrologists often recommend it earlier, that is at a higher eGFR than in nondiabetic people. Clinical considerations should dominate the decision, including uraemic symptoms (especially anorexia and cachexia), but also hypervolaemia and hypertension.

Type 1 diabetes

Dialysis

Dialysis in Type 1 patients has a poor outlook. Mortality, already high in patients with lesser degrees of CKD, increases to 11–13 per 100 person-years; in the early 2000s nearly 40% died within five years of starting dialysis, mostly from cardiovascular disease. Patients receiving a pre-emptive renal transplant, that is, before they need dialysis, have a mortality of only 0.9 per 100 person-years. The current trend is to start dialysis at a lower serum creatinine (e.g. mean value was 663 µmol/l in 1996 but 380 µmol/l in 2007), though there is no evidence for mortality or morbidity benefit (Pavlakis, 2012). Most importantly, there should be an agreed management plan and awareness of the variability of the impact of uraemic symptoms. Most patients receive haemodialysis, but dialysis mode varies between countries and centres; for example, in Sweden 40% of Type 1 patients use peritoneal dialysis, a much higher proportion than in Type 2 patients. The impact of dialysis on the patient and family is enormous, and routine diabetes care can be sidelined; this may contribute to the very high hospital admission rate of dialysis patients. Outcomes are better if patients are transplanted shortly after the start of dialysis.

Renal transplantation

The treatment for ESRD in Type 1 diabetes is transplantation. The benefits in these younger people are unequivocal; the under-40s gain on average 17 additional years of life and the benefits are similar in those up to 60. The options for transplantation are wider than before and there has been a recent rapid increase in the rate of living donors, mostly related, but occasionally Good Samaritan. Ten-year graft survival outcomes are much as one would expect:

- pre-emptive living transplants – 75%
- pre-emptive deceased – 69%
- non-pre-emptive live – 49–62%
- non-pre-emptive deceased – 39–49%.

All Type 1 patients should be actively considered for pancreas transplantation, either simultaneous or after renal transplant (see **Chapter 7**).

Type 2 diabetes

Dialysis (Rossing et al., 2015)

Although criteria for initiation of dialysis in Type 2 patients are still not established and uniform, UK trends are numerically encouraging. Initiation of renal replacement therapy doubled in the 15 years up to 2009. Over the same period, survival improved and the proportion of patients 'crash landing' – requiring dialysis within three months of first presentation to nephrologist – fell from 23% of patients to 11% (Hill and Fogarty, 2012). This is fortunate: the prognosis after renal crash landing is grim, in part associated with the need to haemodialyse through a catheter, rather than the more efficient A-V fistula, graft, or peritoneal dialysis.

There are major differences in the mode of dialysis between and within countries; even where there is evidence physician preference and logistics dominate the decision. In the USA, around 95% of patients use peritoneal dialysis. There has been a sharp decline in the use of peritoneal dialysis in the United Kingdom, partly related to concerns about the complication of sclerosing encapsulating peritonitis. Peritoneal dialysates have high glucose concentrations and patients absorb 100–150 g glucose daily via this route, which contributes to weight gain, but there are still sound grounds for recommending it:

- Survival in the first two years of treatment is higher than with haemodialysis, though survival advantage is greater with haemodialysis after four years; one study found that patients who started with peritoneal dialysis, and then moved to haemodialysis once renal function had further deteriorated, had improved survival than those haemodialysed throughout. The improved outcomes with peritoneal dialysis may, in part, be due to some renal function persisting. Patients can, therefore, maintain urine output for years, in comparison with haemodialysis patients who are usually anuric within six months of starting treatment. This allows greater flexibility in oral intake.
- Sclerosis of forearm vessels, which makes it difficult to create a fistula.
- Peritoneal dialysis is slower and more sustained compared with haemodialysis and reduces the risk of changes in volume, blood pressure and cardiac strain.
- Renal transplantation is not contraindicated in people who have had peritoneal dialysis.

General physicians and diabetologists frequently encounter diabetic patients on dialysis in the emergency or ward setting:

- *Blood pressure*
  Diabetic patients on dialysis are more hypertensive than non-diabetic patients. Their blood pressure is highly volume-dependent and they are prone to hypotension during dialysis sessions (intradialytic hypotension), while being hypertensive and often requiring multiple antihypertensive medications at other times (contributory factors include advanced autonomic neuropathy and impaired left ventricular function). Omission of antihypertensives before dialysis sessions, longer dialysis sessions, more frequent dialysis at home are recommended strategies; intradialytic hypotension carries a threefold increased risk of cardiac death.
- *Cardiovascular disease*
  Patients awaiting the start of their dialysis programmes are at exceptionally high risk of cardiac events, with an especially high prevalence of congestive heart failure. Sudden cardiac death during and between dialysis sessions is high. Angiotensin

blocking treatments are often continued but, in view of the sympathetic neuropathy, β-blockers, especially the metabolically neutral agents, are probably not sufficiently used (Rossing *et al.*, 2015).

- *Malnutrition in dialysis patients*
  Dialysis patients have lower than recommended energy and protein intake. The obesity paradox operates: a higher body mass index is associated with reduced mortality in people of all ages (but especially those under 65) and overall duration of dialysis treatment (Vashistha *et al.*, 2014). At the least we should be aiming to maintain weight. Unfortunately renal nutritionists are in very short supply in many units and data specific to people with diabetes is sparse (though they have a higher body mass index than non-diabetic patients).
- *Infections and foot ulceration* (see **Chapter 3**)

Renal transplantation

Not very long ago, Type 2 diabetes was considered an absolute contraindication to transplantation (in much the same way as coronary bypass surgery), but between 1995 and 2009 the proportion of transplants in patients with diabetes increased by one-half to 12.5% of all new transplants. Graft survival in diabetes is similar to that in non-diabetic renal disease but mortality is still higher, interestingly more so in the under 40s compared with the over 55s, and mortality has not improved since the mid-1990s (Lim *et al.*, 2017). However, transplantation carries a better outlook than dialysis, even in the elderly. For example, in the over 70s, mortality was nearly 60% lower in transplanted compared with patients on dialysis who were on the waiting list for transplantation. After transplantation, cardiovascular events are common, especially in the three months after surgery, highlighting the need for careful pre-operative cardiovascular testing. The ethical issues of transplanting older Type 2 patients when there is inevitably a general shortage of donor organs are considerable; live-related donation and using higher risk kidneys, including expanded criteria donors, donation after cardiac death and cold ischaemia time >24 hours, have addressed some of the shortfall in older patients.

ESRD in the elderly

Dialysis is increasingly offered to elderly people but the evidence base for the complex decisions involved is very slim. Even technical decisions – haemodialysis or peritoneal dialysis – and where dialysis is optimally delivered – home or hospital unit – are difficult for both patient and practitioner. In practice, most patients receive haemodialysis in dedicated dialysis centres, whereas home peritoneal dialysis, at least up to three years, may be preferable for many older patients (no travel, no need for vascular access, continuous slow ultrafiltration).

The very difficult area of conservative – that is, non-dialytic – care in older ESRD patients is, fortunately, starting to be actively addressed (Raghavan and Holley, 2016). This new subspecialty is based on:

- Recognizing the immense personal, physical and mental toll that dialysis can place on patients, especially the frail and elderly and their carers.
- Recognizing that older people starting dialysis have a poor outlook; for example, fewer than 50% of 75+-year olds will survive a year. In the 70–74 year age group in the USA life expectancy is four years compared with 12 years for the general population.
- Conservative treatment in the over-75s with multiple comorbidities does not carry a lower life expectancy than haemodialysis (Chandna *et al.*, 2011).

- Structured advanced care planning.
- Active palliation of the many and often severe symptoms associated with ESRD, including pain, fatigue, disturbed sleep, pruritus and anorexia, and in the terminal stages nausea and vomiting, agitation and dyspnoea.

The decision is complex and often counterintuitive; for example, patients find travel to hospital-based facilities a major burden and they may be prepared to forgo survival advantage to be relieved of this, and to have greater freedom to travel themselves. Many dialysis centres are actively developing palliative care teams with specific expertise and interest in this important area of practice.

References

Aiello LP, Ayala AR, Antoszyk AN. Diabetic Retinopathy Clinical Research Network. Assessing the effect of personalized diabetes risk assessments during ophthalmologic visits on glycemic control: a randomized clinical trial. *JAMA Ophthalmol* 2015;133: 888–96 [PMID: 25996263].

Akbari A, Clase CM, Acott P et al. Canadian Society of Nephrology commentary on the KDIGO clinical practice guideline for CKD evaluation and management. *Am J Kidney Dis* 2015;65:177–205 [PMID: 25511161] Free full text.

Atkins RC, Briganti EM, Lewis JB et al. Proteinuria reduction and progression to real failure in patients with type 2 diabetes mellitus and overt nephropathy. *Am J Kidney Dis* 2005;45:281–7 [PMID: 15685505].

Bailey RA, Wang Y, Zhu V, Rupnow MF. Chronic kidney disease in US adults with type 2 diabetes: an updated national estimate of prevalence based on Kidney Disease: Improving Global Outcomes (KDIGO) staging. *BMC Res Notes* 2014;7:415 [PMID: 24990184] PMC4091951.

Bang CN, Greve AM, La Cour M et al. Effect of randomized lipid lowering with simvastatin and ezetimibe on cataract development (from the Simvastatin and Ezetimibe in Aortic Stenosis Study). *Am J Cardiol* 2015;116:1840–4 [PMID: 26602073].

Beauchamp G, Boyle CT, Tamborlane WV et al. T1D Exchange Clinic Network. Treatable diabetic retinopathy is extremely rare among pediatric T1D Exchange Clinic Registry participants. *Diabetes Care* 2016;39:e218–e219 [PMID: 27852686].

Beaulieu WT, Bressler NM, Melia M et al. Diabetic Retinopathy Clinical Research Network. Panretinal photocoagulation versus ranibizumab for proliferative diabetic retinopathy: patient-centered outcomes from a randomized clinical trial. *Am J Ophthalmol* 2016;170:206–13 [PMID: 27523491].

Bilo H, Coentrao L, Couchoud C et al. Clinical practice guideline on management of patients with diabetes and chronic kidney disease stage 3b or higher (eGFR <45 mL/min). *Nephrol Dial Transplant* 2015;30(Suppl 2):ii1–142 [PMID: 25940656].

Bilous R, Chaturvedi N, Sjølie AK et al. Effect of candesartan on microalbuminuria and albumin excretion rate in diabetes: three randomized trials. *Ann Intern Med* 2009;151:11–20 [PMID: 19451554].

Chandna SM, Da Silva-Gane M, Marshall C et al. Survival of elderly patients with stage 5 CKD: comparison of conservative management and renal replacement therapy. *Nephrol Dial Transplant* 2011;26:1608–14 [PMID: 21098012] PMC3084441.

Chaturvedi N, Porta M, Klein R et al.; DIRECT Programme Study Group. Effect of candesartan on prevention (DIRECT-Prevent 1) and progression (DIRECT-Protect 1) of retinopathy in type 1 diabetes: randomised, placebo-controlled trials. *Lancet* 2008;372:1394–402 [PMID: 18823656].

Chen PM, Lai TS, Chen PY et al. Multidisciplinary care program for advanced chronic kidney disease: reduces renal replacement and medical costs. *Am J Med* 2015;128: 68–76 [PMID: 25149427].

DCCT Research Group. The effect of intensive treatment of diabetes on the development and progression of long-term complications in insulin-dependent diabetes mellitus. The Diabetes Control and Complications Trial Research Group. *N Engl J Med* 1993;329:977–86 [PMID: 8366922] Free full text.

DCCT/EDIC Research Group; Aiello LP, Sun W, Das A et al. Intensive diabetes therapy and ocular surgery in type 1 diabetes. *N Engl J Med* 2015;372:1722–33 [PMID: 25923552] Free full text.

Diabetic Retinopathy Clinical Research Network; Wells JA, Glassman AR, Ayala JR et al. Aflibercept, bevacizumab, or ranibizumab for diabetic macular edema. N Engl J Med 2015;372;1193–203 [PMID: 25692915] PMC4422053.

Ekinci EI, Jerums G, Skene A et al. Renal structure in normoalbuminuric and albuminuric patients with type 2 diabetes and impaired renal function. Diabetes Care 2013;36:3620–6 [PMID: 23835690] PMC3816854.

Emanuele N, Moritz T, Klein R et al. Veterans Affairs Diabetes Trial Study Group. Ethnicity, race, and clinically significant macular edema in the Veterans Affairs Diabetes Trial (VADT). Diabetes Res Clin Pract 2009;86:104–10 [PMID: 1920420].

English E, Idris I, Smith G et al. The effect of anaemia and abnormalities of erythrocyte indices on HbA1c analysis: a systematic review. Diabetologia 2015;58:1409–21 [PMID: 25994072].

Ficociello LH, Perkins BA, Silva KH et al. Determinants of progression from microalbuminuria to proteinuria in patients who have type 1 diabetes and are treated with angiotensin-converting enzyme inhibitors Clin J Am Soc Nephrol 2007;2:461–9 [PMID: 17699452].

Fox CS, Matsushita K, Woodward K et al. Chronic Kidney Disease Prognosis Consortium. Associations of kidney disease measures with mortality and end-stage renal disease in individuals with and without diabetes: a meta-analysis. Lancet 2012;380:1662–73 [PMID: 23013602] PMC3771350.

Fried LF, Emanuele N, Zhang JH et al.; VA NEPHRON-D Investigators. Combined angiotensin inhibition for the treatment of diabetic nephropathy. N Engl J Med 2013; 369: 1892–903 [PMID: 24206457] Free full text.

Gaede P, Lund-Anderson H, Parving HH, Pederson O. Effect of a multifactorial intervention on mortality in type 2 diabetes. N Engl J Med 2008;358:580–91 [PMID: 18256393] Free full text.

Gæde P, Oellgaard J, Carstensen B et al. Years of life gained by multifactorial intervention in patients with type 2 diabetes mellitus and microalbuminuria: 21 years follow-up on the Steno-2 randomised trial. Diabetologia 2016;59:2298–307 [PMID: 27531506].

Hackam DG, Spence JD, Garg AX, Textor SC. Role of renin-angiotensin system blockade in atherosclerotic renal artery stenosis and renovascular hypertension. Hypertension 2007;50:998–1003 [PMID: 17923585] Free full text.

Haller H, Ito S Izzo JL Jr et al. ROADMAP Trial Investigators. Olmesartan for the delay or prevention of microalbuminuria in type 2 diabetes. N Engl J Med 2011;364:907–17 [PMID: 1388309] Free full text.

Harindhanavudhi T, Mauer M, Klein R. Renin Angiotensin System Study (RASS) group. Benefits of renin-angiotensin blockade on retinopathy in type 1 diabetes vary with glycemic control. Diabetes Care 2011;34:1838–42 [PMID: 21715517] PMC3142059.

Hayreh SS, Podhajsky A, Zimmerman MB. Central and hemicentral retinal vein occlusion: role of anti-platelet aggregation agents and anticoagulants. Ophthalmology 2011;118:1603–11 [PMID: 21704382] PMC3150626.

Hill CJ, Fogarty DG. Changing trends in end-stage renal disease due to diabetes in the United Kingdom. J Ren Care 2012;38 Suppl 1:12–22 [PMID: 22348360].

Jeppesen, Bek T. The occurrence and causes of registered blindness in diabetes patients in Arhus County, Denmark. Acta Ophthalmol Scand 2004;82:526–30 [PMID: 15453847] Free full text.

Keech A, Simes RJ, Barter P et al. FIELD study investigators. Effects of long-term fenofibrate therapy on cardiovascular events in 9795 people with type 2 diabetes mellitus (the FIELD study): randomised controlled trial. Lancet 2005;366:1849–61 [PMID: 16310551].

Lane M, Matthewson PA, Sharma HE et al. Social deprivation as a risk factor for late presentation of proliferative diabetic retinopathy. Clin Ophthalmol 2015;9:347–52 [PMID: 25733801] PMC4337620.

Lewis EF, Claggett B, Parfrey PS et al. Race and ethnicity influences on cardiovascular and renal events in patients with diabetes mellitus. Am Heart J 2015;170:322–9 [PMID: 26299230].

Liew G, Michaelides M, Bunce C. A comparison of the causes of blindness certifications in England and Wales in working age adults (16–64 years), 1999–2000 with 2009–2010. BMJ Open 2014;4:e004015 [PMID: 24525390] PMC3927710.

Lim WH, Wong G, Pilmore HL et al. Long-term outcomes of kidney transplantation in people with type 2 diabetes: a population cohort study. Lancet Diabetes Endocrinol 2017;5:26–33 [PMID: 28010785].

Mauer M, Zinman B, Gardiner R *et al.* Renal and retinal effects of enalapril and losartan in type 1 diabetes. *N Engl J Med* 2009;361:40–51 [PMID: 19571282] Free full text.

Miras AD, Chuah LL, Khalil N *et al.* Type 2 diabetes mellitus and microvascular complications 1 year after Roux-en-Y gastric bypass: a case-control study. *Diabetologia* 2015;58:1443–7 [PMID: 25893730] PMC4473013.

Moist LM, Troyanov S, White CT *et al.* Canadian Society of Nephrology commentary on the 2012 KDIGO Clinical Practice Guideline for Anemia in CKD. *Am J Kidney Dis* 2013;62:860–73 [PMID: 24054466].

Molitch ME, Steffes M, Sun W *et al.* Epidemiology of Diabetes Interventions and Complications Study Group. Development and progression of renal insufficiency with and without albuminuria in adults with type 1 diabetes in the Diabetes Control and Complications Trial and the Epidemiology of Diabetes Interventions and Complications Study. *Diabetes Care* 2010;33:1536–43 [PMID: 20413518] PMC2890355.

Niranen TJ, Johansson JK, Reunanen A, Jula AM. Optimal schedule for home blood pressure measurement based on prognostic data: the Finn-Home Study. *Hypertension* 2011;57:1081–6 [PMID: 21482956].

Orchard TJ, Secrest AM, Miller RG, Costacou T. In the absence of renal disease, 20 year mortality risk in type 1 diabetes is comparable to that of the general population: a report from the Pittsburgh Epidemiology of Diabetes Complications Study. *Diabetologia* 2010;53:2312–9 [PMID: 20665208] PMC3057031.

Packham DK, Alves TP. Dwyer JP *et al.* Relative incidence of ESRD versus cardiovascular mortality in proteinuric type 2 diabetes and nephropathy: results from the DIAMTRIC (Diabetes Mellitus Treatment for Renal Insufficiency Consortium) database. *Am J Kidney Dis* 2012;59:75–83 [PMID: 22051245].

Papademetriou V, Lovato L, Doumas M *et al.*; ACCORD Study Group. Chronic kidney disease and intensive glycaemic control increase cardiovascular risk in patients with type 2 diabetes. *Kidney Int* 2015;87:649–59 [PMID: 25229335].

Park J, Lertdumrongluk P, Molnar MZ *et al.* Glycemic control in diabetic dialysis patients and the burnt-out syndrome. *Curr Diab Rep* 2012;12:432–9 [PMID: 22638938].

Parving HH, Lehnert H Brochner-Mortensen J *et al.* Irbesartan in Patients with Type 2 Diabetes and Microalbuminuria Study Group. The effect of irbesartan on the development of diabetic nephropathy in patients with type 2 diabetes. *N Engl J Med* 2001;345:870–8 [PMID: 11565519] Free full text.

Pavlakis M. The timing of dialysis and kidney transplantation in type 1 diabetes. *Diabetes Obes Metab* 2012;14:689–93 [PMID: 22239150].

Perrin NE, Torbjörnsdotter T, Jaremko GA, Berg UA. Risk markers of future microalbuminuria and hypertension based on clinical and morphological parameters in young type 1 diabetes patients. *Pediatr Diabetes* 2010;11:305–13 [PMID:19761528].

Pfeffer MA, Burdmann EA, Chen CY *et al.* TREAT Investigators. A trial of darbopoeitin alfa in type 2 diabetes and chronic kidney disease. *N Engl J Med* 2009;361:2019–32 [PMID: 19880844] Free full text.

Porta M, Hainer JW, Jansson SO *et al.* DIRECT Study Group. Exposure to candesartan during the first trimester of pregnancy in type 1 diabetes: experience from the placebo-controlled DIabetic REtinopathy Candesartan trials. *Diabetologia* 2011;54:1298–303 [PMID: 21225259].

Pugliese G, Solini A, Zoppini G *et al.* Renal Insufficiency and Cardiovascular Events (RIACE) Study Group. High prevalence of advanced retinopathy in patients with type 2 diabetes from the Renal Insufficiency And Cardiovascular Events (RIACE) Italian Multicenter Study. *Diabetes Res Clin Pract* 2012;98:329–37 [PMID: 23020932].

Raghavan D, Holley JL. Conservative care of the elderly CKD patient: a practical guide. *Adv Chronic Kidney Dis* 2016;23:51–6 [PMID: 26709063].

Rasmussen ML, Broe R, Frydkjaer-Olsen U *et al.* Microaneursym count as a predictor of long-term progression in diabetic retinopathy in young patients with type 1 diabetes: the Danish Cohort of Pediatric Diabetes 1987 (DCPD1987). *Graefes Arch Cin Exp Ophthalmol* 2015;253:199–205 [PMID: 24898428].

Rossing P, Fioretto P, Feldt-Rasmussen B, Parving, HH. Diabetic nephropathy, in Skorecki K, Chertow GM, Marsden PA *et al.* (eds): Brenner and Rector's The Kidney, 10th edn. Elsevier, 2015, pp.1283–320.

Roy Chowdhury S, Thomas RL, Duseath GJ et al. Diabetic retinopathy in newly diagnosed subjects with type 2 diabetes mellitus: contribution of β-cell function. *J Clin Endocrinol Metab* 2016;101:572–80 [PMID: 26652932].

Sag AA, Sos TA, Benli C et al. Atherosclerotic renal artery stenosis in the post-CORAL era part 2: new directions in Transcatheter Nephron Salvage following flawed revascularization trials. *J Am Soc Hypertens* 2016;10:368–77 [PMID: 26996432].

Salardi S, Balsamo C, Zucchini S et al. High rate of regression from micro-macroalbuminuria to normoalbuminuria in children and adolescents with type 1 diabetes treated or not with enalapril: the influence of HDL cholesterol. *Diabetes Care* 2011;34:424–9 [PMID: 21216861] PMC3024361.

Sala-Vila A, Diaz-López A, Valls-Pedret C et al. Prevención con Dieta Mediterránea (PREDIMED) Investigators. Dietary marine ω-3 fatty acids and incident sight-threatening retinopathy in middle-aged and older individuals with type 2 diabetes: prospective investigation from the PREDIMED trial. *JAMA Ophthalmol* 2016;134:1142–9 [PMID: 27541690].

Sander B, Larsen M, Andersen EW, Lund-Andersen H. Impact of changes in metabolic control on progression to photocoagulation for clinically significant macular oedema: a 20 year study of type 1 diabetes. *Diabetologia* 2013;56:2359–66 [PMID: 23989773] PMC3824341.

Schjoedt KJ, Astrup AS, Persson F et al. Optimal dose of lisinopril for renoprotection in type 1 diabetic patients with diabetic nephropathy: a randomised crossover trial. *Diabetologia* 2009;52:46–9 [PMID: 18974967].

Sharma SG, Bomback AS, Radhakrishnan J et al. The modern spectrum of renal biopsy findings in patients with diabetes. *Clin J Am Soc Nephrol* 2013;8:1718–24 PMID: 23886566] Free full text.

Stoycheff N, Stevens LA, Schmid CH et al. Nephrotic syndrome in diabetic kidney disease: an evaluation and update of the definition. *Am J Kidney Dis* 2009;54:840–9 [PMID: 19556043] PMC4036614.

Strutton R, Du Chemin A, Stratton IM, Forster AS. System-level and patient-level explanations for non-attendance at diabetic retinopathy screening in Sutton and Merton (London, UK): a qualitative analysis of a service evaluation. *BMJ Open* 2016;6:e010952 [PMID: 27194319] PMC4874146.

Thomas RL, Dunstan FD, Luzio SD et al. Prevalence of diabetic retinopathy within a national diabetic screening service. *Br J Ophthalmol* 2015;99:64–8 [PMID: 25091950].

Toppe C, Möllsten A, Schön S et al. Renal replacement therapy due to type 1 diabetes: tie trends during 1995–2010 – a Swedish population based register. *J Diabetes Complications* 2014;28:152–5 [PMID: 24332762].

Vashistha T, Mehrotra R, Park J et al. Effect of age and dialysis vintage on obesity paradox in long-term-hemodialysis patients. *Am J Kidney Dis* 2014;63:612–22 [PMID: 24120224] PMC3969454.

Wanner C, Tonelli M; Kidney Disease: Improving Global Outcomes Lipid Guideline Development Work Group Members. KDIGO Clinical Practice Guideline for Lipid Management in CKD: summary of recommendation statements and clinical approach to the patient. *Kidney Int* 2014;85:1303–9 [PMID: 24552851].

Wei N, Zheng H, Nathan DM. Empirically establishing blood glucose targets to achieve HbA1c goals. *Diabetes Care* 2014;37:1048–51 [PMID: 24513588] PMC3964488.

Wong TY, Mwamburi M, Klein R et al. Rates of progression in diabetic retinopathy during different time periods a systematic review and meta-analysis. *Diabetes Care* 2009;32:2307–13 [PMID: 19940227] PMC 2782996.

Zhang L, Long J, Jiang W et al. Trends in chronic kidney disease in China. *N Engl J Med* 2016;375:905–6 [PMID: 27579659].

Further reading

Kidney Disease: Improving Global Outcomes (KDIGO): CKD Work Group. KDIGO 2012 Clinical Practice Guidelines for the evaluation and management of chronic kidney disease. *Kidney Int Suppl* 2013; Suppl 3(1):1–150. http://www.kdigo.org/clinical_practice_guidelines/pdf/CKD/KDIGO_2012_CKD_GL.pdf; last accessed 9 August 2017.

Rossing P, Fioretto P, Feldt-Rasmussen B, Parving, HH. Diabetic nephropathy, in Skorecki K, Chertow GM, Marsden PA et al. (eds): Brenner and Rector's The Kidney, 10th edn. Elsevier, 2015, pp.1283–320.

Key points

- Peripheral neuropathy can be detected with simple techniques but there are no specific treatments for many of its features
- The most effective treatments for painful neuropathy are pregabalin/gabapentin, duloxetine/venlafaxine and tricyclic antidepressants
- Carpal tunnel syndrome is common, often accompanied by other components of the 'diabetic hand'
- Syndromes of clinical autonomic neuropathy (upper and lower gastrointestinal, postural hypotension) need specialist assessment and management but drug treatments are unsatisfactory
- Alert anaesthetists to patients with suspected or known autonomic neuropathy
- The skin is a frequent target for a wide variety of manifestations of diabetes
- Both Type 1 and Type 2 patients are at increased risk of fractures

NEUROPATHY

Because there is no simple standard way to measure neuropathy (compare fully-quantitative albumin:creatinine ratio in renal disease, rigorous scoring of retinal photography), epidemiological data are difficult to interpret. Some neuropathic syndromes, especially 'amyotrophy' (proximal motor neuropathy, diabetic neuropathic cachexia) and painful diabetic neuropathy, seem to have become less frequent over the past decades, and since these are both associated with Type 2 diabetes, improved multimodal management in many patients may be responsible. However, neuropathic foot ulceration in both Type 1 and Type 2 remains prevalent and is still the commonest reason for hospital admission for diabetic complications. Sensory symptoms short of full-blown painful neuropathy are a major burden for patients, as are the consequences of autonomic neuropathy, especially erectile dysfunction and gastrointestinal symptoms.

Decades of basic and clinical research have not resulted in any useful prophylactic treatment for the common sensorimotor polyneuropathy of diabetes, the most powerful determinant of foot ulceration, other than vigorous attempts to improve glucose control in Type 1 diabetes (Diabetes Control and Complications Trial (DCCT); **Chapter 7**), and Steno-2-type multimodal intervention in Type 2 diabetes; **Chapters 4 and 10**). Drug treatments have been developed and trialled over nearly 40 years. The supposedly specific aldose reductase inhibitors of the 1970s and 1980s were designed to reduce neuronal accumulation of sorbitol, resulting from conversion of glucose, but in several large-scale trials they turned out to be either ineffective or toxic. Interest in them persists. Supplementation with recombinant nerve growth factor was ineffective too, another salutary example of 'obvious' treatment not helping. The antioxidant α-lipoic (thioctic)

Practical Diabetes Care, Fourth Edition. David Levy.
© 2018 John Wiley & Sons Ltd. Published 2018 by John Wiley & Sons Ltd.

acid has been extensively trialled and alleviates symptoms, and is well tolerated, but is only available in some countries.

Because it is difficult and time consuming to detect and measure neuropathy, it was not extensively studied in the important group of glycaemic trials in Type 2 diabetes reporting in the mid-2000s. However, there is no doubt that neuropathy is common, and not just in older patients. Nearly 50% of young people aged 6–18 years with Type 1 diabetes had at least one clearly abnormal result on a nerve conduction study – widely considered the 'gold standard' indicator of neurological deficit, but in spite of numerous similar cross-sectional studies, we still have almost no prospective studies using any validated neuropathy measurement that will help predict the onset of the worst outcomes, especially recurrent foot ulceration (Hirschfeld *et al.*, 2015). Recall the high rate of spontaneous resolution of even marked degrees of albuminuria in the DCCT; we are likely seeing the same temporary abnormalities in neurophysiology and only prospective studies – difficult to envisage – will help us do more than scratch the surface of peripheral nerve abnormalities in diabetes.

Practice point

The natural history of diabetic neuropathy is not as well understood as that of the other, more easily quantifiable, microvascular complications, retinopathy and kidney disease.

The most devastating complications of neuropathy – recurrent foot ulceration and amputation – may not be amenable to pharmacology but are significantly reduced by intensive education, high-quality and prompt podiatric care and provision of footwear (Monami *et al.*, 2015). In reality, this level of care is delivered much less than it is advocated or promised. Painful syndromes can be helped by judicious combinations of medication, and the management of erectile dysfunction was transformed by the introduction of PDE5 inhibitors. The more uncommon but more easily recognizable autonomic syndromes are also yielding to focused pharmacology.

Diagnosis of neuropathy
The common neuropathy of diabetes is 'distal sensorimotor polyneuropathy'.

Symptoms
The earliest symptom of neuropathy, though a manifestation of autonomic, not somatic neuropathy, is erectile dysfunction; when present it is associated with widespread endothelial dysfunction and in Type 2 patients a high cardiovascular risk profile. Somatic neuropathy usually presents as insidious and often unnoticed numbness of the toes, with or without paraesthesiae, slowly progressing proximally to involve the feet and shins. Type 2 patients often describe intermittent relapsing and remitting symptoms before the clinical diagnosis of diabetes. This question will probably never be addressed through a prospective study but metabolic syndrome subjects (and probably prediabetic subjects too) were at higher risk of carefully-defined polyneuropathy in a cross-sectional study (Callaghan *et al.*, 2016). This situation may be analogous to the specific renal lesions associated with obesity (see **Chapter 4**).

The Michigan Neuropathy Screening Instrument includes the following positive and negative symptoms:

- *Negative*: numbness of legs and/or feet; inability to distinguish hot and cold water; sensing feet on walking (joint position sense)
- *Positive*: burning; hypersensitivity of the feet; cramps in legs/feet; prickling; pain when bedcovers touch the skin; nocturnal worsening of symptoms; dry, cracked skin on feet.

Bear in mind a differential diagnosis when patients present with symptoms, especially if there is pain. Practitioners are still inclined to attribute symptoms to 'arthritis', degenerative joint disease, gout, peripheral vascular disease or the aches and pains of old age. Even when the symptoms are truly neuropathic, there is a range of different causes, broader even than the better recognized non-diabetic diagnoses in renal disease with proteinuria (see **Chapter 4**). Perhaps 10–50% of diabetic patients have another cause of peripheral neuropathy (neurotoxic medications, alcohol, vitamin B$_{12}$ deficiency, uraemia, vasculitis, chronic inflammatory demyelinating neuropathy or inherited neuropathy) (Freeman, 2009).

Signs

Classically there is a stocking distribution of sensory loss, starting at the tips of the toes, progressing proximally. Loss is usually to all sensory modalities, with large and small nerve fibres all involved:

- light touch
- pain (pinprick)
- temperature
- vibration
- proprioception.

In some people, small fibre-mediated modalities (pain and temperature) are more affected, while in others the large-fibre modalities (touch, vibration and proprioception) are primarily involved. In a fortunately very small group, there is severe loss of proprioception, resulting in a 'pseudo-tabetic' variant, with instability when standing or walking, especially on uneven surfaces. Occasionally this is further exacerbated by postural hypotension caused by sympathetic neuropathy. Motor neuropathy leads to wasting of the small foot muscles, causing clawing of the toes and increased exposure of pressure areas on the soles.

Signs can be subtle (**Figure 5.1**). Hair loss on the dorsum of the foot is usually stated to be due to 'trophic' neuropathic changes but it is more unreliable than atrophy of the fibrofatty tissue of the heel pad. High-risk clinical features include:

- Guttering on the dorsum of the feet, caused by small muscle wasting, often combined with high arches, atrophy of the heel pad and the important protective fatty pads overlying the heads of the first and fifth metatarsals.
- Callus, which always precedes neuropathic ulceration, and is not benign in the diabetic foot, as it increases focal pressure. It recurs quickly and requires frequent active removal by a podiatrist. Callus at the tip of a toe may conceal an abscess or osteomyelitis. Bleeding into callus needs urgent attention.

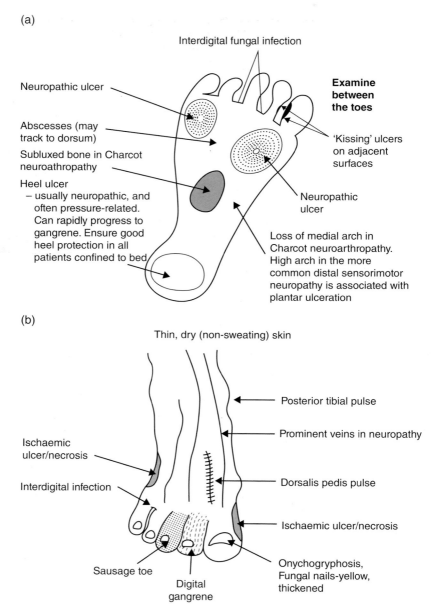

Figure 5.1 Features of the high-risk foot. (a) Plantar view. Neuropathic ulceration always occurs at areas of high pressure, under the first and fifth metatarsal heads, and less commonly the heel. (b) Dorsal view. *Source*: Levy, 2016. Reproduced with permission of John Wiley & Sons.

- Deeply fissured dry skin, often on the heels, is a portal for infection. Advise frequent use of hydrating agents containing urea (e.g. Flexitol preparations) on the skin – but not between the toes, which must be kept meticulously dry.
- Interdigital fungal infections, another portal for infection.
- Ingrowing toenail, especially if infected; subungual haematoma.
- Cellulitis.
- Ankle reflexes are usually absent in established neuropathy. Absent knee reflexes in the absence of other neuromuscular disorders suggests advanced neuropathy.

Practice point

Callus is evidence of high pressure and should be regularly removed by podiatrists. Advise maintaining regular skin hydration using urea-containing emollients.

Identifying the high-risk foot

A 2008 consensus suggested using one, preferably two, of the following five tests to detect loss of protective sensation and thereby identify the high-risk foot (Boulton et al., 2008):

- 10 g monofilament
- vibration perception threshold (neurothesiometer)
- 128 Hz tuning fork
- pinprick sensation
- ankle reflexes.

In practice, the 10 g monofilament is the most widely available test for neuropathy (**Figure 5.2**). Formally, 10 trials are required: eight or more correct responses is normal, 1–7 indicates reduced sensation. The performance characteristics of this (and all the other tests) are fiercely debated, but even simpler tests can be just as reliable, for example the Ipswich Touch Test, which requires no equipment (Rayman et al., 2011). Lightly touch the tips of the first, third and fifth toes on each foot: the presence of two or more insensate digits is as reliable as a negative monofilament test – at least compared with a 'gold standard' test (vibration perception threshold 25 volts or more using the neurothesiometer). In practice, foot assessment is a particularly depressing example of perfection (not attained in many years) being the enemy of the good (or even adequate): we can all agree any examination focused on detecting abnormalities in the foot or peripheral nerves is meaningfully better than no examination at all.

Practice point

10 g monofilament testing is simple and takes little time. An abnormal result is associated with future foot ulceration: act on the result.

Vibration perception threshold

Vibration is the simplest sensory modality to quantify. Nowadays it is as difficult to find a tuning fork as it is to track down a fully charged and functioning ophthalmoscope, but if you can locate one of the correct frequency (128 Hz) and use it on the pulp of the great

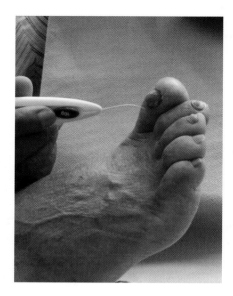

Figure 5.2 Monofilament. In practice the 10 g monofilament is the simplest semi-quantitative method to detect clinical neuropathy. Apply the monofilament perpendicularly to the skin of the distal great toe, between the nail fold and the distal interphalangeal joint, until it just buckles, ensuring a relatively constant applied pressure. Note the typical neuropathic features of the foot: thickened dystrophic nails, which always require podiatry to keep them neat, the high arch, slight wasting of the intrinsic muscles, and prominence of the high pressure areas under the great and fifth toes.

toe, inability to detect the vibration is a reliable but insensitive indicator of neuropathy. With the neurothesiometer the operator gradually increases the amplitude of vibration (arbitrarily measured in volts) applied by a probe to the great toe pulp. The patient is asked to indicate when they can feel the vibration. These are reliable devices and their output is quantitative, reproducible and prognostic – inability to feel vibration above 25 volts indicates lack of protective sensation and predicts a greatly increased risk of progression to ulceration – but they are rarely used.

Nerve conduction studies ('EMG')

Formal nerve conduction studies are rarely used to diagnose diabetic polyneuropathy outside the research setting but they can be useful in differentiating diabetic from other neuropathies. Median nerve studies are routinely performed in patients with suspected carpal tunnel syndrome and the neurophysiologist will usually do supplementary tests to establish the presence and severity of coexistent polyneuropathy in the upper limb, as this may modify the prognosis of carpal tunnel release (see later). Lower limb studies are not usually done, but if asking for an upper limb study, request a sural nerve sensory action potential amplitude and common peroneal motor nerve conduction velocity. An absent sural nerve sensory action potential is a good indicator of polyneuropathy, as is a reduced peroneal nerve conduction velocity. Because of the length-dependency of diabetic neuropathy, upper limb studies are likely to show less severe involvement than the legs.

Box 5.1 Key elements of education for patients with high-risk feet.

- Where possible, request a formal specialist podiatry review (this will include assessment of peripheral vascular disease and footwear).
- Regular routine podiatry for nails and callus, regrettably low priority in most healthcare systems. Regularly reinforce advice to patients not to attempt to cut their own toenails, still a depressingly frequent precipitant of infection and ulceration in insensitive feet. In the general population poor nail care is associated with increased falls.
- Emphasize simple strategies for avoiding exposing feet to painless injury:
  - Always wear footwear (even, perhaps especially, when going to the toilet in the night).
  - Use the elbow to pretest bathwater. Fortunately, thermal injury to the feet from hot water is now much less of a risk with widespread use of showers.
  - Never go barefoot outside (and do not wear open-toed sandals), especially on holiday when walking on hot sand, marble floors or temple steps. Soles of the feet are also at risk when sunbathing.
  - Feel inside shoes and shake them out before putting them on to avoid penetrating injuries from gravel and other objects.
  - In severely neuropathic feet, suggest seamless socks.
  - Try to check feet every day, including between the toes.
  - Ensure there are secure lines of communication between the patient and specialist podiatry services so that patients with acute problems, especially early ulceration and injury to neuropathic feet can have access to urgent specialist review within 24 hours.

Education

The link between insidious progression of numbness in the feet, lack of protective sensation and subsequent painless damage resulting in foot ulceration is not always evident to professionals. It is widely accepted that focused education reduces the incidence of foot lesions, but this is not the conclusion of several systematic reviews when considering either short single education sessions (e.g. 1 hour) or even complex interventions (Dorresteijn et al., 2014) Trial numbers are small and bias widespread, so these findings need to be taken with the usual pinch of meta-analytical salt, and it would be remiss of professionals not to emphasize important preventive strategies when seeing high-risk individuals and their carers (**Box 5.1**).

Foot ulceration

This is covered in detail in **Chapter 3**.

Pharmacological treatment of diabetic polyneuropathy

Of vitamins and antioxidants

Old habits die very hard indeed and patients are still given useless vitamin supplements (recall that there is still evidence for harm of pharmacological doses of some vitamins, though fortunately not the B-group vitamins that are usually prescribed in this situation). However, benfotiamine, a vitamin B_1 derivative, has been widely promoted, though had no effect on peripheral nerve function in long-standing Type 1 diabetes (Fraser et al., 2012). Alpha-lipoic acid is also widely used and there is some clinical trial information. In a long double-blind study there were no objective improvements, but interestingly there was no significant deterioration in the placebo-controlled group. Post hoc analysis found some improvements in neuropathic measures in those with worse baseline neuropathy but, similar to Steno-2, patients with normal body mass index and blood pressure seemed to do better and autonomic function improved in people taking ACE inhibitors, all consistent with data from other trials and observational studies (Ziegler *et al.*, 2016). Benfotiamine and α-lipoic acid are not available for prescription in the United Kingdom.

Practice point

Vitamin supplementation for people with diabetic neuropathy does not help.

Aldose reductase inhibitors and other agents

One aldose reductase inhibitor (epalrestat) is available but only in Japan, where clinical trials showed improvement in electrophysiological measurements and some symptoms. There are no large-scale double-blind placebo-controlled studies, which would be necessary for licensing in Europe and the USA. The protein kinase C β-isoform antagonist ruboxistaurin was extensively investigated for many years in diabetic retinopathy and appeared to benefit other microvascular complications. However, the research agenda has moved away from the search for 'specific' agents for prevention of individual complications, given the overwhelmingly important role of hyperglycaemia in complications of Type 1 diabetes and the recognition that a multimodal approach is the most effective in Type 2. An 'obvious' treatment, subcutaneously injected recombinant nerve growth factor, has not been revisited since the early years of the millennium and work on monoclonal antibodies against nerve growth factors, potentially valuable in painful neuropathy, has also stopped.

Painful diabetic neuropathy

A distressing and unexplained syndrome of distal foot and leg pain that occurs in 5–7% of a clinic population, though some estimates are as high as 1 in 5 patients (Javed *et al.*, 2015). It is difficult to believe that this is the current prevalence in countries with advanced healthcare, and the clinical impression is that painful neuropathy is seen less frequently than in the past. Because it is often associated with Type 2 diabetes, improved multimodal intervention over a long period might be responsible for this (undocumented and speculative) fall. However, it also means that its diagnosis is likely to be even further delayed than at present. Characteristic clinical features are shown in **Box 5.2**. Its association with Type 1 diabetes, noted particularly in young women with eating disorders, especially anorexia, was well described nearly 30 years ago (Steel *et al.*, 1987), though there are no systematic modern studies. The pathology may lie in the spinal cord and not in the peripheral nerves, hence the success of implantable spinal cord stimulation in severe and refractory cases. Poor glycaemic control is usual. Unfortunately, pain resolves in only a minority of cases and many patients have debilitating symptoms lasting several years. Pain often co-exists with the typical distal numbness of polyneuropathy, giving rise to a combination, understandably perplexing to a patient, of excruciating lancinating pains emanating from an insensitive foot. The diagnosis is a clinical one; always consider other painful syndromes in diabetes.

Practice point

Painful neuropathy occurs in the feet and lower legs and is worse – much worse – at night. Distinguish it from other painful syndromes, especially rest pain due to ischaemia.

Box 5.2 Features of painful diabetic neuropathy.

Clinical features
- Confined to feet and lower legs; more or less symmetrical (compare sciatica).
- Not exacerbated by exercise (compare ischaemic symptoms).
- Pain much worse at night (mandatory for diagnosis).
- No systemic involvement (weight loss, inflammatory markers normal).

Lower limb symptoms
- Stabbing/shooting/burning pains, often described in graphic terms e.g. red-hot pokers or needles, electric shocks.
- Contact hypersensitivity, especially to bedclothes.
- Altered sensation (allodynia): pain elicited by stimuli that are normally not painful, for example light touch or shower water.
- Heightened awareness of sensation (hyperaesthesiae).
- Cold feet (not always subjectively supported by partners).
- 'Tight skin'.

Other painful neuromyopathic states in diabetes

- *Diabetic amyotrophy* is also known by a bewildering variety of other terms, including proximal motor neuropathy, femoral neuropathy and lumbosacral plexopathy. It characteristically occurs in older Type 2 males who present with deep, burning pain in the thighs, accompanied by dramatic muscle wasting and precipitous weight loss, usually with profound depression. Patients are usually taking oral agents and may not be in poor control, possibly as a result of the systemic upset and anorexia. It responds dramatically and gratifyingly to insulin treatment, but a hunt for an underlying malignancy is understandably an accompaniment of this syndrome. It seems to have become much less common over the past 20 years, probably because of improved management of Type 2 diabetes in primary care.

- *Meralgia paraesthetica* (compression neuropathy of the lateral cutaneous nerve of the thigh, L2–L3) is more common in diabetes but occurs in non-diabetic people too, and may be associated with simple obesity. There is typical burning neuropathic pain in the expected distribution over the anterolateral thigh, associated with numbness and variable decreased sensation on examination. Symptoms are sometimes aggravated by standing or walking and, in distant times, when very low-slung trousers were common, by fashion. Nerve conduction studies can confirm the diagnosis. Local steroid injection preceded by confirmatory nerve block is reported to help, as is nerve block and neurectomy; but, as with many compression neuropathies, time may heal just as surely (Khalil *et al.*, 2012).

- *Insulin neuritis and oedema.* Insulin neuritis (treatment-induced neuropathy) is an uncommon acute neuropathy affecting the lower limbs, and occurs where there are dramatic improvements in glycaemia (e.g. >2–4% over about 3 months). It is, therefore, characteristic of people who are starting or intensifying insulin treatment. Fortunately, severe symptoms are rare but milder forms, with pain and some autonomic features may go undiagnosed. Warn susceptible patients about the possibility of these symptoms and reassure them that they are not a 'side effect' of insulin but a response to rapid establishment of blood glucose control. Like other acute neuropathic syndromes, it resolves, but it may take a few months (Gibbons and Freeman, 2015). *Insulin oedema* is also induced by rapid improvement in glycaemic control. It is usually confined to the lower limbs, but more generalized oedema with shortness of breath sometimes occurs. Recall that rapid falls in HbA$_{1c}$ can also temporarily worsen retinopathy (see **Chapter 4**).

- *Rest pain associated with peripheral vascular disease/critical limb ischaemia.*

Management of painful neuropathy

Your pain management team can be helpful, as they deal with a wide variety of neuropathic pain syndromes, but ensure that patients remain under regular diabetes review: opiate misuse is a concern and, although pain is the dominant symptom, patients are likely to have other associated diabetes complications that need continuing input. Improved glycaemic control, never definitively associated with improvement in pain, is a real challenge in these patients, some of whom, understandably, have given up on diabetes, on the people who help them look after it and – through its firm link with depression – on life itself.

Practice point

Try to keep in contact for general diabetes care with patients who have painful neuropathy.

Trials of analgesia for painful neuropathy are hampered by the usual lack of statistical power, a powerful placebo effect and bias. Vitamins, again, do not help, unless there is documented deficiency. Simple analgesics (paracetamol, NSAIDs where not contraindicated) are not supported by meta-analysis, but it would be remiss not to suggest them to start with, especially at bedtime if there are nocturnal symptoms.

A systematic review and meta-analysis (Finnerup *et al.*, 2015) was valuable because it developed recommendations based on an analysis that included some unpublished studies (**Table 5.1**). Combination treatment was previously recommended as part of the stepped-therapy approach but a large trial of duloxetine and pregabalin showed that the combination was no more effective than monotherapy with either agent, though the combination was as well tolerated (Tesfaye *et al.*, 2013).

Practice point

Gabapentin and pregabalin are often the most effective drugs in painful neuropathy, but titrate doses carefully and slowly.

Mononeuropathies

Carpal tunnel syndrome and ulnar nerve entrapment

Carpal tunnel syndrome is very common and equally prevalent in Type 1 and 2 diabetes; it occurs at a younger age in Type 1, where there is a 50% lifetime incidence. It is related to age and duration but not with microvascular complications (Singh *et al.*, 2005). As with all neuropathies, it may present atypically, since it is often superimposed on polyneuropathy, or can co-exist with other mononeuropathies and cervical disc disease. Consider it in any patient with pain or ache in the forearm or hand, especially at night. Request median nerve conduction studies (and always check thyroid function in Type 1 and Type 2) and refer. Outcomes of open surgical release are as good in diabetes as in other subjects, so long as there is no associated neuropathy, when the symptomatic results are not as good (Zimmerman *et al.*, 2017). No trials of steroid injection therapy or other approaches have been reported in diabetes; outcomes are again likely to be modified by the presence of polyneuropathy. Ulnar neuropathy is also associated with diabetes.

Entrapment occurs at the elbow or in the forearm, causing pain in the ring and little fingers, and although it is frequently detected on nerve conduction studies it is much less likely to cause symptoms than median nerve compression (Rota and Morelli, 2016).

Practice point

Think of carpal tunnel syndrome if there is pain in the hand or lower arm. Outcomes of intervention are good so long as there is no upper-limb polyneuropathy.

Truncal neuropathy

An unusual mononeuropathy involving one or more intercostal nerve, and presenting with acute pain in a dermatomal distribution. Cutaneous hyperaesthesia is characteristic and it is very occasionally associated with herniation of the intercostal or abdominal

Table 5.1 Recommendations for drug treatment of neuropathic pain (after Finnerup *et al.*, 2015).

	Drug regimen	Comments
Strong recommendations		
Gabapentin	1200–3600 mg daily in three divided doses	
Pregabalin	300–600 mg daily in two divided doses	
SNRI (serotonin-noradrenaline reuptake inhibitor)	Duloxetine: 60-120 mg once daily m/r venlafaxine 150–225 mg once daily	
Tricyclic antidepressants	Amitriptyline, imipramine, clomipramine up to 75 mg daily in two divided doses	Higher doses associated with increased risk of anticholinergic and arrhythmic side effects Subantidepressant doses of amitriptyline, e.g. 10 mg are effective in neuropathic pain
Weak recommendations		
Topical preparations		
Lidocaine 5% patches	1–3 patches to the painful area once a day up to 12 hours	Not approved in diabetic neuropathy
(Capsaicin 8% patches)		
Tramadol	m/r 200–400 mg daily in two or three divided doses	
Strong opioids	Individual titration	Use with caution
Other topical treatments with limited trial evidence for benefit		
OpSite dressing or spray		Non-pharmacological, and may reduce contact discomfort and allodynia
Isosorbide dinitrate spray	e.g. Isocard spray, 30 mg/dose, one spray to each leg at bedtime	Acts through local vasodilatation or possibly nitric oxide donation
Capsaicin cream (0.075%)	Needs 3–4 applications daily	The value of capsaicin cream is reduced by the need for frequent application, but this is required to manage the initial exacerbation in pain caused by neuropeptide depletion

muscles. Spinal osteoporosis or malignancy would be the usual primary diagnoses; shingles would soon become apparent. It usually recovers spontaneously over a few months.

Cranial mononeuropathies

About 40% of oculomotor nerve palsies occur in people with diabetes. Lateral rectus sixth and painful third nerve palsy with pupillary sparing are common, especially in Type 1 diabetes (Wilker *et al.*, 2009). Brain MRI is usually done, as there are rare non-diabetic causes (compressive and inflammatory). Ophthalmological and orthoptist input is needed. They resolve spontaneously over several months. Bear in mind the very rare association between myasthenia gravis with Type 1 diabetes that can present with features suggesting an oculomotor neuropathy.

Nonarteritic anterior ischaemic optic neuropathy

This rare but serious condition first came to the attention of diabetologists after the introduction of the PDE5 inhibitors for erectile dysfunction. Its dramatic clinical features include acute onset of blurred vision or visual field loss, and in the PDE5-associated cases was reported occurring a few hours after taking the medication. After years of data-crunching, it is still not clear if the drugs are implicated; a recent synthesis concluded that diabetes and its associated vascular risk factors dominated. Longer-term visual outcomes are similar in people with and without diabetes (Chen *et al.*, 2013).

Autonomic neuropathy and its cardiovascular consequences

Much as in sensorimotor polyneuropathy, there are countless studies emphasizing the high prevalence of autonomic neuropathy in diabetes, especially if sensitive methods are used, but only a small proportion of patients develop significant symptoms beyond erectile dysfunction. Like sensorimotor neuropathy, the manifestations and detection methods vary widely and the reported prevalences vary accordingly. But asymptomatic autonomic neuropathy in both Type 1 and 2 diabetes has a sinister prognosis not shared by peripheral neuropathy. Cardiovascular events were nearly threefold greater after the DCCT closeout in Type 1 patients with abnormal cardiovascular autonomic function and were related to long-term HbA_{1c} and its legacy effect (Pop-Busui *et al.*, 2017).

In the ACCORD study, Type 2 patients with established cardiovascular autonomic neuropathy were on average 63 years old, with 11–13 years of diagnosed diabetes, and nearly 50% used insulin. Abnormal cardiovascular autonomic reflexes were associated with a one-and-a-half to twofold increased risk of all-cause and cardiovascular death at four years follow-up. Good glycaemic control in Type 1 diabetes reduced the risk of progression to autonomic neuropathy in DCCT and multimodal treatment in Steno-2 reduced the risk in Type 2, but once autonomic neuropathy is established ACCORD found that tight control did not reduce mortality (Pop-Busui *et al.*, 2010).

Diagnosis

Cardiovascular autonomic reflexes are the only tests routinely available for diagnosing early autonomic neuropathy (**Table 5.2**). Because there is no simple treatment, they are required only when there is a clinical problem, for example investigating the cause of gastrointestinal symptoms or in preoperative assessment. The easiest test is measuring heart rate variation with deep breathing (sinus arrhythmia). Run an ECG rhythm strip while the patient takes slow deep breaths – five seconds each in inspiration and expiration. Heart rate variation is the difference between the fastest heart rate during inspiration and the slowest during expiration. Systolic blood pressure fall after standing will detect orthostatic hypotension and after exclusion of other causes is diagnostic of sympathetic neuropathy. Other tests of vagal function (heart rate response to the Valsalva manoeuvre and the heart rate response to lying and standing) are too complicated for use outside research.

Practice point

Abnormal heart rate variation with deep breathing is a reliable indicator of autonomic (vagal) neuropathy. Significant postural hypotension (sympathetic) occurs late.

Table 5.2 Autonomic function tests.

	Normal	Borderline	Abnormal
Heart rate variation to deep breathing (beats/min)	≥15	11–14	≤10
Systolic BP fall two minutes after standing (mm Hg)	≤10	11–29	≥30 (>20 according to some guidelines)

Source: after Ewing *et al.*, 1985.

Management of autonomic neuropathy syndromes

Erectile dysfunction (ED)

Erectile dysfunction is the most frequent neuropathic complication of diabetes: in the UKPDS around 20% of men had ED at diagnosis, increasing to 34% at 12 years. In primary care, the prevalence may be as high as 50%. The relationship between peripheral neurological function and potency is weak. However cardiovascular risk factors and the metabolic syndrome are strongly linked to ED through impaired endothelial function, and silent myocardial ischaemia is very commonly reported in patients with ED. It is not surprising, therefore, that in men between 55 and 88 years in the ADVANCE study, baseline erectile dysfunction was associated with an increased five-year risk of all cardiovascular disease and cerebrovascular disease. In men reporting chronic ED over the first two years, cardiovascular risk increased by 30–50%; there was also a strong association with cognitive decline and dementia (Batty *et al.*, 2010).

The association between ED and coronary artery disease reinforces the case for cardiovascular risk factor control; intensive lifestyle management in the Look AHEAD study had only a mildly beneficial effect on erectile function (Wing *et al.*, 2010). Urinary incontinence improved, but not troublesome nocturia or daytime frequency. Cardiovascular drugs (statins and angiotensin blockade) do not themselves improve ED.

A brief history and examination are wise because there are other causes of ED and other contributory factors in people with diabetes.

History

Distinguish between ED and loss of libido; the latter may be psychogenic or, more rarely, endocrine in origin (usually hypogonadism, but there are rarer conditions, for example hyperprolactinaemia). Peyronie's disease, resulting in pain, and significantly more common in diabetes, may be another factor. Remember the link between genetic haemochromatosis, hypogonadism and Type 1 diabetes. The duration of ED is no longer thought to be a reliable indicator of aetiology.

Drug history

- Antihypertensives (thiazides more likely to cause ED than β-blockers).
- Psychotropics of all kinds (SSRIs are associated with ED, reduced libido and delayed ejaculation; antipsychotics with hyperprolactinaemia).
- Alcohol, tobacco, cannabis.

Practice point

Erectile dysfunction is associated with a higher risk of all cardiovascular events. Vigorous secondary prevention is needed, but unfortunately does not improve the erectile dysfunction.

Investigations and treatment

Serum testosterone, gonadotrophins (LH and FSH) and prolactin levels are generally requested, and it is important to exclude significant hypogonadism especially in middle-aged Type 2 patients presenting with ED. Always consider non-diabetic causes of primary and secondary hypogonadism, associated with respectively low and elevated gonadotrophin levels. The specific hypogonadism of Type 2 diabetes is now well recognized but its aetiology is complex and there is no consistent pattern of gonadotrophins. There has been much discussion about diagnostic cut-points for serum testosterone levels. A large placebo-controlled study of long-acting intramuscular testosterone undecanoate found that erectile dysfunction, sexual desire and satisfaction with intercourse improved after 30 weeks of treatment, but only in those with severe biochemical hypogonadism (total serum testosterone ≤8.0 nmol/l or free testosterone ≤0.18 nmol/l); those with milder hypogonadism (total testosterone 8.1–12 nmol/l or free testosterone 0.18–0.25 nmol/l) did not benefit (Hackett et al., 2016). Given the lack of consensus on treatment criteria, testosterone replacement treatment is firmly in the hands of specialists in andrology.

Treatment

The PDE5 inhibitors, of which four are available (sildenafil is generic), increase the availability of vasodilatory nitric oxide by inhibiting cyclic AMP. The only absolute contraindication to treatment is nitrate therapy (including nicorandil). They should not be taken at the same time as potent CYP3A4 inhibitors (erythromycin, ketoconazole, various antiretrovirals, grapefruit juice). Sildenafil should be taken about an hour before intercourse; the others are effective within 30 minutes. Daily use of tadalafil (5 mg daily), in contrast to on-demand usage, is effective both for ED and lower urinary tract symptoms and nocturnal urinary frequency due to benign prostatic disease. It may also be effective in ED patients who did not respond fully to on-demand treatment. ED improves in patients with obstructive sleep apnoea treated with CPAP.

Andrologists use other agents singly or in combination. Intraurethral alprostadil is effective and can be used in patients not responding to PDE5 inhibitors or in whom they are contraindicated. Intracavernosal injections are still used. Vacuum tumescence devices and surgical implants need specialist consideration.

Practice point

In erectile dysfunction do routine investigations (serum testosterone, LH/FSH, prolactin). Testosterone replacement therapy is effective where serum testosterone level is very low (≤8.0 nmol/l); otherwise suggest a trial of PDE5 inhibitors.

Symptomatic postural hypotension

A late sympathetic autonomic complication that can be disabling but is fortunately very uncommon. Symptoms are often worse in the morning and correlate notoriously weakly with measured postural falls in blood pressure. Advanced neuropathy is often accompanied by established proteinuric diabetic kidney disease, so it is difficult to balance renal protection with angiotensin blockade and the resulting postural symptoms, especially with ACE inhibitors. Ambulatory blood pressure monitoring will not detect postural drops, which occur over minutes, but may highlight the classical finding of recumbent (nocturnal) hypertension (modest head-up of bed, around 10 cm, may reduce this). Minimize the use of diuretics (though many of these patients have troublesome multifactorial dependent oedema), vasodilators, tricyclics and α-blockers prescribed for prostatic symptoms. Supine hypertension is difficult to manage but older short-acting antihypertensives may be of help, for example the prototype ACE-inhibitor captopril, overnight nitroglycerine patch, clonidine or hydralazine, but few physicians have contemporary experience of using these drugs.

Simple manoeuvres may help (Low and Tomalia, 2015). Ensure patients drink enough water (1.25–2.5 litres) through the day, especially in warm weather; this is one situation where generous salt supplementation of food is important. Drinking boluses of water in quick succession (e.g. two large glasses of cold water) is also helpful and elevates standing systolic blood pressure by about 20 mm Hg for 1–2 hours. Doing this on waking might help counteract the early morning exacerbation of hypotension. Manoeuvres involving contraction of groups of muscle for about 30 seconds, relaxing and then repeating, may also help (standing on tips of toes, crossing legs and squeezing, clenching buttocks and upper thigh muscles).

Mechanical aids and devices are too troublesome for these often disabled patients.

No drug apart from fludrocortisone is licensed in the United Kingdom for postural hypotension (0.1–0.2 µg daily), but it is a long-acting agent, so exacerbates hypertension during the night, and worsening peripheral oedema would not be welcome either.

A specific short-acting pressor α1-adrenoceptor agonist, midodrine, is unfortunately not widely available in the United Kingdom and is unlicensed, but is licensed in the USA. Potential side effects are paraesthesias (including tingling of the scalp), goose-bumps and bladder pain or inability to pass urine, but the short duration of action of this drug means that if it can be sourced locally it is well worth a brief trial.

Practice point

Practical treatments for symptomatic postural hypotension include adequate general hydration through the day, bolus drinks of cold water, regular bouts of contracting lower limb muscles and, if available, midodrine.

Gastrointestinal dysfunction

Advanced autonomic neuropathy can affect any part of the gastrointestinal tract. Visceral pain sensation is decreased and symptoms often atypical or blunted. They are also intermittent, have a complex relationship with prevailing blood glucose levels and are difficult to distinguish from other functional and structural problems. They often occur in the fortunately rare cases of severe eating disorders in young Type 1 females.

Gastroparesis

Gastroparesis accompanies advanced somatic neuropathy and other features of autonomic neuropathy. The pathogenesis is complex and includes contributions from vagal neuropathy, reduction in gastric pacemaker cells and neurohormonal changes. Acute elevations of blood glucose delay gastric emptying. Although retained gastric contents are sometimes observed during incidental upper gastrointestinal endoscopy, troublesome clinical symptoms are fortunately very uncommon. When they do occur, they can be dreadful. Early symptoms are subtle and include slight fullness or early satiety after eating; in more advanced cases there is episodic nausea and vomiting, characteristically 30–120 minutes after eating, with the risk of recurrent diabetic ketoacidosis. However, early morning vomiting is uncommon and suggests a non-neuropathic cause (Camilleri, 2007). Gastric emptying is unpredictable and hypoglycaemia frequent because of poor coordination between eating, insulin injection and glucose absorption. Most patients are in poor long-term glycaemic control and have the attendant problem of hypoglycaemia unawareness. Weight loss and malnutrition are real risks. Pancreas or islet transplantation should be seriously considered in Type 1 patients.

Investigations

Upper gastrointestinal endoscopy will diagnose concurrent pathologies or retained food residue (pharyngeal/oesophageal candidiasis occasionally causes significant upper gastrointestinal symptoms). The delay in gastric emptying can be quantified with a nuclear medicine study; retention of >40% of a standard solid meal at two hours or >10% at four hours is considered abnormal. Treatment is complex. The only pro-motility agent currently considered sufficiently safe is metoclopramide, 10 mg three times daily before meals (only in those over 19 years of age, and preferably as a solution rather than tablets), but low dose erythromycin, 125 mg twice daily in oral form, is effective and well-tolerated, though there is tachyphylaxis after prolonged courses (caution is required when given with other potent CYP3A4 inhibitors).

Nutritional assessment is important in these patients and they often benefit from enteral feeding, for example through percutaneous endoscopic jejunostomy; gastrostomies with jejunal extensions are less difficult to place but tubes tend to migrate into the stomach. In intractable cases, there is gastric electrical stimulation using a 'gastric pacemaker' (Enterra system), though gastric emptying is still constrained, and gastrojejunostomy is currently advised (Sarosjek et al., 2015). Total or subtotal gastrectomy with gastrojejunostomy is sometimes recommended; the anatomy and physiology are sound,

---

Practice point

Be alert to subtle symptoms of gastroparesis (bloating, nausea, episodic diarrhoea). Upper gastrointestinal endoscopy and formal nuclear medicine gastric emptying studies will help confirm the diagnosis.

---

and again symptom relief can be dramatic. In the era of 'evidence-based' medicine, it is difficult for patients to obtain surgical treatment, as it is unlikely definitive clinical trials in sufficiently large numbers of patients can be performed.

Large bowel involvement

Intermittent constipation, caused by large bowel atony, is common. Diarrhoea is characteristic and usually lasts a few days, then remits, but it can be persistent, frequent and distressing. There is sometimes faecal incontinence. Exclude coeliac disease in Type 1. In Type 2 diabetes pancreatic exocrine sufficiency is increasingly recognized, usually in thin insulin-requiring people, and there is a hint, though no formal comparative studies, that it is more common in people of Indian origin (Shivaprasad *et al.*, 2015). Diarrhoea, progressive weight loss and increasingly frequent hypoglycaemia in the face of decreasing insulin requirements are clinical pointers. Laboratory evidence for exocrine insufficiency is described in countless studies, with reported prevalence levels from 5 to 30%. There is no point hunting for this syndrome in the absence of symptoms. Initial investigations should include plain abdominal radiograph or abdominal CT scan for pancreatic calcification, and possibly faecal elastase measurement. If there is diagnostic doubt after initial investigations, a short trial of pancreatic enzyme replacement therapy is worthwhile.

In large-bowel autonomic neuropathy, the diarrhoea is usually attributed to small intestinal bacterial overgrowth; a hydrogen breath test may help diagnose it. There are no adequate clinical trials and treatment is based on anecdote. Tetracycline, 250 mg qds for one week, has often been given but metronidazole (e.g. 750 mg daily) and ciprofloxacin (e.g. 1000 mg daily) have also been used. Rifaximin is a broad-spectrum non-absorbed antibiotic beneficial in non-diabetic bacterial overgrowth syndromes and is licensed for use in uncomplicated travellers' diarrhoea. It is, therefore, neither more nor less studied than other agents, and because bacterial resistance and systemic side effects are likely to be less of a problem, it may be worth a therapeutic trial of 7–10 days at 1200–1600 mg/day.

Practice point

In suspected large-bowel autonomic neuropathy a trial of short-term antibiotics is worthwhile, for example metronidazole 750 mg daily or the non-absorbable rifaximin 1200–1600 mg daily.

Perioperative care of patients with autonomic neuropathy

There are no prospective studies of perioperative complications in people with established autonomic neuropathy, though they are well discussed in reviews (McGrane *et al.*, 2014). At induction of anaesthesia there can be abrupt falls in blood pressure and heart rate, and previously unsuspected or undetected gastroparesis with retained gastric contents poses an aspiration risk. Greater pressor support is often needed because of inadequate peripheral vasoconstriction, but vasoactive drugs can have unpredictable effects; denervation hypersensitivity is the proposed culprit. Thermal dysregulation can lead to hypo- or hyperthermia. There may be an increased tendency to arrhythmias on account of prolonged QTc intervals and other complex abnormalities of ECG wave dispersion seen in autonomic neuropathy. Hypoglycaemia is probably pro-arrhythmic and, while this will be diligently avoided during surgery, it is also a risk after major surgery during the period when patients need continuous intravenous insulin infusions. A continuous glucose monitoring study identified a high risk of hypoglycaemia 10 and 30 hours after abdominal surgery (Joseph *et al.*, 2009).

Practice point

Patients with long-standing diabetes can have asymptomatic, undiagnosed autonomic neuropathy. Ensure meticulous anaesthetic and perioperative care, avoid hypoglycaemia and pay special attention to blood pressure and electrolytes.

MUSCULOSKELETAL

Cheiroarthropathy: limited joint mobility, the 'diabetic hand' (Smith et al., 2003)

Apart from the autoimmune association between Type 1 diabetes and rheumatoid arthritis, there are no other specific rheumatological conditions identifiable through serological tests. However in long-standing Type 1 diabetes, even when there are no associated microvascular complications (but especially when there are) there is progressive thickening and stiffening of connective tissues, probably due to accumulation of advanced glycation end products. Biopsy evidence of periarticular collagen thickening, similar to that seen in scleroderma, was reported in the 1980s. The structural consequences are widespread and highly troublesome in both Type 1 and Type 2 diabetes, but limited joint mobility and the prayer sign (the observer can see clear space between the patient's opposed hands) are more prevalent in Type 1 diabetes.

Terms and definitions are unclear. Cheiroarthropathy was previously defined as stiffening of the hands (leading to limited joint mobility) and characterized by the positive prayer sign. The DCCT/EDIC group broadened the definition to include several upper limb disorders that impair functionality (Larkin et al., 2014). In decreasing order of prevalence after a mean duration of 30 years of Type 1 diabetes:

- adhesive capsulitis of the shoulder ('frozen' shoulder) (31%)
- carpal tunnel syndrome (30%; see previously)
- flexor tenosynovitis (trigger finger) (28%)
- positive prayer sign (22%)
- Dupuytren's contracture (9%).

While clinically significant upper limb polyneuropathy is uncommon except in patients with advanced peripheral and autonomic neuropathy, light touch perception is reported to be reduced and progressive in patients with long-standing diabetic hand syndromes. The combination most frequently encountered was carpal tunnel syndrome with flexor tenosynovitis, often involving multiple digits. The frequent occurrence together of carpal tunnel syndrome, tenosynovitis, a positive prayer sign and Dupuytren's contracture warrants the term the 'diabetic hand'. In a long-term study of the DCCT cohort, 24 years after the start of the trial, the prevalence of cheiroarthropathy was the same – and very high (66%) – in both intensive and conventional treatment groups but worse glycaemia through the study was associated with a higher prevalence and, not surprisingly, retinopathy and neuropathy were associated with the presence of cheiroarthropathy (Larkin et al., 2014). Each individual component requires detailed assessment and individualized treatment by specialist upper limb surgeons: disability can be significant, even to the extent of difficulty with injections and blood glucose monitoring.

Adhesive capsulitis

A disabling musculoskeletal problem that causes progressive and painful restriction of shoulder movements, especially external rotation and abduction. It is at least three times commoner in people with diabetes and overall prevalence is nearly 15% (Zreik et al., 2016). It occurs at a younger age in diabetic patients and is associated with less pain but lasts longer and is more resistant to treatment. Even in people without diabetes there is no meaningful evidence base for the best approaches to management. Analgesia and intra-articular steroid injections are the mainstay of pragmatic treatment but, as with all steroid therapy in diabetes, it often results in significant deterioration in glucose control for 24–48 hours. Surgery is sometimes needed.

Flexor tenosynovitis (trigger finger)

Trigger finger is very common in diabetes and usually responds well to steroid injection of the flexor tendon sheath. Multiple digits can be involved.

Dupuytren's contracture

Thickening of palmar or digital tissues resulting in tethering or contracture. In diabetes the third and fourth digits are usually affected, compared with the fifth finger in non-diabetic patients, but contracture is often milder in diabetes and only very rarely requires surgery.

Practice point

Patients can develop significant disability from multiple abnormalities of the hand and upper limb in long-standing diabetes. Refer to a rheumatologist or orthopaedic surgeon with a specialist upper limb interest.

Diffuse idiopathic skeletal hyperostosis (DISH)

New bone formation, especially in the thoracolumbar spine, and with a characteristic radiological appearance of new 'flowing' bone. It is associated with both diabetes/impaired glucose tolerance and obesity, and with calcification of tendons and ligaments elsewhere (e.g. skull, pelvis, heels or elbows), and is more prevalent in Type 1 diabetes. Symptoms are not usually severe,and it is often an incidental radiological finding, but there is sometimes mild early-morning stiffness of the spine, and dysphagia has been reported.

Gout

This is discussed in more detail in **Chapter 13**.

Fracture risk

The broad topic of bone health in diabetes was more one of mechanistic interest than clinical relevance until evidence accumulated of the increased risk of fractures with the thiazolidinedione drugs (**Chapter 10**). But there is generally more interest in fracture risk and bone health overall, and studies have attempted to unpick the factors contributing to changes in bone density and fracture risk in diabetes.

Type 1 diabetes

There is broad agreement that fracture risk in Type 1 diabetes is elevated across the lifespan, though poor glycaemic control and the presence of microvascular complications are probably more important than disease duration. The risk seems to be lower in recent studies than in older and smaller ones, which quoted a 10- to 12-fold increased fracture risk, but there is at least a threefold increased risk of hip fractures, with a strikingly high risk in men (Hotherstall *et al.*, 2014). Individual patients with associated endocrine disorders, especially hyperthyroidism and coeliac disease should be considered at especially high risk, though there are no systematic studies of these groups. There are no intervention studies but, until there are, careful vitamin D replacement in deficient people would be sound.

Type 2 diabetes

The factors contributing to bone density in Type 2 diabetes are complex and studies are confounded by the unknown duration of hyperglycaemia in many patients. It was widely imagined that increased body weight associated with Type 2 diabetes would protect against fractures, but bone fragility itself is probably increased and, in addition, there is an increased risk of falls and serious fractures and hospitalization, due a combination of multiple factors, including neuropathy, visual impairment from retinopathy and orthostatic hypotension. Type 2 diabetes is now included in the FRAX algorithm as a cause of secondary osteoporosis, indicating an increased risk when bone density data is not available. However, because the increased risk is not related to reduced bone mineral density, use of standard drugs for osteoporosis may be not be of value in many patients (Dede *et al.*, 2014).

Practice point

Type 1 patients and, to a lesser extent, Type 2 patients are at increased risk of fractures. Ensure optimum glycaemia and vitamin D supplementation.

Effects of antidiabetic agents on bones

The dramatically increased risk of all fractures in postmenopausal women taking glitazones, though not in men, is of less concern now that these drugs are little used. Other agents are either neutral or protective for bones. Sulfonylureas and metformin are both associated with a lower fracture risk, the former possibly through an anabolic effect. At least in vitro metformin has a direct osteogenic effect. Incretins are directly involved in bone turnover. In clinical studies, GLP-1-receptor agonists are probably bone-neutral, though study durations are short. DPP-4 inhibitors have, likewise, not been adequately studied but there is no signal of harm. Data on the SGLT2 inhibitors are awaited. They increase tubular phosphate reabsorption and may lead to some degree of secondary hyperparathyroidism, but bone and fracture outcomes will not be known for some time (Meier *et al.*, 2016).

SKIN

The skin is a target of multiple insults in diabetes: there are infections (see **Chapter 3**), conditions specific to diabetes and, given the large number of medications taken by many patients, a high burden of cutaneous drug reactions.

Specific skin conditions

Necorobiosis lipoidica diabeticorum (Figure 5.3)

Necrobiosis, a hallmark cutaneous indication of Type 1 diabetes, is uncommon and its aetiology mysterious. A national survey from Germany found it in about 0.25% of patients, around two-thirds female. It usually affects the shins but other areas of the legs can be affected. Lesions elsewhere are uncommon. It starts as asymptomatic dull red plaques, irregular in shape but well demarcated. Small satellite lesions are common.

(a)

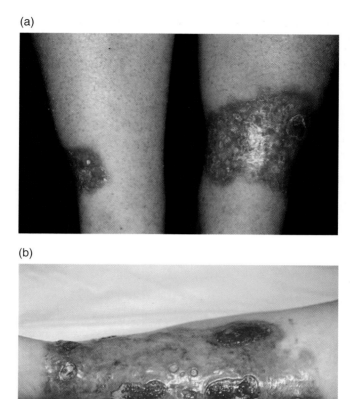

(b)

Figure 5.3 (a) Non-ulcerated necrobiosis in its typical distribution on the anterior shin(s); (b) ulcerated lesions of necrobiosis. *Source*: Ahn *et al.*, 2016. Reproduced with permission of Elsevier.

When chronic it becomes indurated with areas of waxy-looking atrophy, and crossed by prominent telangiectasiae. Chronic disfiguring ulceration occurs in about 25%, which is slow to heal and tends to recur. The diagnosis is clinical and biopsy risks causing or aggravating ulceration. Its cause is unknown but it tends to be clustered with the 'auto-immune' associations of Type 1 diabetes. However, the German study found only a marginal increase in the prevalence of thyroid autoimmunity, though formally diagnosed coeliac disease was three times as frequent. There have been hints of an association with established microvascular complications but there was no excess either of retinopathy or microalbuminuria. There is a clinical association with insulin resistance: insulin doses were higher in necrobiosis patients, though body mass index was similar (some of this may be mediated by the higher rate of smoking noted in necrobiosis patients). Several studies have shown worse glycaemic control, but hardly dramatically so (HbA$_{1c}$ 8.7 vs 8.3%, 72 vs 67) (Hammer *et al.*, 2017).

All manner of treatments have been used, including steroids, either topical under occlusion or intralesional, and they may be helpful in early lesions. Individual dermatologists may have experience with other agents, for example TNF-α antagonists, mycophenolate and topical psoralen ultraviolet A therapy.

Practice point

Necrobiosis usually occurs in female Type 1 patients, and is associated with smoking, higher insulin requirements and an increased prevalence of coeliac disease.

Diabetic dermopathy (shin spots)

Common, especially in middle-aged males with established complications of diabetes. Oval red papules, about 1 cm across become scaly and brown, and tend to fade in 1–2 years.

Acanthosis nigricans (Figure 5.4)

A specific cutaneous hallmark of insulin resistance and hyperinsulinaemia: velvety epidermal overgrowth with a papillomatous feel and usually hyperpigmented. It usually involves the neck, axilla, the inguinal region and the inframammary region, but can occur on the

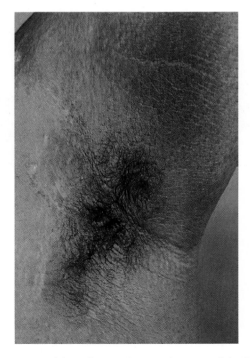

Figure 5.4 Acanthosis nigricans of the axilla. Acanthosis can be a very subtle clinical sign. *Source:* Ahn *et al.*, 2016. Reproduced with permission of Elsevier.

extensor surfaces, including the knuckles and elbows. In its milder forms it is not always noticed by the patient. In the USA, the highest prevalence is seen in Native Americans (about one-third), followed by African-Americans, Hispanics, then white subjects. Since the millennium it has been used in Texas school health screening to identify children at high risk of dysglycaemia and hypertension (Otto *et al.*, 2010) (see **Chapter 1**).

Polycystic ovarian syndrome (PCOS)

Hirsutism and acne, the cutaneous manifestations of hyperandrogenism, are prominent in the definitions and presentations of PCOS, which is very common in both types of diabetes, though the underlying mechanisms are different. The other components are chronic anovulation and appearance of polycystic ovaries on ultrasound. In Type 2 diabetes, hyperinsulinaemia/insulin resistance leads to gonadotrophic stimulation of both ovarian and adrenal steroidogenesis. Acanthosis nigricans is associated with, but not part of the definition of PCOS. The most severe manifestation of insulin resistance in the skin is hidradenitis suppurativa, a chronic, painful and disfiguring chronic inflammatory skin disease, characterized by recurrent nodules and abscesses in the axillae, groin and perineum. It is probably underdiagnosed and is difficult to treat, but requires specialist dermatological care. There is an isolated case report of improvement after liraglutide treatment leading to weight loss (Jennings *et al.*, 2016).

Practice point

Polycystic ovarian syndrome, probably caused by hyperinsulinaemia and insulin resistance, is common in both Type 1 and Type 2 diabetes. Metformin is of variable benefit.

PCOS, according to the definition used, is present in 20–40% of Type 1 women, compared with 5–10% in the background population. Hirsutism is present in about 30%. Supraphysiological systemic hyperinsulinaemia is assumed to be the underlying reason, hence the increased risk of PCOS in patients intensively treated with insulin and those taking high insulin doses. This is confirmed by the finding of a similar phenotype in Type 1 women age- and body mass index-matched with non-diabetic individuals. PCOS is strongly associated with the cluster of metabolic syndrome features that carry a high cardiovascular risk, so all patients with PCOS must be assessed for hypertension and dyslipidaemia. Metformin is widely used to treat PCOS and its associated anovulation and infertility in both Type 1 and 2 diabetes, with variable benefit on the individual phenotypic characteristics. As in Type 2 diabetes, there is no convincing evidence that it reduces cardiovascular events. It is safe in women of child-bearing age, but in non-obese subjects can cause mild hypoglycaemia; advise a mid-morning snack in the early stages of treatment.

References

Ahn CS, Yosipovitch G, Huang WW. Diabetes and the skin, in: Callen J, Jorizzo JL, Zone JJ et al. (eds), *Dermatological Signs of Clinical Disease*. Elsevier, 2016, pp.205–14.

Batty GD, Li Q, Czernichow S et al.; ADVANCE Collaborative Group. Erectile dysfunction and later cardiovascular disease in men with type 2 diabetes: prospective cohort study based on the ADVANCE (Action in Diabetes and Vascular Disease: Preterax and Diamicron Modified-Release Controlled Evaluation) trial. *J Am Coll Cardiol* 2010;56:1908–13 [PMID: 21109113] PMC4170755.

Boulton AJ, Armstrong DG, Albert SF et al. Comprehensive foot examination and risk assessment: a report of the task force of the foot care interest group of the American Diabetes Association, with endorsement by the American Association of Clinical Endocrinologists. Diabetes Care 2008;31:1679–85 [PMID: 18663232] Free full text.

Callaghan BC, Xia R, Reynolds R et al. Association between metabolic syndrome components and polyneuropathy in an obese population. JAMA Neurol 2016;73:1468–76 [PMID: 27802497].

Camilleri M. Diabetic gastroparesis. N Engl J Med 2007;356:820–9 [PMID: 17314341].

Chen T, Song D, Shan G et al. The association between diabetes mellitus and nonarteritic anterior ischemic optic neuropathy: a systematic review and meta-analysis. PLoS One 2013;8:e76653 [PMID: 24098798] PMC3786911.

Dede AD, Tournis S, Dontas I, Trovas G. Type 2 diabetes mellitus and fracture risk. Metabolism 2014;63:1480–90 [PMID: 25284729].

Dorresteijn JA, Kriegsman DM, Assendelft WJ, Valk GP. Patient education for preventing diabetic foot ulceration. Cochrane Database Syst Rev 2014;12:CD001488 [PMID: 25514250].

Ewing DJ, Martyn CN, Young RJ, Clarke BF. The value of cardiovascular autonomic function tests: 10 years experience in diabetes. Diabetes Care 1985;8:391–8 [PMID: 4053936].

Finnerup NB, Attal N, Haroutounian S et al. Pharmacotherapy for neuropathic pain in adults: a systematic review and meta-analysis. Lancet Neurol 2015 14:162–73 [PMID: 25575710] PMC4493167.

Fraser DA, Diep LM, Hovden IA et al. The effects of long-term oral benfotiamine supplementation on peripheral nerve function and inflammatory markers in patients with type 1 diabetes: a 24-month, double-blind, randomized, placebo-controlled study. Diabetes Care 2012;35:1095–7 [PMID: 224466172] PMC3329837.

Freeman R. Not all neuropathy in diabetes is of diabetic etiology: differential diagnosis of diabetic neuropathy. Curr Diab Rep 2009;9:422–31 [PMID: 19954686].

Gibbons CH, Freeman R. Treatment-induced neuropathy of diabetes: an acute, iatrogenic complication of diabetes. Brain 2015; 138(Pt 1):43–52 [PMID: 25392197] PMC4285188.

Hackett G, Cole N, Saghir A et al. Testosterone undecanoate improves sexual function in men with type 2 diabetes and severe hypogonadism: results from a 30-week randomized placebo-controlled study. BJU Int 2016;118:804–13 [PMID: 27124889].

Hammer E, Lilienthal E, Hofer SE et al.; DPV Initiative and the German BMBF Competence Network for Diabetes Mellitus. Risk factors for necrobiosis lipoidica in Type 1 diabetes mellitus. Diabet Med 2017;34:86–92 [PMID: 27101431].

Hirschfeld G, von Glischinski M, Knop C et al. Difficulties in screening for peripheral neuropathies in children with diabetes. Diabet Med 2015;32:786–9 [PMID: 25640325].

Hothersall EJ, Livingstone SJ, Looker HC et al. Contemporary risk of hip fracture in type 1 and type 2 diabetes: a national registry study from Scotland. J Bone Miner Res 2014;29:1054–60 [PMID: 24155126] PMC4255308.

Javed S, Petropoulos IN, Alam U, Malik RA. Treatment of painful diabetic neuropathy. Ther Adv Chronic Dis 2015;6:15–28 [PMID: 25553239] PMC4269610.

Jennings L, Nestor L, Molloy O et al. The treatment of hidradenitis suppurativa with the glucagon-like peptide-1 agonist liraglutide. Br J Dermatol 2016 [PMID: 27943236] Epub ahead of print.

Joseph JI, Hipszer B, Mraovic B et al. Clinical need for continuous glucose monitoring in the hospital. J Diabetes Sci Technol 2009;3:1309–18 [PMID: 20144385] PMC2787031.

Khalil N, Nicotra A, Rakowicz W. Treatment for meralgia paraesthetica. Cochrane Database Syst Rev 2012;12:CD004159 [PMID: 23235604].

Larkin ME, Bernie A, Braffett BH et al.; Diabetes Control and Complications Trial/Epidemiology of Diabetes Interventions and Complications Research Group. Musculoskeletal complications in type 1 diabetes. Diabetes Care 2014;37:1863–9 [PMID: 24722493] PMC4067398.

Levy D. The Hands-on Guide to Diabetes Care in Hospital, John Wiley & Sons Ltd, Chichester, 2016.

Low PA, Tomalia VA. Orthostatic hypotension: mechanisms, causes, management J Clin Neurol 2015;11:220–6 [PMID: 26174684] PMC4507375.

McGrane S, Atria N, Barwise JA. Perioperative implications of the patient with autonomic dysfunction. Curr Opin Anesthesiol 2014;27:365–70 [PMID: 24722004].

Meier C, Schwartz AV, Egger A, Lecka-Czernik B. Effects of diabetes drugs on the skeleton. Bone 2016;82:93–100 [PMID: 25913633].

Monami M, Zannoni S, Gaias M et al. Effects of a short educational program for the prevention of foot ulcers in high-risk patients: a randomized controlled trial. *Int J Endocrinol* 2015 [PMID: 26448748] PMC4581554.

Otto DE, Wang X, Tijerina SL et al. A comparison of blood pressure, body mass index, and acanthosis nigricans in school-age children. *J Sch Nurs* 2010;26:223–9 [PMID: 20335230].

Pop-Busui R, Evans GW, Gerstein HC et al. Effects of cardiac autonomic dysfunction on mortality risk in the Action to Control Cardiovascular Risk in Diabetes (ACCORD) Trial. *Diabetes Care* 2010;33:1578–84 [PMID: 20215456] PMC2390862.

Pop-Busui R, Braffett BH, Zinman B et al.; DCCT/EDIC Research Group. Cardiovascular autonomic neuropathy and cardiovascular outcomes in the Diabetes Control and Complications Trial/Epidemiology of Diabetes Interventions and Complications (DCCT/EDIC) Study. *Diabetes Care* 2017;40:94–100 [PMID: 2780312] PMC5180458.

Rayman G, Vas PR, Baker N et al. The Ipswich Touch Test: a simple and novel method to identify inpatients with diabetes at risk of foot ulceration. *Diabetes Care* 2011;34:1517–8 [PMID: 21593300] PMC3120164.

Rota E, Morelli N. Entrapment neuropathies in diabetes mellitus. *World J Diabetes* 2016;7:342–53 [PMID: 27660694] PMC5027001.

Sarosjek I, Davis B, Eichler E, McCallum RW. Surgical approaches to treatment of gastroparesis: gastric electrical stimulation, pyloroplasty, total gastrectomy and enteral feeding tubes. *Gastroenterol Clin North Am* 2015;44:151–67 [PMID: 25667030].

Shivaprasad C, Pulikkal A, Kumar KM. Pancreatic exocrine insufficiency in type 1 and type 2 diabetics of Indian origin. *Pancreatology* 2015;15:616–9 [PMID: 26549275].

Singh R, Gamble G, Cundy T. Lifetime risk of symptomatic carpal tunnel syndrome in type 1 diabetes. *Diabet Med* 2005;22:625–30 [PMID: 15842519].

Smith LL, Burnet SP, McNeil JD. Musculoskeletal manifestations of diabetes mellitus. *Br J Sports Med* 2003;37:30–5 [PMID: 12547740] PMC 1724591.

Steel JM, Young RJ, Lloyd GG, Clarke BF. Clinically apparent eating disorders in young diabetic women: associations with painful neuropathy and other complications. *Br Med J (Clin Res Ed)* 1987;294:859–62 [PMID: 3105777] PMC1245924.

Tesfaye S, Wilhelm S, Lledo A et al. Duloxetine and pregabalin: high-dose monotherapy or their combination? The "COMBO-DN study" – a multinational randomized, double-blind, parallel-group study in patients with peripheral neuropathic pain. *Pain* 2013;154:2616–25 [PMID: 23732189] Free full text.

Wilker SC, Rucker JC, Newman NJ et al. Pain in ischaemic ocular motor cranial nerve palsies. *Br J Ophthalmol* 2009;93:1657–9 [PMID: 19570771] PMC2998753.

Wing RR, Rosen RC, Fava JL et al. Effects of weight loss intervention on erectile function in older men with type 2 diabetes in the Look AHEAD trial. *J Sex Med* 2010: 7(1 Pt 1);156–65 [PMID: 19694925] PMC4461030.

Ziegler D, Low PA, Freeman R et al. Predictors of improvement and progression of diabetic polyneuropathy following treatment with α-lipoic acid for 4 years in the NATHAN 1 trial. *J Diabetes Complications* 2016;30:350–6 [PMID: 26651260].

Zimmerman M, Dahlin E, Thomsen NO et al. Oucome after carpal tunnel release: impact of factors related to metabolic syndrome. *J Plast Surg Hand Surg* 2017; 51(3):165–71 [PMID: 27467092].

Zriek NH, Malik RA, Charalambous CP. Adhesive capsulitis of the shoulder and diabetes: a meta-analysis of prevalence. *Muscles Ligaments Tendons J* 2016;6:26–34 [PMID: 27331029] PMC4915459.

6 Diabetes and the cardiovascular system

Key points

- In Type 2 diabetes cardiovascular events have decreased because of widespread comprehensive secondary prevention and improved interventional techniques, but they still pose a major threat to all people with diabetes
- The historical very high rates of ischaemic heart disease in South Asian people in the United Kingdom may have dramatically improved in the past twenty years
- Premenopausal protection against macrovascular events is eradicated in diabetic women
- There is a high risk of premature coronary disease in longstanding Type 1 diabetes patients in their 40s, especially females
- Patients may have attenuated or atypical symptoms of cardiac ischaemia, but they should be investigated vigorously
- Screening asymptomatic Type 2 patients, for example with myocardial perfusion scans, is not of proven value
- Patients with multivessel coronary artery disease should be offered bypass surgery; they are likely to do less well with multiple stents
- Vigorous control of risk factors reduces mortality and events in secondary prevention patients; target smoking in particular

INTRODUCTION

Back in 1996, Miles Fisher made the prescient statement that '[Type 2] diabetes is a state of premature cardiovascular death, which is associated with chronic hyperglycaemia and may also be associated with blindness and renal failure' (Fisher, 2009). He was making a powerful point. The emphasis on blood glucose levels and concern with the microvascular complications of Type 2 diabetes had obscured the terrible toll of cardiac and cerebrovascular disease at the time. In the succeeding 20 years emphases have changed: blindness is mercifully much less common and, in some countries, the burden of end-stage renal disease in Type 2 diabetes may have passed its peak (very definitely so in many advanced countries in people with Type 1 diabetes; see **Chapter 4**). Devastating extensive transmural myocardial infarctions are also much less common and stroke incidence has also steadily fallen. Thrombolysis in acute myocardial infarction has been succeeded by immediate invasive management; stent technology has changed, and the skill of cardiologists in placing them has improved impressively (though perhaps with the unintended consequence of reducing coronary artery bypass grafting (CABG) in some people who would benefit from surgery rather than multiple stent placement); and secondary prevention is a world away from the 1990s, when statins were exciting new

Practical Diabetes Care, Fourth Edition. David Levy.
© 2018 John Wiley & Sons Ltd. Published 2018 by John Wiley & Sons Ltd.

drugs and experts were still arguing with earnest seriousness over apparently contradictory evidence on the association between LDL cholesterol and coronary heart disease, and the benefits of reducing it.

In Type 1 diabetes, patients' fears about end-stage renal disease, blindness and amputations can more easily be assuaged, but macrovascular disease continues to emerge as a significant risk to younger people in their 40s and 50s, that is, usually about 30–40 years after developing diabetes. Identifying at-risk patients in both Type 1 and Type 2 diabetes has been relatively unsuccessful, though certainly not through lack of trying, nor indeed of good clinical trial data.

Yet, although in the most optimistic studies cardiovascular events and mortality in Type 2 diabetes are tantalisingly close to those of non-diabetic people, the excess of events in most studies is still substantial. The nature of those events, though, has changed and there is growing awareness that the decrease in acute coronary syndromes is being replaced with a more insidious increase in less acute and headline-grabbing outcomes such as chronic heart failure.

Practice point

Acute coronary syndromes have become less frequent in Type 2 patients but there is still an increased risk compared with non-diabetic people. Macroalbuminuria remains the most powerful risk factor.

In this chapter, although heart disease will be emphasized, the data and clinical approaches to cerebrovascular and peripheral vascular disease will also be discussed.

TYPE 1 DIABETES

Macrovascular disease in Type 1 diabetes has not only been neglected, but is still considered to be no different from that of Type 2 diabetes. Two factors have been responsible: first, it was underrepresented in the young cohort (average age 27 years) recruited into the Diabetes Control and Complications Trial (DCCT), for many years the only prospective study of Type 1 diabetes; second, it was also considered to be mostly linked to the very high morbidity associated with advanced diabetic kidney disease (see **Chapter 4**). However, while diabetic nephropathy has fallen over time, coronary artery disease in Type 1 patients has not. More up to date and representative cohort studies have elaborated these important points. For example, the long-term Pittsburgh Epidemiology of Diabetes Complications study found that in Type 1 patients coronary atherosclerosis was markedly accelerated, by some 10–15 years in males compared with an age-matched non-diabetic group (Orchard and Costacou, 2010). The factors accounting for this are not clear but analysis of the DCCT cohort after 27 years follow-up confirm the powerful effect of HbA$_{1c}$ (1% increase was associated with a 30–40% increased risk of macrovascular events), with less important factors including blood pressure, lipids and non-use of ACE inhibitors also contributing (DCCT/EDIC, 2016). The 30-year DCCT follow-up confirmed many other studies that macroalbuminuria constitutes a very powerful risk factor for adverse cardiovascular outcomes (approximately 50-fold increase) and that microalbuminuria carries a weaker but still significant approximately twofold increased risk, but against expectation found that there was no reduction in this risk if microalbuminuria resolved, casting further doubt on the primacy of ACE inhibitor treatment in microalbuminuric Type 1 patients (de Boer et al., 2016).

Although the DCCT did not find gender a risk factor, most studies have found that females are particularly at risk, even when they are premenopausal, usually a strongly protective factor in non-diabetic women. The reasons for this striking difference are not really known. One view is that female fat distribution is associated with increased insulin resistance in Type 1 patients, which, in turn, is linked to the increased coronary artery calcification found in women. However, setting aside these interesting mechanistic speculations, clinicians should be persistently alert for the presence of clinical coronary artery disease in Type 1 patients in their 30s and 40s, recognizing that even in the contemporary Pittsburgh study, the median age of those having a first cardiovascular event was just under 40 years.

> **Practice point**
>
> Premature coronary artery disease is common in Type 1 patients in their 40s, especially in females. Symptoms may be vague, transient and non-specific.

Early functional and structural changes in large vessels in Type 1 patients

A raft of changes is described in people with less than five years of Type 1 diabetes. Structural abnormalities found after even this short duration include increased arterial stiffness and carotid intima-media thickness; functional abnormalities loosely related to the structural abnormalities include impaired flow-mediated vasodilatation. Inflammatory markers (perhaps also mediators) such as high-sensitivity C-reactive protein (hsCRP) are increased, albeit only slightly, and factors reflecting an increased thrombotic tendency, for example PAI-1, also rise. Finally, there is great interest in the reduction in endothelial progenitor cells seen in Type 1 diabetes, where levels are maintained in the ultra-long Type 1 survivors of the Joslin Medalist cohort compared with age-matched controls (see **Chapter 14**) (Hernandez et al., 2014), perhaps explaining some of their resistance to cardiovascular events. Poor vitamin C status may be a nutritional contribution. Fascinating though these early changes are, no prospective studies have enlightened us on their specific role or, more importantly, of any useful intervention. We are left with active glycaemic control to the DCCT-recommended levels, which will at least help optimize certain factors, especially increased carotid intima-media thickness, which in the DCCT was strongly associated with increased atherothrombotic risk. Most important, traditional risk factors – hypertension, smoking and dyslipidaemia – operate in this group as in everyone else.

Later changes

Autonomic neuropathy

Autonomic neuropathy contributes to abnormal heart rate variation and blood pressure responses and, in turn, may be associated with coronary ischaemia. The traditional view is that there is impaired perception of ischaemic pain, again through autonomic neuropathy, which may contribute to the late presentation of patients with definite coronary events. Proteinuria is associated with an exaggerated inflammatory response that impairs endothelial function broadly in line with its severity.

Coronary calcification

Coronary calcification in the arterial intima is different from the medial calcification easily visible on plain radiography of the lower legs and feet, but is simple to quantify on CT scan. Its quantity (volume) is broadly associated with cardiovascular risk and in the long-term EDIC follow up of the DCCT patients, at an average age of 42 years and duration 21 years, those in the original tight glycaemia group had a lower prevalence of any coronary calcification than the conventional group (Cleary *et al.*, 2006). Frustratingly for clinical implementation of this investigation, which can now be carried out at low radiation exposure, there are still no studies of cardiovascular events in diabetic patients in relation to baseline coronary calcification.

Prevalence of coronary artery disease in Type 1 diabetes

By the time patients, still only in their 40s, reach 30 years or thereabouts of Type 1 diabetes, many will have significant coronary disease but, as in Type 2, symptoms are uncommon, and even when present can be diffuse, non-specific and misleading, both to patients and professionals, and the results of simple non-invasive tests, for example routine exercise stress testing, often unhelpful. In Norwegian subjects with long-duration diabetes (mean 30 years, age 40) one-third had a 50% stenosis in one or more main coronary arteries and one in ten patients (3 of 29) had asymptomatic triple vessel disease. Although about one-third were smokers, long-term mean HbA_{1c} was fairly good at 8.2% (66) (Larsen *et al.*, 2002). Another study in patients of similar long duration without diabetic kidney disease planned for islet-cell transplantation uncovered significant stenosis of at least one coronary artery in nearly 50% (Senior *et al.*, 2005). In the presence of proteinuric diabetic kidney disease, the prevalence is much higher.

Practice point

Clinically silent coronary artery disease is common in Type 1 patients in their 40s, even in the absence of conventional cardiovascular risk factors.

Risk prediction in Type 1 diabetes (Box 6.1)

Predicting risk in a Type 1 individual is difficult and most risk prediction models are not helpful. Not surprisingly, the United Kingdom Prospective Diabetes Study (UKPDS) Risk Engine underestimated risk in the Pittsburgh Type 1 cohort (it has not been updated since 1997, is valid only in people between 25 and 65, and included only tiny numbers

---

Box 6.1 Identifying CAD in Type 1 diabetes.

High-risk clinical situations
- Diabetic nephropathy, renal replacement therapy.
- Established cardiac autonomic neuropathy.
- Patients for renal and/or pancreatic transplantation.
- Patients with advanced retinopathy.

Clinical factors
- Long duration, e.g. >20–30 years, even in the absence of microvascular complications.
- Female gender, obesity, increased waist–hip ratio.
- Smoking.
- Multiple insulin-resistance characteristics.
- Symptoms, especially atypical ones, for example chest discomfort, new-onset shortness of breath, reduced exercise tolerance, fatigue (heart failure).

of ethnic minority people). The Framingham risk score, still recommended by some, did not include any Type 1 subjects. The UK-based QRISK2 is preferable, as it included around 5000 Type 1 patients in its validation cohort. It underestimates risk in some females but is reliable in males with any risk profile. It is probably the best current screening tool, though the Steno Type 1 Risk Engine, which in addition takes into account glycaemic control, eGFR and albuminuria, may be an important development once it is user-friendly (Vistisen *et al.*, 2016). These simple scoring systems may be preferable even to advanced imaging techniques, such as computed tomographic angiography (CTA), the use of which in high-risk individuals did not reduce cardiac outcomes in either Type 1 or 2 patients up to four years after appropriate intensive intervention (Muhlestein *et al.*, 2014). While the elective 12-lead ECG is now widely regarded as obsolete and is certainly insensitive (for example, it was abnormal in only 3% of the Pittsburgh cohort), it is relatively specific. However, because of its low-tech reputation it is infrequently requested – and routine ECGs, at least in the hospital setting, may not be as readily available as before.

Practice point

QRISK2 (UK) is probably currently the most reliable risk predictor for people with Type 1 diabetes (www.qrisk.org).

Practice point

The 12-lead ECG is still a valuable investigation in both Type 1 and Type 2 diabetes, though a normal tracing does not exclude significant coronary artery disease.

Management

Patients identified with multivessel disease should be offered coronary bypass grafting: mortality and risk of myocardial infarction up to three years are significantly lower. Multiple stents, while always tempting, are associated with a high rate of re-intervention and increased major cardiac and cerebrovascular events up to 3–5 years.

The outcomes of CABG in Type 2 diabetes now approach those of non-diabetic people, but they are significantly worse in Type 1 patients. The differences are substantial and clinically meaningful. For example, compared with a 10-year mortality of 20% in Type 2 and non-diabetic subjects, there is a two- to threefold increased mortality rate in Type 1 diabetes (Holtzman *et al.*, 2015). Poor pre-operative glycaemic control is a significant factor. The 5-year risk of death or major cardiovascular events after CABG increased by 18% (confidence interval 6–32%) for each 1% increase in preoperative HbA_{1c}; at a value of 8–9% (64–75) the risk increased by nearly three-quarters (Nyström *et al.*, 2015). This striking relationship is not seen in Type 2 patients. One technical factor contributing to poor outcomes in Type 1 diabetes may be the extent of medial coronary calcification. This is a common finding and it is tempting to regard it as characteristic of coronary artery disease in Type 1 diabetes, but there are no systematic studies of this potentially important feature. In practice, however, extensive calcification can prevent surgeons forming proximal anastomoses, resulting in distal grafting with less complete revascularization.

Peripheral vascular disease and stroke

Peripheral vascular disease

Even at the end of long-term projects, such as EDIC and Pittsburgh, participants are still relatively young people with a low incidence of new vascular disease. Most clinicians now mostly encounter peripheral vascular disease in Type 1 patients with advanced diabetic kidney disease. Although at this stage, glycaemia is probably only a minor factor, in the long term it is important. For example, in the DCCT, intensive treatment reduced peripheral vascular calcification but not occlusion (Carter *et al.*, 2007). As in coronary artery disease, it is assumed that the natural history of early peripheral vascular disease and its distribution in the arterial tree are the same as in Type 2 diabetes, but this does not seem to be the case. In Type 2 diabetes, arterial disease is concentrated in the infrapopliteal (trifurcation) region below the knee. In Type 1 diabetes proximal lesions with associated heavy calcification may occur even in lifelong non-smokers. Like coronary artery disease, it seems to occur after 30 or more years of diabetes. Some degree of sensory neuropathy is common at this stage, even in people with good long-term glycaemia, and this may delay presentation with symptoms. Interventional radiology techniques continue to improve, and proximal lesions are often successfully treated with transluminal angioplasty and stents.

Stroke

Stroke is also a rather neglected area, though cerebral infarction is about twice as common in Type 1 compared with Type 2 diabetes, at least in women (Janghorbani *et al.*, 2007). Cerebral haemorrhage is probably also more common. The gender distribution of stroke is changing over time. It was much commoner in females diagnosed between the 1970s and early 1990s, but in the more recent FinnDiane study 60% of cerebral infarction and haemorrhage patients were male. There is a strikingly high risk of stroke in younger Type 1 patients under 50, not surprisingly in those with established renal disease, but less obviously in non-nephropathic subjects with laser-treated retinopathy. Lacunar infarcts, possibly a microvascular complication, are also commoner in Type 1 diabetes (Hägg *et al.*, 2013). The key message is always to bear in mind the risk of large vessel disease in Type 1 diabetes, even in those who are not very old and are free of established renal disease, but who may – even at some remote time – have had laser-treated retinopathy. Viewing the retinal vasculature is well-known to be the only direct non-invasive way of viewing blood vessels, but it may also be a wider window into the state of the whole vasculature in people with both Type 1 and Type 2 diabetes; meta-analysis confirms three- to fourfold increased all-cause and cardiovascular risk in patients with any degree of retinopathy (Kramer *et al.*, 2011).

> **Practice point**
>
> Always be alert to non-typical symptoms of macrovascular disease in Type 1 patients – minor chest symptoms, unilateral lower limb discomfort and transient cerebral ischaemia.

TYPE 2 DIABETES

The clinical impression that fewer patients now have acute coronary syndromes compared with the past is based on fact. Over the period 1990–2010 acute myocardial infarction rates in diabetic patients in the USA have shown a dramatic and progressive fall

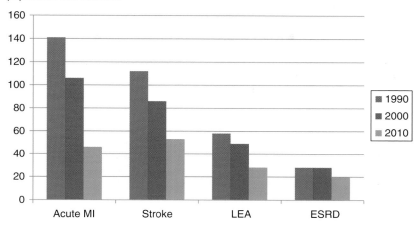

Events per 10 000 adult population with diabetes

Figure 6.1 Changes in the risks of major diabetes complications in Type 2 patients in the USA. *Source*: Gregg *et al.*, 2014. Reproduced with permission of Massachusetts Medical Society.

(Gregg *et al.*, 2014) (**Figure 6.1**). These changes have been much more marked in diabetic patients than in the general population and are especially notable in people aged 75 or over. Furthermore, myocardial infarction rates narrowed between males and females. A large study in the Netherlands found that in a white population first myocardial infarctions present at an older age in people with diabetes compared with non-diabetic individuals; prior vigorous LDL reduction (mean 2.5 mmol/l compared with 3.4 mmol/l) was a significant explanatory factor (Kasteleyn *et al.*, 2016). Non-ST elevation outnumber ST elevation myocardial infarctions.

Practice point

There have been dramatic reductions in myocardial infarction rates in Type 2 diabetes. Probably as a result of vigorous lipid lowering, non-diabetic people have an initial cardiac event at a younger age than people with Type 2 diabetes.

A similar pattern, though less dramatic, was seen in both amputation and stroke (**Figure 6.1**). A combination of improved interventional techniques, reducing the risk of further events, and widespread implementation of primary and secondary prevention are probably responsible. It is critically important to convey this information to individuals concerned about complication risks, because the rise in diabetes cases overall (the frequently-cited 'diabetes epidemic') has obscured the reduction in risk in the individual.

Coronary artery disease

About ten years ago, it was fashionable to quote the 'coronary equivalent' thesis of Type 2 diabetes: the risk of acute myocardial infarction in someone with diabetes was thought to be similar to that of a non-diabetic individual who had already suffered a myocardial infarction. It is clear from more recent studies that this is no longer generally the case and in the general diabetes population the risk may be only about one-half of that of people with coronary heart disease. However, the risk equivalence story seems still to hold good for people with more than 10 years of diagnosed Type 2 diabetes (Rana *et al.*, 2016). People with Type 2 diabetes nevertheless still run significantly increased risks of vascular disease compared with the background population. A major meta-analysis (Emerging Risk Factors Collaboration, 2010) found a twofold increase for myocardial infarction in diabetes, slightly lower for stroke (and non-significant for haemorrhagic stroke), but only studies up to 2010 were included, some were very old and few ethnic minority subjects were included.

Practice point

Type 2 patients have a generally lower risk of heart attack than non-diabetic patients with a previous event, especially those with under 10 years of diagnosed diabetes. The concept of the 'coronary equivalence' of Type 2 diabetes is no longer generally valid.

Ethnicity

Ethnic minority groups with diabetes, especially South Asians, who contribute around 4% of the UK population, were found many years ago to have considerable excess vascular disease, especially coronary artery disease. The 11-year follow-up of the original Southall Study confirmed the poor vascular outlook: diabetes conferred a twofold increased risk of cardiovascular death compared with European people. In the same population followed up after another decade, the excess burden of cardiovascular mortality in diabetes became startlingly clear. Nearly half of coronary deaths in South Asians occurred in people with diabetes, compared with 13% in the European population (Forouhi *et al.*, 2008). In spite of extensive epidemiological study, there is no convincing explanation for this dramatic excess incidence and mortality. Lower activity levels and differences in diet remain popular – but unconfirmed – explanations. For example, clarified butter, ghee, much less used now, is still widely blamed, as is low fruit and vegetable intake, though it is most unlikely that these components on their own could account for such a high risk. When objectively measured South Asians have the same activity levels as white participants, though they markedly underestimate the levels compared with white subjects (Yates *et al.*, 2015).

There is still concern that South Asians and Africans/African-Caribbeans continue to be at a cardiovascular disadvantage compared with white UK people with diabetes, as there is evidence from local studies that both ethnicities are less likely to meet targets for glycaemia, blood pressure and total cholesterol. However, a large study from England is broadly reassuring. Younger South Asians with diabetes lost considerably fewer years of life than white subjects and, strikingly, Asians over 65 with diabetes had a longer life expectancy than those without diabetes (their reduced mortality applied to cardiovascular disease, but also cancer and respiratory disorders). There were similar findings in blacks with diabetes. This study confirms remarkable improvements in primary care over the years in ethnic minority people in England (Wright *et al.*, 2017).

In diagnostic categories, congestive heart failure may be more common in South Asians. Stroke is less commonly due to major vessel disease than haemorrhage or lacunar infarction, even though hypertension is overall no more frequent than in the background population. Peripheral vascular disease is much less common.

Practice point

South Asian people with diabetes have historically had a markedly increased risk of coronary heart disease, but the outlook in the UK seems to have improved dramatically.

Symptoms

Silent coronary ischaemia: identification and management

The primary symptom of coronary ischaemia, exertional chest pain, is often attenuated, blunted or absent in diabetic people even with severe obstructive coronary disease. The supposed reasons for this frequent clinical observation (autonomic neuropathy and the presence of diffuse distal multivessel coronary disease without typical localised typical proximal stenosis) have surprisingly limited evidence to support them. Studies have mostly focused on identifying significant asymptomatic coronary disease in people with diabetes and, more importantly and difficult, conducting randomized therapeutic trials to evaluate outcomes in people with such 'silent' ischaemia. The striking and almost certainly continuing decrease in acute coronary syndromes in people with diabetes adds a historical difficulty, the lack of agreement on optimum detection techniques a host of others.

Silent myocardial infarction is common in the general population, more so in diabetes, and myocardial perfusion scanning (SPECT) detected it in over one-third of people with diabetes in a large validation study, compared with one-quarter of non-diabetic people (Arenja et al., 2013). On average, around 10% of the left ventricle was involved and left ventricular ejection fraction significantly reduced in those with silent infarctions (47% compared with 60%).

Given the high prevalence, is routine screening of this large asymptomatic population justified? Two studies came to different conclusions. In the DIAD study (Young et al., 2009), Type 2 patients were randomized to either a screening myocardial perfusion scan or no scan. Subsequent management decisions were left to physicians and patients. At five-years follow-up, the overall cardiac event rate was very low at 0.6% (again certainly not supporting the 'coronary equivalent' thesis) and myocardial infarction, cardiac death and coronary revascularization were no different in the two groups, despite intensification of medical prevention treatment in both groups. The investigators concluded that routine screening with myocardial perfusion scanning was not of value.

In contrast, the BARDOT study of asymptomatic patients recruited older people than DIAD, with diabetes of longer duration; nearly all had more than one definite micro- or macrovascular complication (Zellweger et al., 2014). All patients had myocardial perfusion scans at baseline and two years, and those with abnormal scans had medical or medical/invasive management in a small randomized treatment arm of the trial. Patients with abnormal scans had more ischaemia or evidence of new scarring at the two-year follow-up, though there was no difference in the small number of events.

Taking the results of these trials together, it seems worthwhile considering myocardial perfusion scan in patients with long duration Type 2 diabetes (e.g. 13 years or longer) who have evidence of other complications, though it is still not clear whether invasive action following a positive scan reduces long-term cardiac outcomes.

Practice point

Routine screening for asymptomatic coronary disease in diabetes is of unproven value, but discuss it in people with longstanding diabetes who have established microvascular complications.

ACUTE MYOCARDIAL INFARCTION

Abnormalities of glucose tolerance

Data on the prevalence of various degrees of glucose intolerance in acute cardiac patients require cautious interpretation because of selection criteria and changes in criteria for assessing glucose intolerance and diabetes, but all studies show that a high proportion of patients with acute myocardial infarction or stroke have abnormal glucose levels. The situation is complicated by the temporary hyperglycaemia induced by acute illness itself (so-called 'stress hyperglycaemia') that then remits spontaneously after the acute event. A widely-quoted study in the early 2000s from Scandinavia (Norhammer *et al.*, 2002) found that results of glucose tolerance tests performed on admission and three months later were broadly similar, that is 50% had normal glucose tolerance, 20% diabetes and 30% impaired glucose tolerance. Admission random glucose levels, average 6.1 mmol/l, were unremarkable and the mean HbA_{1c} at 5.0% (31) was strictly normal. In an ethnically mixed population in the United Kingdom, comprising 30% South Asians, mean admission glucose levels were higher (6.9 mmol/l) but still nowhere near levels diagnostic of diabetes (11.1 mmol/l or higher).

> **Practice point**
>
> Around 20% of patients with ST-segment acute coronary syndromes will have 'stress hyperglycaemia' that will settle to normal levels within three months of the event.

In a more recent study in patients with ST-segment elevation myocardial infarction the prevalence of any degree of glucose intolerance (impaired fasting glucose, impaired glucose tolerance and diabetes) fell from around 50% when inpatients to 25% at three months after the event (Knudsen *et al.*, 2009). An admission HbA_{1c} >5.7% (39) carried a fourfold increased risk of abnormal glucose levels at follow-up and admission glucose >7.7 mmol/l at least a twofold increased risk. The prevalence of 'stress hyperglycaemia' was around 20% in this study. Indicative values are shown in **Box 6.2**.

Management of hyperglycaemia in patients with acute coronary syndromes

The acute management of hyperglycaemia is the same for all patients but, importantly, the era of ultra-tight glucose management should be considered over. It was heralded decades ago by the mechanistic demonstration of increased efficiency of myocardial

---

Box 6.2 Diagnosing abnormal glucose levels in ACS patients.

Diagnosis of diabetes

Fasting glucose	≥11.1 mmol/l
HbA_{1c}	≥6.5% (48 mmol/mol)

High risk for subsequent abnormal glucose levels

Random glucose	>7.7 mmol/l
HbA_{1c}	>5.7% (39 mmol/mol)

Source: Modified after Knudsen *et al.*, 2009.

energy metabolism of glucose compared with fatty acids, a process improved by glucose/insulin/potassium (GIK). The key clinical study was the now old DIGAMI study published in 1997 when thrombolysis was the immediate treatment for myocardial infarction and there is still lingering hope that normoglycaemia in acute coronary syndromes might improve outcomes; it did so in a limited sense in DIGAMI, in which coronary death, but critically not recurrent myocardial infarction, was reduced at one year in patients treated acutely with intravenous glucose in a GIK combination, followed by subcutaneous basal-bolus insulin (Malmberg, 1997). While there is no modern-era trial of stringent glucose control, other studies have raised sufficient concerns about the risks of intensive glucose control that the widely-accepted target for blood glucose control in all inpatients, that is 7–10 mmol/l, is appropriate for cardiac patients, itself quite a challenge in acute clinical practice.

DIGAMI's successor study, DIGAMI 2, attempted to separate the roles of acute intravenous GIK treatment (relatively simple and practicable) and the much more difficult problem of starting and maintaining subcutaneous insulin therapy. Recruitment faltered and the trial was terminated without a clear answer. In a 20-year follow-up of the original DIGAMI patients, intensively insulin-treated patients had a legacy reduction in long-term mortality, again hinting at prolonged benefit of short-term glycaemic improvement, especially in patients with poor glycaemic control on admission (mean HbA_{1c} in DIGAMI was 8.2%, 66). But the entire picture of presentation, and immediate and long-term management of acute events means that two decades on, early intervention and subsequently striving for optimum multifactor intervention has outweighed the single available modifiable factor explored in DIGAMI (Bonds, 2014).

After DIGAMI, subsequent studies suggested that reasonable blood glucose control with or without insulin is a sound strategy; insulin is not mandatory, and large infusion volumes are to be avoided:

- In the acute phase, two large studies using GIK infusions in STEMI, CREATE-ECLA study and OASIS-6 GIK (both 2007), achieved only modest glucose levels (mean values 8–10 mmol/l) but found an increased risk of hyperkalaemia and of heart failure and death in the first two days, attributed to fluid overload.
- In chronic treatment, the BARI 2D study (2009) did not find an advantage in insulin-providing treatments (insulin itself or sulfonylureas) over insulin-resistance lowering treatment (metformin and glitazones).
- The small HI-5 study of insulin/dextrose for 24 hours did not reduce mortality up to six months but there was a lower risk of heart failure and reinfarction up to three months. Clinically more relevant, perhaps, is the observation that patients achieving blood glucose levels ≤8 mmol/l had a lower mortality, broadly consistent with current guidance (Cheung *et al.*, 2006).

Practices differ widely between hospitals but most advocate a variable rate intravenous insulin infusion (VRIII; previously 'sliding scale' (UK) or insulin drip (USA)) if blood glucose levels in the acute phase are consistently higher than the diagnostic level for diabetes, >11 mmol/l, with a target of 7–10 mmol/l.

Non-insulin agents

Non-insulin agents can remain unchanged if the patient is eating but discontinue the now little-used pioglitazone because of its risk of fluid retention. Metformin usually causes anxiety, but it should not, bearing in mind:

- The dose should be modified (see **Chapter 10**) if renal function deteriorates.
- Discontinue if eGFR <30 ml/min.

- Discontinue for 48 hours after angiography but reinstate so long as serum creatinine has not risen by >25%.
- Metformin is an effective drug and blood glucose levels can rise rapidly after reducing or discontinuing it. A temporary intravenous insulin infusion or improvised subcutaneous basal-bolus regimen may be needed. No other oral agents have a rapid enough action and acutely sulfonylureas carry a high risk of hypoglycaemia.
- Oher agents, for example the DPP-4 inhibitors, the injected GLP-1-receptor agonists and SGLT2 inhibitors (see **Chapter 10**) are probably safe in the post-ACS phase (but do not start these agents in the acute setting: they have a relatively slow onset of action and patients are often already being exposed to several or many new drugs, some of which, for example high-dose statins, have immediate benefits that have never been demonstrated for similar attention to blood glucose control).

Practice point

Use intravenous insulin treatment in ACS patients with blood glucose >11 mmol/l. Continue non-insulin agents but observe for renal and contrast contraindications for metformin and withdraw sulfonylureas (with careful monitoring) because of hypoglycaemia risk.

Interventional strategies

Acute coronary syndromes

Practice is moving towards early intervention in diabetic patients with non-ST-segment elevation acute coronary syndromes (NSTE-ACS). The collaborative meta-analysis of O'Donoghue *et al.* (2012) found that while early intervention did not reduce total cardiovascular events more in diabetes, recurrent myocardial infarction was reduced by around 30% compared with non-diabetic patients.

Stable coronary disease

Since the first BARI study (1996) there has been a suspicion that people with diabetes and complex coronary artery disease have a better prognosis for future events and survival after coronary bypass compared with other interventions. The FREEDOM trial (Farkouh *et al.*, 2012) endorsed this approach. Patients with two or more coronary stenoses greater than 70% but sparing the left main coronary were randomized to drug-eluting stents (three on average) or CABG, followed by high adherence to intensive medical treatment in all patients. The majority of patients (82–85%) had triple-vessel disease. Even allowing for an increase in stroke in CABG patients (most events occurred in the first 30 postoperative days), the combined absolute rate of cardiovascular events at five years was nearly 8% lower, and all-cause mortality 5.5% lower. At five years NSTEMIs were reduced by over 50% in the CABG patients.

Practice point

In patients with triple vessel disease CABG is the preferred intervention.

The COURAGE trial (Sedlis *et al.*, 2015) studied patients with a similar average age to those in the FREEDOM trial (63 years old), but with less severe coronary artery disease (only 30% had triple-vessel disease). They were randomized to intensive medical treatment with or without percutaneous intervention. In a long-term follow-up of the small number of diabetic patients, there was no difference in survival. Intensive sub-group analysis could not distinguish any groups that would gain more benefit from percutaneous intervention. Careful judgments, based on individual coronary anatomy and the overall clinical picture, are needed in disease that is less severe than triple vessel and all patients require careful follow-up. The continuing ISCHEMIA trial (results due 2019) may help some of these difficult decisions.

South Asian ethnicity carries a higher risk of multivessel coronary disease. A large UK study found that outcomes with percutaneous intervention after three years were no different from those in their Caucasian counterparts (Jones et al., 2014). While these reports reassure that case-fatality rates for interventions are now no different, South Asians were on average four years younger at the time of intervention and thereafter have higher rates of restenosis and CABG. Ultra-vigorous secondary prevention is prob-ably key in these subjects.

Secondary prevention

It cannot be overstated how important it is to successfully implement a comprehensive package of secondary prevention measures in patients who have either had an acute event or have chronic stable ischaemic heart disease. A headline estimate is that deaths deferred by secondary prevention packages are equivalent to the number of deaths averted by acute hospital treatment. However, in real life implementation of secondary prevention deviates considerably from copious best-practice advice.

Practice point

Successful secondary prevention prevents at least the same number of cardiovascular deaths as acute hospital treatment.

Lifestyle adjustments

Portfolios of substantive lifestyle changes are increasingly reported, often in popula-tions with high proportions of people with diabetes. For example, the REGARDS study (2014) in a very high-risk population in the Southern USA found that after the acute postrehabilitation phase, an intensive programme focusing on smoking cessation, phys-ical activity four or more times a week and the highest level of Mediterranean diet score reduced recurrent coronary events and mortality by about 40% over 4½ years. These are profoundly important effects, quantitatively similar to the impact of pharmacologi-cal intervention (Booth et al., 2014).

Cardiac rehabilitation

The benefits of cardiac rehabilitation in the general population are undisputed. Exercise-based rehabilitation in secondary prevention patients (myocardial infarction, coronary bypass, percutaneous intervention, angina or angiographically-defined coronary artery disease) reduces total mortality by 13% and cardiovascular mortality by about 25%, and hospital readmission by 40% (Heran et al., 2011) but recommendations are onerous. For example, in the COURAGE trial there were 30–45 minutes of moderate intensity exercise five times a week and a recommended increase in daily lifestyle activity. There is no dif-ference in outcomes between home- and group-based programmes, and individual pref-erences should be taken into account. Health-related quality of life improves equally in diabetic and non-diabetic participants; in a large one-year randomized study, intensively rehabilitated patients in Denmark had meaningful reductions in HbA_{1c} (~0.5%) and BP (8/5 mm Hg) and showed objective improvements in exercise capacity (Soja *et al.*, 2007) (**Figure 6.2**).

> **Practice point**
>
> Cardiac rehabilitation in diabetes is probably as beneficial as in non-diabetic subjects, and may have meaningful metabolic outcomes.

Smoking cessation

While we expend great efforts managing blood glucose levels after acute coronary events, until recently the same could not be said for smoking cessation. Inpatient smoking cessation counselling after acute myocardial infarction significantly reduces mortality (Van Spall *et al.*, 2007) and persistence with smoking cessation reduces recurrent coronary events and mortality by about 50% in non-diabetic subjects; though there is no comparative trial data, relative risk reductions are likely to be similar in people with diabetes, with an accordingly higher absolute risk reduction. For example, if the high-risk cardiovascular patients in the ADVANCE trial stopped smoking, there was a 30% reduction in all-cause mortality over five years (Blomster *et al.*, 2016).

Fortunately, practice has changed substantially over the past decade. In the DANSUK rehabilitation study from 2007, at one year the proportion of smokers had barely changed (from 27 to 24%; Soja *et al.*, 2007) while in more recent randomized trials smoking cessation rates at one year are much higher (see later). The benefit of smoking cessation is much greater than that of any other single secondary intervention measure.

> **Practice point**
>
> Focus smoking cessation interventions on all patients but especially in patients with diabetes, as they are at the highest cardiovascular risk.

Diet

The benefit of adhering to a full Mediterranean diet has been known for many years (see **Chapter 9**). In the Lyon heart study in the 1990s, a Mediterranean diet after myocardial infarction reduced cardiac events independently of other traditional risk factor modification. In view of the results of the REGARDS study, in which maximum adherence to the Mediterranean diet reduced the risk of recurrent coronary events and death by 15–25% (though the benefit was more marked for smoking cessation and activity and was not itself statistically significant), it is likely to be further emphasised in future (Booth *et al.*, 2014). The widespread guidance targeting weight loss of 5–10% in this situation, ultimately aiming for BMI <25 is not strongly supported by evidence and in the REGARDS study waist circumference was not associated with recurrent ischaemic events or mortality. However, out of the acute situation, a post hoc analysis of the Look AHEAD study detected meaningful mortality reductions in those who lost 10% or more body weight during the first year, but increases in fitness did not seem to have the same benefit (Look AHEAD Research Group, 2016). We await the definitive trial of intensive compared with routine multi-interventions in people who have had an acute coronary syndrome.

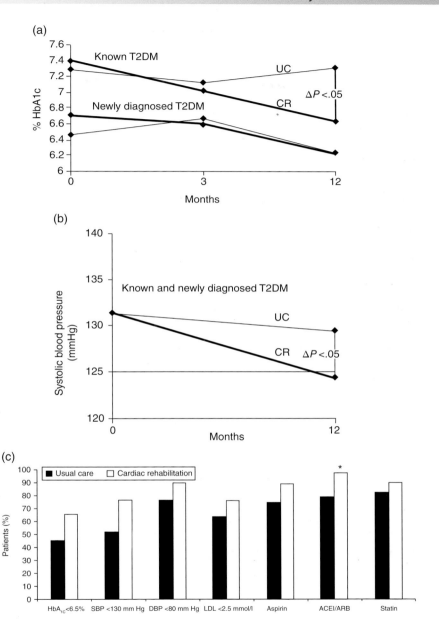

Figure 6.2 The benefit of formal cardiac rehabilitation up to one year on biomarkers in Type 2 diabetes. CR: cardiac rehabilitation; UC: usual care. In comparison with UC, glycaemia improved in both known and newly-diagnosed Type 2 patients (a), blood pressure fell (b) and prescription of secondary prevention medication and achievement of treatment goals was higher (c). *Source*: Soja *et al.*, 2007. Reproduced with permission of *American Heart Journal*.

> **Practice point**
>
> Good adherence to a Mediterranean diet, and possibly 10% or more body weight loss, can reduce postinfarction mortality.

Secondary prevention medication

The portfolio of secondary prevention medication and associated targets for intermediate outcomes is now well-established, and its prognostic benefits were confirmed in BARI 2D (**Box 6.3, Figure 6.3**). In this study, the number of risk factors at optimal levels was linearly related to risk reduction during a five-year follow-up, though there was a signal of harm in patients where systolic blood pressure was either lower (<110 mm Hg) or higher (>140 mm Hg) than the optimum defined range (see **Chapter 11**). Optimal medical therapy in recent trials comprises:

- Treatment with a statin to reduce LDL-cholesterol <2.6 mmol/l for all secondary prevention patients, and to <1.8 in people at very high risk; or use evidence-based

---

Box 6.3 Risk factor control in BARI 2D (Type 2 patients with stable, confirmed ischaemic heart disease).

Subjects: mean age 62 years, mean duration 10 years

Target levels for risk factors (maximum 6):

SBP	<130 mm Hg
DBP	<80 mm Hg

Non-smoking

HbA$_{1c}$	<7.0% (53)
Triglycerides	<1.7 mmol/L
Non-HDL-C	<3.4 mmol/l (optimal goal <2.6)

Source: Modified after Bittner *et al.*, 2015.

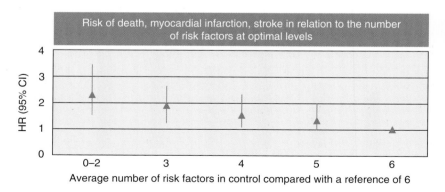

Figure 6.3 Risk factor control in BARI 2D. There is a clear gradient of decreasing risk with increasing numbers of risk factors in the optimum range. *Source*: Bittner *et al.*, 2015. Reproduced with permission of Elsevier.

high-potency statins at recommended doses e.g. atorvastatin 80 mg daily (see **Chapter 12**).

- BP <130/80 mm Hg.
- Antiplatelet treatment.
- β-blockade
- Angiotensin blockade } independent of drugs needed for BP control.
- Good glycaemic control (undefined, but HbA$_{1c}$ <7.0% (53) without hypoglycaemia is reasonable in these high risk patients, though there is no evidence base).

Statins

Patients are routinely started on a high-dose statin when in hospital, which of itself improves adherence. Statins work quickly in this situation and reduce mortality and cardiovascular events after only four months of treatment. Most trials have used atorvastatin 80 mg daily, which has a good safety record in this situation, and although side-effects are likely to emerge in a significant proportion of patients only after discharge, adherence to statins is no lower than to other medications after a myocardial infarction. No additional lipid-modifying drugs are prognostic either acutely or in the long-term. The benefits of pharmacological doses of omega-3 fatty acids have not been seen in trials since the now-old GISSI Prevenzione Study (1999) and they are no longer recommended for secondary prevention (see **Chapter 12** for their continued role in lowering triglycerides).

β-blockers

A β-blocker started at a low dose in hospital may not be uptitrated in the community. They have been in use for decades, long after the original myocardial infarction trials were reported, where they were used with none of the current adjuncts. They are conventionally prescribed in much lower doses compared with those used in the early trials. There have been no recent trials, nor are there likely to be, but a registry study (Goldberger *et al.*, 2015) found that most patients were discharged taking between 12.5 and 25% of the target doses (e.g. metoprolol 25–50 mg daily, compared with 200 mg daily; carvedilol 6.25–12.5 mg daily, compared with 50 mg daily), and that only about one-half of patients continued to take them beyond 1–2 years. Nevertheless, β-blockers given at any dose significantly reduced mortality risk over two years. Angiotensin blocking agents (in patients without heart failure) may also be given in lower than recommended doses, but there is little modern-era trial data; patients with pre-existing diabetes are likely already to be taking higher doses because of their routine use in hypertension.

Secondary prevention: how well are we doing, and can we do better?

Given the clear benefits of reaching as many of the recognized targets as possible, it is disappointing that we are not achieving these apparently relatively simple aims. Even in clinical trials adherence is variable. An analysis combining results of three trials (COURAGE, BARI 2D and FREEDOM) – which probably indicate best achievable practice in the modern era from the late 1990s onwards – found the following (Farkouh *et al.*, 2013):

- *LDL target (<2.6 mmol/l)* at one year was achieved in about 75% of patients in all three trials (but in the FREEDOM trial the more stringent target <1.8 mmol/l was only reached in 42%).
- *SBP target (<130 mm Hg)* was achieved by only 40–50%.
- *HbA$_{1c}$ <7% (53)*: 45–50% achieved target.
- *Smoking cessation*: good results here, with 86–94% continuing smoking cessation at one year.

Real-life versus the clinical trials

In the 2012–2013 EUROASPIRE IV survey of diabetic patients with cardiovascular disease, about 80% of patients were taking β-blockers, angiotensin blocking agents and statins, and >90% aspirin; however, only around 60% were taking all four and 70% reported low physical activity (Gyberg et al., 2015), though 97% stated that they always or very nearly always took their medication. The route from aspiration to clinical target and outcome is clearly not smooth: only about 30% of patients had systolic blood pressure <130 mm Hg and LDL <1.8 mmol/l – as expected, substantially lower attainments in real life compared with clinical trials. While these studies were all based in the USA, payment for medication was probably not a significant barrier (adherence rates improved only marginally in a study when medications were provided free of charge, though in another study private insurance and payment assistance programmes were associated with significantly improved persistence up to 6 months). In limited studies, fixed-dose combinations of several of these important agents – the 'polypill' – may reduce the rate of rehospitalization for ischaemic heart disease or stroke within a year, but the low commercial incentives for producing these agents mean that the polypill will likely progress beyond an academically sound and potentially promising idea in only a handful of countries.

The reasons for poor adherence are manifold and vary between and within countries, healthcare systems, cultures and beliefs. However, every healthcare professional interacting with diabetes patients must become more engaged with the importance and the details of multiple medications, which are, after all, a fundamental tool of diabetes management. Medication reviews must be a process of actively engaging with the patient.

Practice point

Frequently engage patients in adhering to all secondary prevention medication in the long-term. Do this enthusiastically but recognize how arduous it is for patients: healthcare professionals should happily believe in the unequivocal evidence in this instance.

STROKE

The burden of cerebrovascular disease in Type 2 diabetes is still not sufficiently recognized compared with the high profile of coronary heart disease. Between 10 and 20% of stroke patients have diabetes, and the rate is rising. Diabetes approximately doubles the risk of ischaemic stroke and transient ischaemic attack, especially in younger people (**Figure 6.4**), but there is no excess of intracerebral haemorrhage and subarachnoid haemorrhage is significantly less common (Shah et al., 2015). There is no agreement on whether Type 2 women are at higher risk of stroke, in comparison with the consistent findings in coronary heart disease.

Acute management

Given within six hours of the onset of the acute stroke event, thrombolysis using t-PA is standard practice, but clinical outcomes are worse in people with previously unknown hyperglycaemia (intracranial haemorrhage, life-threatening haemorrhage and in-hospital mortality). In stroke patients with known diabetes, in-hospital mortality and intracranial haemorrhage climb with increasing admission glucose and HbA$_{1c}$ (Masrur et al., 2015). These potential adverse effects of thrombolysis in hyperglycaemic patients are compelling reasons for a successful trial of blood glucose lowering strategies in acute

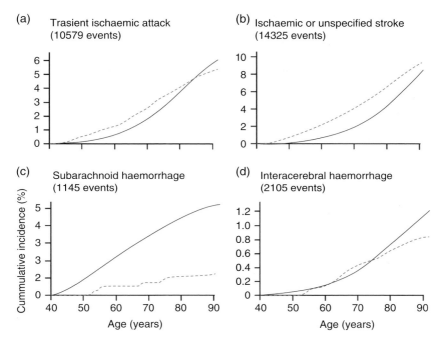

Figure 6.4 Cumulative incidence of cerebrovascular events in Type 2 diabetes in the UK. Dotted red line: diabetes. Blue line: non-diabetic subjects. *Source*: Shah *et al.*, 2015. Reproduced with permission of Elsevier.

stroke, but at present hyperglycaemic patients must be thrombolysed because of the potential benefits.

Blood glucose control

As with acute coronary syndromes there is no shortage of experimental and theoretical data that near-normoglycaemia, usually achieved with a combined glucose–potassium–insulin infusion in the acute ischemic phase, may improve outcomes by preserving the metabolic function of penumbral ischaemic tissue. However, the practicalities of demonstrating clinical benefit in stroke are even more formidable than in the acute coronary situation because of the clear hazards of hypoglycaemia, and theoretical targets outweigh practical guidance for clinicians. The GIST-UK trial (Gray *et al.*, 2007) fell by the recruitment wayside much as DIGAMI 2 did and failed to demonstrate a treatment effect on 90-day mortality using a GIK infusion in patients with admission blood glucose >6 mmol/l. However, it illuminated several important points. Mean admission glucose was not dramatically elevated (8.4 mmol/l) and, as several studies have shown, the level falls spontaneously during the first day even when insulin is not used. The insulin-treated group had a mean glucose level only 1.4 mmol/l lower than the saline-treated group, and there was no difference after 24 hours (**Figure 6.5a**). It is asking quite a lot of a marginal and transient reduction in blood glucose level to reduce stroke mortality. A further trial (SHINE) is randomizing patients to stringent glucose control (4.4–7.2 mmol/l) compared with standard care (<10 mmol/l) and investigating whether near-normoglycaemia reduces the risk of subarachnoid haemorrhage due to intravenous t-PA.

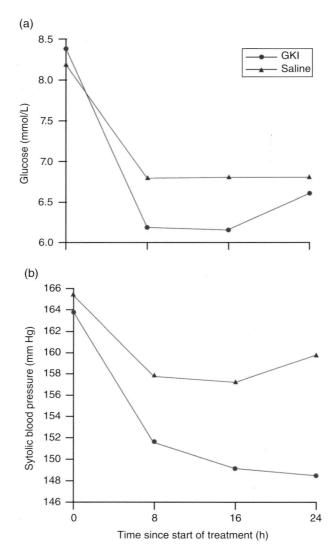

Figure 6.5 Blood glucose (a) and systolic blood pressure (b) in the first 24 hours of ischaemic stroke in the GIST-UK trial, demonstrating the major spontaneous falls in both measurements with saline infusion only. The mean difference in achieved blood glucose was 1.5 mmol/l. *Source:* Gray *et al.*, 2007. Reproduced with permission of Elsevier.

Blood pressure control

There are no randomized trials of blood pressure control in acute ischaemic stroke. There is widespread concern about the wisdom of reducing elevated admission blood pressure, especially in view of the spontaneous fall in systolic blood pressure that occurs in the first eight hours. However, observational data from the IST-3 trial indicate that high baseline blood pressure and blood pressure variability in the first 24 hours are associated with worse early outcomes, and the use of BP-lowering treatment during this phase improved the outcome at six months (Berge *et al.*, 2015). Antihypertensive treatment in acute stroke seems safe if the clinical scenario demands it, but the ENCHANTED trial (NCT01422616) is formally randomizing patients to current target levels (<180–185 mm Hg) or to intensive BP lowering (130–140 mm Hg).

Practice point

There is no evidence for a specific blood glucose target in the acute phase of stroke. Maintain blood glucose at <10 mmol/l, avoiding hypoglycaemia.

There are also few studies of blood pressure control in secondary prevention. However, in nearly four years of follow-up in the SPS3 study of lacunar strokes (see later) there was a consistent trend of 15–30% risk reduction in all stroke, disabling or fatal stroke, myocardial infarction or vascular death, and intracerebral haemorrhage in intensively treated patients with target SBP <130 mm Hg (achieved mean 127 mm Hg). Effects were similar in diabetic and non-diabetic patients (SPS3 Study Group, 2013).

Practice point

In secondary prevention after stroke, target systolic blood pressure <130 mm Hg.

Lacunar strokes

Lacunar strokes of deep brain structures, caused by small vessel occlusion (though they are much larger vessels than those affected in microvascular disease), are common in diabetes, disabling and have a poor outlook because of the presence of other cardiovascular disease. In the important SPS3 (Secondary Prevention of Small Subcortical Strokes Study) (Palacio *et al.*, 2014) nearly 40% of the patients recruited had diabetes. They were more likely than non-diabetic people to have intracranial arterial stenosis, and posterior circulation involvement of the brain stem or cerebellum, and about twice as likely to have a recurrent and disabling or fatal stroke. All measures of cardio- and cerebrovascular disease were more prevalent, including a higher burden of white matter abnormalities on MRI. Dual platelet therapy with clopidogrel did not improve the outlook and there was a higher risk of bleeding. Especially vigorous secondary prevention is needed in these patients.

PERIPHERAL VASCULAR DISEASE

This subject is discussed in more detail in **Chapter 5**.

HEART FAILURE

Heart failure is about three times as common in people with diabetes than the general population and, with the likely continued fall in acute coronary syndromes, it may already be the most frequent presentation of ischaemic heart disease in diabetes. The prognosis is not good: even with refined drug therapy median survival is only about four years. The risk of hospital admission from heart failure is at least as great in Type 1 diabetes as in Type 2 and, although the risk of heart failure progressively increases with glycaemia and albuminuria, it is probably elevated even in Type 1 patients with no evidence of renal disease and in reasonable control (HbA$_{1c}$ 7.0–7.8%, 53–62), pointing again to processes related to longstanding hyperglycaemia and their effects on the myocardium (Rosengren et al., 2015). Dyspnoea short of clinically diagnosed heart failure is emerging as an important symptom. Nearly 25% of middle-aged Type 1 people with an average of 26 years diabetes but who had no history of cardiovascular disease reported some degree of dyspnoea (using the standard New York Heart Association classification); its severity was closely linked to global longitudinal strain on speckle-tracking echocardiography (Jensen et al., 2016). Cardiac magnetic resonance imaging in the DCCT/EDIC cohort uncovered a small number of patients with non-ischaemic scars. These are probably caused by long-term exposure to known risk factors (age, male gender, smoking history, obesity, lower HDL cholesterol and higher average HbA$_{1c}$) and were associated with circumferential strain. It is possible these may predict diffuse myocardial fibrosis and heart failure (Armstrong et al., 2017). In the ADVANCE trial, among a range of biomarkers N-terminal pro-B-type natriuretic peptide (NT-proBNP) was the only one to emerge as a strong predictor of both incidence and progression of clinical heart failure (Ohkuma et al., 2017), though (see later) serum BNP cannot be used to diagnose heart failure with preserved ejection fraction.

Although most clinical trials have been done in patients with systolic heart failure and reduced ejection fraction (HFrEF), the most prevalent form of heart failure now is characterized by a preserved ejection fraction (HFpEF), which carries an even higher risk of hospitalization and mortality.

Practice point

Dyspnoea in otherwise well Type 1 patients signals impaired myocardial function.

Heart failure with preserved ejection fraction

HFpEF is a restrictive form of cardiomyopathy, characterized by a small left ventricle, thickened left ventricular (LV) walls, a preserved LV ejection fraction (≥50%), normal end-diastolic volume index (≤97 ml/m^2), elevated LV filling pressure, and a large left atrium. A common clinical phenotype is an obese elderly Type 2 diabetic female. The clinical presentation is usually with tiredness, fatigue and fluid retention, but symptoms can be non-specific. HFpEF should now be added to the differential diagnosis of tiredness in Type 1 patients (with among others obstructive sleep apnoea, poor glycaemic control, depression).

BNP is not diagnostic in HFpEF and values are lower than those in HFrEF, especially in outpatients presenting with limited exercise tolerance. Echocardiography is the only reliable diagnostic modality.

Practice point

Think of HFpEF in diabetic patients who present with non-specific fatigue. Echocardiography, not serum BNP, is the diagnostic test.

Glycaemia cannot be the sole driving factor: meta-analysis has not uncovered a link between glycaemic control and heart failure. Postulated additional factors include increased myocardial stiffness caused by accumulated advanced glycation end-products, microvascular rarefaction and occlusion, cardiomyocyte hypertrophy in response to hyperinsulinaemia, and interstitial fibrosis, processes that are especially prominent in subjects with preserved ejection fraction. In HFpEF there is interest in a peripheral component affecting skeletal muscle, perhaps linked to the complex processes underlying sarcopenia, and this is plausible in a syndrome where exercise intolerance dominates. This change of focus from cardiac to skeletal muscle may eventually bear fruit in improvement in HFpEF using structured aerobic training (Maurer and Schulze, 2012).

Mortality from heart failure is especially high in women and people younger than the mid-60s. Studies consistently identify a 50% higher mortality rate than in non-diabetic people, but there is up to a twofold increased risk in those with HFpEF. Dyspnoea is associated with hospitalization and higher mortality; fatigue is a risk factor for hospitalization.

Management

Heart failure with reduced ejection fraction

HFrEF should be managed in diabetic subjects in the same way as in non-diabetic people. All established treatments including β-blockers are equally effective in both groups (Girerd et al., 2015). Angiotensin blockade treatment reduces the relative risk of death by about 15% (both ACE-inhibitors and angiotensin receptor blockers have similar beneficial effects) but people with diabetes benefit particularly from the reduction in hospitalization associated with angiotensin blockade. In practice, dose escalation or even initiation of angiotensin blocking agents is often limited by hyperkalaemia and deteriorating renal function (see **Chapter 4**). There are no contraindications to β-blockers or the mineralocorticoid receptor antagonists eplerenone and spironolactone, though hyperkalaemia is a real risk with the latter group of drugs. Ivabradine and digoxin can also be used in the recommended stepped therapy. In black patients, the combination of hydralazine plus isosorbide dinitrate is equally effective in diabetic and non-diabetic people, but it is not used in the United Kingdom.

Endocrinologists do not usually initiate or uptitrate heart failure medication either in clinic or inpatients, but the guidelines are established and relatively simple, and they should. At the very least, diabetes teams should form close links with their local heart failure/heart support teams given that they will share many patients.

> **Practice point**
>
> Heart failure is very common in diabetes. Heart failure teams are a key component of the wider diabetes team.

Highly specialist procedures – implantable defibrillators and cardiac resynchronization therapy – are probably equally effective. Girerd et al. (2015) believed it would be simple for diabetologists to refer patients with LVEF <35% for specialist cardiac advice on ICD/CRT therapy. Though diabetes doubles the risk of a device infection, patients with non-diabetic long-term conditions, such as chronic obstructive pulmonary disease and renal impairment, share a similar increased risk.

Heart failure with preserved ejection fraction

Current recommendations are to control hypertension and to use diuretics appropriately. Beta-blockers are of no value and may be harmful, especially in women. Exercise training may be of benefit in improving exercise capacity and physical measures of quality of life, but a formal randomized trial is needed.

Practice point

Heart failure patients with preserved ejection fraction do not benefit from specific medication other than diuretics. Increased aerobic activity might help.

Glycaemic treatments and heart failure (Chapter 10)

Metformin is not harmful in heart failure, even with reduced ejection fraction, and should not be withheld unless there are other contraindications. There is some evidence from cohort studies that it confers mortality and hospitalization benefits, especially in comparison with sulfonylureas (Eurich et al., 2013). However, it does not improve left ventricular stiffness and, therefore, probably does not help HFpEF. Although sulfonylureas in current use do not cross-react with cardiac ATP-sensitive potassium channels, thereby reducing ischaemic resistance, minimize doses where possible.

DPP4-inhibitors and GLP-1receptor agonists

The DPP4-inhibitor saxagliptin was associated with an increased risk of heart failure but it was not seen in the very large TECOS study using sitagliptin. The safety of this class of drugs in heart failure is still not clear. Small studies of GLP-1-receptor agonist drugs in patients with heart failure or at increased risk of it have been reported over several years, exploring the hope that their cellular action might improve cardiac function. In large placebo-controlled Phase IV studies, lixisenatide, liraglutide and semaglutide did not increase the risk of heart failure, but liraglutide up to 1.8 mg daily for six months in diabetic and non-diabetic patients recently hospitalized with heart failure did not improve clinical and laboratory measures of heart failure (Margulies et al., 2016). GLP-1-receptor agonists consistently increase heart rate. Given that a key aim of heart failure treatment is to reduce sympathetic drive, primarily through β-blockade, do not initiate this group of drugs in people with known heart failure.

Practice point

Drugs acting through the incretin system probably do not increase the risk of heart failure in Type 2 patients but they should not be initiated in patients with diagnosed or suspected known heart failure.

SGLT2 inhibitors

Of the several cardiovascular benefits seen in the EMPA-REG OUTCOME three-year phase IV study of empagliflozin in Type 2 patients at high cardiovascular risk, the heart failure outcomes were striking, especially as they were predefined. New-onset heart failure, and hospitalization and death from heart failure, were reduced by 35–40%; hospitalization for any reason – primarily, of course, cardiovascular – was reduced by 10% (Fitchett et al., 2016). Patients already taking effective heart failure medication – angiotensin blocking drugs, diuretics and β-blockers – and those with eGFR <60 ml/min benefited to the same degree; improved outcomes were seen shortly after starting the medication, confirming a drug effect and not one of longer-term benefits on cardiovascular disease. How this drug exerts its beneficial effects on heart failure, seemingly in addition to those of established heart failure medication, is not known, and although empagliflozin is safe in patients with heart failure formal trials are needed to establish whether it has a specific role in heart failure treatment.

ARRHYTHMIAS

People with diabetes often have two additional factors associated with an increased risk of arrhythmias: hypertension and obstructive sleep apnoea. However, the literature is sparse.

Atrial fibrillation

The risk of atrial fibrillation (AF) in people with diabetes is about twice that of the general population (Movahed *et al.*, 2005). There are many reasons. Accelerated atrial fibrosis with a contribution from excess advanced glycation end products is likely to be important but autonomic imbalance with sympathetic excess and abnormal atrial electrophysiology contribute, at least in animal models.

In the general population, AF is related to glycated haemoglobin levels. In patients with impaired glucose tolerance, a 1 mmol/l increase in fasting glucose is associated with a one-third increase in the risk of developing AF. This is reflected in the presence of diabetes in the $CHADS_2$ and CHA_2DS_2-VASc scoring systems for AF risk. The converse therapeutic outcomes are, as usual, less clear-cut. Even very tight glycaemic control in the large ACCORD study did not improve the incidence or outcomes of AF, but tight blood pressure control (target systolic blood pressure <120 mm Hg) reduced the incidence of AF combined with P-wave indices that are considered precursors of AF (Chen *et al.*, 2015). However, good control in patients undergoing ablation is important; the recurrence rate in patients with paroxysmal AF was higher (70% vs 50%) in people with HbA_{1c} levels ≥6.9% (52) (Lu *et al.*, 2015).

> **Practice point**
>
> Ensure the best possible glycaemic control (HbA_{1c} <7.0%, 53) in patients having ablation therapy for AF.

In the Framingham Study obesity (BMI >30) was associated with a 50% increased risk of AF compared with normal weight people (BMI <25), raising the possibility that obesity is a modifiable risk factor for the development of AF. However, while significant weight loss in the Look AHEAD study did not reduce the risk of developing AF, 10% or greater weight loss in the well-controlled LEGACY study (Pathak *et al.*, 2015) reduced symptoms, AF burden on ambulatory monitoring and duration of freedom from AF, with or without rhythm control strategies. This benefit was significantly reversed by weight fluctuations exceeding 5%. There are no studies of patients with AF undergoing bariatric surgery. Although this population is at high risk of arrhythmias, they are relatively young and only about 2% are in AF.

There has been much hope that specific cardiac medication (especially statins, angiotensin receptor blockers and omega-3 fatty acids) may reduce the risk of developing AF through mechanisms underlying its pathology, for example inflammation. None has been substantiated in individual clinical trials, though there is some evidence that angiotensin blocking agents might reduce the recurrence rate, but probably not the onset, of AF.

Ventricular arrhythmias

Diabetes carries a high risk of ventricular arrhythmias, increasing the risk of sudden cardiac death. While the most powerful factor is ischaemic heart disease, a multitude of other factors may contribute, including autonomic neuropathy, microvasculopathy and, as in atrial fibrillation, diabetes-induced structural and electrophysiological abnormalities in the ventricle itself. The role of prolonged QTc interval on ECG has been extensively investigated.

While there is no firm link with hyperglycaemia, there is increasing concern about hypoglycaemia and significant arrhythmias. Hypoglycaemia detected on continuous glucose monitoring (interstitial glucose <3.1 mmol/l) is strongly linked to the number of severe ventricular arrhythmias on Holter monitoring in Type 2 patients with established coronary artery disease, especially in the presence of low TSH levels, perhaps indicating subclinical hyperthyroidism. Causality and even a link between hypoglycaemia and cardiac events will be difficult to establish, but the reach of the clinical consequences of hypoglycaemia is now potentially much greater, and adds to the growing concern around it (Pistrosch *et al.*, 2015).

Calcific aortic valve disease is a growing problem in the elderly. In USA veterans, diabetes doubled the risk of non-rheumatic valve disease, but this is in a male population, and the risk in females is not known. In addition it is not clear whether diabetes is a risk factor for progression of calcific aortic valve disease. However, it is well-described in the metabolic syndrome in association with fatty liver.

ASPIRIN IN PRIMARY PREVENTION

It was not very long ago that aspirin therapy was a target for all people with diabetes, in the hope that a very cheap treatment would make a meaningful impact on cardiovascular outcomes. It was assumed that benefit was large and risk small. There is no argument in secondary prevention but there is only selective benefit in primary prevention, for example non-fatal myocardial infarction in men and stroke in women. Repeated meta-analyses find that cardiovascular events are reduced slightly and non-significantly by approximately 9–10%, while bleeding, primarily gastrointestinal, is increased about twofold. This meta-analytic effort results in consensus only: consider low-dose aspirin in those with a 10-year cardiovascular risk of 10% or more and who do not have an increased risk of bleeding. Even weaker evidence is used in the same guidelines to propose aspirin in those at intermediate risk (5–10% 10-year risk) – but this itself is preciously close to all-inclusiveness (Fox *et al.*, 2015).

> **Practice point**
>
> Aspirin may be of value in primary prevention if 10-year cardiovascular risk is 10% or greater and there are no risk factors for increased bleeding.

REFERENCES

Arenja N, Mueller C, Ehl NF *et al*. Prevalence, extent, and independent predictors of silent myocardial infarction. *Am J Med* 2013;126:515–22 [PMID: 23597799].

Armstrong AC, Ambale-Venkatesh B, Turkbey E *et al*. DCCT/EDIC Research Group. Association of cardiovascular risk factors and myocardial fibrosis with early cardiac dysfunction in type 1 diabetes: the Diabetes Control and Complications Trial/Epidemiology of Diabetes Interventions and Complications Study. *Diabetes Care* 2017;40:405–411 [PMID: 27986796] PMC5319473.

Berge E, Cohen G, Lindley RI *et al*. Effects of blood pressure and blood pressure-lowering treatment during the first 24 hours among patients in the third International Stroke Trial of thrombolytic treatment for acute ischemic stroke. *Stroke* 2015;46:3362–9 [PMID: 26486868] Free full text.

Bittner V, Bertolet M, Barraza Felix R *et al*. BARI 2D Study Group. Comprehensive cardiovascular risk factor control improves survival: The BARI 2D Trial. *J Am Coll Cardiol* 2015;66:765–73 [PMID: 26271057] PMC4550809.

Blomster JI, Woodward M, Zoungas S et al. The harms of smoking and benefits of smoking cessation in women compared with men with type 2 diabetes: an observational analysis of the ADVANCE (Action in Diabetes and Vascular Disease: Preterax and Diamicron modified release Controlled Evaluation) trial. *BMJ Open* 2016;6:e009668 [PMID: 26747037] PMC4716176.

de Boer IH, Gao X, Cleary RA et al. Diabetes Control and Complications Trial/Epidemiology of Diabetes Interventions and Complications (DCCT/EDIC) Research Group. Albuminuria changes and cardiovascular and renal outcomes in type 1 diabetes: the DCCT/EDIC Study. *Clin J Am Soc Nephrol* 2016;11:1969–77 [PMID: 27797889] PMC5108190.

Bonds DE. DIGAMI 1: 20 years later. *Lancet Diabetes Endocrinol* 2014;2:603–4 [PMID: 24831991].

Booth JN 3rd, Levitan EB, Brown TM et al. Effect of sustaining lifestyle modifications (nonsmoking, weight reduction, physical activity, and Mediterranean diet) after healing of myocardial infarction, percutaneous intervention, or coronary bypass (from the Reasons for Geographic and Racial Differences in Stroke Study). *Am J Cardiol* 2014;113:1933–40 [PMID: 24793668] PMC4348576.

Carter RE, Lackland DT, Cleary PA et al.; Diabetes Control and Complications Trial/Epidemiology of Diabetes Interventions and Complications (DCCT/EDIC) Study Research Group. Intensive treatment of diabetes is associated with a reduced rate of peripheral arterial calcification in the diabetes control and complications trial. *Diabetes Care* 2007;30:2646–8 [PMID: 17623823] PMC2655324.

Chen LY, Bigger JT, Hickey KT et al. Effect of intensive blood pressure lowering on incident atrial fibrillation and P-wave indices in the ACCORD blood pressure trial. *Am J Hypertens* 2015;11:1276–82 [PMID: 26476086].

Cheung NW, Wing VW, McLean M. The Hyperglycaemia: Intensive Insulin Infusion in Infarction (HI-5) study: a randomized controlled trial of insulin infusion therapy for myocardial infarction. *Diabetes Care* 2006;29:765–770 [PMID: 16567812].

Cleary PA, Orchard TJ, Genuth S et al. Diabetes Control and Complications Trial/Epidemiology of Diabetes Interventions and Complications (DCCT/EDIC) Research Group. The effect of intensive glycemic treatment on coronary artery calcification in type 1 participants of the Diabetes Control and Complications Trial/Epidemiology of Diabetes Interventions and Complications (DCCT/EDIC) Study. *Diabetes* 2006;55:3556–65 [PMID: 17130504] [PMC2701297].

DCCT/EDIC (Diabetes Control and Complications Trial/Epidemiology of Diabetes Interventions and Complications Research Group, Nathan DM, Bebu I, Braffett BH et al. Risk factors for cardiovascular disease in type 1 diabetes. *Diabetes* 2016;65:1370–9 [PMID: 26895792] PMC4839209.

Emerging Risk Factors Collaboration, Sarwar N, Gao P, Seshasai SR et al. Diabetes mellitus, fasting blood glucose concentrations, and risk of vascular disease: a collaborative meta-analysis of 102 prospective studies. *Lancet* 2010;375:2215–22 [PMID: 20609967] PMC2904878.

Eurich DT, Weir DL, Majumdar SR et al. Comparative safety and effectiveness of metformin in patients with diabetes mellitus and heart failure: systematic review of observational studies involving 34,000 patients. *Circ Heart Fail* 2013;6:395–402 [PMID: 23508758] Free full text.

Farkouh ME, Domanski M, Sleeper LA et al. FREEDOM Trial Investigators. Strategies for multivessel revascularization in patients with diabetes. *N Engl J Med* 2012;367:2375–84 [PMID: 23121323] Free full text.

Farkouh ME, Boden WE, Bittner V et al. Risk factor control for coronary artery disease secondary prevention in large randomized trials. *J Am Coll Cardiol* 2013;61:160–15 [PMID: 23500281] Free full text.

Fisher M (ed). *Heart Disease and Diabetes (Oxford Diabetes Library)*. Oxford University Press, 2009. ISBN: 978-0-19-954372-4.

Fitchett D, Zinman B, Wanner C et al. EMPA-REG OUTCOME® trial investigators. Heart failure outcomes with empagliflozin in patients with type 2 diabetes at high cardiovascular risk: results of the EMPA-REG OUTCOME® trial. *Eur Heart J* 2016;37:1526–34 [PMID: 26819227] PMC4872285.

Forouhi NG, Sattar N, Tillin T et al. Do known risk factors explain the higher coronary heart disease mortality in South Asian compared with European men? Prospective follow-up of the Southall and Brent studies, UK. *Diabetologia* 2008;49:2580–8 [PMID: 16972045].

Fox CS, Golden SH, Anderson C et al. American Heart Association Diabetes Committee of the Council on Lifestyle and Cardiometabolic Health; Council on Clinical Cardiology, Council on

Cardiovascular and Stroke Nursing, Council on Cardiovascular Surgery and Anesthesia, Council on Quality of Care and Outcomes Research; American Diabetes Association. Update on prevention of cardiovascular disease in adults with type 2 diabetes mellitus in light of recent evidence: a scientific statement from the American Heart Association and the American Diabetes Association. *Diabetes Care* 2015;38:1777–803 [PMID: 26246459] PMC 4876675.

Girerd N, Zennad F, Rosssignol P. Review of heart failure treatment in type 2 diabetes patients: It's at least as effective as in non-diabetic patients! *Diabetes Metab* 2015;41:446–55 [PMID: 26249760].

Goldberger JJ, Bonow RO, Cuffe M et al. OBTAIN Investigators. Effect of beta-blocker dose on survival after myocardial infarction. *J Am Coll Cardiol* 2015;66:1431–44 [PMID: 26403339] PMC4583654.

Gray CS, Hildreth AJ, Sandercock PA et al. GIST Trialists Collaboration. Glucose-potassium-insulin infusions in the management of post-stroke hyperglycaemia: the UK Glucose Insulin in Stroke Trial (GIST-UK). *Lancet Neurol* 2007;6:397–406 [PMID: 17434094].

Gregg EW, Li Y, Wang J et al. Changes in diabetes-related complications in the Unites States, 1990–2010. *N Engl J Med* 2014;370:1514–23 [PMID: 24738668] Free full text.

Gyberg V, De Bacquer D, De Backer G et al.; EUROASPIRE Investigators. Patients with coronary artery disease need improved management: a report from the EUROASPIRE IV survey: a registry from the EuroObservational Research Programme of the European Society of Cardiology. *Cardiovasc Diabetol* 2015;14:133 [PMID: 26427624] PMC4591740.

Hägg S, Thorn LM, Putaala J et al. FinnDiane Study Group. Incidence of stroke according to presence of diabetic nephropathy and severe diabetic retinopathy in patients with type 1 diabetes. *Diabetes Care* 2013;36:4140–6 [PMID: 24101700] PMC3836162.

Heran BS, Chen JM, Ebrahim S et al. Exercise-based cardiac rehabilitation for coronary heart disease. *Cochrane Database Syst Rev* 2011;CD001800 [PMID: 21735386] PMC4229995.

Hernandez SL, Gong JH, Chen L et al. Characterization of circulating and endothelial progenitor cells in patients with extreme-duration type 1 diabetes. *Diabetes Care* 2014;37:2193–201 [PMID: 24780357] PMC4113171.

Holtzman MJ, Rathsman B, Eliasson B et al. Long-term prognosis in patients with type 1 and 2 diabetes mellitus after coronary artery bypass grafting. *J Am Coll Cardiol* 2015;65:1644–52 [25908069].

Janghorbani M, Hu FB, Willett WC et al. Prospective study of type 1 and type 2 diabetes and risk of stroke subtypes: the Nurses' Health Study. *Diabetes Care* 2007;30:1730–5 [PMID:17389335].

Jensen MT, Risum N, Rossing P, Jensen JS. Self-reported dyspnoea is associated with impaired global longitudinal strain in ambulatory type 1 diabetes patients with normal ejection fraction and without known heart disease – The Thousand & 1 Study. *J Diabetes Complications* 2016;30:928–34 [PMID: 26944814].

Jones DA, Gallagher S, Rathod KS et al. NICOR. Mortality in South Asians and Caucasians after percutaneous coronary intervention in the United Kingdom: an observational cohort study of 279,256 patients from the BCIS (British Cardiovascular Intervention Society) National Database. *JACC Cardiovasc Interv* 2014;7:362–71 [PMID: 24742942] Free full text.

Kasteleyn MJ, Vos RC, Jansen H, Rutten GE. Differences in clinical characteristics between patients with and without type 2 diabetes hospitalized with a first myocardial infarction. *J Diabetes Complications* 2016;30:830–3 [PMID: 27134032].

Knudsen EC, Seljeflot I, Abdelnoor M et al. Abnormal glucose regulation in patients with acute ST-elevation myocardial infarction – a cohort study on 224 patients. *Cardiovasc Diabetol* 2009;8:6 [PMID: 19183453] PMC2646717.

Kramer CK, Rodrigues TC, Canani LH et al. Diabetic retinopathy predicts all-cause mortality and cardiovascular events in both type 1 and 2 diabetes: meta-analysis of observational studies. *Diabetes Care* 2011;34:1238–44 [PMID: 21525504] PMC3114518.

Larsen K, Brekke M, Sandvik L et al. Silent coronary atheromatosis in type 1 diabetic patients and its relation to long-term glycemic control. *Diabetes* 2002;51:2637–41 [PMID:12145181] Free full text.

Look AHEAD Research Group, Gregg EW, Jakicic JM, Blackburn G et al. Association of the magnitude of weight loss and changes in physical fitness with long-term cardiovascular disease outcomes in overweight or obese people with type 2 diabetes: a post-hoc analysis of the Look

AHEAD randomised clinical trial. *Lancet Diabetes Endocrinol* 2016;4:913–21 [PMID: 27595918] PMC5094846.

Lu ZH, Liu N, Bai R *et al*. HbA1c levels as predictors of ablation outcome in type 2 diabetes mellitus and paroxysmal atrial fibrillation. *Herz* 2015;40(Suppl 2):130–6 [PMID: 25336239].

Malmberg K. Prospective randomised study of intensive insulin treatment on long term survival after acute myocardial infarction in patients with diabetes mellitus. DIGAMI (Diabetes Mellitus, Insulin Glucose Infusion in Acute Myocardial Infarction) Study Group. *BMJ* 1997;314:1512–5 [PMID: 9169397] PMC2126756.

Margulies KB, Hernandez AF, Redfield MM *et al*. NHLBI Heart Failure Clinical Research Network. Effects of liraglutide on clinical stability among patients with advanced heart failure and reduced ejection fraction: a randomized clinical trial. *JAMA* 2016;316:500–8 [PMID: 27483064] PMC5021525.

Masrur S, Cox M, Bhatt DL *et al*. Association of acute and chronic hyperglycemia with acute ischaemic stroke outcomes post-thrombolysis: findings from Get with the Guidelines – Stroke. *J Am Heart Assoc* 2015;4:e002193 [PMID: 26408015] PMC4845108.

Maurer MS, Schulze PC. Exercise intolerance in heart failure with preserved ejection fraction: shifting focus from the heart to peripheral skeletal muscle. *J Am Coll Cardiol* 2012;60:129–31 [PMID: 22766339] PMC3391741.

Movahed MR, Hashemzadeh M, Jamal MM. Diabetes mellitus is a strong, independent risk for atrial fibrillation and flutter in addition to other cardiovascular diseases. *Int J Cardiol* 2005;105;315–8 [PMID: 16274775].

Muhlestein JB, Lappé DL, Lima JA *et al*. The FACTOR-64 randomized clinical trial Effect of screening for coronary artery disease using CT angiography on mortality and cardiac events in high-risk patients with diabetes: the FACTOR-64 randomized clinical trial. *JAMA* 2014;312:2234–43 [PMID: 25402757].

Norhammer A, Tenerz A Nilsson G *et al*. Glucose metabolism in patients with acute myocardial infarction and no previous diagnosis of diabetes mellitus: a prospective study. *Lancet* 2002;359: 2140–4 [PMID: 12090978].

Nyström T, Holtzmann MJ, Elizasson B *et al*. Glycemic control in type 1 diabetes and long-term risk of cardiovascular events or death after coronary bypass grafting. *J Am Coll Cardiol* 2015;66:535–43 [PMID: 26227192].

O'Donoghue ML, Vaidya A, Afsal R *et al*. An invasive or conservative strategy in patients with diabetes mellitus and non-ST-segment elevation acute coronary syndromes: a collaborative meta-analysis of randomized trials. *J Am Coll Cardiol* 2012; 60:106–11 [PMID: 22766336] Free full text.

Ohkuma T, Jun M, Woodward M *et al*. ADVANCE Collaborative Group. Cardiac stress and inflammatory markers as predictors of heart failure in patients with type 2 diabetes: the ADVANCE trial. *Diabetes Care* 2017:40:1203–9 [PMID: 28684396].

Orchard TJ, Costacou T. When are type 1 diabetic patients at risk for cardiovascular disease? *Curr Diab Rep* 2010;10:48–54 [PMID: 20425067].

Palacio S, McClure LA, Benavente OR *et al*. Lacunar strokes in patients with diabetes mellitus: risk factors, infarct location, and prognosis: the secondary prevention of small subcortical strokes study. *Stroke* 2014;45:2689–94 [PMID: 25034716] PMC4146755.

Pathak RK, Middeldorp ME, Meredith M *et al*. Long-term effect of goal-directed weight management in an atrial legacy cohort: a long-term follow-up study (LEGACY). *J Am Coll Cardiol* 2015; 65:2159–69 [PMID: 25792361].

Pistrosch F, Ganz X, Bornstein SR *et al*. Risk of and risk factors for hypoglycaemia and associated arrhythmias in patients with type 2 diabetes and cardiovascular disease: a cohort study under real-world conditions. *Acta Diabetol* 2015;52:889–95 [PMID: 25749806].

Rana JS, Liu JY, Moffet HH *et al*. Diabetes and prior coronary heart disease are not necessarily risk equivalent for future coronary heart disease events. *J Gen Intern Med* 2016;31:387–93 [PMID: 26666660].

Rosengren A, Vestberg D Svensson AM *et al*. Long-term excess risk of heart failure in people with type 1 diabetes: a prospective case-control study. *Lancet Diabetes Endocrinol* 2015;3:876–85 [PMID: 26388415].

Sedlis SP, Hartigan PM, Teo KK *et al*. COURAGE Trial Investigators. Effect of PCI on long-term survival in patients with stable ischemic heart disease. *N Engl J Med* 2015;373:1937–46 [PMID: 26559572] Free full text.

Senior PA, Welsh RC, McDonald CG *et al*. Coronary artery disease is common in nonuremic, asymptomatic type 1 diabetic islet transplant candidates. *Diabetes Care* 28:866–72 [PMID: 15793187].

Shah AD, Langenberg C, Rapsomaniki E *et al*. Type 2 diabetes and incidence of cardiovascular diseases: a cohort study in 1.9 million people. *Lancet Diabetes Endocrinol* 2015;3:105–13 [PMID: 25466521] PMC4303913.

Soja AM, Zwiser AD, Frederiksen M *et al*. Use of intensified comprehensive cardiac rehabilitation to improve risk factor control in patients with type 2 diabetes mellitus or impaired glucose tolerance – the randomized DANish StUdy of impaired glucose metabolism in the settings of cardiac rehabilitation (DANSUK) study. *Am Heart J* 2007;153:621–8 [PMID: 17383302].

SPS3 Study Group; Benavente OR, Coffey CS, Conwit R *et al*. Blood-pressure targets in patients with recent lacunar stroke: the SPS3 randomised trial. *Lancet* 2013;382:507–15 [PMID: 23726159] PMC3979302.

Van Spall HG, Chong A, Tu JV. Inpatient smoking-cessation counselling and all-cause mortality in patients with acute myocardial infarction. *Am Heart J* 2007;154:213–20 [PMID:17643569].

Vistisen D, Andersen GS, Hansen CS *et al*. Prediction of first cardiovascular disease event in type 1 diabetes mellitus: the Steno type 1 risk engine. *Circulation* 2016;133;1058–66 [PMID: 26888765].

Wright AK, Kontopantelis E, Emsley R *et al*. Life expectancy and cause-specific mortality in type 2 diabetes: a population-based cohort study quantifying relationships in ethnic subgroups. *Diabetes Care* 2017; 40:338–45 [PMID: 27998911].

Yates T, Henson J, Edwardson C *et al*. Differences in levels of physical activity between white and south Asian populations within a healthcare setting: impact of measurement type in a cross-sectional study. *BMJ Open* 2015;5:e006181 [PMID: 26204908] PMC4513447.

Young LH, Wackers FJ, Chyun DA *et al*.; DIAD Investigators. Cardiac outcomes after screening for asymptomatic coronary artery disease in patients with type 2 diabetes: the DIAD study: a randomized controlled trial. *JAMA* 2009;301:1547–55 [PMID: 19366774] PMC2895332.

Zellweger MJ, Maraun M, Osterhues HH *et al*. Progression to overt or silent CAD in asymptomatic patients with diabetes mellitus at high coronary risk: main findings of the prospective multicentre BARDOT trial with a pilot randomized treatment substudy. *JACC Cardiovasc Imaging* 2014;7: 1001–10 [PMID: 25240454].

Web sites

Cardiovascular risk prediction (UK)
QRISK®2. https://qrisk.org

7 Type 1 diabetes: glycaemic control

Key points

- Glycaemic control determines the outcome of all complications in Type 1 diabetes
- HbA_{1c} values consistently <7.0% (53) carry a very low risk of microvascular complications in the long term, and this is a widely agreed target
- Nearly all patients with advanced microvascular complications have had HbA_{1c} values >9% (75) for many years; in the DCCT similar levels were associated with long-term increased mortality
- Many population studies have shown steady improvements in HbA_{1c} values over the past 10–15 years, falling at approximately 0.01–0.04% per year, and several have also demonstrated continuing decreases in severe hypoglycaemia rates
- Generalists need to know how to safely help a patient with Type 1 diabetes to manage their insulin regimen
- Teams must be knowledgeable and experienced in multiple dose (basal-bolus) regimens
- Education, and inspiring confidence through knowledge and experience, are more important than small differences in insulin action between different preparations
- Type 1 diabetes demands continuous presence of insulin

INTRODUCTION

Insulin treatment in Type 1 diabetes is completely different from insulin treatment in Type 2 diabetes: the physiology is different, especially overnight, and in practice insulin treatment is often more difficult in Type 1 because of the effective absence of endogenous insulin production, which in the non-diabetic person maintains astonishingly stable blood glucose levels (**Figure 7.1a**). Overall insulin treatment requires a much more delicate touch than in Type 2 diabetes, self-monitoring needs to be more intensive, dosage variation is higher and much more of the variation of blood glucose control is unexplained by conventional factors. Basal insulin treatment has become more sophisticated in the past fifteen years but there have been no meaningful improvements in injected prandial insulin for nearly two decades; postprandial glucose control is often very difficult in Type 1 patients, even in patients using insulin pumps. Practitioners who are expert in insulin introduction in Type 2 patients failing on non-insulin agents (see **Chapter 10**) are likely to find advising a Type 1 patient more difficult. People with Type 1 diabetes have usually used insulin for several or many years and have unique insights into factors that affect their individual blood glucose control.

Practical Diabetes Care, Fourth Edition. David Levy.
© 2018 John Wiley & Sons Ltd. Published 2018 by John Wiley & Sons Ltd.

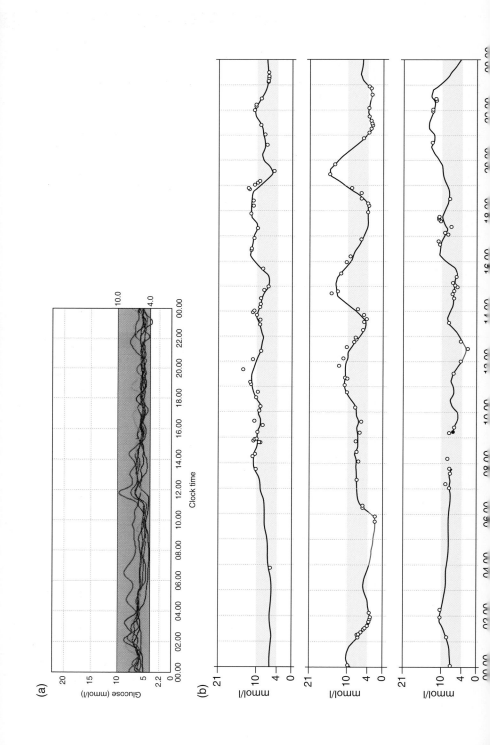

Practice point

Helping patients with insulin treatment in Type 1 diabetes is more complex than in Type 2, and requires experienced practitioners.

The introduction of the fully-automated (closed-loop) insulin pump (artificial pancreas) has been predicted for many years, but progress is now rapid (see **Chapter 8**). In the meantime, careful use of conventional insulin replacement therapy, usually with multiple daily injections or, increasingly, insulin pumps, can often ensure very good glycaemic control (**Figure 7.1b**). But hard work, intensive and informed discussion, education and recognition that changes in insulin doses must be subtle and targeted are all needed to ensure optimum outcomes.

NOMENCLATURE: INSULIN REGIMENS

While to the non-specialist even the reduced numbers of insulin preparations is difficult to remember (see later), the number of terms used to describe different insulin regimens is almost as complex. An international proposal in 2015 to tidy up the various terms (Neu *et al.*, 2015) is unlikely to bear fruit soon, but the framework is valuable (**Table 7.1**).

INSULIN PREPARATIONS: HISTORICAL

From 1922, when insulin was first used, until the mid-1930s, short-acting soluble insulin was the only preparation available and patients needed multiple injections, up to five times a day – including during the night. Multiple dose insulin is, therefore, not a recent innovation. Attempts to prolong insulin action, by combining with the fish protein protamine, began in the 1930s but the prototype intermediate-acting insulin, NPH (Neutral Protamine Hagedorn, isophane) was not introduced until 1946. Multiple variants of insulin zinc preparations, aiming for a basal insulin that would last 24 hours or more, were launched in the 1950s. Other than the ultra-long-acting protamine zinc insulin, PZI, they faded out of use and many patients continued to use twice-daily NPH (free-mixed with twice-daily soluble insulin) until the long-acting analogue (modified human) insulins were introduced: the first was insulin glargine in 2000.

Highly purified soluble pork insulin preparations in the 1970s reduced the risk of disfiguring immune-mediated lipoatrophy. Insulins with a shorter action than the animal-derived

---

◄

Figure 7.1 Continuous glucose monitoring studies. (a) Non-diabetic profile obtained with the blinded Medtronic iPro2 system. *x*-axis, clock time, midnight-to-midnight; *y*-axis, interstitial glucose readings (shaded range 4-10 mmol/l). Glucose levels after meals can transiently reach 10 mmol/l but most values are between 4 and 7 mmol/l. (b) Type 1 diabetes, >30 years duration, multiple daily injections (basal × 2, mealtime × 4–6). Established microvascular complications (laser-treated retinopathy, mildly increased albuminuria, definite hypertension and mild symptomatic neuropathy) had provoked a determined effort to improve control (usual HbA$_{1c}$ ~9.0%, 75). Profiles on three consecutive days obtained with the Abbot FreeStyle Libre ambulatory glucose system (unblinded). HbA$_{1c}$ at the time was 7.2% (55). This is 'near-normoglycaemia' and represents about the best control that can be obtained with current insulin therapy. Note the marked day-to-day variability. Postprandial excursions are low, partly due to multiple dosing with meals and snacks, but also because he was making efforts to reduce his carbohydrate intake. There is early morning hypoglycaemia on the second day (glucose ~2.2 mmol/l), which woke the patient.

Table 7.1 Classification and definitions of insulin regimens.

Proposed term	Usual current term	Synonyms	Definition
Fixed insulin dose regimens	—	Basal insulin only (rare in adult practice) Premixed insulin only Free-mixed insulin combinations	Fixed insulin dosage, at most minimally adjusted for meals. Insulin dosage (particularly the morning dose) determines the timing of meals later on in the day and their carbohydrate content.
Glucose and meal-adjusted injection regimens	Basal-bolus regimen	Intensified conventional insulin therapy Multiple daily injections (MDI) Flexible insulin therapy (FIT)	No set dose. Insulin given according to self-monitored glucose values and varying meal times. Insulin dose is adjusted according to likely carbohydrate content of meal.
Pump therapy	—	CSII	Continuous subcutaneous insulin infusion (CSII). Insulin dosing as for 'basal-bolus' regimen.

Source: Neu *et al.*, 2015. Reproduced with permission of John Wiley & Sons.

products were inadvertently introduced when biosynthetic insulin was announced in 1982. Thought to be identical in action to highly purified insulins, they were introduced without formal randomized trials and it quickly became apparent that they had a more rapid onset (and offset) of action, leading to an increased risk of severe hypoglycaemia. Modified biosynthetic fast-acting insulin analogues have been the object of attention since the late 1990s. The aim here was to inhibit the natural formation of insulin hexamers and promote monomer formation, so that insulin absorption was more rapid and possibly more predictable. Insulin lispro was introduced in 1997 and two further fast-acting analogues since then, but none since the mid-2000s.

The classification and naming of insulin preparations has always been complicated but recently insulin manufacturers have dramatically 'rationalized' their product lines and there are only about a dozen preparations available in the United Kingdom, of which about six are in widespread use. **Table 7.2** lists them, emphasizing those likely to be encountered in routine practice. Patents on the first wave of analogue insulins are expiring and as well as completely new products there will be increasing numbers of biosimilar insulins or 'branded generics'. Contentiously, fully generic insulin is not available, and preparations must be prescribed by brand name.

INSULIN ANALOGUES

In general chemistry the term 'analogue' refers to a molecule that has been modified in one of its components. In this case, the parent molecule is biosynthetic human insulin, which has been modified, usually in more than one amino acid, in order to change its physicochemical characteristics and thereby change the duration of its action. Most insulin prescribed in the United Kingdom is analogue but human insulin preparations are widely used in Type 2 diabetes (see **Chapter 10**). They are still of value in Type 1 diabetes, though much less used in high-expenditure health economies. For example, in a survey of

Table 7.2 Insulin preparations available in the United Kingdom.

Short acting	Basal insulin (intermediate or long acting)	Biphasic insulin mixtures (fixed mixtures of short and intermediate acting)
Taken 10–30 minutes before meals Clear insulin	Taken at bedtime (or morning, or twice daily about 12 hours apart) independent of mealtimes. Human preparations are cloudy, analogues clear	Taken twice or three times daily before meals Cloudy
NovoRapid (aspart, A) Humalog (lispro, A) Humulin S (H) Insuman Rapid (H) Apidra (glulisine, A) Fiasp (faster-acting insulin aspart, A)	Lantus (glargine, A) Levemir (detemir, A) Humulin I (H) Insuman Basal (H) Insulatard (H) Tresiba (degludec, U100, U200, A) Abasaglar (biosimilar glargine) (A) Toujeo (U300 glargine) (A)	NovoMix 30 (A) Humulin M3 (H) Humalog Mix25 (A) Humalog Mix50 (A) Insuman Comb (15, 25 and 50) (H) Ryzodeg (degludec 70%, aspart 30%) [long-acting analogue combination]

A: analogue insulins (modified human insulins)
H: synthetic recombinant human insulins

paediatric practice in Germany and Austria, approximately 20% of patients in 2014 were using soluble and NPH insulins, representing a substantial minority (Bohn *et al.*, 2016); glycaemic control in Germany is, nevertheless, the best in Europe (McKnight *et al.*, 2015). HbA_{1c} was maintained at about 7% (53) in the intensively-treated cohort of the Diabetes Control and Complications Trial (DCCT) years before analogue insulins were introduced.

Long-acting analogue insulins

Early clinical trials established that new long-acting analogues and the older human preparations (NPH) had identical effects on HbA_{1c}, but hinted at a reduced risk of severe, especially overnight, hypoglycaemia. The assumption was that the smoother pharmacokinetic profile of long-acting analogues, especially glargine, would allow fasting glucose values to be targeted more precisely at a lower value. This hope turned out not to be consistently the case in the small number of trials conducted in Type 1 patients. The more recent HypoAna trial confirmed that hypoglycaemia-prone subjects benefited from a clinically meaningful reduction (around 50%) in both severe and non-severe nocturnal hypoglycaemia when taking an analogue basal-bolus regimen of detemir and aspart compared with a regimen of NPH and human soluble insulin (Pedersen-Bjergaard *et al.*, 2014), but this has long been recognized clinically, and the majority of Type 1 patients have been using long-acting insulin analogues for many years (the first, glargine, was introduced way back in 2000); the marked peak effect of NPH insulin occurring 4–6 hours after injection was well-known to cause recurrent nocturnal hypoglycaemia, especially in young people, and accounted for the rapid and widespread adoption of long-acting analogues in Type 1 diabetes even in the absence of watertight evidence.

> **Practice point**
>
> Nocturnal hypoglycaemia – severe and non-severe – is reduced in studies using basal long-acting analogue insulin compared with NPH. Most Type 1 patients have used long-acting analogues for many years.

Current clinical trials comparing differences between long-acting analogues repeatedly show no difference in overall glycaemic control and the focus has been on uncovering differences in hypoglycaemia. Global statements on 'reduced hypoglycaemia' with a specific insulin preparation must be critically assessed before recommending changes in treatment (Owens *et al*., 2014), bearing in mind that only about 10% of severe hypoglycaemic episodes are nocturnal (Heller *et al*., 2016). The time period over which nocturnal hypoglycaemia is recorded in trials varies (e.g. 11:00 p.m. to 6:00 a.m., 1:00 a.m. to 6:00 a.m.) and, as seen with insulin degludec compared with glargine in Type 1 diabetes, a slightly lower nocturnal rate of hypoglycaemia was accompanied by an overall increased rate throughout the day. The rigorous trial protocols for basal insulin titration may exaggerate differences between nocturnal hypoglycaemia rates that would not be apparent in clinical practice where titration regimens are more gentle and individualized. For example, many studies aim for fasting glucose levels of about 4–5 mmol/l, lower than the NICE recommendation of 5–7 mmol/l (see later), and escalate basal insulin doses more rapidly than in clinical practice, for example by four units if fasting glucose is 10–15 mmol/l and six units if >15 mmol/l (Birkeland *et al*., 2011). A study of degludec vs glargine in Type 1 patients reported achieved fasting glucose levels for both insulins that were much higher than the target – about 8 mmol/l (Heller *et al*., 2016). Finally, the variable timing of basal insulin in trials probably adds further uncertainty to the relevance of statements about hypoglycaemia reduction with specific insulin products.

The higher-concentration insulin preparations (e.g. U200 degludec, U300 glargine) are intended for use in Type 2 diabetes, though U300 glargine gave results indistinguishable from U100 glargine in people with long-duration Type 1 diabetes, and these preparations may be of practical help in the unusual case of a Type 1 person requiring high basal insulin doses (Home *et al*., 2015). It is striking that in contemporary comparative studies continuous glucose monitoring (see **Chapter 8**), now long-established and reliable in clinical practice, has not been used even in subgroups of Type 1 patients in clinical trials; they would enhance and objectify analyses of hypoglycaemia.

> **Practice point**
>
> Long-acting insulin analogues in Type 1 diabetes have virtually indistinguishable clinical profiles.

Short-acting analogues: 'eat-and-inject'

The benefits of the short-acting prandial insulin preparations (lispro, aspart and glulisine) were even less apparent; trials, meta-analyses and the HypoAna studies agree that daytime hypoglycaemia is no different when using analogue or human prandial insulin, and achieved HbA$_{1c}$ levels are the same. Many of the studies of the latest short-acting analogue to be approved (glulisine, mid-2000s) were devoted to exploring the pharmacokinetics of this especially rapid-acting insulin, but there were no comparative studies with other insulin analogues (Home, 2012). A faster-acting aspart preparation (fiasp) was introduced in 2017, coincidentally the same year the patent expired on aspart itself. It is not a new analogue, but standard aspart in a diluent containing several new excipients thought to inhibit insulin hexamer formation (nicotinamide, L-arginine and trometamol). It may marginally improve glycaemia by reducing postprandial glucose excursions compared with standard aspart but there are no clinically meaningful advantages.

Practice point

The short-acting analogues are now old: their advantages over human soluble insulin preparations are more assumed than supported by clinical trials.

An additional proposed advantage of short-acting prandial insulin was the possibility of postprandial injection ('flexibility', 'eat-and-inject'), which is widely advised. However, studies supporting this practice were not performed as part of the clinical trial programme and there is very little to support it. In the best trial, using lispro, all measures of glycaemia were significantly and probably clinically meaningfully worse with immediate postmeal compared with immediate premeal injection (Schernthaner *et al.*, 2004).

Practice point

Fast-acting analogues should not be injected after meals, even immediately, as glycaemic control is worse than when taken before meals. The current advice is wherever possible to inject prandial insulin 15 minutes before the start of a meal.

GLYCAEMIC TARGETS AND EVIDENCE FOR THEM

Current United Kingdom and USA recommendations are shown in **Table 7.3**. The NICE Guidelines Development Group (2015) justified its HbA$_{1c}$ target of 6.5% (48) or lower by judging that the risk of retinopathy developing in the DCCT and other studies was minimal at that level, with no appreciable benefit at lower values. Mean HbA$_{1c}$ in the DCCT intensive group was quoted as just under 7% (53), though the median value quoted by the DCCT itself was 7.2% (55). A further justification was that, in practice, 7% or lower would be more likely achieved if the guideline target value were set at 6.5%, an assumption that itself is not evidence-based. Finally, there is a bias in guidelines to quote self-monitored blood glucose levels associated with specific HbA$_{1c}$ values that are lower than would be

Table 7.3 Current recommendations for glycaemic targets in Type 1 diabetes and associated derived values from the ADAG study.

	NICE (2015)	ADA (2015)	ADAG (2014)
HbA$_{1c}$	≤6.5% (48)	≤7.0% (53)	6.5–6.99% (48–52)
Fasting glucose (mmol/l)	5–7	–	8.4
Preprandial (mmol/l)	4–7	4–7	7.1 (prelunch)
Postprandial (mmol/l)	5–9 (≥90 mins after meal)	<10 (1–2 hours after meal)	7.9 (postevening meal)

Sources: NICE NG17 (2015); American Diabetes Association (2015).

mathematically predicted. The ADAG study (Wei *et al.*, 2014) established the best available estimates; it can be seen that for desired HbA$_{1c}$ levels between 6.5% (48) and 7.0% (53), which span the UK and USA recommendations, the average blood glucose levels needed to achieve this level are considerably higher (and probably safer from the point of view of hypoglycaemia risk) than the quoted numbers. They are also more realistic given the limitations of current injected insulin therapy and congruent with clinical trial data showing, for example, optimum achieved fasting glucose levels about 8 mmol/l (see previously).

Glycaemic control in real life

The ultra-low targets enshrined in aspirational documents are far removed from actual glycaemic control reported in whole countries, regions and individual clinics. However, there are encouraging trends emerging in reports from some countries where data has been systematically collected over many years. For example, in Germany and Austria, population HbA$_{1c}$ levels in children and adolescents have fallen consistently over nearly 20 years. Changes, averaging out at −0.04% HbA$_{1c}$ per year were the same for all modes of treatment (conventional – 1–3 injections a day; multiple dose – four or more injections; and insulin pump), strongly implicating system-wide factors and not innovations in insulin products in these striking and consistent improvements (Rosenbauer *et al.*, 2012). Examples of non-insulin factors include increased frequency of home glucose monitoring, intensive diabetes education, multiprofessional teams and collaborative quality improvement programmes, such as the German DPV initiative itself. Remarkably, rates of serious hypoglycaemia have simultaneously fallen too (Karges *et al.*, 2017), an achievement that was not predicted by the results of the DCCT where there was a close inverse relationship between the rates of severe hypoglycaemia and HbA$_{1c}$. The encouraging lack of correlation between low HbA$_{1c}$ and increased rates of severe hypoglycaemia has also been reported in under-18s in cross-sectional studies from Western Australia and the USA (Haynes *et al.*, 2016). The situation is not as well documented in older age groups. Hospitalization resulting from severe hypoglycaemia fell in the over-16s in Denmark between 2006 and 2012 (Ishtiak-Ahmed *et al.*, 2017), but more data is needed on changes in HbA$_{1c}$ in older people before generalized self-congratulation is justified.

Glycaemic control in individuals over long periods of time: glycaemic 'tracking'

There are also trends in glycaemia over the lifetime of people with Type 1 diabetes, with the expected peak in HbA$_{1c}$ during adolescence and early adulthood, and a gradual downwards drift through middle age and beyond (**Figure 7.2**); this is associated with decreased risks of diabetic ketoacidosis, but an increased tendency to hypoglycaemia (see **Chapter 14**). Within these trends is the phenomenon of glycaemic 'tracking', which defines groups of people whose glycaemic control, seemingly independent of treatments, remains poor and fixed, often for many years, and which predisposes them to microvascular complications. Groups of young people tracking at the highest levels (often ethnic minority patients, those at socioeconomic disadvantage and in single-parent households) need identifying for particularly intensive educational and medical attention.

Insulin regimens and glycaemic control in real-life studies

A study of children and adolescents attending a French diabetes camp between 2009 and 2014 found that HbA$_{1c}$ was the same (8.1–8.3%, 65–67) whether patients were using pumps, multiple dose insulin or 2–3 injections a day (though not solely biphasic insulin). Mean HbA$_{1c}$ was much higher, 9.0% (75) in biphasic users, but there are likely to be other factors contributing to less good control in this group (Keller *et al.*, 2017).

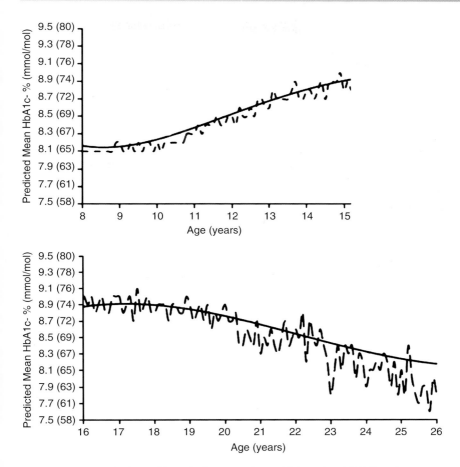

Figure 7.2 Changes in HbA$_{1c}$ with age in the T1D Exchange Clinic Registry (USA).There is a consistent climb in values from later childhood through adolescence, peaking at 16–18 years, then gradually falling during the 20s. There is a further slow fall from 40 years onwards, with an associated decreased risk of diabetic ketoacidosis, but increased hypoglycaemia. *Source*: Clements *et al.*, 2016. Reproduced with permission of John Wiley and Sons.

Notably, these results are very similar to the Hvidøre study reporting on glycaemic control in young people, mostly European, in the early years of the millennium. Mean HbA$_{1c}$ was 8.1–8.2% (65–66) in subjects using insulin pumps, basal-bolus regimens and hybrid regimens, higher in those taking twice-daily premix insulin (8.6%, 70), but at least as good (7.9%, 63) in children on the now much-less used twice daily free-mixed regimen of NPH and soluble insulin (de Beaufort *et al.*, 2007). Control with any insulin regimen was good in those centres with overall low HbA$_{1c}$ values. The team educating and implementing insulin in conjunction with the individual patient is far more important than the brand, or even – with some exceptions – the insulin regimen.

> **Practice point**
>
> Good glycaemic control in Type 1 diabetes does not depend on the insulin regimen or insulin type used (analogue/human or different analogues) but on the team supervising and coordinating care and whole-system support for patients.

FIXED INSULIN DOSE REGIMENS: BIPHASIC MIXTURES

The consistently worse control associated with twice-daily biphasic insulin taken before breakfast and the evening meal means this regimen has almost disappeared from use in some countries, for example Germany and Austria (Bohn *et al.*, 2016), and some centres. In the SEARCH study in young people in the USA, although HbA$_{1c}$ increased in all subjects with time, the rise was smaller in people who had intensified their insulin regimen, compared with those who remained on once or twice-daily biphasic insulin (Pihoker *et al.*, 2013). Individualization is, as always, of paramount importance. Some patients, perhaps for practical reasons, prefer or insist on biphasic insulin, and since there is no evidence that pushing these patients to change to multiple dose insulin results in improved glycaemic control, the approach should be continual explanation and guidance; many patients will at some stage volunteer to move to multiple dose insulin. There is a pragmatic case for using biphasic insulins during short periods of personal or psychological difficulties that prevent patients focusing on their diabetes. Thereby they can at least avoid an insulin-free period in the middle of the day, while accepting the difficulty of reliably taking insulin in the middle of a fraught working day at a lunchtime that may vary by two hours or more (or may not happen at all for many people in the current work environment). Consider how reliably you would take a tablet or injection at lunchtime as part of a four-times daily ritual. None of these important practical considerations have been explored in clinical studies and it is not even known how frequently people in education or in employment take their prelunch dose of insulin.

Paediatricians sometimes use three-times daily insulin as a bridge between twice-daily biphasic insulin and multiple dose insulin. This manoeuvre is nearly always used to avoid the mid-day injection, but the regimen is complicated and requires three different insulin preparations: a biphasic mixture before breakfast, fast-acting before the evening meal, and basal insulin at bedtime. A better three-injection regimen may be one injection of the coformulation of the ultra-long-acting analogue degludec and aspart with one meal, and two further injections of aspart with the other two meals – a trial found that it was non-inferior to multiple dose insulin (Hirsch *et al.*, 2017).

> **Practice point**
>
> Twice-daily biphasic insulin rarely gives good glycaemic control in Type 1 diabetes; gently encourage patients to consider moving to multiple-dose insulin.

BASAL-BOLUS INSULIN (MULTIPLE DOSE INSULIN, FLEXIBLE INSULIN THERAPY)

The standard for injected insulin regimens in Type 1 diabetes, comprising multiple daily doses of insulin that includes a basal (background) insulin preparation and variable numbers of bolus (short-acting, prandial) doses (**Figure 7.3**). The introduction of

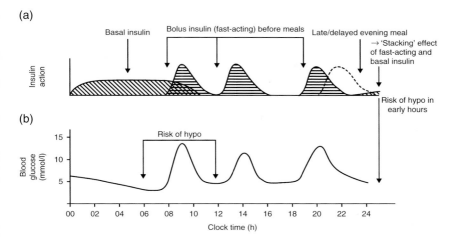

Figure 7.3 Basal-bolus insulin regimen. (a) Standard insulin action schematic; (b) typical resulting blood glucose profile, emphasizing likely times of hypoglycaemic reactions. Bedtime long-acting analogue insulin may cover long lie-ins and missed breakfasts, but in patients who eat dinner late in the evening and then go to bed shortly afterwards, there is a risk of insulin 'stacking' and hypogly-caemia in the middle of the night. See text for discussion of this problem and possible solutions.

basal-bolus insulin therapy was driven by progress in the technology of injection pens from the 1980s onwards. Practitioners who wish to manage Type 1 patients must be confident with this regimen and be able to work closely with patients to adjust dosing and timing of injections to optimize glycaemic control and reduce the risks of severe hypoglycaemia. There should also be access to some form of carbohydrate counting course, for example DAFNE.

In general, the more boluses given during the day the better the glycaemic control. Most studies have been done in people using insulin pumps, as the detailed bolus history can be retrieved. In general they have shown that omitting one or more mealtime boluses each week is the most important reason for suboptimal control and can account for up to 1% difference in HbA$_{1c}$ (Burdick *et al.*, 2004).

Initial insulin strategy

- Basal insulin dose is approximately 0.3–0.4 U/kg/day. In the United Kingdom the most widely used basal insulin is glargine (e.g. Lantus [Sanofi], Abasaglar [Lilly]).
- Prandial insulin approximately 0.45 U/kg/day, resulting in a basal:prandial insulin ratio around 40%:60% (King *et al.*, 2012). Initially, prandial insulin can be divided up approximately according to carbohydrate intake at each meal, so, for example, 30% with breakfast, 30% with lunch and 40% with evening meal.

Basal insulin

Glargine and degludec are widely used once a day, while NPH and detemir are usually given twice daily. Few systematic studies are available to help clinicians and patients optimize the timing of basal analogue insulin. Glargine is widely believed to be a true

24-hour basal insulin, but blood glucose levels rise around the time of once-daily injection whatever time it is given (Ashwell *et al.*, 2006). Given the importance of basal insulin to overall glycaemic control, it is assumed, rather than known, that bedtime injection allows more precise titration against fasting glucose values. In the more recent trials of degludec compared with glargine, degludec was consistently taken at dinner time, while glargine was given at bedtime (Owens *et al.*, 2014); the reasons for this discrepancy were not given and the actual times at which the different insulin were given is not known. It was hoped that the long action of degludec would permit dosing less often than once daily, but trials of degludec taken three times weekly showed worse control and more hypoglycaemia compared with once daily glargine. The optimum timing of twice-daily detemir is unknown in Type 1 diabetes.

Potencies of basal insulin preparations

Long-acting insulin analogues do not have identical potencies. The least potent, unit for unit, is detemir; the number of units required to give the same fasting glucose levels is considerably higher than glargine, and up to 30% more in Type 1 children (Abali *et al.*, 2015). Glargine and NPH are similar in potency, degludec around 10% more potent than either. The corresponding figures for higher-concentration insulin (e.g. U300 glargine) are not known but overall these differences may have clinically meaningful consequences and practitioners must exercise great caution when suggesting changes to long-acting insulin preparations, especially when glycaemic control is already good. Because there are no differences in achieved glycaemic control or overall or severe hypoglycaemia between these preparations, there should be little need to recommend changes, and certainly not frequent changes.

Practice point

Detemir (and NPH) are usually given twice daily, glargine and degludec once daily. There is no evidence to guide the best times for injecting basal insulin in Type 1 patients. For equal glycaemic efficacy detemir consistently requires higher doses than other long-acting analogues.

Dosage adjustment

Optimizing basal insulin treatment requires intensive blood glucose monitoring associated with frequent small changes in insulin doses. Good overnight and peri-breakfast glucose control is more important than daytime control for reducing HbA$_{1c}$ values (Maahs *et al.*, 2014), so this should be the initial focus for intensive management when control is suboptimal, though it is difficult to see how this can be precisely managed if patients are using twice-daily basal insulin taken – as often is the case – first thing in the morning and 12 hours later in the early evening. Neglect of overnight control results in a tendency for the night-time:daytime insulin ratio to fall, indicating disproportionate attempts to control (often amounting to 'chasing') prandial glucose levels, though this hazardous situation, which often results in daytime hypoglycaemia, is much better recognized and less often encountered. Diagnosis and treatment can be helped in the individual by diagnostic continuous glucose monitoring (CGM) studies, usually conducted over 5–7 consecutive days. Unfortunately, there are no studies of the effects of food, alcohol and exercise on basal insulin requirements, so suggestions on adjusting doses are pragmatic and no doubt idiosyncratic.

Prandial insulin

Control of postprandial glucose excursions is a real problem in many patients. Increasing use of continuous glucose monitoring systems often highlights profound rises in glucose levels after high carbohydrate intake, and in response some patients voluntarily curb carbohydrate. In pharmacodynamic studies, rapid-acting analogues consistently mimic normal mealtime insulin excursions more closely than older soluble insulin preparations, and show a faster rise (as designed), higher peak insulin levels and a slightly more rapid offset, though even three hours after injection there is no meaningful difference in insulin levels compared with human soluble insulin (see example in **Figure 7.4**). These encouraging findings stimulated the still widespread practice of injecting prandial analogues during or even after a meal, a practice based on highly tenuous evidence; this may have contributed in part to the weak evidence that quality of life measures were better compared with older soluble insulin (Home, 2012). Glucose control is better if rapid-acting analogues are taken about 15 minutes before a meal (Luijf *et al.*, 2010). As long- and short-acting analogues are nearly always now used in combination, separating their effects on glycaemic control and rates of hypoglycaemia is no longer possible and their use in preference to human soluble insulin is a matter of habit rather than evidence.

Standard dose-titration against a postprandial glucose measurement is still used, but carbohydrate counting is preferred as a way of adjusting prandial insulin doses. Carbohydrate counting systems using, for example DAFNE (Dose Adjustment For Normal Eating) in the United Kingdom, modified from a highly successful programme in

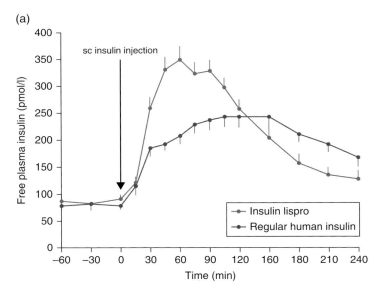

Figure 7.4 Pharmacokinetics of lispro insulin compared with human soluble insulin. The rapid rise of serum insulin levels, with higher peak values, was the aim of the development of the rapid-acting analogues. The offset of action, however, is not especially rapid and in clinical practice postprandial hypoglycaemia is not meaningfully reduced. *Source*: Heinemann *et al.*, 1996. Reproduced with permission of John Wiley & Sons.

Germany, aim to increase patients' confidence in adjusting prandial insulin according to carbohydrate load and preprandial glucose results. The results of a comprehensive evaluation of DAFNE in the United Kingdom were mixed: confidence was certainly gained, especially in people with high levels of diabetes stress and elevated HbA$_{1c}$ but the dose calculations are complex, estimations of carbohydrate content of food became less accurate with time, and many patients experienced waning confidence in their ability to adjust doses. Effects on glycaemia are not consistent (Heller *et al.*, 2014). Patients can be relieved of much of the arithmetic burden by using glucose meters with in-built automated bolus calculators, though whether they improve glycaemia is a question that studies have not yet definitively answered (Colin and Paris, 2013).

Practice point

Formal carbohydrate counting systems, for example DAFNE, may boost confidence and reduce diabetes-related stress in some people but they do not consistently improve glycaemic control.

Adherence to insulin injections

There is little population data on adherence to insulin treatment in Type 1 diabetes, though groups of patients where this is known to be a particular problem (for example, young women with disordered eating, or those with brittle diabetes) have been studied extensively. In insulin-taking patients, many of whom will be Type 2, data linkage with prescriptions consistently shows adherence of less than 80%, and this may not be too different in Type 1 diabetes. Older and more recent studies report high levels of insulin omission, especially after overeating (increasing in one study from 8% in 11–13 year olds to nearly 40% in 17–19 year olds) (Wisting *et al.*, 2013), and this practice may continue until middle-age and beyond.

In general the more boluses given during the day the better the glycaemic control, and given the effort involved in taking extra injections, especially with snacks, this relationship is probably causal (Patton *et al.*, 2014).

Practice point

Sensitive discussion can elicit patterns of insulin omission, and managing this problem is probably more productive than moving to a more intensive insulin regimen with a risk of even lower adherence.

Practical considerations

Injection sites

Always examine them. In comparison with animal insulins, analogues cause lipoatrophy very infrequently, but it has been reported (Babiker and Datta, 2011). However, lipohypertrophy is common, especially in patients with long-standing diabetes who understandably habitually inject in the same sites. Fibrosis and other changes in the subcutaneous tissues are evident even when there is no clinical lipohypertrophy. Clinically patients often notice that previously good control has slipped over the course of about a year, with associated and puzzling changes in HbA$_{1c}$. They may also notice that mealtime injections are slower to act or are increasingly unpredictable in their effects. These clinical observations are supported by an elegant crossover study. Insulin absorption was reduced by injecting into lipohypertropic sites, with a lower risk of hypoglycaemia, but postprandial glucose variability was higher and peak glucose levels were about one-quarter higher and occurred later (Famulla *et al.*, 2016). Advise on using extensive injection sites and encourage injections in the abdomen, and not in the limbs. Resolving this can lead to restoration of previous good control.

Practice point

Subclinical lipohypertrophy caused by repeated injections into the same area is a frequent reason for otherwise puzzling deterioration in glycaemic control.

Mixing techniques

In the small number of patients still using cloudy insulin preparations (isophane, biphasics), ensure that mixing technique is sound, that is 15 gentle rolls of the pen or vial before each injection.

Injection technique and blood glucose meters

Not usually as big a problem as failure to rotate injection sites. There is a great deal of agonizing about optimum needle length and angle of injection. Perpendicular injection after a routine air-shot of two units using a 4- or 5-mm needle is recommended. It is not clear that ultra-short needles are meaningfully more comfortable than slightly longer needles and insulin given even slightly carelessly through a very short needle may result in intracutaneous injection. Blood glucose meters may be many years older than patients think they are. Encourage them to get an up-to-date meter if there is any hint of the old one not working or giving imprecise measurements.

Practice point

Regularly review injection sites and technique. If insulin does not get to the correct place (subcutaneous fat) in the intended dose it has no chance of working properly.

Trouble-shooting glucose control problems in patients taking multiple dose insulin

Establish patterns of glucose control

Request a spread of blood glucose measurements throughout the day over a week or two. DAFNE courses encourage only preprandial glucose testing, but postprandial levels are important. Even more important is overnight control and access to continuous glucose monitoring (CGM). It is impossible to overestimate the importance of detecting and reducing hypoglycaemia, especially severe episodes, which have a long prognostic reach: for example in a large Taiwanese cohort all-cause and cardiovascular mortality continued to be elevated for five years after an episode of severe hypoglycaemia (relative risk 1.7), though the highest risk (relative risk 2.7) occurred in the first year (Lu *et al.*, 2016).

Overnight and fasting control

Even with long-acting analogues nocturnal hypoglycaemia is common; a CGM study in Type 1 patients in their mid-40s with an average of 20 years diabetes discovered hypoglycaemia (glucose <3.9 mmol/l between midnight and 6:00 a.m.) in nearly 30% of nights. When hypoglycaemia occurred it went on for a long time – a median of nearly two hours (Desjardins et al., 2013). The situation may be worse in younger people. Hypoglycaemia is no less profound or extensive in patients using pumps than multiple dose insulin. There is no clear relationship between the carbohydrate content of a bedtime snack and whether rapid-acting insulin is taken. Even with careful CGM analysis in individuals it is often very difficult to work out a consistent link.

The dawn phenomenon – fasting and postbreakfast hyperglycaemia – is common in Type 1, especially in poorly-controlled pubertal patients, where surges in insulin antagonist growth hormone levels may contribute. CGM is the only technique that will help distinguish between persistent hyperglycaemia overnight due to inadequate long-acting insulin and the dawn phenomenon, which will not respond to increasing the dose of basal insulin. If the dawn phenomenon is marked and persistent, insulin pump treatment with programmed increased basal rates in the latter part of the night is the best option. Persistent overnight hyperglycaemia will often respond to relatively small increases in basal insulin doses or larger doses of short-acting insulin with late meals. Patients who are anxious about nocturnal hypoglycaemia are reluctant to increase their basal insulin, and CGM may reassure them.

Practice point

Suspicion of nocturnal hypoglycaemia (measured low fasting glucose, erratic fasting levels, symptomatic events) is best analysed by diagnostic continuous glucose monitoring.

Daytime hypoglycaemia

Hypoglycaemia during the day is as common with fast-acting analogues as with soluble insulin preparations. The focus should be activity levels and meal timing. Missed or delayed lunch and highly variable midday meals are increasingly difficult to manage in the modern workplace; healthcare professionals have an important role in educating employers that they are obliged to make allowances for insulin-taking patients, especially over meal breaks, and facilities for blood glucose testing and injection. However, because of the risk of discrimination, Type 1 patients are often reluctant to disclose their diabetes to employers (Ruston et al., 2013).

OTHER ROUTES OF INSULIN ADMINISTRATION

The failure of the first inhaled insulin preparation (Exubera) during its short commercial life (2006–2007) confirmed that injections are not as troublesome to patients as they are to focus groups of pharmaceutical companies. Another system (Afrezza, Sanofi/Mannkind), less cumbersome to use, was quietly launched in 2015. Injected basal insulin is still needed. It may be of very occasional value in the truly needle-phobic. Although inhaled insulin is absorbed rapidly, its clinical action is similar to that of fast-acting analogue insulin, though there may be less hypoglycaemia. It is unlikely that further products will come to market. Other non-injected routes are regularly announced and some (e.g. oral) raise excitement levels in biotech circles and the media, but if they are ever introduced they are unlikely to be satisfactory for Type 1 patients.

NEW INSULIN PREPARATIONS

Peglispro had a long half-life and was relatively hepatoselective but development was discontinued in 2015 after adverse hepatic and liver effects were uncovered in Phase 3 trials. Given the failure of alternate day degludec, further long- and ultra-long acting analogues may be slow to arrive. Several attempts are being made to inhibit insulin hexamer formulation to generate ultra-fast acting insulin. The first new preparation to emerge since glulisine was the faster-acting insulin aspart (Fiasp), which was introduced in 2017. Postprandial glucose levels were numerically slightly lower compared with aspart, but HbA_{1c} levels similar. Overall, hypoglycaemia was identical but there was more hypoglycaemia in the first postprandial hour, a concern with all fast-acting analogues, though not highlighted in the original trials of lispro, aspart and glulisine.

GLYCAEMIC CONTROL IN VERY LONG DURATION TYPE 1 DIABETES

Gratifyingly, increasing numbers of patients are surviving into healthy older age with long duration diabetes. Three important studies of patients surviving 50 or more years of Type 1 diabetes have been published. In the UK Golden Years Cohort, studied at an average age of 69, mean HbA_{1c} was 7.6% (60). Long-term glycaemic trajectory was not known: did this group show glycaemic tracking so that their lifetime HbA_{1c} was not meaningfully different from that in their mid-70s? The USA Joslin Medalist Study participants were strikingly similar to their trans-Atlantic companions, with an even lower HbA_{1c} (7.0%, 53) at the time of examination. Importantly, around one-third of Joslin subjects had never had retinopathy more severe than mild non-proliferative, and more than half had never had proliferative retinopathy; only 5% had proteinuria, confirming the very poor prognosis of diabetic nephropathy, 40% had no clinical evidence of neuropathy and 50% had no cardiovascular disease. The largest cohort reported to date is from Sweden, comprising 1000 patients. Phenotypically they are similar to the USA and UK cohorts (e.g. BMI low at 25, triglycerides 1.1 mmol/l and very high mean HDL levels – 1.7 mmol/l) but mean blood pressure was not notably low (144/71 mm Hg). Importantly, however, patients of all diabetes durations were followed up for 10 years; the risks of microvascular complications increased by 10–25% for an HbA_{1c} increase of 0.5%, though the strength of this association was much less powerful beyond 40 years' duration. (Interestingly, being married, divorced or widowed was a significant protective factor against microvascular disease, suggesting a legacy effect of ever being married; Adamsson Eryd et al., 2017.)

NON-INSULIN DRUGS FOR GLYCAEMIC CONTROL IN TYPE 1 DIABETES

Several agents used in Type 2 diabetes have been studied in combination with insulin to exploit pathways that indirectly enhance insulin action. Pramlintide (synthetic amylin) is the only licensed agent and is available only in the USA. Other drugs are summarized in **Table 7.4**. Trials resulted in small effects, confirming that mechanisms apart from insulin deficiency in Type 1 diabetes are not significant. Metformin is widely prescribed in Type 1 patients, but in the patients most likely to benefit (overweight or obese adolescents) glycaemic control did not improve in a 6-month randomised study using 2 g daily. Only about one-quarter of patients showed an improvement in BMI and insulin doses (Libman et al., 2015). Metformin does not help Type 1 patients. The extra-pancreatic effects of

Table 7.4 Non-insulin glycaemic agents trialled in Type 1 diabetes.

Drug	Actions	Dose and glycaemic impact	Other effects	Comments
Metformin	Decreased hepatic glucose output and intestinal glucose metabolism; weight loss	HbA$_{1c}$ ↓ 0.1% Weight ↓ 2 kg	Possible ↑hypoglycaemia; gastrointestinal side-effects ↓insulin dose (~7 units)	In widespread use, and probably overused. Unlicensed. Not effective in overweight adolescents
Synthetic amylin (pramlintide)	Cosecreted with insulin from β-cells. Inhibits glucagon secretion, ↓hepatic glucose production; stimulates satiety; delays gastric emptying. Prandial effect only	30–60 µg s/c before meals 3–4 times daily HbA$_{1c}$ ↓0.3–0.5%	Weight ↓1 kg ↑hypoglycaemia, including severe events Prominent nausea during first few weeks of treatment	In limited use (additional injections, nausea and hypoglycaemia, and limited glycaemic impact). Licensed in Type 2 diabetes for use with prandial insulin in the USA since 2005
GLP-1-receptor agonists	Enhanced glucose-induced insulin secretion; inhibition of glucagon secretion; increased satiety; delayed gastric emptying	Exenatide: 10 µg bd or qds, 2.0 mg weekly. Liraglutide: 1.2, 1.8 mg daily HbA$_{1c}$ ↓0.2–0.4%; most studies report no change in HbA$_{1c}$	Weight ↓5% Insulin doses (basal and prandial) ↓by up to 40% ↑symptomatic hypoglycaemia, but no changes in severe hypoglycaemia ↑risk of ketosis with liraglutide 1.8 mg	Adverse effects as in Type 2 diabetes, predominantly nausea, constipation and vomiting, and tending to diminish with continued treatment
DPP-4 inhibitors	Inhibition of glucagon secretion; enhance insulin secretion in those with residual β-cell function	Sitagliptin: 100 mg daily Vildagliptin: 100 mg bd HbA$_{1c}$ ↓0.3% No change in weight	Insulin doses slightly ↓; no increase in hypoglycaemia	Well tolerated, as in Type 2 diabetes, but of limited value: the DPP-4 inhibitors are active on the incretin mechanism, and not on the satiety or gastric emptying effects
SGLT2 inhibitors	Increased renal glucose excretion. Possibly some effect on gut hormones (GLP-1, PYY) – incretin effect and satiety	Empagliflozin: 10, 25 mg daily. HbA$_{1c}$ ↓0.4–0.5%. Weight ↓1.5–2.0 kg. Canagliflozin: 100 mg, 200 mg daily. HbA$_{1c}$ ↓0.3%. Weight ↓1.5 kg	Insulin doses slightly ↓	Significant risk of diabetic ketoacidosis. Fasting β-OH butyrate levels were consistently ↑ with empagliflozin SGLT1 is a major pathway for intestinal glucose absorption. Dual SGLT1/2 inhibitors, e.g. sotagliflozin, are under investigation

Source: Frandsen *et al.*, 2016. Reproduced with permission of Elsevier.

GLP1-RA drugs are of interest, especially weight reduction. In a large placebo-controlled trial, liraglutide 1.2 mg daily reduced weight by ~4 kg, but HbA_{1c} reduction was modest, 0.2%. Symptomatic hypoglycaemia was more frequent at the 1.2 mg dose, and the highest dose, 1.8 mg daily increased the frequency of hyperglycaemia with ketosis (>1.5 mmol/l) (Ahrén et al., 2016). Adjunctive non-insulin treatments are of no value in Type 1 diabetes.

Practice point

All Type 2 drugs are unlicensed and of very limited help in Type 1. Metformin, widely used, helps neither glycaemia nor weight.

EXERCISE

People with Type 1 diabetes are no more or less inactive than the general population, which is itself encouraging, given the challenges of exercise while maintaining glucose control and avoiding hypoglycaemia. Whether any long-term benefits of exercise are mediated through reductions in HbA_{1c} is not known. Physiological and mechanistic studies are too short to demonstrate any consistent effects on glucose control (Kennedy et al., 2013) but in a large German study of young people, 3–18 years old, those exercising three or more times a week had an HbA_{1c} ~0.3% lower than their inactive peers. There were also measurable benefits on diastolic blood pressure and dyslipidaemia was less frequent in the older group (15–18 years) (Herbst et al., 2007). However, the important prospective FinnDiane study should shift our focus from inconsistent evidence of short-term metabolic effects to the increasing evidence for long-term reduction in vascular complications: moderate or high intensity exercise was associated with a lower risk of progression of albuminuria and new cardiovascular events were reduced in those doing longer and more intensive exercise (Tikkanen-Dolenc et al., 2017).

Aerobic exercise (e.g. cycling, running) tends to induce hypoglycaemia in Type 1 patients within 45 minutes. This trend is more pronounced in highly-trained people, probably because their work load intensity is higher. The recommendation is to increase carbohydrate intake or reduce insulin (or both) before exercise. Recommended glucose levels during aerobic exercise are between 7 and 10 mmol/l but higher levels are sound if they reduce hypoglycaemia risk. An episode of severe hypoglycaemia (e.g. blood glucose ≤2.8 mmol/l or hypoglycaemia requiring assistance) in the 24 hours before aerobic exercise is a contraindication to exercise, because of the greatly increased risk of a more severe episode, especially if the activity is intrinsically hazardous (e.g. downhill skiing, swimming, trekking alone). Anaerobic exercise (e.g. weights, martial arts) does not usually cause pronounced falls in glucose, and resistance exercise can increase glucose levels (**Figure 7.5**).

Strategies for maintaining safe glucose levels during exercise are complex but expert consensus is available (**Box 7.1**) (Riddell et al., 2017). Many expert patients are well aware of the extended reach of the risk of hypoglycaemia after exercise, which may continue for up to 48 hours.

ORGANIZATION OF CARE FOR TYPE 1 PATIENTS

There is remarkably little evidence on the best ways to engage Type 1 patients in the clinic system. The important transition from paediatric to adult clinic is often poorly handled, largely because the best way to achieve a smooth transition satisfactory for young

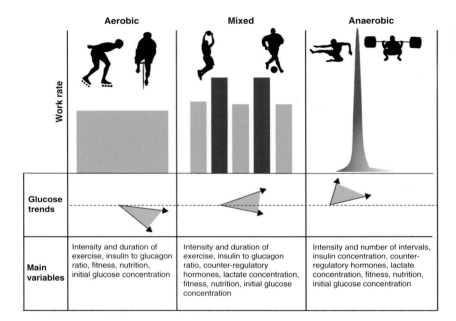

Figure 7.5 Outline of blood glucose responses to different forms of exercise in Type 1 diabetes. *Source*: Riddell *et al.*, 2017. Reproduced with permission of Elsevier.

Box 7.1 Outline strategies for glucose management before and during exercise.

- **Blood glucose levels before exercise**
  <5.0 mmol/l: take 10–20 g glucose; do not start exercise until blood glucose >5 mmol/l.
  5.0–6.9 mmol/l: take 10 g glucose before aerobic exercise but start anaerobic or high-intensity interval training without supplementation.
  7–15 mmol/l (i.e. at or slightly above target): start aerobic or anaerobic exercise; glucose levels may rise during anaerobic exercise.
  >15 mmol/l: if due to a recent meal, start exercise. If not, check blood ketones and do not exercise if >1.4 mmol/l; lower than this, restrict to light exercise for <30 minutes.
- **Carbohydrate supplementation for aerobic exercise**
  Meal taken before exercise: ≥1 g carbohydrate per kg body weight (adjust for particular exercise).
  Meal after exercise: 1.0–1.2 g carbohydrate per kg body weight.
- **Recommended carbohydrate supplementation for different exercise durations**:
  Up to 30 minutes: no carbohydrate needed for performance.
  30–60 minutes: carbohydrate at 10–15 g/h may improve performance.
  60–150 minutes: take carbohydrate at 30–60 g/h.
  >150 minutes: carbohydrates at 20–30 g every 20 minutes. Take a mixture of carbohydrates e.g. glucose and fructose.

- **Reducing the risk of late hypoglycaemia after exercise**
  - Nocturnal hypoglycaemia is common after exercise, especially if taken during the afternoon. Where possible, recommend exercise earlier in the day.
  - Reduce bolus insulin for a meal after exercise of 50%.
  - Pump patients: suggest a temporary reduction in basal insulin rate from bedtime of about 20% for six hours.
  - A bedtime snack alone without reduction in basal insulin is not enough to prevent nocturnal hypoglycaemia.
  - Strictly avoid alcohol.

Source: Modified after Riddell *et al.*, 2017.

people is unknown. Significant numbers of patients are lost to follow-up during transition, characterized by their already high risk (Mistry *et al.*, 2015):

- Diagnosis before the age of 12.
- Those taking twice or three times daily insulin (compared with multiple dose insulin or pump).
- High HbA$_{1c}$.
- Fewer clinic visits in the previous year.
- Patients who did not ask questions at the diabetes transition clinic visit.

Another critical transition period for young people is their time at university. Since this is the period after peak HbA$_{1c}$ has been reached (see earlier), it is a good opportunity to engage in improving control. In some countries, care is fully transferred to the local university hospital. In the United Kingdom and USA university health services will often be responsible, but in a US survey only one-half of college health facilities felt confident dealing with Type 1 patients (Monaghan *et al.*, 2015). In a UK survey from the mid-2000s, glycaemic control did not improve during time at university.

Outside the United Kingdom, adult Type 1 patients are seen only in teaching hospital clinics. The picture in the United Kingdom is not consistent. Type 1 patients, and certainly those with any complications, should be offered regular reviews in a hospital clinic. The geographical mobility of young people, probably combined with other factors seems to have left significant numbers of urban Type 1 patients without specialist support. This has been recognized and more intensive community programmes for education and advanced dietetics have been established. Their impact on diabetes care overall is unknown but glycaemic control in young people in the United Kingdom is consistently worse than in other advanced healthcare systems, with a mean population HbA$_{1c}$ of nearly 9% (75) (McKnight *et al.*, 2015). Using approximations from the DCCT, this could represent an approximately 30% increased risk of developing significant microvascular complications, and 9% is at or near the threshold where mortality begins to rise rapidly in a very long-term DCCT follow-up (DCCT/EDIC, 2016).

The physical locus of care has been overemphasized; the important factor is not so much where patients are seen but whether their care teams have extensive experience in managing Type 1 patients and whether the organization of care is appropriate, especially for the younger patients and those at university. It is important to recognize the quite different spectrum of concerns in Type 1 and 2 patients, some of which are outlined in **Table 7.5**.

Table 7.5 The different focus of Type 1 and Type 2 diabetes.

Clinical feature	Type 1 diabetes	Type 2 diabetes
Glycaemic control	Primary and paramount	Significant, but probably no more important than management of macrovascular risk factors, hypertension and lipids
Day to day glycaemic management	24 hour	Predominantly controlling fasting glucose levels
Obesity	Increasingly important, but weight loss is not a focus	Primary
Macrovascular disease	Rarely apparent until 20 years after diagnosis, but stage is set early on (essential hypertension, albuminuria, sustained hyperglycaemia) Premature vascular disease occurs at a relatively young age even in the absence of classical risk factors	Often apparent at presentation and still the commonest complication and cause of death
Microvascular disease	Driven nearly entirely by hyperglycaemia	Hyperglycaemia is only one of several factors involved
Insulin treatment	Primary therapy. Requires subtle and continuous adjustment	Secondary therapy, rarely needed in the early stages, and less so even in the later stages
Hypoglycaemia	A continuous threat and still a common cause of morbidity and mortality in the under 40s	Rare but serious. Usually a manageable concern
Technology	Continually changing, advanced and complicated, and a potential major contributor to improved control (e.g. insulin pump treatment, CGM, artificial pancreas; Chapter 8)	Limited importance compared with sustained lifestyle intervention, clinical care and management of cardiovascular risk factors
Education	Aim: improved management over short time periods with focus on anticipating and avoiding hypoglycaemia Flexible insulin dosing of major importance	Aim: improved management over longer time-frame (e.g. weight loss, activity)
Prepregnancy and pregnancy; contraception	Type 1 diabetes is a condition of young people Prepregnancy counselling should be a routine part of care	Although pre-existing Type 2 diabetes is becoming more important, it is much less common than in Type 1 diabetes, but represents a high risk group for perinatal complications (see Chapter 14)

References

Abali S, Turan S, Atay Z et al. Higher insulin detemir doses are required for the similar glycemic control: comparison of insulin detemir and glargine in children with type 1 diabetes mellitus. *Pediatr Diabetes* 2015;16:361–6 [PMID: 25039448].
Adamson Eryd S, Svensson AM, Franzén S et al. Risk of future microvascular and macrovascular disease in people with Type 1 diabetes of very long duration: a national study with 10-year follow-up. *Diabet Med* 2017;34:411–8 [PMID: 27647178].

Ahrén B, Hirsch IB, Pieber TR *et al*. ADJUNCT TWO Investigators. Efficacy and safety of liraglutide added to capped insulin treatment in subjects with Type 1 diabetes: the ADJUNCT TWO Randomized Trial. *Diabetes Care* 2016;39:1693–701 [PMID: 27493132] Free full text.

American Diabetes Association. Standards of medical care in diabetes – 2015. *Diabetes Care* 2015;38(Suppl 1): S33–S40.

Ashwell SG, Gebbie J, Home PD. Optimal timing of injection of once-daily insulin glargine in people with Type 1 diabetes using insulin lispro at meal-times. *Diabet Med* 2006;23:46–52 [PMID: 16409565].

Babiker A, Datta V. Lipoatrophy with insulin analogues in type 1 diabetes. *Arch Dis Child* 2011;96:101–2 [PMID: 20570843].

de Beaufort CE, Swift PG, Skinner CT *et al*. Hvidoere Study Group on Childhood Diabetes 2005. Continuing stability of center differences in pediatric diabetes care: do advances in diabetes treatment improve outcome? The Hvidoere Study Group on Childhood Diabetes. *Diabetes Care* 2007;30:2245–50 [PMID: 17540955].

Birkeland KI, Home PD, Wendisch U *et al*. Insulin degludec in type 1 diabetes: a randomized controlled trial of a new-generation ultra-long-acting insulin compared with insulin glargine. *Diabetes Care* 2011;34:661–5 [PMID: 21270174] PMC3041203.

Bohn B, Karges B, Vogel C *et al*. DPV Initiative. 20 years of pediatric benchmarking in Germany and Austria: age-dependent analysis of longitudinal follow-up in 63,967 children and adolescents with type 1 diabetes. *PLoS One* 2016;11:e0160971/ [PMID: 27532627] PMC4988648.

Burdick J, Chase HP, Slover RH *et al*. Missed insulin meal boluses and elevated haemoglobin A1c levels in children receiving insulin pump therapy. *Pediatrics* 2004;113(3 Pt 1):e221–4 [PMID: 14993580].

Clements MA, Foster NC, Maahs DM *et al*. T1D Exchange Clinic Network. Hemoglobin A1c (HbA1c) changes over time among adolescent and young adult participants in the T1D exchange clinic registry. *Pediatr Diabetes* 2016;17:327–36 [PMID: 26153338].

Colin IM, Paris I. Glucose meters with built-in automated bolus calculator: gadget or real value for insulin-treated diabetic patients? *Diabetes Ther* 2013;4:1–11 [PMID: 23250633] PMC36877095.

DCCT/EDIC (Diabetes Control and Complications Trial/Epidemiology of Diabetes Interventions and Complications) Study Research Group. Mortality in type 1 diabetes in the DCCT/EDIC versus the general population. *Diabetes Care* 2016;39:1378–83 [PMID: 27411699] PMC4955932.

Desjardins K, Brazeau AS, Strychar I *et al*. Association between post-dinner dietary intakes and nocturnal hypoglycemic risk in adult patients with type 1 diabetes. *Diabetes Res Clin Pract* 2013;106:420–7 [PMID: 25451901].

Famulla S, Hövelmann U, Fischer A *et al*. Insulin injection into lipohypertrophic tissue: blunted and more variable insulin absorption and action and impaired postprandial glucose control. *Diabetes Care* 2016;39:1486–92 [PMID: 27411698].

Frandsen CS, Dejgaard TF, Madsbad S. Non-insulin drugs to treat hyperglycaemia in type 1 diabetes mellitus. *Lancet Diabetes Endocrinol* 2016;4:766–80 [PMID: 26969516].

Haynes A, Hermann JM, Miller KM *et al*. T1D Exchange, WACDD and DPV registries. Severe hypoglycaemia rates are not associated with HbA1c: a cross-sectional analysis of 3 contemporary pediatric diabetes registry databases. *Pediatr Diabetes* 2016 [Epub ahead of print] [PMID: 27878914].

Heinemann L, Kapitza C, Starke AA, Heise T. Time-action profile of the insulin analogue B28Asp. *Diabet Med* 1996;13:683–4 [PMID: 8840108].

Heller S, Lawton J, Amiel S *et al*. Improving management of type 1 diabetes in the UK; the Dose Adjustment For Normal Eating (DAFNE) programme as a research test-bed. *Southampton (UK): NIHR Journals Library*; 2014 Dec [PMID: 25642502] Free full text.

Heller S, Mathieu C, Kapur R *et al*. A meta-analysis of rate ratios for nocturnal confirmed hypoglycaemia with insulin degludec vs insulin glargine using different definitions for hypoglycaemia. *Diabet Med* 2-16;33:478-87 [PMID: 26484727] PMC5064738.

Herbst A, Kordonouri O, Schwab KO *et al*. Impact of physical activity on cardiovascular risk in children with type 1 diabetes: a multicenter study of 23,251 patients. *Diabetes Care* 2007;30:2098–100 [PMID: 17468347].

Hirsch IB, Franek E, Mersebach H *et al*. Safety and efficacy of insulin degludec/insulin aspart with bolus mealtime insulin aspart compared with standard basal-bolus treatment in people with Type

1 diabetes: 1-year results from a randomized controlled trial (BOOST® T1). *Diabet Med* 2017;34:167–73 [PMID: 26773446] PMC26773446.

Home PD. The pharmacokinetics and pharmacodynamics of rapid-acting insulin analogues and their clinical consequences. *Diabetes Obes Metab* 2012;14:780–8 [PMID: 22321739].

Home PD, Bergenstal RM, Bolli GB *et al*. New insulin glargine 300 units/mL versus glargine 100 U/mL in people with type 1 diabetes: a randomized, phase 3a, open-label clinical trial (EDITION 4). *Diabetes Care* 2015;38:2217–25 [PMID: 26084341].

Ishtiak-Ahmed K, Carstensen B, Pedersen-Bjergaard IJ, Jørgensen ME. Incidence trends and predictors of hospitalization for hypoglycemia in 17.230 adult patients with type 1 diabetes: a Danish register linkage cohort study. *Diabetes Care* 2017;40:226–32 [PMID: 27899494].

Karges B, Kepellen T, Wagner VM *et al*.; DPV Initiative. Glycated hemoglobin A1c as a risk factor for severe hypoglycaemia in pediatric type 1 diabetes. *Pediatr Diabetes* 2017;18:51–8 [PMID: 26712064].

Keller M, Attia R, Beltrand J *et al*. Insulin regimens, diabetes, knowledge, quality of life, and HbA1c in children and adolescents with type 1 diabetes. *Pediatr Diabetes* 2017;18:340–7 [PMID: 27161814].

Kennedy A, Nirantharakumar K, Chimen M *et al*. Does exercise improve glycaemic control in type 1 diabetes? A systematic review and meta-analysis. *PLoS One* 2013;8:e58861 [PMID: 23554942] PMC3598953.

King AB, Clark D, Wolfe GS. How much do I give? Dose estimation formulas for once-nightly insulin glargine and premeal insulin lispro in type 1 diabetes mellitus. *Endocr Pract* 2012;18:382–6 [PMID: 22440988].

Libman IM, Miller KM, DiMeglio LA *et al*. T1D Exchange Clinic Network Metformin RCT Study Group. *JAMA* 2015;314:2241–50 [PMID: 26624824].

Lu CL, Shen HN, Hu SC *et al*. A population-based study of all-cause mortality and cardiovascular disease in association with prior history of hypoglycaemia among patients with type 1 diabetes. *Diabetes Care* 2016;39:1571–8 [PMID: 27385329].

Luijf YM, van Bon AC, Hoekstra JB, Devries JH. Premeal injection of rapid-acting insulin reduces postprandial glycemic excursions in type 1 diabetes. *Diabetes Care* 2010;33:2152–5 [PMID: 20693354] PMC2945151.

Maahs DM, Chase HP, Westfall E *et al*. The effects of lowering nighttime and breakfast glucose levels with sensor-augmented pump therapy on hemoglobin A1c levels in type 1 diabetes. *Diabetes Technol Ther* 2014;16:284–91 [PMID: 24450776].

McKnight JA, Wild SH, Lamb MJ *et al*., Glycaemic control of Type 1 diabetes in clinical practice early in the 21st century: an international comparison. *Diabet Med* 2015;32: 1036–50 [PMID: 25510978].

Mistry B, Van Blyderveen S, Punthakee Z, Grant C. Condition-related predictors of successful transition from paediatric to adult care among adolescents with Type 1 diabetes. *Diabet Med* 2015;32:881–5 [PMID: 25764182].

Monaghan M, Helgeson V, Wiebe D. Type 1 diabetes in young adulthood. *Curr Diabetes Rev* 2015;11:239–50 [PMID: 25901502] PMC4526384 [comprehensive review].

Neu A, Lange K, Barrett T *et al*.; Hvidoere Study Group. Classifying insulin regimens – difficulties and proposal for comprehensive new definitions. *Pediatr Diabetes* 2015;16:402–6 [PMID: 25865149].

Owens DR, Matfin G, Monnier L. Basal insulin analogues in the management of diabetes mellitus: what progress have we made? *Diabetes Metab Res Rev* 2014;30:104–19 [PMID: 24026961].

Patton SR, DeLurgio SA, Fridlington A *et al*. Frequency of mealtime insulin bolus predicts glycated haemoglobin in youths with type 1 diabetes. *Diabetes Technol Ther* 2014;16:519–23 [PMID: 24773597] PMC4172563.

Pedersen-Bjergaard U, Kristensen PL, Beck-Nielsen H *et al*. Effect of insulin analogues on risk of severe hypoglycaemia in patients with type 1 diabetes prone to recurrent severe hypoglycaemia (HypoAna trial): a prospective, randomised, open-label, blinded-endpoint crossover trial. *Lancet Diabetes Endocrinol* 2014;2:553–61 [PMID: 24794703].

Pihoker C, Badaru A, Anderson A et al. SEARCH for Diabetes in Youth Study Group. Insulin regimens and clinical outcomes in a type 1 diabetes cohort: the SEARCH for Diabetes in Youth Study. Diabetes Care 2013;36:27–33 [PMID: 22961571] PMC3526205.

Riddell MC, Gallen IW, Smart CE et al. Exercise management in type 1 diabetes: consensus statement. Lancet Diabetes Endocrinol 2017;5:377–90 [PMID: 28126459].

Rosenbauer J, Dost A, Karges B et al. DPV Initiative and the German BMBF Competence Network Diabetes Mellitus. Improved metabolic control in children and adolescents with type 1 diabetes: a trend analysis using prospective multicenter data from Germany and Austria. Diabetes Care 2012;35:80–6 [PMID: 22074726] PMC3241332.

Ruston A, Smith A, Fernando B. Diabetes in the workplace: diabetic's perceptions and experiences of managing their disease at work: a qualitative study. BMC Public Health 2013;13:386 [PMID: 23617727] PMC3649948.

Schernthaner G, Wein W, Shnawa N et al. Preprandial vs. postprandial insulin lispro – a comparative crossover trial in patients with Type 1 diabetes. Diabet Med 2004;21:279–84 [PMID: 15008840].

Tikkanen-Dolenc H, Wadén H, Forsblom C et al.; FinnDiane Study Group. Frequent and intensive physical activity reduces risk of cardiovascular events in type 1 diabetes. Diabetologia 2017;60:574–80 [PMID: 28013340].

Wei N, Zheng H, Nathan DM. Empirically establishing blood glucose targets to achieve HbA1c goals. Diabetes Care 2014;37:1048–51 [PMID: 24513588] PMC3964488.

Wisting L, Frøisland DH, Skrivarhaug T et al. Disturbed eating behaviour and omission of insulin in adolescents receiving intensified insulin treatment: a nationwide population- based study. Diabetes Care 2013;36:3382–7 [PMID: 23963896] PMC 3816868.

8 Type 1 diabetes: technology and transplants

Key points

- Microvascular complications of Type 1 diabetes can be reliably prevented if HbA$_{1c}$ can be maintained in the long-term at <7% (53)
- This can be achieved in a substantial proportion of patients using multiple dose insulin and routine home (self) blood glucose monitoring
- Insulin pump treatment improves quality of life, may improve glycaemia in many patients and overall reduces severe hypoglycaemia
- Continuous subcutaneous glucose monitoring (CGM) improves glycaemic control in a variety of different situations if there is high adherence; diagnostic CGM is educationally valuable
- These intermediate-level technologies are used to widely different extents even in countries that spend a lot on healthcare
- Eventually the artificial pancreas may be available widely enough to prevent most end-stage complications
- The results of islet and whole pancreas transplants continue to improve. Always consider whether patients fulfil the continually developing criteria for transplantation

INTRODUCTION

Most technology now routine in Type 1 diabetes is relatively low level and not high cost, for example insulin injection pens and finger-prick blood glucose monitoring, but there are wide variations in their use. For example, traditional insulin vials and syringes are widely used in the USA because of cost, while elsewhere they are almost never encountered. Simple devices have contributed to the improved glycaemic control and reduced rates of end-stage microvascular complications documented in many countries over the past 10–15 years. Overall, however, glycaemia at the population level is still not consistently low enough to minimize microvascular events, but there is confidence that emerging technology, culminating in a commercially-available artificial pancreas, will further improve these outcomes. The challenge for the foreseeable future will be to integrate increasingly sophisticated technology into routine care in cost-constrained times.

Practice point

Impressive though technology is for Type 1 diabetes, it requires patients and clinicians to use it critically and with sensitivity.

Practical Diabetes Care, Fourth Edition. David Levy.
© 2018 John Wiley & Sons Ltd. Published 2018 by John Wiley & Sons Ltd.

GLUCOSE METERS AND HOME BLOOD GLUCOSE MONITORING (HBGM; SELF-MONITORING OF BLOOD GLUCOSE, USA – SMBG)

While there is still an active debate over the benefit of routine home capillary blood glucose monitoring in Type 2 diabetes (see **Chapter 10**), there is less argument in Type 1 diabetes, though the association between increased frequency of blood glucose testing and lower HbA_{1c} has not been shown to be causal and is better considered as a marker of good self-management. In the large but not fully representative T1D Exchange cohort in the USA, in all age groups and in both pump and multiple daily injection users there was a fall in HbA_{1c} across the spectrum of testing frequency, from 0–2 up to >13 tests per day. The most marked fall was in the 13–26 year age group and between the groups testing 0–2 and 5–6 times daily, associated with approximately 1.5% HbA_{1c} reduction in patients using multiple daily injections and 1.0% in pump users. These data were robust for extensive statistical correction for ethnicity and a variety of socioeconomic factors (Miller *et al.*, 2013). Testing up to six times daily should be encouraged and healthcare professionals should make the case for Type 1 patients to be prescribed sufficient glucose test strips (up to 1 container of 50 strips a week); test strips are a traditional area for pharmacy cost-cutting (though the burden of cost is in Type 2 patients not treated with insulin where the value of HBGM is not established).

Glucose results have traditionally been laboriously written in record books. In a small formal crossover trial in pump patients glucose control was meaningfully better (including less hypoglycaemia) when a proprietary electronic information management system was used (Reichel *et al.*, 2013). We should encourage patients to use electronic uploads – even if the information may be more difficult for healthcare professionals to immediately interpret.

Practice point

Glucose testing up to six times a day is associated with progressive improvements in HbA_{1c}. Patients should have access to sufficient test strips if they wish to test intensively.

Bolus advisers

Improvements in technology have led to the introduction of affordable blood glucose meters with electronic bolus advisers that suggest prandial dosing. Calculations are based on carbohydrate-to-insulin ratio, glucose-correction factor, duration of insulin action and correction target. These are quantitative measures that pump patients know; multiple dose insulin patients are less likely to be familiar. Some trials show that electronic bolus advisers improve control in multiple dose insulin users (Ziegler *et al.*, 2013) without increasing hypoglycaemia rates or the numbers of test strips used. They should probably be used more frequently but currently there is no evidence that they uniformly improve glycaemia. Concerns that they de-skill people with Type 1 diabetes have no basis; accurate carbohydrate counting is a skill that few patients can acquire and once education has finished the accuracy of the estimates falls with time (see **Chapter 7**). Systems can only take into account carbohydrate intake at meals: there are many other important factors, for example the impact of physical exercise, and acute insulin resistance induced by hypoglycaemia. There are no internationally accepted standards for development of the software and there is concern about potential risk through inaccuracy, though in reality this is likely to be less than patients relying on their own calculations.

INSULIN PUMP TREATMENT (CONTINUOUS SUBCUTANEOUS INSULIN INFUSION, CSII)

The aim of pump treatment, developed in the mid-1970s, is to deliver a continuous low level of subcutaneous rapid-acting insulin to mimic physiological background (basal) insulin production; it replaces the one or two injections of long-acting insulin. Superimposed on this are self-administered boluses of the same rapid-acting insulin that aim to mimic prandial insulin secretion. Rapid-acting analogue insulin is now universally used in pumps, though good glycaemic control was achieved with animal and human soluble insulin preparations in pump-treated patients in the Diabetes Control and Complications Trial (DCCT). Continuous refinements now permit basal infusion rates to be temporarily changed as often as necessary and in tiny increments, for example 0.025 U/h. In practice adjustable basal rates are valuable and they can be set to help manage scenarios that are difficult with patients using multiple dose insulin, for example postexercise hypoglycaemia and the dawn phenomenon. One concern has emerged from the German/Austrian DPV study: patients employing a wider range of basal rates ('variability index') had a higher rate of both severe hypoglycaemia and diabetic ketoacidosis (Laimer et al., 2016). This may be association and not causal, but multiple basal rate changes instead of more precise bolus dosing may be used to correct overall glucose variability, leading to increased hypoglycaemia. Bolus doses are determined and adjusted using the calculated or estimated carbohydrate content of food. Various meal-time bolus delivery curves are built in but it is not clear that this technology delivers better glycaemia or reduces hypoglycaemia (Heinemann, 2009; see **Chapter 7**).

IMPACT OF PUMP TREATMENT ON TYPE 1 DIABETES

Glycaemic control

Insulin pump treatment is a notable example of advanced technology that was introduced without the support of substantive clinical trials. Convincing evidence is very recent, and the first large comparative study of pumps and multiple dose insulin treatments was not reported until 2010 (Bergenstal et al., 2010). The insulin pumps were sensor-augmented by integrated continuous glucose monitoring (see later), so this study aimed to maximize the difference between the two groups. HbA_{1c} fell by a sustained 0.6% in both children and adults, but the improvement nearly doubled in those using continuous glucose monitoring more than 80% of the time. Less intensive studies, and a Cochrane systematic review, calculate a likely mean reduction in HbA_{1c} of approximately 0.3%. Even using this modest improvement in glycaemia, overall insulin pump treatment emerges as cost effective (Roze et al., 2015).

Acute metabolic disturbances – hypoglycaemia and diabetic ketoacidosis

Overall hypoglycaemia rates are similar with pumps and multiple dose insulin, but severe hypoglycaemia is less frequent with pump treatment, especially in people with the most severe hypoglycaemia while using multiple dose insulin and those with the longest duration of diabetes (Pickup and Sutton, 2008). Hypoglycaemia in children is probably also reduced with pump treatment. In the early years of pump treatment, the risk of diabetic ketoacidosis increased, due to both imperfect technology (pump failure) and poor education (the need to revert immediately to multiple dose insulin in case of pump failure – and ensuring patients have the kit to do this). There is no longer an increased risk of diabetic ketoacidosis in pump users.

Non-metabolic complications

Technical problems with pumps are still common (Pickup *et al.*, 2014). About one-half of insulin pumps are referred back to the manufacturer in the first year of use – though in the majority of cases no fault is found after mandatory extensive investigation. Local problems are frequently reported. Infusion tubing, especially if used for more than the recommended maximum of three days, is still prone to blocking. Skin reactions are common. Lipohypertrophy is reported in 25% of patients, especially people who have used them for a long time, and about the same proportion have had a skin infection.

Quality of life (QoL)

The benefits of insulin pump treatment are only in part captured by its benefit on acute metabolic disturbances and severe hypoglycaemia; there is a consistent benefit on many quality of life measures. However, benefits are not apparent immediately and may not be evident in the first year of treatment (Misso *et al.*, 2010). This is intuitively sound: starting pump treatment is an important life-event for people with diabetes and inevitably will require significant adjustments to self-management. Confidence and associated improvement in quality of life, therefore, may take a while to emerge and continued encouragement and support is needed during this early phase. General satisfaction is high with pump treatment and few patients discontinue. In a group up to young adult age in Germany only 5% discontinued, though the rate was higher in 10–15 year olds and in females (Hofer *et al.*, 2010). The important clinical question that has not been answered is whether or not patients using multiple dose insulin with poor quality of life (diabetes-specific or otherwise) benefit from a trial of pump treatment.

Long-term outcomes

A remarkable follow-up – average seven years' treatment – of a large Swedish registry found that insulin pump treatment was associated with a significantly lower risk of fatal coronary and cardiovascular disease and all-cause mortality, even though there was no difference in glycaemic control between patients using pumps or multiple daily injections (8% [64] in both groups). The mortality benefit may be associated with a reduction in severe hypoglycaemic episodes, but other factors acting over the longer term, such as education, may be more relevant (Steineck *et al.*, 2015). Using current measures, this major real-life study, showing no difference in HbA_{1c} between pump and multiple dose treatments in a high-resource healthcare environment, would probably not emerge as 'cost effective', but if these results are replicated in other studies it would render these traditional considerations largely irrelevant.

Indications for insulin pump treatment

Insulin pumps are routinely used in some countries. For example, in Norway every newly-diagnosed patient is offered pump treatment. About 70% of Type 1 children use them and about 25% of adults. In the USA, a wholly different healthcare system, about 40% of patients use pumps. The corresponding figure in the United Kingdom is 7%, though this increases to nearly 20% in the under 18s. The indication in some countries, therefore, is minimal – being a person with Type 1 diabetes – and therefore encourages maximum use of pumps. In more constrained systems, non-evidence-based consensus indications are used (**Box 8.1**).

Box 8.1 Indications for insulin pump treatment (after Pickup, 2012).

Primary indications
- Persistently raised HbA_{1c} (e.g. ≥8.5%, 69) despite optimized multiple dose insulin; criteria vary between and often within countries.
- The same criterion would be appropriate for children but additionally if MDI is not considered suitable or appropriate.
- Pregnancy.

Additional indications
- Wide glycaemic fluctuations even in the presence of 'good' HbA_{1c} values.
- Hypoglycaemia unawareness (see later).
- People prone to ketosis (insulin pump treatment will ensure continuity of basal insulin supply sufficient to suppress ketosis).
- Poor control with potentially reversible microvascular complications, for example moderate or severe background retinopathy, established microalbuminuria.
- Problematic overnight control, for example prominent dawn phenomenon.
- Irregular shift patterns or frequent long-haul flights.
- Some patients requiring either very high doses of insulin, for example >200 units/day, or very small doses where the minimum increments delivered by insulin pens (0.5 or 1 unit) may be too large.
- Continuing severe or disabling hypoglycaemia despite optimized multiple dose insulin.

Practice point

Insulin pump treatment is cost effective, improves quality of life, reduces the risk of hypoglycaemia and may carry long-term cardiovascular benefits.

Many of these indications may be refined through further clinical studies. For example, the rise in glucose levels in the early morning (the dawn phenomenon) would seem ideal for pump treatment, using programmed increases in basal insulin rates. However, early morning glucose control was no better in people who used such a programmed increase and, moreover, hypoglycaemia was more frequent (Bouchonville *et al.*, 2014). Do patients with established hypoglycaemia unawareness benefit from pump treatment? There is no evidence that pump-alone treatment helps but continuous glucose monitoring in people using pumps or multiple dose insulin is definitely of value (see later).

Insulin pumps: rapidly-developing technology

Around eight different systems are available in the United Kingdom and they share a library of features (**Figure 8.1**). Several have remote wireless control devices that avoid the inconvenience of accessing the pump itself to adjust settings. Disposable 'patch pumps' are either tubing-free or have very short tubes. They are more expensive than traditional pump designs and there are reports of insulin leakage from the skin insertion site. But many share important features and individual choice – and local availability and funding – will, in combination, determine the device eventually chosen. Clinically more important is the addition of integrated continuous glucose monitoring (sensor-augmented pump), with or without threshold suspend (insulin infusion is automatically stopped for

(a)   (b)

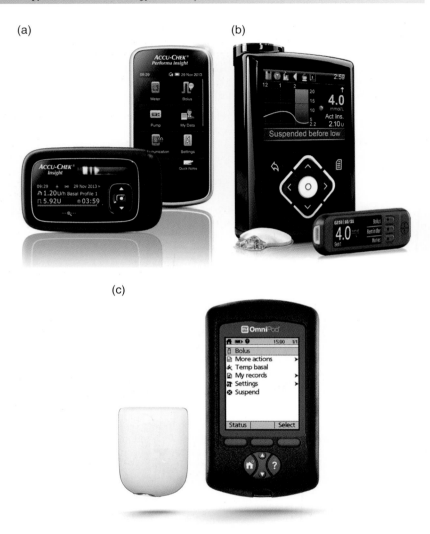

(c)

Figure 8.1 Some insulin pumps. (a) Pump with remote control device (AccuChek Insight [Roche]); (b) sensor-augmented pump (MiniMed 640G®) with SmartGuard® – software that pauses insulin delivery if hypoglycaemia is predicted low (low-glucose suspend); (c) Patch pump (mylife OmniPod [Ypsomed]).

a specific period when detected glucose levels reach a prespecified low values). Threshold-suspend pumps have been shown to reduce nocturnal hypoglycaemia (Bergenstal *et al.*, 2013) and in a long-term follow-up of nearly four years in hypoglycae-mia-prone patients, HbA$_{1c}$ and the incidence of hypoglycaemia and of hypoglycaemia unawareness fell within the first year and was maintained thereafter (Gómez *et al.*, 2017).

Many years after insulin pump treatment was first used, it has become one of the very few areas of diabetes practice where technology itself has beneficial effects with notably few downsides. This does not, of course, mean that it should be used uncritically.

CONTINUOUS INTRAPERITONEAL INSULIN INFUSION (CIPII)

Another example of insulin delivery technology being introduced (about 30 years ago) before clinical trials, and it still has no formal evidence base. Infusion of insulin directly into the peritoneum gives more physiological insulin levels than subcutaneous injection, though it is not known whether it improves glycaemia. The device requires surgical implantation under general anaesthetic; it is controlled by a standard insulin pump (AccuCheck Spirit Combo [Roche]). It is only rarely used, but may be of value in difficult individual cases of, for example, lipoatrophy/hypertrophy, severe skin reactions to insulin, insulin allergy, erratic insulin absorption and 'brittle' diabetes with persisting severe hypo-glycaemia despite all attempts at subcutaneous insulin therapy (van Dijk *et al.*, 2014).

CONTINUOUS GLUCOSE MONITORING (CGM)

Continuous subcutaneous sensing of interstitial glucose levels has been practical since the late 1990s. There are several types currently available:

- Blinded diagnostic systems where data cannot be viewed until uploaded (e.g. iPro2, Medtronic, sensor life up to 7 days).
- Stand-alone unblinded systems for personal use, for example Dexcom G4 Platinum.
- Systems integrated with insulin pumps, for example Animas and Medtronic pumps.

Interstitial glucose levels take time to equilibrate with blood; this, together with the time needed to process output in the device, leads to a cumulative delay up to about 12–15 minutes before the data is viewable. Clinically the delay seems to show quite high interindividual variation. This is not a problem in diagnostic systems but must be taken into account in current real-time CGM systems. Predictive algorithms are being developed for use in the artificial pancreas but many current systems have simple alerts when glucose levels are moving towards preset high or low values.

The FreeStyle Libre personal glucose device (Abbott) is not strictly CGM but is significantly cheaper, and is affordable for personal use. Sensors last up to 14 days and they are factory calibrated and therefore do not require finger-prick blood glucose tests for calibration. The device displays instantaneous glucose readings only when the sensor is scanned (hence 'flash glucose monitoring system', rather than CGM); there are no alarms but there are screen displays of recent trends and long-term data are fully downloadable. Sensor delay is around five minutes for this device and performance characteristics are good (Bailey *et al.*, 2015). However, even this delay may be significant in certain circumstances, for example before driving, where standard instantaneous finger-prick values are mandatory.

Practice point

Because of the delay in registering glucose levels, continuous glucose monitoring devices must not be used before or during driving.

Therapeutic use

An important series of meticulous studies published between 2010 and 2012 in pump-treated patients established the value of CGM in improving diabetic control. The main conclusions were:

- HbA$_{1c}$ improves by about 0.5%; improvement was noticeable by three months, and was maximum at six months.
- Glycaemia improves in patients with moderately poor control (Battelino *et al.*, 2012).
- Glycaemia returned to baseline within about three months of discontinuing CGM; it has no significant 'legacy' effect and must be used continuously for sustained benefit (**Figure 8.2**).
- There was a variable effect on severe hypoglycaemia, which at baseline was already infrequent in these well-controlled patients, but one study reported a near-50% reduction.
- Patients using CGM also used more of the specialized pump features, for example, daily boluses, temporary basal rates and manual insulin suspends.
- Higher persistence in use (>70% of the time) was associated with better glycaemic control. It is not known whether there is rapidly-fading novelty value for these devices in clinical practice, as there is for other appealing health-related technology devices (see **Chapter 9**).
- In SWITCH, quality of life was not impaired by using CGM, and some meaningful measures improved, for example treatment satisfaction and school days, so long as there was >70% persistence with use. Telephone consultations did not increase in children and the numbers fell in adults (Hommel *et al.*, 2014).

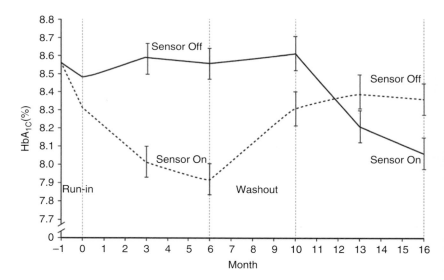

Figure 8.2 Crossover study (SWITCH) of continuous glucose monitoring in moderately poorly controlled Type 1 diabetes (mean baseline HbA$_{1c}$ 8.6% [70]). Control improves promptly but the effect does not persist after stopping CGM. No 'legacy' here. *Source*: Battelino *et al.*, 2012.

Table 8.1 Characteristics of the patients in the GOLD continuous glucose monitoring study (Lind *et al.*, 2017). Monitoring system was Dexcom G4 Platinum.

Mean age (years)	47
Mean duration of diabetes (years)	23
Body mass index	27.0
HbA$_{1c}$	8.7% (72)
Median number of daily insulin injections	5

Are the benefits of therapeutic CGM generalizable? It seems so: for example, two elegant crossover studies in a much more familiar group of patients (older, long duration, taking multiple dose insulin; **Table 8.1**) showed an overall HbA$_{1c}$ reduction of 0.4–0.6% while using CGM. There is still, of course, no 'legacy' effect; during the four-month washout period, HbA$_{1c}$ values in both groups returned to baseline, reinforcing the established evidence that persistent use of this method of real-time feedback (and high adherence too) are required for sustained glycaemic improvements.

In the GOLD study exploratory analyses found that fear of hypoglycaemia was lower during CGM and, although hypoglycaemia was rare, episodes of severe hypoglycaemia were numerically lower (five compared with one during non-CGM periods). In the DIAMOND study the time spent at glucose levels <3.9 mmol/l was reduced during CGM by about 50% from an average of 80 minutes per day to 43 minutes (Beck *et al.*, 2017)).

In spite of these largely encouraging studies, clinical CGM is still in its early phase. Currently costs are not reimbursed, except selectively in the USA, and therefore only small numbers of patients likely to benefit will have access to it. With the accumulating and consistent evidence for its value in different groups (age, prior glycaemic control, treatment modality) the situation should change.

Hypoglycaemia unawareness

Hypoglycaemia should improve in people with hypoglycaemia unawareness if they persist with CGM. This was demonstrated in the IN CONTROL Trial (van Beers *et al.*, 2016) in a group typically affected by this troublesome and hazardous condition, that is middle-aged people (mean age 49 years) with long duration of diabetes (mean 31 years). About one-half of the participants used insulin pumps. Patients were randomized to CGM or standard self-blood glucose monitoring and crossed over to the other monitoring system after four months. CGM was associated with substantial reductions in severe hypoglycaemic events, whether defined clinically or using different glucose cut-off values (**Figure 8.3**). The improvement was the same for patients whether using multiple dose insulin or insulin pumps. Interestingly, time spent in the normoglycaemic range (defined as 4–10 mmol/l) was the same whether or not patients used carbohydrate counting. Subjective measures of hypoglycaemia unawareness did not change, in contrast to classical early studies that showed restoration of hypoglycaemia awareness after rigorous avoidance of clinical hypoglycaemia for around four months (Cranston *et al.*, 1994), but ascertainment of hypoglycaemia is likely to be more complete in the recent study.

Practice point

Good adherence to continuous glucose monitoring (~90% of the time) reduces hypoglycaemic events in people with hypoglycaemia unawareness.

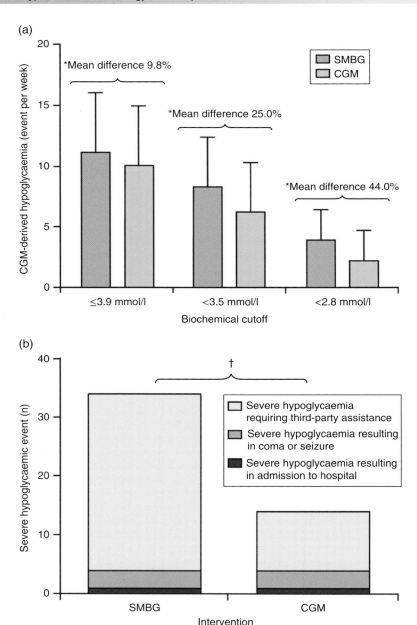

Figure 8.3 Reduction in biochemical (a) and clinical (b) hypoglycaemia with high (~90%) adherence to continuous glucose monitoring over 16–18 weeks in people with long-standing Type 1 diabetes and hypoglycaemia unawareness. The more severe the biochemical hypoglycaemia the greater the reduction in events, but CGM did not reduce the risk of seizure or hospital admission. *Source*: van Beers *et al.*, 2016.

Diagnostic use

Currently CGM is widely used over short periods – usually for the duration of one sensor, therefore 4–5 days up to two weeks – to diagnose hypoglycaemia unawareness, nocturnal hypoglycaemia, the dawn phenomenon and postprandial peaks, and potentially to correct them. Although analysing the output is primarily the responsibility of the healthcare professional, it must be done in close consultation with the patient because they know the factors contributing to day-to-day variability of the output. The quantity of data is huge and data overload with confusion for patients and professionals alike can be a significant barrier to interpretation. Agreement on a standardized format is emerging, for example, presenting median glucose values together with 25th to 75th and 10th to 90th percentile values, though daily tracings are of help in order to learn from more exceptional events (**Figure 8.4**). Because it has to take into account many variables, CGM diagnosis is complicated and time-consuming, and strangely – or perhaps not so strangely – there are no reports of outcomes for patients when CGM is used in this way. By contrast, as we have seen, the benefit of therapeutic CGM in improving glycaemic outcomes is more or less settled.

Practice point

When used as an occasional diagnostic system CGM requires experienced clinicians to help patients interpret the output.

ARTIFICIAL PANCREAS

The components of the fully-automated closed-loop insulin pump (artificial pancreas) – the insulin pump and continuous glucose monitoring system – already exist in sophisticated forms. Integrating the two via software to control compact portable devices that will ensure fully-automated delivery of insulin (or the bi-hormonal pump delivering both insulin and glucagon) was the challenge issued to researchers in 2006 when the Juvenile Diabetes Research Foundation (JDRF) Artificial Pancreas Project was inaugurated (**Figure 8.5**). More than a decade on, the practical artificial pancreas is not yet here, but there has been astonishing progress, especially over the past few years, and incremental improvements are regularly reported. The components of the artificial pancreas will include developments of:

- *Sensor-augmented insulin pumps.* A term that refers to wireless transmission of interstitial glucose measurements made by CGM devices to an insulin pump, where they can be used by patients to track changes in glucose levels and manually adjust basal rates and mealtime boluses.
- *Threshold suspend.* Software that temporarily interrupts insulin delivery when sensor-detected glucose levels approach a predetermined low value. The first device was introduced in the United Kingdom in 2009 and in the USA in 2015. It reduces the risk of nocturnal hypoglycaemic events in people with baseline HbA$_{1c}$ <7–8% (53–64) and those experiencing a fall in HbA$_{1c}$. Intensification of treatment in pump patients is therefore more secure (Weiss et al., 2015).
- *Trials of bihormonal and closed-loop systems.* Proof-of-concept studies were first reported in 2014. A bihormonal pump ('bionic pancreas' delivering both insulin and glucagon) was successfully trialled over five days in a rigorously controlled study in adolescents and adults and a closed-loop insulin-only system controlled by a modified mo-

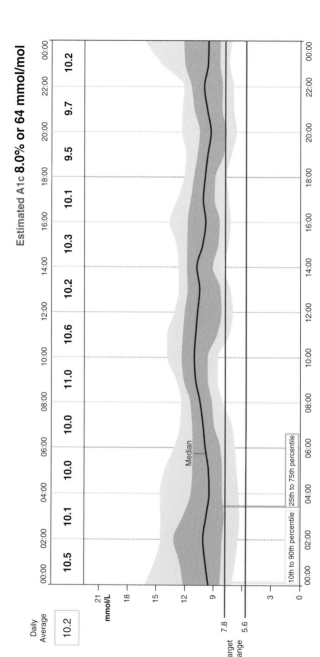

Figure 8.4 Standardized format for continuous glucose monitoring display, showing median and 25th–75th and 10th–90th percentile values (FreeStyle Libre, Abbott). The variability of glucose measurements at any time of day can be immediately appreciated. Individual daily tracings allow specific events to be carefully analysed. A rough automated calculation of HbA$_{1c}$ was 8.0% (64). The simultaneous laboratory measurement was much lower, 70% (53). There is almost no hypoglycaemia and glucose ranges are narrow during the day, slightly wider during the night. Male Type 1 patient, duration four years, basal-bolus regimen (aspart and glargine). He used low doses of prandial insulin with a very low carbohydrate diet, which accounts for the almost peakless median tracings during the day.

1970s ——→ 2000 ——————— 2017–18 ——————— → 2020–5

Associated technological developments

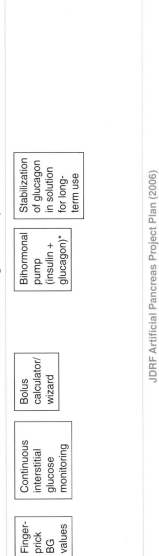

| Finger-prick BG values | Continuous interstitial glucose monitoring | Bolus calculator/wizard | Bihormonal pump (insulin + glucagon)* | Stabilization of glucagon in solution for long-term use |

JDRF Artificial Pancreas Project Plan (2006)

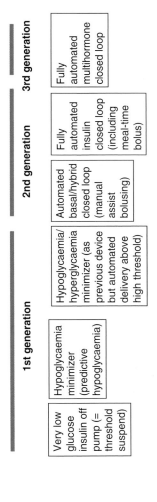

1st generation		2nd generation	3rd generation
Very low glucose insulin off pump (= threshold suspend)	Hypoglycaemia minimizer (predictive hypoglycaemia)		
	Hypoglycaemia/hyperglycaemia minimizer (as previous device but automated delivery above high threshold)	Automated basal/hybrid closed loop (manual assist bolusing)	
		Fully automated insulin closed loop (including meal-time bolus)	
			Fully automated multihormone closed loop

Figure 8.5 Developing the artificial pancreas: the Juvenile Diabetes Research Foundation Artificial Pancreas Project.

bile phone interface reduced the time spent in hypoglycaemia (Kovatchev *et al.*, 2014). The technical challenges of developing stable glucagon solutions for use in the artificial pancreas will no doubt rapidly be overcome. There are no differences overall in glycaemia with insulin-only and bihormonal pumps, except there is less time spent in hypoglycaemia with the bihormonal systems. Hypoglycaemic blood glucose levels rise only slowly after suspending an insulin infusion, but much more quickly when glucagon is given.

In 2017 a quartet of large-scale clinical trials was announced by the NIH to start in 2017–2018. These will likely lead to the introduction of FDA-approved artificial pancreas devices towards the end of the decade.

ISLET AND WHOLE PANCREAS TRANSPLANTATION

Transplantation is currently the only way to ensure consistent and long-term normoglycaemia. Until 2000, only whole-pancreas transplantation was available, with its formidable attendant surgery, but the Edmonton Protocol for donor islet preparation and transplantation held out the hope of a much less invasive – indeed outpatient – procedure with less immunosuppression.

Clinicians in diabetes practice should always consider whether Type 1 patients might be suitable for transplantation; although the acceptance rate, especially for islet transplantation, is low, for example 20%, all potentially suitable patients should have the opportunity to be evaluated. An important and pioneering study from Edinburgh (Forbes *et al.*, 2015) established that the benefits of islet transplantation can be extended to socioeconomically deprived people (nearly three-quarters of their eighteen patients had this background and around 90% were neither in work nor had a driver's licence).

> **Practice point**
>
> Repeatedly evaluate whether long-standing Type 1 patients might benefit from a whole pancreas or islet transplantation.

Islet transplantation

Initial enthusiasm for islet transplantation was stimulated by good results in the original Edmonton studies, though this was tempered by lower success rates in achieving insulin-independence and continued insulin secretion indicated by C-peptide positivity in a global study (Shapiro *et al.*, 2006). However, results continue to improve as islet yields from donor pancreas increase and immunosuppression regimes are further refined (**Table 8.2**); however, worldwide the number of procedures is currently only about one-tenth that of whole-pancreas transplants (200–250 compared with 2500 per year). Primary indications for islet transplantation include:

- severe glycaemic lability
- recurrent severe hypoglycaemic episodes
- hypoglycaemia unawareness.

Patients are reliably protected from severe hypoglycaemia after transplantation even if they do not remain fully insulin-independent, as counterregulation by glucagon and noradrenaline is restored. Normal or near-normal blood glucose levels after transplantation are likely to retard or reverse progression of early microvascular complications; these are now emerging as indications, though patients with established diabetic nephropathy

Table 8.2 Progressive improvements in islet transplantation between 1999 and 2010 (from Barton *et al.*, 2012). Insulin-independence rates have increased in the face of increasing age and diabetes duration of recipients.

	Period 1 1999–2002	Period 2 2003–2006	Period 3 2007–2010
Number	214	255	208
Age at baseline (years)	42	45	48
Insulin-independence at 3 years (%)	27	37	44
Islet reinfusion for graft failure or falling C-peptide (%)	60–65	—	48
Donor age (years)	42	43	44
Immunosuppression regime	Edmonton Protocol: Induction: IL-2 receptor antagonist, e.g. daclizumab Maintenance: mTOR inhibitor (e.g. sirolimus) + calcineurin inhibitor (e.g. tacrolimus)		Induction: T-cell depleting antibody + TNF-α inhibitor, e.g. etanercept Maintenance: mTOR inhibitor or inosine monophosphate dehydrogenase inhibitor (e.g. mycophenolic acid) + tacrolimus

require combined pancreas-kidney transplantation. The procedure itself is relatively straightforward: currently nearly all islet transplantations are performed with intrahepatic islet infusion via the portal vein. The results of islet transplantation are now comparable with those of pancreas-alone transplantation in non-uraemic patients. While the aim is single-donor transplants, a high proportion of patients are transplanted with islets from more than one donor pancreas. Scoring systems do not yet reliably predict the characteristics of either donors or donor pancreases that give the best clinical outcomes. Encouragingly, a failed islet transplantation does not jeopardize a subsequent whole pancreas transplant; outcomes up to five years are identical compared with a primary pancreas transplant cohort (Gruessner and Gruessner, 2016). Islet transplantation in people with impaired hypoglycaemia awareness and severe hypoglycaemic events was dramatically successful in a large multicentre trial: nearly 90% of patients remained hypoglycaemia-free for one year and 70% for two years with normal HbA_{1c} values (mean 5.6%, 38) (Hering *et al.*, 2016).

Practice point

After islet transplantation the majority of patients with intractable hypoglycaemic events and hypoglycaemia unawareness remit for at least two years with non-diabetic HbA_{1c} levels.

WHOLE PANCREAS TRANSPLANTATION

Pancreas transplantation in its varying forms has been a standard, if formidable, operation for 50 years; the total number of procedures performed worldwide to 2010 was about 25 000. Two of the procedures – combined simultaneous kidney-pancreas transplantation

(SPK) and pancreas-after kidney (PAK), comprising respectively 72% and 17% of procedures in the USA – are widely undertaken in patients with established CKD due to diabetic renal disease. Pancreas-alone operations account for only about 7% of procedures. In the USA, where the large majority of pancreas transplants are carried out, the numbers of all these transplants fell between 2004 and 2011, especially PAK and pancreas-alone. In part this may be due to a decrease in end-stage renal disease but less positive factors, including lack of acceptance by the diabetes care community, inadequate training opportunities and increasing risk aversion due to regulatory scrutiny probably also contribute (Stratta *et al.*, 2016). Surgical techniques continue to be refined and re-transplantation is becoming commoner. There is a small but increasing number of segmental living donor procedures, often combined with a simultaneous kidney transplant from the same donor.

Clinical indications for pancreas transplantation are wide. Most patients have established diabetic renal disease and are often on dialysis, with unremitting severe hyperglycaemia, or frequent severe hypoglycaemia, usually with hypoglycaemia unawareness. However, patients with progressing CKD not yet warranting renal transplantation and not requiring dialysis are nowadays more often considered for a pre-emptive renal transplant or SPK.

Outcomes
Remarkable in experienced centres. More than 95% of patients survive more than a year, up to 90% five years and >70% 10 years. Because patients having pancreas-alone transplants are not uraemic, their survival is even better, around 80% at 10 years. Graft failure, highest in the first year, falls thereafter to about 4% per year for both pancreas and renal grafts, though as the overall outlook has been transformed for patients, concern is emerging about the risk of malignancy, which accounts for around 7% of deaths after the first posttransplant year. The complications of immunosuppression are ever-present and specialist follow-up is intensive and lifelong.

Impact on complications
Assessing the effect of pancreas transplantation on microvascular complications is confounded by the presence of high rates of advanced retinopathy and neuropathy in transplanted patients, neither of which can be expected to improve with even prolonged normoglycaemia. Epidermal nerve fibre loss – probably not surprisingly – shows no sign of reversal up to eight years after simultaneous pancreas and kidney transplantation (Havrdova *et al.*, 2016). However, erectile function is reported to improve meaningfully after simultaneous pancreas-kidney transplants, though not after kidney-alone transplantation (Salonia *et al.*, 2011). Diabetic kidney disease slowly but surely improves with prolonged near-normoglycaemia. In non-uraemic patients the histological appearance of even advanced nephropathy improves between five and ten years after establishing normoglycaemia, and microalbuminuria regressed too (Mauer and Fioretto, 2013). Nephrotic-range proteinuria in Type 1 patients with normal renal function is reported to resolve a few months after simultaneous kidney-pancreas transplantation (Sedlak *et al.*, 2007).

Macrovascular outcomes and quality of life
Intermediate indicators of macrovascular disease, for example, carotid intima-media thickness and quantitative coronary angiography, improve within a few years, but cardiovascular outcomes are still relatively uncommon and have not been reported until recently. In a large study of patients transplanted between 1983 and 2012, and followed up for a median eight years, cardiovascular mortality was higher in those transplanted in the early part of this era (1983–1999); the risk of cardiovascular mortality was about

40% lower after a combined transplant compared with living donor kidney-alone trans-plants (Lindahl *et al.*, 2016). Quality of life outcomes are surprisingly sparse, presumably because it is assumed that freedom from dialysis and insulin treatment will inevitably improve quality of life; while that is likely, the same may not be the case for patients pre-emptively given combined transplants, where, for example, dominant neuropathic symptoms may not improve.

References

Bailey T, Bode BW, Christiansen MP *et al*. The performance and usability of a factory-calibrated flash glucose monitoring system. *Diabetes Technol Ther* 2015;17:787–94 [PMID: 26171659] PMC4649725.

Barton FB, Rickels MR, Alejandro R *et al*. Improvement in outcomes of islet transplantation: 1999–2010. *Diabetes Care*, 2012;35:1436–45 [PMID: 22723582] PMC3379615.

Battelino T, Conget I, Olsen B *et al*. SWITCH Study Group. The use and efficacy of continuous glucose monitoring in type 1 diabetes treated with insulin pump therapy: a randomised controlled trial. *Diabetologia* 2012;55:3155– 62 [PMID: 22965294] PMC3483098.

Beck RW, Riddlesworth T, Ruedy K *et al*. DIAMOND Study Group. Effect of continuous glucose moni-toring on glycemic control in adults with type 1 diabetes using insulin injections: the DIAMOND randomized clinical trial. *JAMA* 2017;317:371–8 [PMID: 28118453].

van Beers CA, DeVries JH, Kelijer SJ *et al*. Continuous glucose monitoring for patients with type 1 diabetes and impaired awareness of hypoglycaemia (IN CONTROL): a randomised, open-label, crossover trial. *Lancet Diabetes Endocrinol* 2016;4:893–902 [PMID: 27641781].

Bergenstal RM, Tamborlane WV, Ahmann A *et al*. STAR 3 Study Group. Effectiveness of sensor- aug-mented insulin-pump therapy in type 1 diabetes. *N Engl J Med* 2010;363:311–20 [PMID: 20587585] Free full text.

Bergenstal RM, Klonoff DC, Garg SK *et al*.; ASPIRE In-Home Study Group. Threshold-based insulin-pump interruption for reduction of hypoglycemia. *N Engl J Med* 2013;369:224–32 [PMID: 23789889] Free full text.

Bouchonville MF, Jaghab JJ, Duran-Valdez E *et al*. The effectiveness and risks of programming an insulin pump to counteract the dawn phenomenon in type 1 diabetes. *Endocr Pract* 2014;20:1290–6 [PMID: 25533134].

Cranston I, Lomas J, Maran A *et al*. Restoration of hypoglycaemia awareness in patients with long-duration insulin-dependent diabetes. *Lancet* 1994;344:283–7 [PMID: 7914259].

van Dijk PR, Logtenberg SJ, Gans RO *et al*. Intraperitoneal insulin infusion: treatment option for type 1 diabetes resulting in beneficial endocrine effects beyond glycaemia. *Clin Endocrinol (Oxf)* 2014;81:488–97 [PMID: 25041605].

Forbes S, McGowan NW, Duncan K *et al*. Islet transplantation from a nationally funded UK centre reaches socially deprived groups and improves metabolic outcomes. *Diabetologia* 2015;58:1300–8 [PMID: 25810037] PMC4415991.

Gómez AM, Marin Carrillo LF, Muñoz Velandia *et al*. Long-term efficacy and safety of sensor aug-mented insulin pump therapy with low-glucose suspend feature in patients with type 1 diabetes. *Diabetes Technol Ther* 2017;19:109–14 [PMID: 28001445].

Gruessner RW, Gruessner AC. Pancreas after islet transplantation: a first report of the International Pancreas Transplant Registry *Am J Transplant* 2016;16:688–93 [PMID: 26436323].

Havrdova T, Boucek P, Saudek F *et al*. Severe epidermal nerve fiber loss in diabetic neuropathy is not reversed by long-term normoglycaemia after simultaneous pancreas and kidney transplantation. *Am J Transplant* 2016;16:2196–201 [PMID: 26751140].

Heinemann L. Insulin pump therapy: what is the evidence for using different types of boluses for coverage of prandial insulin requirements? *J Diabetes Sci Technol* 2009;3:1490–500. [PMID: 20144405] PMC2787051.

Hering BJ, Clarke WR Bridges ND *et al*. Clinical Islet Transplantation Consortium. Phase 3 trial of transplantation of human islets in type 1 diabetes complicated by severe hypoglycemia. *Diabetes Care* 2016;39:1230–40 [PMID: 27208344].

Hofer SE, Heidtmann B, Raile K et al. DPV-Science-Initiative and the German working group for insulin pump treatment in pediatric patients. Discontinuation of insulin pump treatment in children, adolescents, and young adults. A multicenter analysis based on the DPV database in Germany and Austria. Pediatr Diabetes 2010;11:116–21 [PMID: 19566740].

Hommel E, Olsen B, Battelino T et al. SWITCH Study Group. Impact of continuous glucose monitoring on quality of life, treatment satisfaction, and use of medical care resources: analyses from the SWITCH study. Acta Diabetol 2014;51:845–51 [PMID: 25037251] PMC4176956.

Kovatchev BP, Renard E, Cobelli C et al. Safety of outpatient closed-loop control: first randomized crossover trials of a wearable artificial pancreas. Diabetes Care 2014;37:1789–96 [PMID: 24929429] PMC4067397.

Laimer M, Melmer A, Mader JK et al. Variability of basal rate profiles in insulin pump therapy and association with complications in type 1 diabetes mellitus. PLoS One 2016;11:e0150604 [PMID: 26938444] PMC4777503.

Lind M, Polonsky W, Hirsch IB et al. Continuous glucose monitoring vs conventional therapy for glycemic control in adults with type 1 diabetes treated with multiple daily insulin injections: the GOLD randomized clinical trial. JAMA 2017;317:379–87 [PMID: 28118454].

Lindahl JP, Hartmann A, Aakhus S et al. Long-term cardiovascular outcomes in type 1 diabetic patients after simultaneous pancreas and kidney transplantation compared with living donor kidney transplantation. Diabetologia 2016;59:844–52 [PMID: 26713324].

Mauer M, Fioretto P. Pancreas transplantation and reversal of diabetic nephropathy lesions. Med Clin North Am 2013;97:109–14 [PMID: 23290733] PMC3646375.

Miller KM, Beck RW, Bergenstal RM et al. T1D Exchange Clinic Network. Evidence of a strong association between frequency of self-monitoring of blood glucose and hemoglobin levels in T1D exchange clinic registry participants. Diabetes Care 2013;36:2009–14 [PMID: 23378621] PMC3687326.

Misso ML, Egberts KJ, Page M et al. Continuous subcutaneous insulin infusion (CSII) versus multiple insulin injections for type 1 diabetes mellitus. Cochrane Database Syst Rev 2010;20:CD005103 [PMID: 20091571].

Pickup JC, Sutton AJ, Severe hypoglycaemia and glycaemic control in Type 1 diabetes: meta-analysis of multiple daily insulin injections compared with continuous subcutaneous insulin infusion. Diabet Med 2008;25:765–74 [PMID: 18644063].

Pickup JC. Insulin-pump treatment for type 1 diabetes mellitus. N Engl J Med 2012; 366:1616– 24 [PMID: 22533577].

Pickup JC, Yemane N, Brackenridge A, Pender S. Nonmetabolic complications of continuous subcutaneous insulin infusion: a patient survey. Diabetes Tech Ther 2014;16:145–9 [PMID: 24180294].

Reichel A, Rietzsch H, Ludwig B et al.Self-adjustment of insulin dose using graphically depicted self-monitoring of blood glucose measurements in patients with type 1 diabetes. J Diabetes Sci Technol 2013;7:156–62 [PMID: 23439172] PMC3692228.

Roze S, Smith-Palmer J, Valentine W et al. Cost-effectiveness of continuous subcutaneous insulin infusion versus multiple daily injections of insulin in Type 1 diabetes: a systematic review. Diabet Med 2015;32:1415–24 [PMID: 25962621].

Salonia A, D'Addio F, Gemizzi C et al. Kidney-pancreas transplantation is associated with near-normal sexual function in uremic type 1 diabetic patients. Transplantation 2011;92:802–8 [PMID: 21822170].

Sedlak M, Biesenbach G, Margreiter R. Proteinuria disappears promptly after simultaneous kidney-pancreas transplantation in nephrotic diabetic patients with near-normal GFR. Clin Nephrol 2007;68:330–4 [PMID: 18044267].

Shapiro AM, Ricordi C, Hering BJ et al. International trial of the Edmonton protocol for islet transplantation. N Engl J Med 2006;355:1318–30 [PMID: 17005949] Free full text.

Steineck I, Cederholm J, Eliasson B et al. Swedish National Diabetes Register. Insulin pump therapy, multiple daily injections, and cardiovascular mortality in 18,168 people with type 1 diabetes: observational study. BMJ 2015;350:h334 [PMID: 26100640] PMC4476263.

Stratta RJ, Fridell JA, Gruessner AC et al. Pancreas transplantation: a decade of decline. Curr Opin Organ Transplant 2016;21:386–92 [PMID: 270965564].

Weiss R, Garg SK, Bode BW *et al.* Hypoglycemia reduction and changes in haemoglobin A1c in the ASPIRE In-Home Study. *Diabetes Technol Ther* 2015;17:542–7 [PMID: 26237308] PMC4528987.

Ziegler R, Cavan DA, Cranston I *et al.* Use of an insulin bolus advisor improves glycemic control in multiple daily insulin injection (MDI) therapy patients with suboptimal glycemic control: first results from the ABACUS trial. *Diabetes Care* 2013; 36:3613–9 [PMID: 23900590] PMC3816874.

Further reading

Continuous glucose monitoring

Fonseca VA, Grunberger G, Anhalt H *et al.* Consensus Conference Writing Group. Continuous glucose monitoring: a consensus conference of the American Association of Clinical Endocrinologists and American College of Endocrinology. *Endocr Pract* 2016;22:1008–21 [PMID: 27214060].

9 Type 2 diabetes: weight loss, exercise and other 'lifestyle' interventions

Key points

- 'Lifestyle' is a vague term. In prediabetes there is evidence for long-term cardiovascular benefits of formal prolonged interventions with weight loss, exercise or both
- The traditional high carbohydrate, low saturated fat diet probably does not carry benefits that matter to people with diabetes
- A traditional Mediterranean diet improves cardiovascular and probably cancer outcomes; additional daily extra-virgin olive oil or nuts add to this benefit
- Higher protein diets are associated with a better chance of maintaining weight loss
- Very-low-calorie diets can reverse some of the abnormalities underlying Type 2 diabetes, especially fat overload
- Only extreme exercise can cause meaningful weight loss, but moderate exercise improves glycaemia and non-alcoholic fatty liver and can reduce weight gain after dieting; in Type 1 diabetes it is associated with a lower risk of microvascular complications

INTRODUCTION

'Lifestyle' is a catch-all term for non-pharmacological interventions that – properly – displaced the instructional, top-down and dogmatic approach of instructing patients in 'diet', 'exercise' and other aspects of self-management. However, its vague colloquial use may prove to be no more helpful than the old approach. For example, in the area of diet it does not make the critical distinction between quantitative calorie restriction and qualitative changes to dietary components or specific foods, nor between activity that is part of everyday life (inevitably termed 'lifestyle' activity) and more structured exercise. All these important components can now be separated. There is widespread awareness of the relatively recent demonstration that intensive weight loss using very low calorie diets can reverse some of the fundamental deficits of Type 2 diabetes – something that no current drug treatment can do. The spectrum of 'lifestyle' intervention has broadened significantly; the American Diabetes Association includes diabetes self-management education, diabetes self-management support and psychosocial care under its lifestyle rubric (American Diabetes Association, 2017).

LEGACY EFFECT OF NON-PHARMACOLOGICAL INTERVENTIONS

Good glycaemic control using drugs carries beneficial legacy effects in both Type 1 and 2 diabetes; good blood pressure control, on the other hand, does not. What is the

Practical Diabetes Care, Fourth Edition. David Levy.
© 2018 John Wiley & Sons Ltd. Published 2018 by John Wiley & Sons Ltd.

evidence for long-term effects of non-pharmacological interventions? Follow-up studies of a series of trials conducted 15–20 years ago are beginning to supply some answers. However, it may be that these studies have set themselves unrealizable goals, especially reduction in cardiovascular events; the number of modern-era trials of any treatment modality that have shown cardiovascular benefit in primary prevention is vanishingly small.

INTERVENTIONS IN IMPAIRED GLUCOSE TOLERANCE: WEIGHT LOSS AND EXERCISE ARE BETTER THAN MEDICATION

A flurry of impressive studies reporting in the late 1990s and early 2000s investigated large groups of patients with 'prediabetes', more precisely impaired glucose tolerance (IGT) and who were therefore at high risk of progression to Type 2 diabetes. They concluded that comprehensive weight loss and increased intervention reduced the risk of progression to Type 2 diabetes by up to 45%. The delay in onset of Type 2 in the Diabetes Prevention Program amounted to an average of about four years with non-pharmacological intervention compared with two years for treatment with metformin, but the randomized trials were too short to demonstrate whether or not significant diabetes outcomes were affected. Long-term follow-up has now been reported in all the major studies.

Da Qing (start/report1986/1997)

This pioneering study, in Chinese people, intervened for six years with diet only, exercise only or diet-plus-exercise, each of which reduced the risk of progression to Type 2 diabetes to approximately the same degree, 30–45%. Uniquely among these studies, exercise alone had a significant effect.

At 23 years follow-up, there was a remarkable disease-preventing legacy effect, which has either not been found or not reported in the other prevention studies (see later). In the Da Qing study, all-cause mortality was reduced by 30% (absolute reduction about 10%), cardiovascular mortality by 40% (8% absolute) and diabetes itself by 45% (18% absolute). Women benefited more than men. While this study was in Chinese people, whose relatively lean phenotype contrasts with that of Western people (see **Chapter 1**), the results are very striking for the possible sustained cardiovascular legacy effect using rigorous lifestyle intervention alone. However, the effect takes a very long time to emerge: differences in cardiovascular mortality became apparent only 12 years after the start of the study and statistically significant differences were not seen until 23 years (Li et al., 2014).

Practice point

Diet, exercise or diet+exercise significantly reduced cardiovascular events in Chinese individuals with prediabetes, though the effect took many years to become apparent.

The Diabetes Prevention Program (DPP, 1996–9/2002)

The best-known study used metformin and placebo in two arms and lifestyle intervention in the third in USA patients with IGT. Lifestyle intervention over three years reduced progression to diabetes by 60%, compared with only 30% in the metformin group.

After the main study finished those in the lifestyle group continued to receive six-monthly lifestyle 'reinforcement' and the metformin group continued to take medication (metformin 850 mg bd). Although metformin and lifestyle intervention continued to be effective in reducing the progression to diabetes (18% and 27% respectively), most subjects still developed diabetes (about 55% in the intervention groups, 62% in placebo). There were no differences in microvascular outcomes between the treatment groups, but overall microvascular complications were less frequent in women and more frequent in people who developed diabetes compared with those who did not; but this latter finding should not surprise, as biochemical diabetes is defined as the level of glycaemia above which microvascular complications (retinopathy) occur (Diabetes Prevention Program Research Group, 2015). Macrovascular events have not been reported.

Practice point

The majority of patients in the Diabetes Prevention Program ultimately developed Type 2 diabetes, though there was a slightly lower prevalence in the active intervention groups.

Because subjects continued to have some input, lifestyle or medication, after the trial end, the Diabetes Prevention Program gives us no insight into legacy effects. Mean HbA_{1c} in the metformin group was not meaningfully different from the other groups (6.3%, 45, compared with 6.1% and 6.2%, 43 and 44); this is indirect evidence that metformin has no effects on microvascular complications independent of glycaemia.

The Finnish Diabetes Prevention Study (1993–8/2001)
The initial results of the three-year intervention were similar to the Diabetes Prevention Program: intensive individual intensive counselling on weight, food components and activity reduced the risk of progression of IGT to diabetes by about 60% compared with control subjects. Outcomes at nine years were similar to Da Qing: 30% overall risk reduction in the formerly intensive group, together with sustained improvements in weight, fasting and two-hour glucose levels, and a healthier diet (Lindström et al., 2013). Throughout the study the degree of adherence to the different components of the intervention was strongly related to reduction in risk of developing diabetes. The longer weight loss ≥5% could be maintained up to three years the greater the risk reduction. Moderate or vigorous leisure time physical activity and a diet high in fibre reduced inflammatory components strongly associated with diabetes (CRP and IL-6). No vascular complications have been reported.

Practice point

Microvascular complications were not reduced in DPP, and macrovascular benefits have not been reported in either the DPP or the Finnish study

---

Ethnic minority subjects
A trial of intensive versus routine dietician-led intervention to reduce weight in UK South Asian people with prediabetes (baseline mean BMI 31) found that there was a net weight loss of 1.6 kg that was maintained over three years, with a trend towards a lower chance of being diagnosed with diabetes. These modest results are still encouraging, since

subjects were in their early 50s when age-associated weight gain may continue for a decade or more; if weight stability were maintained, then the cumulative difference might be highly meaningful after a longer period. (Bhopal *et al.*, 2014).

LIFESTYLE INTERVENTION IN PEOPLE WITH DIABETES

Newly-diagnosed Type 2 diabetes: ADDITION-Cambridge Study (2014)

In this five-year study there was no reduction in cardiovascular events after intensive lifestyle input. However, significant changes in individuals were important. The number of lifestyle changes, especially activity levels and reducing or stopping alcohol, were strongly related to cardiovascular outcomes. Changes in total calorie, saturated fat and fibre consumption did not reduce cardiovascular events (Long *et al.*, 2014), but these, together with reducing sodium intake and increasing fruits and vegetables, had beneficial effects on blood pressure and triglyceride levels independent of other factors, including activity level, smoking and cardio-protective medication. Only small changes are needed, for example replacing a bar of chocolate with a piece of fruit and reducing salt in cooking by half a teaspoon (Cooper *et al.*, 2014).

Established Type 2 diabetes: Look AHEAD Study (2001/2013)

The massively ambitious Look AHEAD (Action for Health in Diabetes) study investigated the effect of intensive multimodal lifestyle intervention on cardiovascular outcomes in people with established Type 2 diabetes compared with non-intensive support and education. It was terminated after 10 years maximum follow-up, showing no difference in the primary outcomes. Mean peak weight loss of 8% (**Figure 9.1**), physical fitness and HbA_{1c} nadir (−0.6%) were seen at one year and progressively deteriorated thereafter. However, they remained significantly better throughout the study. A post hoc analysis found that whether they entered the control or intervention group, those who lost 10% of their body weight or increased their fitness by 2 metabolic equivalent (METs) in the first year had an approximately 20% reduction in cardiovascular events; there was no advantage if changes were less marked. These are difficult targets to achieve but on the limited evidence of this retrospective study we can both incentivise patients and also counsel against the wisdom of suggesting non-specific 'lifestyle' interventions (Look AHEAD Research Group, 2016).

> **Practice point**
>
> Cardiovascular events are reduced if people with known Type 2 diabetes can maintain 10% body weight reduction or increase fitness by 2 METs over at least a year.

So although the heroic attempt to reduce cardiovascular events through diet, weight loss and increased activity did not succeed, at least with only 10 years follow-up (and this is consistent with the previous studies in prediabetes), other important prespecified outcomes in the Look AHEAD study were significantly improved (**Box 9.1**).

> **Practice point**
>
> While active diet and exercise intervention in the Look AHEAD study did not reduce vascular events, it had definite benefits on a spectrum of outcomes meaningful to people with diabetes.

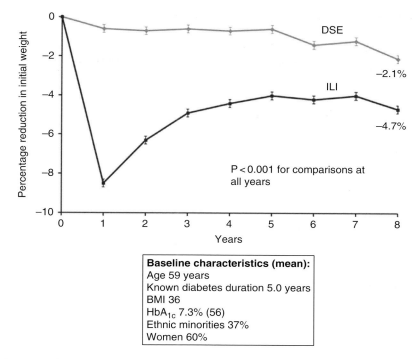

Baseline characteristics (mean):
Age 59 years
Known diabetes duration 5.0 years
BMI 36
HbA$_{1c}$ 7.3% (56)
Ethnic minorities 37%
Women 60%

Figure 9.1 Clinical characteristics of Look AHEAD participants, and weight loss over eight years in the trial. DSE: diabetes support and education; ILI: intensive lifestyle intervention. *Source*: Look AHEAD Research Group, 2014. Reproduced with permission of John Wiley & Sons.

Box 9.1 Interventions and outcomes in Look AHEAD.

Outcomes at year 1 *(with 8 kg weight loss)*
- *Glycaemic control*: fasting glucose ↓1.2 mmol/l, HbA$_{1c}$ ↓0.6%
- *Diabetes medication use*:   ↓10%
- *Blood pressure (systolic/diastolic)*:   ↓7/3 mm Hg
- *Lipid profile*:
  ○ HDL   ↑0.09 mmol/l
  ○ LDL   ↓0.1 mmol/l
  ○ Triglycerides ↓0.3 mmol/l
  ○ Lipid-lowering medication use ↓12%
- *Albumin/creatinine ratio rate of normalization*: ↑15%
- Improved QoL.
- Slight improvement in erectile dysfunction.
- Improvement in resolution of urinary incontinence in men; improvement in incidence of urinary incontinence in women.
- Improvement in measures of obstructive sleep apnoea, especially if weight loss >10 kg.
- Overall reduction in medication cost.
- Reduction in knee pain.

Outcomes at year 4
- Improved fitness.
- Improved physical functioning except in those with cardiovascular disease at baseline.
- Improved apnoea-hypopnoea index, fivefold increased rate of remission of obstructive sleep apnoea.

Outcomes at mean 8 years
- Very high-risk CKD improved (KDOQI classification) (hazard ratio 0.69).
- Hospitalizations and days spent in hospital reduced.
- Medication reduced (including glycaemic, lipid-lowering and blood pressure).
- Depression symptoms reduced.
- No improvement in cognitive function.

EFFECTS OF VERY LOW CALORIE DIETS (VLCD) ON ESTABLISHED TYPE 2 DIABETES: INSIGHTS INTO PATHOPHYSIOLOGY

Over the past few years dramatic improvements in Type 2 diabetes using very low calorie diets (approximately 600 kcal/day), amounting to the reversal that is also seen after bariatric surgery, have been demonstrated in small proof-of-concept studies. Clinical trials assessing the practicality of these challenging diets in routine care settings in the community are now underway. The mechanisms by which very low calorie diets reverse diabetes are becoming clear and are of fundamental importance in understanding Type 2 diabetes itself (**Box 9.2, Figure 9.2**). The key element is fat overload resulting in abnormal insulin-mediated glucose metabolism.

Clinical studies

It is relatively easy to measure hepatic fat with a CT scan, and moderately hypocaloric diets that reduce body weight by 8% can reduce hepatic fat by up to 80%, associated with marked reductions in fasting glucose levels and restoration of insulin sensitivity. The importance of a series of recent studies is that dietary therapy is feasible and may have additional effects that are important in reversing the fundamental processes causing

---

Box 9.2 Insights into the aetiology of Type 2 diabetes from proof-of-concept studies of very low calorie diets.

The twin cycle hypothesis
- Fatty liver results in increased hepatic VLDL triglyceride production.
- Excess triglycerides are exported to all organs, some of which (pancreatic islet cells, kidney, myocardium) are particularly sensitive to their adverse metabolic effects ('lipotoxicity').
- Excess triglycerides impair pancreatic β-cell insulin production.
- Decreased insulin response causes postprandial hyperglycaemia.

- A prolonged hypocaloric diet resulting in weight loss that is not just sufficient to lower blood glucose levels but normalizes pancreatic function should allow established Type 2 diabetes to go into remission by normalizing hepatic and pancreatic fat.
- Regular activity also contributes to reducing liver fat and VLDL secretion, but because exercise does not cause weight loss in middle-aged people with diabetes, calorie restriction is paramount.

Source: Modified after Taylor, 2013.

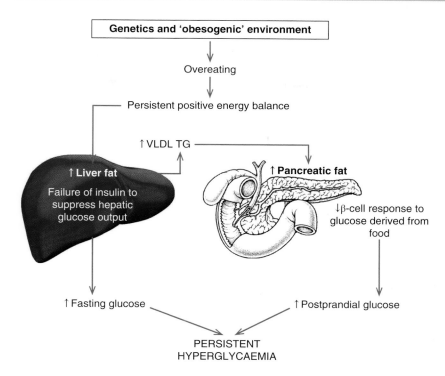

Figure 9.2 Fat overload in the aetiology and treatment of Type 2 diabetes (adapted and modified from Taylor 2008 and others).

Type 2 diabetes. In 2011 it was shown that eight weeks of a severely hypocaloric diet (600 kcal/day) in a group of obese Type 2 patients (mean BMI 34) with less than four years known duration of diabetes:

- normalized fasting glucose levels (6 mmol/l from 9)
- normalized liver fat (from 13% to 3%, where <5% is considered normal)
- resulted in near-normalization of first-phase insulin secretion
- caused a reduction in pancreatic fat (from 8% to 6%) (Lim *et al.*, 2011).

Subsequent questions were: Was the response limited to people with a short duration of diabetes? Was it sustainable? Was it practicable in real life? and What other features were associated with it?

Fasting blood glucose levels normalized after an 8-week VLCD in nearly all patients with less than four years of diabetes, compared with 50% of those with longer duration (more than eight years). About 40% of a small group with duration varying from six months to 23 years maintained normal glucose levels (<7.0 mmol/l) up to six months after a stepped return to an isocaloric diet (Steven *et al.*, 2016). There is meta-analysis evidence that adherence to these diets is good, but only large-scale real-life studies will be able to dispel the intuition that, as with all diets, persistence is low and there is a relentless weight rise after an initial good response. While the overall response rate seems disappointingly low, it may not be very different from the response rate to many medications used in Type 2 diabetes; the results of these studies, and of bariatric surgery in the early stages of diabetes (see **Chapter 10**), should focus further clinical attention on active early intervention. While cross-sectional studies have not consistently found a relationship between pancreatic fat levels and β-cell function (Begovatz *et al.*, 2015), the therapeutic response is, nevertheless, now firmly established.

The excitement generated by these important studies must be tempered by their real-life practicability. The best study so far, the UK Early ACTID study (Andrews *et al.*, 2011), was disappointing in spite of a rigorously conducted trial of newly-diagnosed patients randomized to usual care, diet alone (aiming to lose 5–10% of initial body weight) and diet-plus-exercise (exercise target 30 minutes or more brisk walking five days out of seven, in addition to current activity). HbA_{1c} fell by 0.3% in both intervention groups and antidiabetic agents were used less. There were no changes in blood pressure but there were small changes in the expected direction of triglycerides and HDL cholesterol. At 12 months, weight loss was only about 2.6% in the intervention groups. Critically, the modest increase in activity level did not add to the benefit of diet alone. It is popularly held that in the portfolio of 'lifestyle' changes, exercise can be of metabolic value; this is not confirmed either in the prediabetes intervention trials or in early Type 2 diabetes.

Practice point

The very-low calorie regimen of the Newcastle regimen resulted in near-normal glucose control and improvement in fat levels in the liver and pancreas, which improved insulin action. Whether the diet is practicable in real-life is not known.

CONVENTIONAL DIET THERAPY IN TYPE 2 DIABETES

Nothing stimulates more radical dissension or dogmatic or opinionated views than diet, in general or specifically in diabetes, and to some extent this is because it is supposed there is little evidence. This is no longer the case.

The aims of dietary therapy in Type 2 diabetes are usually stated as follows (ADA, 2013):

- to promote and support healthful eating patterns, emphasizing a variety of nutrient-dense foods in appropriate portion sizes, in order to improve overall health and specifically to:
  - attain individualized glycaemia, blood pressure and lipid goals
  - achieve and maintain body weight goals
  - delay or prevent complications of diabetes
- to address individual nutrition needs
- to maintain the pleasure of eating
- to provide practical tools for day-to-day meal planning rather than focusing on individual macronutrients, micronutrients or single foods.

The last point is widely ignored in the commercial battle to promote the latest 'superfoods'. Even the modest and evidence-based general US dietary recommendations issued in 2015 unleashed a storm of controversy (**Box 9.3**).

> **Box 9.3** 2015 US Dietary Guidelines (Dietary Guidelines Advisory Committee, 2015).
>
> - The upper limit on dietary fat (previously 20–35% of calories) has been abolished, as it may result in a reduction in healthy fats (e.g. nuts, vegetable oils and fish).
> - Replacing fat with carbohydrate does not lower cardiovascular risk.
> - There is therefore no benefit from the traditional 'low fat, high carbohydrate' diet.
> - Reduce refined grain products (e.g. white bread, white rice, crisps, crackers, breakfast cereals and bakery desserts).
> - Increased intake of healthy fats, including the monounsaturated and polyunsaturated fats in the Mediterranean diet (especially olive oil) reduces the risk of cardiovascular disease.
> - Dietary cholesterol intake is irrelevant.

> **Practice point**
>
> Dietary fat should not be restricted, though mono- and polyunsaturated fats should be emphasized. Low dietary cholesterol, often promoted in manufactured food products, is irrelevant.

Dietary therapy in Type 2 diabetes

There are four distinct themes of dietary management in Type 2 diabetes that are of interest and have been studied in recent trials:

1. To modify diet components to reduce the excess burden of cardiovascular disease.
2. To modify the composition of diets to enhance weight loss and to minimize weight regain.
3. To modify the composition of diets to improve glycaemic control.
4. To reduce weight to a degree that will either 'cure' diabetes, that is reduce blood glucose levels to values that no longer require medication, or have an impact on the multiple metabolic targets that if sustained over a long period may delay the onset or slow the progression of diabetic microvascular complications.

To modify diet components to reduce the excess burden of cardiovascular disease: the Mediterranean advantage

Much study and trial attention has focused on the traditional Mediterranean diet characteristic of many regions of southern Europe, especially Spain, Greece and southern Italy. In the Lyon heart study (1999) there was a 50–70% risk reduction in cardiac events (including cardiac deaths and recurrent myocardial infarction) after a heart attack in non-diabetic patients who adhered to a Mediterranean diet over four years (Kris-Etherton *et al.*, 2001). The components emphasized in this early study were bread and green and root vegetables, daily fruit, more fish, less red meat (to be replaced by poultry) and a margarine that more or less mimicked olive oil, though with a higher proportion of linoleic and alpha-linolenic acid. In a non-Mediterranean city, and before its benefits had been generally recognized, olive oil itself was not recommended exclusively except in salads and food preparation, Nevertheless, by the turn of the millennium the importance of this dietary approach was recognized (Kris-Etherton *et al.*, 2001).

PREDIMED (2013): Mediterranean diet plus olive oil or nuts

The most persuasive study was PREDIMED (Estruch *et al.*, 2013), in which Spanish patients at high cardiovascular risk were randomized to an energy-unrestricted control diet, or two Mediterranean-encouraged diets supplemented with either 1 litre extra-virgin olive oil per week, or 30 g mixed nuts daily (**Table 9.1**). About one-half of the recruited cohort had diabetes. Combined, acute myocardial infarction, stroke and cardiovascular death were reduced by 30% in both the supplemented diets, and similar reductions were seen in the patients who had diabetes. Supplementation with nuts seemed to have a particular powerful effect on stroke (risk reduction 55%). The trial was not without controversy. For example, it was argued that the benefits in PREDIMED were primarily due to the supplementary olive oil and nuts, since all participants adhered to the standard precepts of the Mediterranean diet, so the study might better be considered a trial of a Mediterranean-plus diet.

Practice point

Strict adherence to the Mediterranean diet, generously supplemented with extra-virgin olive oil, reduces the risk of cardiovascular events in high cardiovascular risk people with diabetes.

Table 9.1 Components of the recommended Mediterranean diet in the PREDIMED Study.

	Target
Recommended	
Olive oil	≥4 tbsp a day (a further 4 tbsp of extra-virgin olive oil/day in the group assigned to additional olive oil)
Nuts and peanuts	≥3 servings a week (30 g daily in the group assigned to additional nuts: walnuts 15 g, almonds and hazelnuts 7.5 g each)
Fresh fruits	≥3 servings a day
Vegetables	≥2 servings a day
Fish (especially fatty), seafood	≥3 servings a week
Legumes	≥3 servings a week
Sofrito	≥2 servings a week (a traditional Italian base for pasta sauces and soups, comprising carrots, celery and onion, usually cooked slowly in olive oil)
White meat	In place of red meat
Wine	≥7 glasses a week (optional, only people who normally drank alcohol)
Discouraged	
Soft drinks	<1 drink a day
Commercial bakery foods, sweets, pastries	<3 servings a week
Spread fats	<1 serving a day
Red and processed meats	<1 serving a day

Source: Modified after Estruch *et al.*, 2013.
tbsp: tablespoon

This is the only contemporary randomized trial in which adherence to a portfolio of dietary components resulted in meaningful long-term benefits. It also adds to the considerable evidence from careful but non-randomized cohort studies that adherence to the Mediterranean diet is valuable in reducing cardiovascular events and cancer (breast cancer incidence was lower in the PREDIMED group taking supplementary olive oil). While there was no reduction in the incidence of heart failure, high consumption of extra-virgin (but not ordinary) olive oil halved the risk of an osteoporotic fracture over nine years' follow-up in middle-aged and older people (55–80 years old at recruitment) and, also in PREDIMED, measures of fatty liver in older people progressed more slowly in the supplemented groups.

What about the Mediterranean diet in non-Mediterranean countries? There have been no randomized trials since the Lyon heart study but there is some evidence, though less consistent, from cohort studies. In Sweden, higher adherence was associated with lower cardiovascular mortality, but only in women; Australian men benefited; and in Eastern Europe cardiovascular mortality was lower in both men and women, but not ischaemic heart disease or stroke mortality. This is the somewhat unhelpful heterogeneity typical of cohort study outcomes. A huge prospective cohort study in the United Kingdom (EPIC-Norfolk) found a lower incidence of cardiovascular disease and a lower mortality in people with greater Mediterranean adherence (Tong et al., 2016). Given the potential benefit, a trial similar to PREDIMED would be valuable in a genetically and culturally different population and might help address the practicalities of adherence in an environment mostly alien to Mediterranean ingredients and cuisine.

There may be benefits in Type 1 diabetes, too. In Canadian patients, a higher Mediterranean diet score was associated with improved cardiometabolic measures, including lower body mass index, waist circumference, truncal fat and blood pressure (Gingras et al., 2015). Increasing monounsaturated fat intake improves the lipid profile in Type 1 patients.

To modify the composition of diets to enhance weight loss and to minimize weight regain

High(er) protein diets

Another area of great controversy, fuelled by periodic iterations of high or higher protein diet fads, notably, in historical sequence, the extreme Atkins diet, the Dukan diet, and countless variants of the historically dubious 'paleo' diet.

There are no randomized trials in diabetes, but the Diogenes study (2010) investigated the effect of four combinations of lower/higher protein and low/high glycaemic index (GI) over one year in non-diabetic subjects (mean BMI 30) who had already lost at least 8% body weight with a 800 kcal diet (Larsen et al., 2010). The difference in glycaemic index (see later) was modest, around five units, and similarly there was only a 5% increase in protein, accompanied by a 7% decrease in carbohydrate. Despite these, there was a notable difference between the high GI/low protein group, which gained around 1.5 kg over a year, and the low GI/higher protein group, which was the only one to maintain a steady weight. Those taking the high protein diet were also more likely to lose more than 5% body weight. A higher protein diet may be better for weight maintenance after weight loss. These encouraging results were obtained without extreme measures; while very high protein diets, especially those that exclude carbohydrate completely, may be harmful, it is unlikely that a 5% increase in protein intake would be hazardous in the long-term (Larsen et al., 2010).

Lower carbohydrate diets

The elegant 2-year DIRECT study in obese subjects (mean BMI 31) found that weight loss was best maintained with either a calorie-restricted Mediterranean diet or a non-calorie-restricted low-carbohydrate diet compared with a traditional low-fat restricted-calorie diet (Shai *et al.*, 2008). In the small group with diabetes, fasting glucose fell progressively in the Mediterranean group, rose in the low-fat group and remained stable in the low-carbohydrate group. The low-carbohydrate diet used the basic precepts of the Atkins diet, then in vogue: 20 g carbohydrate daily during the induction phase, gradually increased to 120 g. Though not restricted in total calories, fat or protein, the low-carbohydrate group maintained a mean calorie deficit of −370 kcal/day, smaller numerically, but not significantly, compared with the other groups (−550 kcal/day), supporting the view that higher protein, lower carbohydrate diets are more sustainable in practice. A further one-year study in Type 2 patients found that a hypocaloric, very-low-carbohydrate diet (14%), high in polyunsaturated fats and protein (30%), gave similar weight loss and reductions in HbA$_{1c}$, blood pressure and LDL cholesterol as a conventional high-carbohydrate diet (nearly 60%). However, diabetes medication was reduced more in the low-carbohydrate group, as was glycaemic variability and triglycerides; HDL increased more. This confirms the value of the higher protein, low carbohydrate, high polyunsaturated fat diet in Type 2 diabetes, reminiscent of the Mediterranean pattern (Tay *et al.*, 2015).

Type 1 patients are already taking lower carbohydrate diets than recommended (50–60%) and are moving towards low (30–105 g/day) or very low (<30 g/day) intakes. Patients report less hypoglycaemia and less marked hyperglycaemia, especially in those using CGM. However, although blood glucose levels may fall after a high fat meal, they may show a late rise after 2–3 hours, and high-fat/high-protein meals may require more insulin (Bell *et al.*, 2015). However, glycaemia in Type 1 diabetes is paramount and patients should not be discouraged from trying moderate changes that objectively help.

> **Practice point**
>
> Lower carbohydrate diets are sustainable in people with diabetes and do not cause any deterioration in metabolic control or lipid profile compared with conventional low-fat, high-carbohydrate diets. Optimally, these should be integrated into a Mediterranean-type portfolio.

Whole grains

Even if glycaemic index (see later) is a concept whose implementation has equivocal outcomes, there is good evidence for the benefit of wholegrain foods. Non-diabetic subjects in the Nurses Health Study (1984–2010) and the Health Professionals Follow-up Study (1986–2010) had a 10% lower all-cause and cardiovascular mortality in those taking the highest quintile of whole grains, but there was an approximately 2% reduction for each quintile. (Numerically, total wholegrain + bran + germ intake was 46 g/day in the highest quintile of the nurses' study, 67 g/day in the health professionals; compare the lowest quintile: 5 g in nurses, 7 g in health professionals.) Similar benefits were seen in people in the United Kingdom with diabetes, but robustly there was no effect on cancer mortality in either study. In advertising commercially-available products, the wholegrain concept is used with considerable fluidity and translating it into bought food products that have low glycaemic index may not be easy. The British Dietetic Association recommends the following low-glycaemic index wholegrain foods, a notably short list:

- rolled oats and oatmeal
- wholegrain muesli
- bread and crackers (wholegrain with multigrain; seeded, mixed-grain, soya, linseed, rye – pumpernickel)
- wholewheat pasta, whole barley, bulgur (cracked) wheat, quinoa, barley (not pearl).

Modifying dietary components to improve glycaemic control and lipids

Glycaemic index

Glycaemic index (GI) is a quantitative estimate of the effect of eating particular carbohydrates on glucose excursions, defined as the glucose excursion two hours after eating 50 g of the test food, compared with 50 g glucose. It has become a popular qualitative notion of 'good' versus 'bad' carbohydrate – and very heavily promoted by the food industry – but evidence is hard to interpret, as pure carbohydrates are rarely taken on their own and other components of a meal, especially protein, can significantly lower GI. Trials are usually of short duration and factors other than the foods themselves are often studied (e.g. weight, diabetes treatments, fibre content). Meta-analyses of studies in Type 2 diabetes have shown minor benefits in improving glycaemic control (overall effect about -0.4% HbA_{1c}), but such changes cannot be reliably detected in individuals. Mechanistically, the best study is the careful OmniCarb study (2014) in obese non-diabetic adults (mean BMI 32), which compared four different diets: low- and high-carbohydrate, and low- and high-GI in addition to a background DASH diet (see **Chapter 11**). There were no differences in glucose and insulin excursions during glucose tolerance tests, lipid profile or blood pressure (Sacks et al., 2014). The longest study in diabetes (12 months) showed modest lowering of postprandial glucose levels with a high-GI diet and high-sensitivity C-reactive protein (hsCRP) was numerically lower. However, the impact of lower GI on glycaemia and weight seem relatively small compared with portfolio changes, such as the Mediterranean diet, which also has meaningful clinical outcomes.

Practice point

There is more evidence for the benefit of portfolio changes to diets, such as the Mediterranean diet, than for using 'low GI' diets. Encourage carbohydrates that are wholegrain *and* low GI.

Alcohol

Alcoholic drinks contain substantial energy and regular drinkers should have an idea of their calorie content. A simple formula is:

Calories = 0.06 × % alcohol x ml (Rubin and Jarvis, 2011; drinkaware.co.uk)

Some examples are shown on **Table 9.2**.

Alcopops continue to proliferate. While low in alcohol (around 4%), they are high in sugar and calories, for example 180 kcal per bottle, and may contribute to weight gain and weekend hyperglycaemia in young people with Type 1 diabetes. Beer intake is highly relevant: it has a relatively low carbohydrate content (4–5 g/100 ml) but men especially drink large volumes; in the Netherlands, only potatoes, bread, sugar and sugar-sweetened drinks exceeded beer in their contribution to population glycaemic load (Sluik et al., 2016). The lower weekly alcohol limit now promoted in the United Kingdom for

Table 9.2 Calorie content of alcohols.

Alcohol	kcal (units)
1/3 bottle 13% wine (250 ml)	195 (~3.2)
1 pint 5% beer (568 ml)	170 (~2.3)
1 bottle 5% beer (330 ml)	100 (~1.6)
Spirit (40%) – 2 measures (often now 35 ml each)	170 (~3)
1 bottle 4% alcopop (250 ml)	170 (~1.1)

men and women alike – 14 units – was based on a change from emphasizing reduced serious harm to minimizing all-cause risk, but weight loss from substantially reducing alcohol intake is an important potential benefit, although there are no formal studies.

Practice point

Alcoholic drinks are calorific and reducing alcohol intake is likely to help weight loss. Beer is a significant contributor to population glycaemic load in men.

Eggs

Egg consumption is one of the many dietary components around which absent evidence and fear of 'cholesterol' intake has sclerosed to the point where many people with diabetes avoid eating any whole eggs, though most preprepared products contain egg components and eggs are high in mono- and polyunsaturated fatty acids. Epidemiological studies have found some increased cardiovascular risk in Type 2 patients who eat eggs but not in the general population. Clinical studies are sparse but HDL cholesterol levels rose in several studies after increased egg intake. A large six-week trial in Type 2 patients randomized to a high-egg (2 eggs/day) or low-egg diet (<2 eggs/week) but with matched protein intake found that there were no differences in lipid profiles or glycaemia. The high-egg group reported less hunger and greater satiety after breakfast (Fuller *et al.*, 2015).

Practice point

People with diabetes should not fear moderate whole-egg intake.

Superfoods

At the time of writing PubMed contained only 14 references to superfoods, which does not reflect the huge general interest in these products, which emerged as a concept only about 15 years ago Their presence and annual proliferation reflects the widespread belief that individual vegetables and fruits, often exotic, some hitherto barely known, offer a specific treatment for various conditions, including Type 2 diabetes, even if taken in small quantities. The gamut has run from soy, exploring its pro-oestrogenic effects and possible benefits on cardiovascular risk factors (not supported in clinical trials), to rare berries and their extracts. More recently, and with the strong evidence supporting constituents of the Mediterranean diet, the superfood category has snuggled up to mainstream dietary components (functional foods). In discussion, explore patients' own understanding of the idea, but there is no evidence – and probably never will be – that a handful of exotic berries will do anything other than deplete the pocket.

ACTIVITY AND EXERCISE

There is nearly as much confusion about the impact of activity and exercise on diabetes as there is about diet. The lumping of activity into the 'lifestyle' portfolio has blurred the important distinctions between the effect of activity on short- and medium-term glucose control, and its possible long-term benefits on micro- and macrovascular complications. In addition, the distinction between aerobic exercise (e.g. running/jogging, cycling swimming) and resistance exercise (e.g. free weights, weight machines, body weight itself) can be made relatively easily in physiological studies, while in real life they are often combined.

Lack of exercise as a risk factor for Type 2 diabetes is a popular concern at present. Moderate regular exercise, for example 2½ hours or more brisk walking reduces the risk of developing Type 2 diabetes by about 30% (Jeon et al., 2007). This modest activity is more effective in preventing diabetes than reducing the risk of progression from prediabetes to Type 2 diabetes or as a therapeutic intervention in established Type 2 diabetes. Some reports find a linear increase in Type 2 risk with daily duration of TV watching, some that a combination of factors (e.g. a combination of lack of exercise with heavy TV watching >6 hours a day) increases the risk, in this case doubling the risk over the next two years (Smith and Hamer, 2014). Others identify a threshold level, including two meta-analyses that found that three hours or more of TV watching was not only associated with increased diabetes risk but also of fatal cardiovascular disease and all-cause mortality (Grøntved and Hu, 2011). Only the most vigorous exercise can attenuate the mortality effects of prolonged TV watching. There is grave concern that screen-watching time, which now includes time at work and the increasing use of mobile screen technology, may in future increase this risk.

The widely used World Health Organization recommendations for activity have been adopted in the United Kingdom, resulting in the well-known examples of 150 minutes/week of brisk walking or 75 minutes/week running, equivalent to about 600 metabolic equivalent (MET) minutes per week. At this level, risk reduction for diabetes was only about 2%. Increasing activity levels from 600 to 3600 MET minutes per week reduced risk by around 20% and optimum exercise for reduction of risk of diabetes, ischaemic heart disease, stroke and breast and colon cancer is now considered to occur at 3000–4000 (Kyu et al., 2016). The current recommendations are, therefore, minimum for prevention. We need to do much more exercise (**Figure 9.3**).

Technology and exercise

Activity trackers (e.g. Fitbit) are widely used by athletes and it is assumed that similar technology will be of value in improving activity levels in the general population. There are no specific studies in Type 2 diabetes but there is very little evidence that they meaningfully improve activity once the novelty value of the device has worn off; both trained and inactive subjects quickly learn what their activity levels and step counts are. Whether additional measurements or links to social media will improve adherence also remains to be seen. In a large study of working-age people in Singapore only about 10% of subjects used their Fitbit at one year, compared with 90–100% at the start of the trial. Financial incentives maintained slightly increased activity level during the six months they were in place, but rapidly dropped off to levels similar to those in the unincentivized group (Finkelstein et al., 2016). We should not encourage overreliance on technology where there is greater emphasis on its 'lifestyle' attributes rather than the evidence base for its real efficacy.

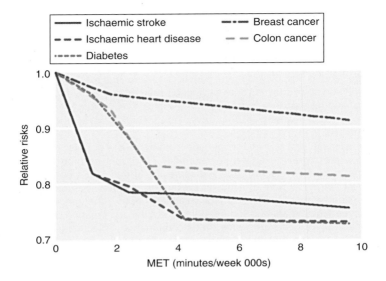

Figure 9.3 Dose-responses for relative risk of reduction in cardiovascular events, Type 2 diabetes and breast and colon cancer with increasing levels of exercise. *Source*: Kyu *et al.*, 2016. Reproduced with permission of BMJ Publishing Group Ltd.

Practice point

The use of activity trackers (e.g. Fitbit) does not increase activity levels in the long term. Financial incentives do not have legacy benefits.

Current levels of exercise in Type 2 diabetes

Little is reported, especially in comparison with non-diabetic populations. In people at high risk of diabetes recruited for UK trials from primary care, objectively studied with pedometers and accelerometers, under 5% took the recommended amount of moderate-to-vigorous activity (more than 30 minutes in bursts of at least 10 minutes, five days a week). Self-reported activity may not be wholly reliable. In the same study, UK South Asians and UK whites had identical levels of activity, even though it is widely believed that South Asians are less active. Although both groups overestimated the amount of moderate-to-vigorous exercise they took, the white population overestimated it by 50 minutes/day, South Asians by 20 minutes (Yates *et al.*, 2015). Similar studies in the USA find that African Americans are as active as white Americans.

Practice point

We all overestimate the amount of moderate-to-vigorous activity we take.

Long-term outcomes of exercise in Type 2 diabetes

Cross-sectional associations are well known and unsurprising: for example, Type 2 patients with higher fitness levels live longer and are at lower risk of cardiovascular events. Moderate or vigorous exercise is associated with a lower risk of cardiac or cerebrovascular disease; meta-analysis demonstrates a hazard ratio of 0.6 for premature death (Sluik *et al.*, 2012). These large effects may be thoroughly undermined by the 'healthy exerciser' effect and cannot be excluded even in large prospective studies that are not randomized.

ADVANCE and Look AHEAD studies

There are some prospective data. A simple baseline exercise score (none, mild and moderate or vigorous activity for more than 15 minutes a week) was recorded in the large prospective five-year ADVANCE study. Mild exercise included easy walking or bowling; moderate exercise fast walking, tennis or dancing; and vigorous exercise jogging or vigorous swimming. There was a consistent approximately 20% risk reduction of cardiovascular events, microvascular events and all-cause mortality in people doing moderate or vigorous activity, but no benefit of mild activity (Blomster *et al.*, 2013). This is a large and clinically significant effect; recall that in the main study (see **Chapters 5 and 10**) HbA_{1c} reduction of 0.7% maintained for five years had no meaningful impact on micro- or macrovascular events.

In contrast, there is the thoroughly negative effect on cardiovascular events of the highly structured exercise regimen in the Look AHEAD study, in which fitness levels were significantly higher in the intervention group during at least the first four years. The absolute differences in activity level between the study groups probably explains the different outcomes. Only 1 MET separated the two groups in Look AHEAD, and although activity was not quantified in ADVANCE, there was probably a much greater difference: for example the moderate-to-vigorous activity group had done more than twice the number of exercise sessions in the previous week compared with the other groups (13 vs 5) (**Box 9.4**).

In people doing moderate-to-vigorous exercise there were minor improvements in cardiometabolic measurements but what they contributed to the beneficial outcomes has not been estimated. Other changes may be more important, for example improved muscle mass and strength through aerobic and resistance exercise, or improved insulin sensitivity, which can persist for up to 14 days after a moderate intensity/long-distance programme (De Feo and Schwarz, 2013). Improved quality of life may also contribute: the mental component predictably increases with any increased level of activity, though only people doing more exercise than 17.5 MET.h/week experienced improved physical measures of quality of life (**Figure 9.4**).

Box 9.4 The MET.

The MET is the ratio of the work metabolic rate to the resting metabolic rate. It is defined as expenditure of 1 kcal/kg/h, similar to the energy expended in resting quietly, and also as a rate of oxygen usage. Example: if someone does 3-MET exercise for 30 minutes, then they have done 90 MET-minutes, that is 1½ MET-hours. MET rating is an indicator of intensity of exercise, and more meaningful than simple measures such as step counts.

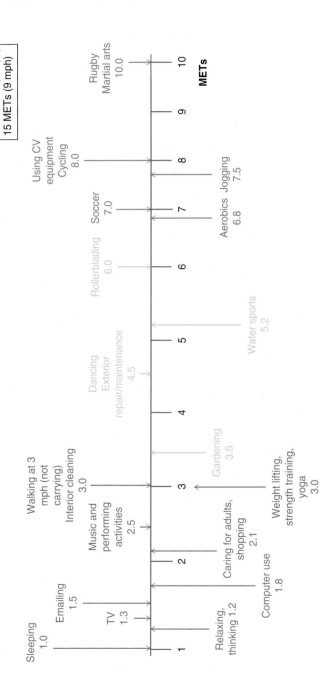

Figure 9.4 Examples of activity and their associated METs. The current recommended level is 600 MET.min/week; current evidence-based values for *reduction* in risk of inactivity-associated diseases is 3000–4000 MET.min/week. Note the marked disparity between resistance training (3.0) and aerobic training (6.8), and the cluster of screen-associated activity that is just above values for sleeping. Activity under 3 METs is considered mild, 3–6 moderate and >6 vigorous. (Data from https://epi.grants.cancer.gov/atus-met/met.php; last accessed 21 August 2017).

Box 9.5 American College of Sports Medicine recommendations for exercise and weight (minutes per week, hours).

Maintaining and improving health: 150 (2½), energy equivalent 1200–2000 kcal per week
Preventing weight gain: 150–200 (2½–3½)
Preventing weight gain after weight loss: 200–300 (3½–5)
Promoting clinically significant weight loss: 225–420 (~4–7)

Exercise, weight loss and fat loss: high-intensity interval training (HIIT)

It is generally agreed that only extended exercise will lead to meaningful weight loss, and the recommended 150 min/week may at most lead to 2–3 kg loss; in clinical discussions it is best to use this guidance on exercise as a recommendation for maintaining, but not losing, weight, and for improving cardiorespiratory fitness (**Box 9.5**). Resistance training alone does not reduce weight. There is more convincing evidence for the benefits of moderate amounts of exercise in the prevention of weight gain, especially after calorie-restricted weight loss. In one study 80 minutes' exercise weekly minimized weight regain, though this is much lower than the recommendations of the American College of Sports Medicine. Aerobic and resistance training were equally effective (Hunter *et al.*, 2010). A recurrent theme is that abnormal fat distribution benefits from exercise independent of total weight loss. One study that matched weight loss caused by diet alone and exercise alone found that total fat mass fell in the exercising subjects, and there is convincing data that exercise is of specific benefit in reducing hepatic steatosis in fatty liver disease (Orci *et al.*, 2016; see **Chapter 13**).

Practice point

Only very high exercise levels will cause weight loss but modest exercise (including high-intensity interval training) improves fatty liver and can prevent weight gain after diet.

This finding is reinforced by a study of a recently-described form of exercise: high-intensity interval training (HIIT), an exercise regimen of around 20 minutes, alternating brief and vigorous activity (usually 1–4 minutes, targeting >90% maximum heart rate) with periods of low activity or rest. Different varieties are described, most popularly sprint interval training, with only a few seconds of maximum activity, but cycling and running, usually on stationary cycles and treadmills, have been studied more rigorously. After 12 weeks, systolic and diastolic function improved and liver fat decreased by 40%; there was only a small reduction in HbA_{1c}. The specific benefits of HIIT are probably due to greater upregulation of muscle GLUT-4 receptors than standard moderate-intensity continuous training, thereby improving insulin resistance. It also increases liver mitochondrial density and boosts catecholamine levels, both of which increase fat oxidation. Standard moderate-intensity exercise may exert its benefit on the liver partly through meaningfully suppressing appetite the day after exercise, amounting to approximately 300 kcal lower intake (Cassidy *et al.*, 2016).

Glycaemic control

As to glycaemia, two good studies, duration six and nine months, compared the effects of resistance, aerobic or combined modalities. They both found that the combination exercise reduced HbA_{1c} more than the individual exercise types, but they inevitably found different absolute reductions compared with a control sedentary group: −0.3% (Church *et al.*, 2010) and −0.9% (Sigal *et al.*, 2007), and in the latter study only those with base-line HbA_{1c} >7.5% (58) showed improvement, similar to the consistent findings in drug trials where absolute HbA_{1c} reductions are greater the higher the baseline value. But these are robust and sustainable results, and there are plenty of drug trials where smaller reductions make the headlines and the guidelines. Cardiorespiratory fitness and glycae-mia therefore meaningfully improve, especially with combined aerobic and resistance training, but blood pressure and lipids do not show consistent improvements.

Practice point

Combined aerobic and resistance training delivers the greatest HbA_{1c} reductions compared with the exercise types individually. With good adherence, anticipate 0.5–1.0% reduction.

Real-life exercise in people with Type 2 diabetes

Most people with Type 2 diabetes are inactive. Thomas *et al.* (2004) found that only 10% of the one-third of patients who took any exercise did sufficient activity to change heart rate or breathing. People do not persist with exercise even when part of a formal pro-gramme and perhaps only 40% will still be doing the prescribed exercise after 12 months. While only one-quarter of patients seem to discontinue for motivational rea-sons, around one-half do because of orthopaedic comorbidities and overuse injuries (Praet and van Loon, 2009).

Low levels of so-called 'lifestyle' exercise do not improve cardiorespiratory fitness or cardiometabolic measures. The popularity of targets for steps taken per day measured by pedometers is not justified by evidence, either. Very small weight losses (<2 kg) and tiny changes in cardiometabolic measurements are all that can be expected, even when rec-ommended steps are doubled from the arbitrary 5000 used to define a sedentary life-style, or increased by 2000–4000 above baseline (Swift *et al.*, 2014). It is not surprising, therefore, that the current vogue for exercise prescription is of no value in weight loss. However, cardiorespiratory fitness is a valuable target for intervention, and improving muscle quality using resistance training as part of an exercise regimen in people with with premature sarcopenia is especially effective.

Practice point

Increased walking (steps) does not cause weight loss, even when measured and motivated by the use of pedometers. There is little evidence that exercise prescriptions have a meaningful impact on daily activity.

Exercise prescription

The concept of exercise prescription for people with Type 2 diabetes patients is intuitively appealing and has gained momentum rapidly since the millennium. National and local schemes, usually short-lived, have proliferated, with associated guidelines, but there is almost no clinical trial evidence that it is beneficial in people without cardiovascular disease (the situation is quite different in people with established vascular disease; see **Chapter 6**). A small but well-controlled two-year study in the Netherlands gave personalized instruc-tion every six weeks with the aim of increasing daily physical activity to 160 min/week or more.

There were similar modest improvements in leisure activity in both intervention and control groups, but no changes in daily activity, and therefore no changes in body composition, glycaemic control or cardiovascular risk factors (Wisse *et al.*, 2010). Further trial evidence is needed before hard-pressed healthcare economies continue these programmes; the more positive data from the studies in prediabetes suggest that broader interventions in diet, weight loss and exercise may be more effective than those exploiting activity alone.

References

American Diabetes Association. 4. Lifestyle management. *Diabetes Care* 2017;40(Suppl 1):S33–S43 [PMID: 27979891] Free full text.

Andrews RC, Cooper AR, Montgomery AA *et al.* Diet or diet plus physical exercise versus usual care in patients with newly diagnosed type 2 diabetes: the Early ACTID randomised controlled trial. *Lancet* 2011;378:129–39 [PMID: 21705068] Free full text.

Begovatz P, Koliaki C, Weber K *et al.* Pancreatic adipose tissue infiltration, parenchymal steatosis and beta cell function in humans. *Diabetologia* 2015;58:1646–55 [PMID: 25740696].

Bell KJ, Smart CE, Steil GM *et al.* Impact of fat, protein, and glycemic index on postprandial glucose control in type 1 diabetes: implications for intensive diabetes management in the continuous glucose monitoring era. *Diabetes Care* 2015;38:1008–15 [PMID: 25998293].

Bhopal RS, Douglas A, Wallia S *et al.* Effect of a lifestyle intervention on weight change in south Asian individuals in the UK at high risk of type 2 diabetes: a family-cluster randomised controlled trial. *Lancet Diabetes Endocrinol* 2014; 2:218–27 [PMID: 24622752] Free full text.

Blomster JI, Chow CK, Zoungas S *et al.* The influence of physical activity on vascular complications and mortality in patients with type 2 diabetes mellitus. *Dabetes Obes Metab* 2013;15:1008–12 [PMID: 23675676].

Cassidy S, Thoma C, Hallsworth K *et al.* High intensity intermittent exercise improves cardiac structure and function and reduces liver fat in patients with type 2 diabetes: a randomised controlled trial. *Diabetologia* 2016;59:56–66 [PMID: 26350611] PMC4670457.

Church TS, Blair SN, Cocreham S *et al.* Effects of aerobic and resistance training on haemoglobin A1c levels in patients with type 2 diabetes: a randomized controlled trial. *JAMA* 2010;304:2253–62 [PMID: 21098771] PMC3174102.

Cooper AJ, Schliemann D, Long GH *et al.* ADDITION-Cambridge study team. Do improvements in dietary behaviour contribute to cardiovascular risk factor reduction over and above cardio-protective medication in newly diagnosed diabetes patients? *Eur J Clin Nutr* 2014;68:1113–8 [PMID: 24801371] PMC4306328.

De Feo P, Schwarz P. Is physical exercise a core therapeutical element for most patients with type 2 diabetes? *Diabetes Care* 2013;36(Suppl 2):S149–54 [PMID: 23882040] PMC3920782.

Diabetes Prevention Program Research Group. Long-term effects of lifestyle intervention or metformin on diabetes development and microvascular complications over 15-year follow-up: the Diabetes Prevention Program Outcomes Study. *Lancet Diabetes Endocrinol* 2015;3:866–75 [PMID: 26377054] PMC4623946.

Dietary Guidelines Advisory Committee (US Department of Health and Human Services/US Department of Agriculture). *Dietary Guidelines for Americans* 2015–2020, 8th edn, 2015, http://health.gov/dietaryguidelines/2015/guidelines/ (last accessed 21 August 2017).

Estruch R, Ros E, Salas-Salvadó J *et al.* PREDIMED Study Investigators. Primary prevention of cardiovascular disease with a Mediterranean diet. *N Engl J Med* 2013;368:1279–90 [PMID: 23432189] Free full text.

Finkelstein EA, Haaland BA, BIlger M *et al.* Effectiveness of activity trackers with and without incentives to increase physical activity (TRIPPA): a randomised controlled trial. *Lancet Diabetes Endocrinology* 2016;4:983–95 [PMID: 27717766].

Fuller NR, Caterson ID, Sainsbury A *et al.* The effect of a high-egg diet on cardiovascular risk factors in people with type 2 diabetes: the Diabetes and Egg (DIABEGG) study – a 3-mo randomized controlled trial. *Am J Clin Nutr* 2015;101:705–13 [PMID: 25833969].

Gingras V, Lreoux C, Desjardins K *et al*. Association between cardiometabolic profile and dietary characteristics among adults with type 1 diabetes mellitus. *J Acad Nutr Diet* 2015;115:1964–75 [PMID: 26052042].

Grøntved A, Hu FB. Television viewing and risk of type 2 diabetes, cardiovascular disease, and all-cause mortality: a meta-analysis. *JAMA* 2011;305:2448–55 [PMID: 21673269] PMC4324728

Hunter GR, Brock DW, Byrne NM *et al*. Exercise training prevents regain of visceral fat for 1 year following weight loss. *Obesity (Silver Spring)* 2010;18:690–5 [PMID: 19816413] PMC2913900.

Jeon CY, Lokken RP, Hu FB, van Dam RM. Physical activity of moderate intensity and risk of type 2 diabetes: a systematic review. *Diabetes Care* 2007;30:744–52 [PMID: 17327354].

Kris-Etherton P, Eckel RH Howard BV *et al*. Nutrition Committee, Population Committee and Clinical Science Committee of the American Heart Association. AHA science advisory: Lyon Diet Heart Study. Benefits of a Mediterranean-style, National Cholesterol Education Program/American Heart Association Step 1 dietary pattern on cardiovascular disease. *Circulation* 2001;103:1823–5 [PMID: 11282918] Free full text.

Kyu HH, Bschman VF, Alexander LT *et al*. Physical activity and risk of breast cancer colon cancer, diabetes, ischemic heart disease, and ischemic stroke events: systematic review and dose-response meta-analysis for the Global Burden of Disease Study 2013. *BMJ* 2016;354:i3857 [PMID: 27510511] PMC4979358.

Larsen TM, Dalskov SM, van Baak M *et al*. Diet, Obesity, and Genes (Diogenes) Project. Diets with high or low protein content and glycemic index for weight-loss maintenance. *N Engl J Med* 2010;363:2102–13 [PMID: 21105792] PMC3359496.

Li G, Zhang P, Wang J *et al*. Cardiovascular mortality, all-cause mortality, and diabetes incidence after lifestyle intervention for people with impaired glucose tolerance in the Da Qing Diabetes Prevention Study: a 23-year follow-up study. *Lancet Diabetes Endocrinol* 2014;2:474–80 [PMID: 24731674].

Lim EL, Hollingsworth KG, Aribisala BS *et al*. Reversal of type 2 diabetes: normalisation of beta cell function in association with decreased pancreas and liver triacylglycerol. *Diabetologia* 2011;54:2506–14 [PMID: 21658330] PMC3168743. *This is widely referred to as the Counterpoint study, though the title and abstract do not include the name*

Lindström J, Peltonen M, Eriksson JG *et al*. Finnish Diabetes Prevention Study (DPS). Improved lifestyle and decreased diabetes risk over 13 years: long-term follow-up of the randomised Finnish Diabetes Prevention Study (DPS). *Diabetologia* 2013;56:284–93 [PMID: 23093136].

Long GH, Cooper AJ, Wareham NJ *et al*. Healthy behaviour change and cardiovascular outcomes in newly diagnosed type 2 diabetic patients: a cohort analysis of the ADDITION-Cambridge study. *Diabetes Care* 2014; 37:1712–20 [PMID: 24658389] PMC4170180.

Look AHEAD Research Group. Eight-year weight losses with an intensive lifestyle intervention: the look AHEAD study. *Obesity (Silver Springs)* 2014;22:5–13 [PMID: 24307184] PMC3904491.

Look AHEAD Research Group. Association of the magnitude of weight loss and changes in physical fitness with long-term cardiovascular disease outcomes in overweight or obese people with type 2 diabetes: a post-hoc analysis of the Look AHEAD randomised clinical trial. *Lancet Diabetes Endocrinol* 2016;4:913–21 [PMID: 27595918] PMC5094846.

Orci LA, Gariani K, Oldani G *et al*. Exercise-based interventions for non-alcoholic fatty liver disease: a meta-analysis and meta-regression. *Clin Gastroenterol Hepatol* 2016; 14:1398–411 [PMID: 27155553].

Praet SF, van Loon LJ. Exercise therapy in type 2 diabetes. *Acta Diabetol* 2009;46:263–78 [PMID: 19479186] PMC2773368.

Rubin AL, Jarvis S. Diabetes diet plan, in: *Diabetes for Dummies*, 3rd edn. Chichester: John Wiley & Sons Ltd, 2011, pp. 149–180.

Sacks FM, Caret VJ, Anderson CA *et al*. Effects of high vs low glycemic index of dietary carbohydrate on cardiovascular disease risk factors and insulin sensitivity: the OmniCarb randomized clinical trial. *JAMA* 2014;312:2531–41 [PMID: 25514303] PC4370345.

Shai I, Shwarzfuchs D, Henkin Y *et al*.; Dietary Intervention Randomized Controlled Trial (DIRECT) Group. Weight loss with a low-carbohydrate, Mediterranean, or low-fat diet. *N Engl J Med* 2008;359:229–41 [PMID: 18635428] Free full text.

Sigal RJ, Kenny GP, Boulé NG et al. Effects of aerobic training, resistance training, or both on glycemic control in type 2 diabetes: a randomized trial. Ann Intern Med 2007;147:357–69 [PMID: 17876019].

Sluik D, Buijsse B, Muckelbauer R et al. Physical activity and mortality in individuals with diabetes mellitus: a prospective study and meta-analysis. Arch Intern Med 2012;172:1285–95 [PMID: 22868663].

Sluik D, Atkinson FS, Brand-Miller JC et al. Contributions to dietary glycaemic index and glycaemic load in the Netherlands: the role of beer. Br J Nutr 2016;115:1218–25 [PMID: 26857156].

Smith L, Hamer M. Television viewing time and risk of incident diabetes mellitus: the English Longitudinal Study of Ageing. Diabet Med 2014;31:1572–6 [PMID: 24975987] PMC4236275.

Steven S, Hollingsworth KG, Al-Mrabeh A et al. Very low-calorie diet and 6 months of weight stability in type 2 diabetes: pathophysiological changes in responders and nonresponders. Diabetes Care 2016;39:808–15 [PMID: 27002059].

Swift D, Johansen NM, Lavie CJ et al. The role of exercise and physical activity in weight loss and maintenance. Prog Cardiovasc Dis 2014;56:441–7 [PMID: 24438736] PMC3925973.

Tay J, Luscombe-Marsh ND, Thompson CH et al. Comparison of low- and high-carbohydrate diets for type 2 diabetes management: a randomized trial. Am J Clin Nutr 2015;102:780–90 [PMID: 26224300].

Taylor R. Pathogenesis of type 2 diabetes: tracing the reverse route from cure to cause. Diabetologia 2008;51:1781–9 [PMID: 18726585].

Taylor R. Type 2 diabetes: etiology and reversibility. Diabetes Care 2013;36:1047–55 [PMID: 23520370] PMC3609491.

Thomas N, Alder E, Leese GP. Barriers to physical activity in diabetes. Postgrad Med J 2004;80:287–91 [PMID: 15138320] PMC1742997.

Tong TY, Wareham NJ, Khaw KT et al. Prospective association of the Mediterranean diet with cardiovascular disease incidence and mortality and its population impact in a non-Mediterranean population: the EPIC-Norfolk study. BMC Med 2016;14:135 [PMID: 27679997] PMC5041408.

Wisse W, Boer Rookhuizen M, de Kruif MD et al. Prescription of physical activity is not sufficient to change sedentary behaviour and improve glycemic control in type 2 diabetes patients. Diabe Res Clin Pract 2010;88:e10–3 [PMID: 20138384].

Yates T, Henson J, Edwardson C et al. Differences in levels of physical activity between White and South Asian populations within a healthcare setting: impact of measurement type in a cross-sectional study. BMJ 2015;5:e006181 [PMID: 26204908] PMC4513447.

Further reading

American Diabetes Association

American Diabetes Association. 4. Lifestyle management. Diabetes Care 2017;40(Suppl 1):S33–S43 [PMID: 27979891] Free full text.

US Department of Health and Human Services/US Department of Agriculture. Dietary Guidelines for Americans 2015–2020, 8th edn, 2015, http://health.gov/dietaryguidelines/2015/guidelines/ (last accessed 21 August 2017).

Calorie content of drinks

Unit & Calorie Calculator. https://www.drinkaware.co.uk/understand-your-drinking/unit-calculator (last accessed 21 August 2017).

10 Type 2 diabetes: glycaemic control

> **Key points**
> - Managing hyperglycaemia in Type 2 diabetes is difficult – hence a long chapter – and wherever possible targets should be realistic, achievable and not based on the outmoded premise of 'lower must be better'
> - Glycaemia does not always show relentless progression
> - Metformin is safe and effective but other than in a subset of UKPDS patients does not confer cardiovascular benefit
> - Liraglutide (GLP-1-receptor agonist) and empagliflozin (SGLT2 inhibitor) may have cardiorenal benefits in high cardiovascular risk patients
> - In long-term treatment GLP-1-receptor agonists are as effective as basal insulin
> - Basal insulin and basal-plus insulin are simple and effective; in general basal-bolus regimens are not
> - Bariatric (metabolic) surgery is an effective diabetes treatment and should form part of the mental map of strategies and considered earlier rather than late or as a last resort

INTRODUCTION

The tenacious focus on the primacy of blood glucose management in Type 2 diabetes has barely wavered, in spite of convincing trial evidence emerging from the mid-2000s onwards that we should be relegating it to second or perhaps third place behind LDL lowering and blood pressure control as a way of reducing the cardiovascular risks that still dominate the prognosis of our patients. 'Lifestyle' measures (**Chapter 9**) are safe, potentially powerful and may reverse important pathophysiological changes that are at the core of the cause of Type 2 diabetes. Drugs cannot yet do this. Although the emphasis of the majority of trials of new agents is still regulatory for establishing safety and efficacy compared with established agents, in the light of the glitazone debacle between 2007 and 2010 the USA Federal Drug Administration (FDA) requires early initiation of cardiovascular safety studies for all new agents, though their long timescale and need to recruit huge patient numbers means that many are still introduced without watertight cardiovascular safety reassurance. Many of these carefully-designed and extended trials (2–4 years in general) have now reported and have provided largely compelling safety data, but they are also revealing potential benefits that could not have been predicted either from their known modes of action or from regulatory trials that run for 6–12 months in most instances. However, it is salutary to recall that between 2006 and 2013 in both privately-insured and Medicare-covered people with diabetes in the USA there have been dramatic changes in the use of hypoglycaemic agents (for

Practical Diabetes Care, Fourth Edition. David Levy.
© 2018 John Wiley & Sons Ltd. Published 2018 by John Wiley & Sons Ltd.

example, reduction in glitazone use from 30% to 6%, but increases in use of metformin, insulin and DPP-4 inhibitors, and presumably GLP-1-receptor agonists), yet overall glycaemic control has not improved. At the same time, end-stage complications from diabetes have decreased, and severe hypoglycaemia rates have remained unchanged (Lipska *et al.*, 2017).

THE PROGRESSIVE NATURE OF TYPE 2 DIABETES

Despite general gloom, there is no reason now to consider Type 2 diabetes a relentlessly progressive disease always requiring complex insulin regimens within a decade or thereabouts of the clinical diagnosis, and characterized by progressive loss of β-cell function with onset shortly before the time of clinical diagnosis of Type 2 diabetes – though this is a widely accepted outline. The United Kingdom Prospective Diabetes Study (UKPDS) provided the paradigmatic tick-configuration of glycaemia both in monotherapy and in patients managed with diet alone (**Figure 10.1a**), in an era when few agents were available, and even metformin was relatively unfamiliar. More recently, the ADOPT study (2006) found that responses to three single agents were similar in shape to the UKPDS tick, but different in gradient, with the sulfonylurea glibenclamide showing the greatest initial effect but the most rapid deterioration in the following five years. Both the UKPDS and ADOPT study used a simple measure, HOMA-β, which is a ratio of fasting insulin to fasting glucose level, as a surrogate for β-cell function. Using this measure, β-cell function was shown to have already substantially fallen at the time of diagnosis of Type 2 diabetes and to fall progressively thereafter. However, HOMA-β may not be as reliable an indicator of β-cell function as, for example, the insulin response to a mixed meal (Reaven, 2009). Regardless of this widely-quoted reason for the inevitability of glycaemic deterioration with time, many trials from the mid-2000s onwards have shown impressive glycaemic flat-lining in both conventionally and intensively treated groups (for example **Figure 10.1b**).

The reasons for this change are not known but are likely to be mostly due to better vigilance of glycaemia. The role of the increasing numbers of drug classes is not clear. For example:

- Stable glycaemia in the PROactive study (**Figure 10.1b**) (Scheen *et al.*, 2009) was observed in the period before the introduction of incretin-associated therapies or SGLT2 inhibitors.
- Careful glycaemic follow-up of patients recruited into the FIELD trial of the lipid-modifying drug fenofibrate (median six years known diabetes) found that glycaemia using the conventional trio of metformin, sulfonylureas and insulin was well maintained over five years, with HbA_{1c} consistently about 0.4% lower in those using insulin compared with oral agents. Weight remained stable in the latter group; insulin-treated patients gained around 4 kg over the same period (Best *et al.*, 2012).

Although there is a group of patients with really troublesome glycaemia that is never adequately brought under control even with complex insulin regimens combined with multiple non-insulin agents, pre-emptively or, worse, 'aggressively', piling up the prescriptions for glycaemia-modifying drugs in anticipation of inevitable glycaemic disaster just round the corner may not be a valuable general strategy. A more nuanced and individualized approach is the key and properly voiced in some current guidelines (NICE Guideline NG28, 2015).

(a)

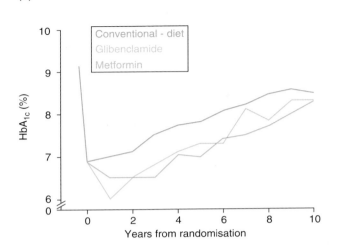

(b)

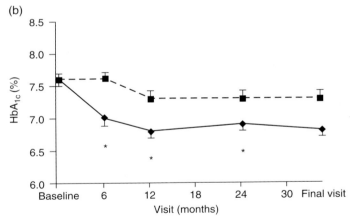

Figure 10.1 The changing face of glycaemia in clinical trials. (a) The UKPDS, showing the not-far-off iconic 'tick' shape of rapidly improving control on diet and monotherapy with oral agents over the first year, followed by progressive slipping of control. *Source*: UK Prospective Diabetes Study Group, 1998. (b) PROActive (2005): the first study to show glycaemic stability over the duration of a long randomized trial (around three years; Scheen *et al.*, 2009. Reproduced with permission of John Wiley & Sons). This pattern was repeated in the major trials in the 2000s and also in recent cardiovascular safety studies. See Figure 10.4 for another example of long-term glycaemic stability.

Practice point:

Used carefully, 'conventional' agents (metformin, sulfonylureas and insulin) can maintain stable glycaemic control for up to five years, even in patients with established Type 2 diabetes.

GLYCAEMIC CONTROL AND COMPLICATIONS IN TYPE 2 DIABETES

This crucial question has exercised researchers and guideline writers now for two decades and the uncertainty shows only limited signs of remitting. The massive DCCT project in Type 1 patients took six years of randomization to arrive at the HbA_{1c} value of 7% (53) or less that would minimize the risks of long-term microvascular complications in Type 1 diabetes, the post-trial EDIC study approximately another 10 years to establish the impact on macrovascular complications, and the population studied had minutely defined retinopathy at recruitment, and no cardiovascular disease. The problems are compounded in Type 2 diabetes, where many patients have evident vascular complications at presentation, and where the known duration of diabetes may bear little relationship to its actual duration. Discussion and meta-analyses have been plagued by a tendency to combine the clear results of the DCCT in Type 1 diabetes with the much more equivocal results of studies in Type 2 diabetes, which presupposes a similar impact of glycaemia on vascular complications in the two forms of diabetes.

Microvascular complications

UKPDS

This iconic-status trial over which only occasional critiques have been aired in the literature (e.g. McCormack and Greenhalgh, 2000) was only the second formal clinical trial in Type 2 diabetes. (The University Group Diabetes Project in the 1960s was the first and investigated the effects on mortality of insulin compared with the early sulfonylurea tolbutamide. It concluded that tolbutamide was harmful and the sulfonylureas have never quite escaped the legacy of the study. However, from the viewpoint of trial design it was clearer than the UKPDS, even if its execution and analysis were flawed; Tattersall, 2009.)

The UKPDS emerged as a study of intensive versus less intensive treatment of newly-diagnosed diabetes but, unlike the later studies, it did not target HbA_{1c} values for either group (the same concern has galvanized a discussion in statin treatment, **Chapter 12**). More intensive glycaemic control with insulin or one of a pair of sulfonylureas commonly used at the time, though not at present (glibenclamide/glyburide and chlorpropamide), was instituted in recently-diagnosed patients when blood glucose levels climbed to >15 mmol/l on diet alone, targeting fasting values <6 mmol/l. This represents a historical approach to Type 2 diabetes that the UKPDS itself did much to eradicate. More intensive treatment resulted in a mean HbA_{1c} 0.9% lower (7.0%, 53) averaged over 10 years follow-up. The reported relative risk reduction in microvascular endpoints of 25% was mostly due to a lower requirement for photocoagulation, a decision taken by ophthalmologists independent of the study and not protocol-defined. Critically, there was no difference in microvascular complications between the sulfonylurea and insulin-treated groups.

In more detailed analyses, the surrogate outcomes of progression of retinopathy and albuminuria were slowed in the intensive group, differences in retinopathy emerging after year 6 of the study and progression of microalbuminuria (defined as urinary albumin concentration >50 mg/l) after year 9. Microvascular outcomes maintained statistically significant reductions in the intensive group in the five years after the main trial had finished (Holman *et al.*, 2008), with HbA_{1c} values between 7.9% and 8.9% (63, 74), varying with the original allocation group. This legacy effect reinforced the guidance that newly-diagnosed patients should maintain HbA_{1c} levels <7.0% (53).

Practice point

After publication of the UKDS (1998), glycaemic target for newly-diagnosed Type 2 patients became <7.0% (53).

VADT, ACCORD, ADVANCE

These massive studies, formulated in part to resolve some of the questions left unanswered by the UKPDS, recruited patients with established Type 2 diabetes (mean duration 8–12 years) including 30–40% of patients with documented macrovascular disease. They all had the same design, included targeted HbA_{1c} values for the intensively treated groups and addressed most of the methodological concerns of the UKPDS, They all started shortly after the UKPDS reported and reported their primary findings between 2008 and 2009.

Glycaemic separation was similar to or wider than in the UKPDS (1.5% in VADT, 1.1% in ACCORD and 0.7% in ADVANCE) and all studies maintained stable control in both groups, unlike the UKPDS. The ACCORD and ADVANCE studies included 10 000–11 000 patients compared with 3000 in the UKPDS, but the VADT was similar in size (1800 patients).

No consistent improvements in microvascular complications were seen after intensive glycaemic control in these studies, though all reported some benefits in some renal outcomes. For example, tight glycaemic control in ADVANCE was associated with a consistent reduction in the risk of developing micro- and macroalbuminuria and a trend to reducing hard renal endpoints (renal replacement therapy or death from renal causes; see **Chapter 4**). In the VADT progression of albuminuria was reduced with intensive control (6.2%, 52) in patients with existing microvascular complications and risk factors.

In the 10-year follow-up (ADVANCE-ON) detailed assessments of microalbuminuria and renal function were not performed but the need for renal replacement therapy was significantly reduced in the previous intensive cohort (though the proportion of patients affected was tiny, about 0.3%); there was no reduction in the need for laser treatment or of diabetes-related blindness either within the study period or the follow-up (Zoungas *et al.*, 2014). In a small subgroup of the ACCORD study, progression of retinopathy was reduced in the previous intensive group at eight years follow-up (ACCORDION, 2016), but the very low HbA_{1c} (6.4%, 46) achieved during the trial was hazardous (see later).

Practice point

Intensive glycaemic control (e.g. sustained HbA_{1c} <7.0%, 53) improves some indicators of retinopathy and kidney disease, but outcomes were inconsistent between trials, and this level of glycaemia may be hazardous.

It had no impact on the clinically important endpoint of moderate visual loss, which occurred at a very high rate, around 30% in both groups.

Macrovascular complications

UKPDS

This vexatious question – does improved glycaemic control reduce the major, macrovascular, complications of diabetes? – has dogged diabetes since the inconclusive UGDP study and 50 years later it is still not fully resolved, but the overall picture is much clearer.

In the UKPDS, more intensive treatment with insulin or sulfonylureas did not significantly reduce the risk of myocardial infarction, though there was a trend towards separation that started within the first few years. However, a very small group of 340 obese patients treated more intensively with metformin had a (just significantly) lower risk of myocardial infarction compared with conventionally treated patients, but there was no effect on stroke or peripheral vascular disease, which is difficult to explain and is a much more limited effect than seen with lipid-lowering or blood pressure control. Diabetes-related deaths and a basket of diabetes-related endpoints were also reduced. These findings, dominated by metformin reducing the risk of myocardial infarction, have not been replicated, but were rapidly translated into guidelines that have remained unchanged for nearly 20 years. In the 10-year UKPDS follow-up, all agents (sulfonylureas, metformin and insulin) were associated with lower risks of cardiovascular and all-cause mortality (Holman et al., 2008), but only around one-third of the original patients were assessed at this stage (Boussageon et al., 2016). The continuation (and statistical increase) of benefit beyond the randomized stage of the study was the first demonstration of a 'legacy' effect of tighter glycaemic control in Type 2 diabetes.

VADT, ACCORD, ADVANCE

Only the ACCORD study found any cardiovascular benefit during the randomized part of the studies, but this was more than offset by increased all-cause (predominantly cardiovascular) death, and the glycaemic arm of the study was stopped early. The possible reasons for this unexpected outcome have been analysed in detail but not identified. Target glycaemia was especially stringent (HbA$_{1c}$ <6.0% 42, achieved 6.4%, 46) and it is clear that values like this when achieved by multiple agents, as in the ACCORD study, should be avoided. There is still suspicion that severe hypoglycaemia may have contributed.

This finding understandably caused widespread concern but there is no doubt of a long-term adverse impact of ultra-tight control: five years after the randomization was curtailed, the excess mortality (relative risk about 1.20) was unchanged, even though mean HbA$_{1c}$ had risen to 7.2% (55) (ACCORD Study Group, 2011).

In the six-year follow-up of the VADT there were no macrovascular benefits (though it was a relatively small study of only 1800 subjects). However, benefit emerged at 10 years' follow-up, with a 17% relative risk reduction. Technically this was not a 'legacy' effect, as the previously intensive group (mean HbA$_{1c}$ 6.9% (52) during the study) remained in slightly better control than the conventional group during most of the follow-up (Hayward et al., 2015). The much larger ADVANCE study found no macrovascular benefits of previous tight glycaemic control at 11 years follow-up (Zoungas et al., 2014).

A plausible synthesis of the results of these trials is that, at best, only minor macrovascular benefits emerge with tight glycaemic control, and these a decade or more after several years of tight control. A reduction in macrovascular events cannot be a plausible reason to persuade patients to maintain tight glycaemic control when lower blood pressure and achieving low LDL levels give similar or greater benefits that become apparent within a much shorter short time (see **Chapters 11 and 12**).

Practice point

Tight glycaemic control (HbA$_{1c}$ maintained <7.0% [53] for several years) cannot be recommended as a strategy for reducing macrovascular events and, if values are very low, higher mortality is a risk.

Multimodal intervention (Steno-2)

Low glycaemic targets in themselves are not sufficient to ensure improved macrovascular outcomes but simultaneous intervention in glycaemia, hypertension and lipids, with lifestyle input, is likely to be more valuable in Type 2 diabetes. However, only one substantial study has been performed – Steno-2 – and that was in patients with slightly elevated albuminuria (78 mg/24 hours; see **Chapter 4**). Glycaemic target in the intensively-treated group was <6.5% (48), though the achieved level after eight years of intervention was much more modest (7.9%, 63). The striking finding was a significant reduction in cardiovascular events. In longer follow-up (13 years) the risk of cardiovascular death was reduced by nearly 60%, and at a median 21 years follow-up, lifespan – predominantly determined by absence of cardiovascular end-points – in the originally intensively-treated group increased by a median eight years (Gæde et al., 2016).

Mean achieved blood pressure in the Steno-2 study was 140/74 mm Hg, LDL 1.8 mmol/l, both eminently reasonable, and using minimal medication; all patients took aspirin and maximum recommended dose of an ACE inhibitor (Gæde et al., 2008). Although again these good outcomes took many years to become apparent, they are more clinically meaningful than any of the pure glycaemia studies, though they have not been demonstrated in people without microvascular complications.

Practice point

In patients with moderately increased albuminuria – and therefore at high cardiovascular risk – moderate multimodal intervention reduces both micro- and macrovascular complications, and prolongs life.

TARGETS FOR GLYCAEMIC CONTROL IN TYPE 2 DIABETES

Having reached some kind of consensus for HbA$_{1c}$ 7% (53) or lower on limited outcome data from the UKPDS, it has been difficult to arrive at further refinements as the trio of trials in the 2000s did not yield meaningful outcomes in their tight glycaemic groups. UK (NICE) and USA (ADA) targets are shown in **Box 10.1**.

Box 10.1 UK (NICE) and USA (ADA) targets for glycaemic control.

NICE

HbA_{1c}: general target <7.5% (58); recommendation for metformin if lifestyle cannot control HbA_{1c} to <6.5% (48) (see text).
Glucose targets: not stated (home/self blood glucose monitoring not recommended).

ADA

HbA_{1c}: general target <7.0% (53), in both Type 1 and 2 diabetes.
Characteristics of people who may warrant more stringent or less stringent glycaemic targets:
More stringent (<6.5%, 48)
- short duration
- long life expectancy
- lifestyle-treated patients with or without metformin
- no significant vascular complications.

Less stringent (<8.0%, 64)
- history of severe hypoglycaemia
- limited life expectancy
- advanced micro- or macrovascular complications (especially diabetic kidney disease, see **Chapter 4**)
- multiple comorbidities
- long-duration diabetes where the general glycaemic target has not been reached despite adequate education and appropriate medication.

Glucose targets: preprandial 4.4–7.2 mmol/l; postprandial <10.0 mmol/l (1–2 hours after start of meal).

SELF-MONITORING OF BLOOD GLUCOSE IN TYPE 2 DIABETES

The question of the value of self-monitoring of blood glucose levels for people with Type 2 diabetes not taking insulin illustrates a long and mostly undistinguished episode with very little supporting evidence. Individual trials are few and far between, and certainly not on the scale that this expensive and probably not entirely benign procedure demands. The topic is therefore muddied by partisan views. Broadly it is agreed that insulin-treated patients should have ready access to blood glucose monitoring, though it is not clear whether it should be as intensive as in Type 1 diabetes. A Cochrane review of blood glucose monitoring in people not treated with insulin concluded that at six months there was a statistically significant benefit on HbA_{1c} (reduction of 0.3%), but that this small reduction dissipated at one year. From the patients' perspective there was no evidence for the impact of self-monitoring on satisfaction, general well-being or health-related quality of life (Malanda *et al.*, 2012). A more recent analysis agreed on the expected improvement in HbA_{1c} (around 0.3%), but detected a more robust effect up to 12 months and beyond and also a slight reduction in body mass index and total cholesterol (Zhu *et al.*, 2016), implicating self-monitoring as a marker of general improved health behaviours. There might be meaningful alternatives. For example in the United Kingdom, routine HbA_{1c} measurements in Type 2 patients are recommended every year; would the feedback resulting from biannual or quarterly measurements be more effective and cheaper than self-monitoring?

Practice point

In Type 2 patients not using insulin, blood glucose self-monitoring has a small effect on HbA$_{1c}$ (e.g. 0.3% reduction), but possibly not beyond about a year.

PHARMACOLOGICAL MANAGEMENT OF HYPERGLYCAEMIA

The total world market for diabetes drugs is estimated to be US$56 billion in 2017. The inevitable focus on newer glycaemic drugs continues to feed the view that glycaemia is the most important target in the management of Type 2 diabetes. We have seen that when given the appropriate educational attention, stringent adherence to weight loss and exercise are at least as effective as drug treatment. The tenuous evidence for the cardiovascular benefits of metformin are still widely believed to be of importance, but there is preliminary and more sound evidence for meaningful cardiorenal benefits of the GLP-1-receptor agonist liraglutide, and cardiovascular benefits of the SGLT2 inhibitor empagliflozin (see **Chapter 4, Table 10.1** and later), though so far only in patients with long-duration diabetes accompanied by severe cardiovascular complications. The calculus for cost effectiveness using these and other drugs is likely to become more complex. The potency of any one antihyperglycaemic agent is limited and multiple drug therapy is the norm, much as it is in hypertension treatment. The challenge for the practitioner now is the art of rational combination therapy to maximize any glycaemic benefit, reduce side-effect risk and minimize the medication burden for the individual.

Table 10.1 Drugs, patents and long-term cardiovascular benefits.

Drug	Patent status	Reduce risk of progression to diabetes	Cardiovascular benefits?
Metformin	Off patent	Yes	In UKPDS; possibly in heart failure
Sulfonylureas	Off patent	No	No; recurrent hint of harm in combination with metformin (though no major prospective study)
Meglitinides (repaglinide, nateglinide)	Off patent	No	No
Acarbose and related drugs	Acarbose off patent	Yes	In STOP-NIDDM, possibly reduced cardiovascular events and new-onset hypertension
Pioglitazone	Off patent	Yes	Yes (PROactive); recurrent stroke (IRIS)
DPP-4 inhibitors	In patent	No	No
GLP-1-receptor agonists	In patent	No	Yes (liraglutide: LEADER; semaglutide: SUSTAIN-6) in people at very high cardiovascular risk
SGLT2 inhibitors	In patent	No	Yes (empagliflozin: EMPA-REG) in people at very high cardiovascular risk

INTENSIFICATION OF TREATMENT IN TYPE 2 DIABETES

A great number of documents urge us to be 'aggressive' in the intensification of glycaemic management of Type 2 diabetes if patients do not achieve agreed targets (see previously). In clinical practice, the opposite is usually seen and the picture is one of 'clinical inertia' or 'delay in treatment intensification'. For example, there was an average of three years delay in increasing treatment from one to two oral agents in UK patients with $HbA_{1c} >7\%$ (53). At least in retrospective cohort studies this may have meaningful consequences. A UK study found that a delay of just one year at the same HbA_{1c} threshold (7%, 53) was associated with an increased risk of myocardial infarction, stroke and heart failure, though this finding is a little difficult to square with the slow effect of improved glycaemia on macrovascular outcomes, and is likely to be related to concomitant 'inertia' with blood pressure- and LDL-lowering treatment. But there is slowness: around one-quarter never had their treatment intensified over two years (Paul et al., 2015). The recommended frequency of HbA_{1c} testing (NICE: six-monthly), with three- to six-monthly measurements until stable should allow timely intensification within a year, but organizationally this remains difficult.

Numerous protocolized approaches to intensification of glycaemic treatment have been advocated, abandoned and reinstated. Currently, individualization of treatment using a wide variety of agents is generally accepted; this compares with the more rigid approach of stepped therapy previously in vogue (though the NICE algorithm, with its sequential stages of intensification is reminiscent of the older approach). The more liberal approach advocated by the American Diabetes Association is in part due to much larger clinical trial programmes of new agents, so that at launch they are licensed for use with most other agents, usually including insulin.

Since the UKPDS metformin has been widely established as the baseline drug treatment for hyperglycaemia (the median dose in the UKPDS was 2250 mg daily). While its impact on vascular outcomes is likely not to be greater than that of any other agents, it has a near-ideal profile of efficacy, safety (very low risk of hypoglycaemia), dose-responsiveness and, at worst, weight-neutrality that only the most recently-introduced classes of drugs have approached.

The algorithms proposed by NICE and ADA/EASD are broadly similar and suggest adding to metformin a drug from any other class of agent as first intensification (dual therapy); the ADA includes basal insulin in its second line recommendation, while it is deferred to the third level of intensification by NICE (second if metformin is contraindicated or not tolerated). NICE also suggests a sulfonylurea or insulin before metformin if there is symptomatic hyperglycaemia (**Figure 10.2**). The ADA guidelines helpfully include a brief profile of each agent to aid clinicians and patients (**Table 10.2**).

GLYCAEMIC EFFICACY (MAGNITUDE OF ANTIHYPERGLYCAEMIC EFFECT) (TABLE 10.2)

It may not be possible to be more precise about glycaemic efficacy beyond the qualitative estimations shown in Table 10.2 (and some, for example classifying the DPP-4 inhibitors as having intermediate glycaemic effects, are open to discussion). There are many reasons. The magnitude of the antihyperglycaemic effect is, as with several other groups of agents, notably antihypertensives, proportionate to the baseline starting HbA_{1c}: the worse the initial control, the greater the absolute fall in glycaemic measures. For example, a variety of sulfonylureas reduce HbA_{1c} by about 0.6–0.8% over a year from a baseline HbA_{1c} of about

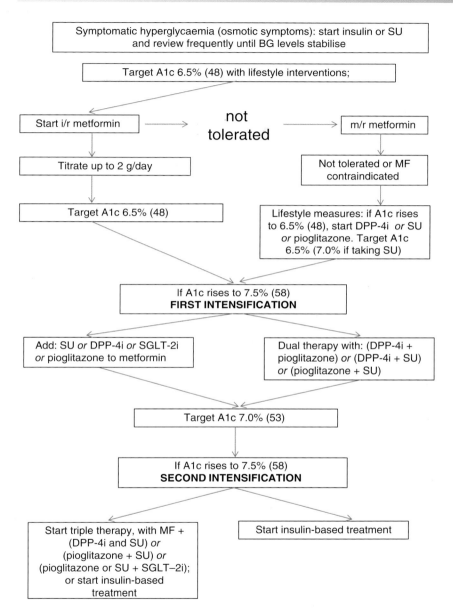

Figure 10.2 Intensification of antihyperglycaemic treatment. *Source*: from NICE guideline NG28, 2015.

Table 10.2 Thumbnail characteristics of diabetes agents (adapted from ADA).

	Metformin	SU	Glitazone	DPP-4 inhibitor	GLP-1-receptor agonist	SGLT2 inhibitor	Basal insulin
Glycaemic efficacy	High	High	High	Intermediate	Intermediate/high	Intermediate/high	High (highest)
Risk of hypos	Low	Moderate	Low	Low	Low	Low	High
Effect on weight	Neutral/loss	Gain	Gain	Neutral	Loss	Loss	Gain
Side effects	GI/lactic acidosis	Hypoglycaemia	Oedema, heart failure, fracture	Rare	GI	GU, dehydration, DKA	Hypoglycaemia
Cost	Low	Low	Low	High	High	High	Variable

GI: gastrointestinal; GU: genitourinary; DKA: diabetic ketoacidosis

7.0% (53), but at a baseline of up to 8.0% (64), the fall over the same period is about 1.1% (Nauck *et al.*, 2007). Older studies recruited patients in worse glycaemic control than more recent studies, so there may be a historical bias towards older agents (this may also contribute to some of the enthusiasm for insulin, which is often still not started until glycaemic control is very poor, while being considered, as in the ADA table, as having the highest glycaemic efficacy). The dose-response relationships of antihyperglycaemic drugs are varied and are not always evident, especially in the more recent drugs.

Durability of effect

Durability is of critical importance and there are comparatively few long-term studies of most agents. Importantly, individual susceptibility to the glycaemic effects of drugs is different. This was most strikingly seen with the thiazolidinediones, which require nuclear receptor switches to activate their many actions, and was widely observed by individual practitioners, though measures of such variability, critical in clinical practice, are not stated in clinical trials. Any differences in glycaemic responses between different compounds within the same class of drugs are nearly always smaller than other reasons for glycaemic variability, though naturally much is made of statistical differences that usually carry no clinical benefit. In mechanistic studies, individual measures of β-cell responsiveness and insulin resistance may help predict responses to particular medications, but these, and other biomarkers – and the field of pharmacogenomics, of which much is promised, but almost nothing delivered – are not yet sufficiently well developed to be of value in clinical practice. For the moment, regular assessment of responses to individual drugs and lifestyle interventions and glycaemic monitoring is the right approach.

METFORMIN

Key practice points

- First line antihyperglycaemic medication, but because of its all-round safety and efficacy, and not because it has more meaningful effects on long-term outcomes than other drugs
- Maximum effective dose 2000 mg daily; titrate gently
- No need to dose more often than twice daily
- Safe down to eGFR 30 ml/min
- Reinstate it promptly after surgery and radiological interventions

Introduction

Metformin is derived from guanidine, found in the plant goat's rue/French lilac, *Galega officinalis*, and has been used clinically since the late 1950s, though its blood glucose lowering properties were identified in the 1920s. Other similar compounds, including phenformin, were clearly associated with a high risk of lactic acidosis, and metformin remains the only biguanide in use. Concerns about lactic acidosis delayed its introduction in the USA until 1995. The benefit of this second, late start is that we have good trial data on its antihyperglycaemic properties, which would not have been available otherwise for such an old compound. There are also data relating to the launch of modified-release metformin about a decade ago.

Mechanism of action

Metformin does not stimulate insulin secretion and has peripheral effects only, but requires some insulin for its action. It suppresses hepatic glycogenolysis and gluconeogenesis, and stimulates insulin-mediated muscle and adipose glucose disposal. Because it does not stimulate insulin secretion it very rarely causes hypoglycaemia in monotherapy. There has always been a suspicion that metformin's effects are strongly linked to the gastrointestinal tract; this is supported by the finding that delayed-release metformin has a more powerful antihyperglycaemic effect than either immediate- or extended-release metformin, even though its bioavailability is significantly lower (Buse *et al.*, 2016). It may have multiple effects on bile acids and even the gut microbiome (McCreight *et al.*, 2016). A few years ago there was much excitement about metformin's possible cancer-reducing properties, based on one of its many molecular targets (AMP-activated protein kinase, AMPK), a component of an intracellular energy-sensing cascade. It may have a modest effect in certain cancers but there are no robust prospective data. This episode is a continuing reminder of the long legacy of premature announcements about properties of diabetes medications beyond blood glucose lowering.

Glycaemic efficiency and durability

Metformin has a good dose-response relationship and in a study of modified-release metformin over the recommended dose range of 500–2000 mg daily, fasting glucose fell by between 1.1 and 4.7 mmol/l and HbA_{1c} by 0.6–1.0% (Fujioka *et al.*, 2005) (**Figure 10.3**). In an early study (Garber *et al.*, 1997) there was a 2% fall with the 2000 g dose, but patients were in poor baseline control (HbA_{1c} about 10%, 86). Even at low doses, for example 500 mg daily, there are glycaemic benefits, and it can be valuable in patients who get side effects at higher doses, or dislike taking many large tablets. Metformin is sometimes prescribed up to 3000 mg daily, but there is no additional glycaemic benefit compared with 2000 mg daily, and side effects are more likely. Immediate-release metformin is usually taken with or just before meals, but there is no need to take it more often than twice-daily, and compliance is bound to be lower with three-times daily dosing. Modified-release preparations, valuable if there are persistent gastrointestinal side effects, can be taken once or twice daily.

Practice point

Metformin has a sound dose-response relationship. Even at low doses (e.g. 500 mg daily) it reduces HbA_{1c} by about 0.4%. Three-times daily dosing is not needed: twice-daily is always fine.

The widespread view that maximum reduction of hyperglycaemia at diagnosis is beneficial, especially because of the purported cardiovascular benefits, means that most patients are encouraged to take maximum or near-maximum doses. It is certainly not clear that low- or high-dose metformin carries any specific long-term effects. In practice, then, slow uptitration is used both to reduce the risk of side effects and to optimize glycaemia. If patients are monitoring fasting glucose levels at home, simple regimens can be used, for example 500 mg twice daily before meals, followed by 500 g before breakfast and 1000 mg before the evening meal, finally 1000 mg twice-daily. Of practical value, patients are more adherent to 1000 mg tablets than 500 mg. Persistence with metformin treatment, as with other OHAs, varies between about 50% and 75% at one year.

Apart from the now little-used thiazolidinediones, metformin has a greater durability of action than other older agents agents (sulfonylureas, meglitinides and DPP-4 inhibitors);

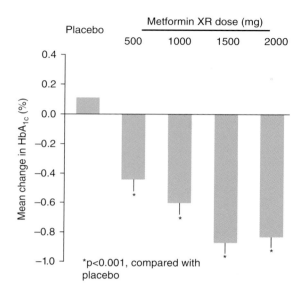

Figure 10.3 Dose-response relationship for extended-release metformin in Type 2 patients poorly controlled on diet and exercise. Mean baseline HbA$_{1c}$ was 7.9–8.4% (63–68). *Source*: Fujioka *et al.*, 2005. Reproduced with permission of John Wiley & Sons.

this was shown in the monotherapy ADOPT study (2006). However, metformin failure is still very common, up to about 60% of patients after five years (failure variously defined as discontinuation, a switch to a new agent, or add-on with a second agent) (Ekström *et al.*, 2015), so the widespread view that metformin maintains its glycaemic effect indefinitely is not correct.

Practice point

Even though it has greater durability than other agents, metformin still has a high failure rate (e.g. 60% after five years).

Effects on weight and risk of hypoglycaemia

Metformin is widely considered to cause weight loss but any effects on weight are modest. Over two years the prediabetic population in the Diabetes Prevention Program lost approximately 2 kg (about 2%) while taking metformin 850 mg bd. Weight loss was directly related to adherence to medication. A balanced view to be conveyed in discussions with patients is the UKPDS data, which over 10 years found that weight gain was moderated to approximately1 kg in patients taking metformin, compared with 4–6 kg in those treated with sulfonylureas or insulin. The weight gain associated with starting antipsychotic therapy is modestly attenuated by metformin, and coprescribing in younger obese patients would be good evidence-based practice, especially if there is already prediabetes (Anagnostou *et al.*, 2016). Hypoglycaemia is very uncommon, only slightly more frequent than patients on diet alone (0.3% per year in the UKPDS, 0.1% of all patients in the ADOPT).

Side effects

Nausea, diarrhoea and flatulence are common in the first 1–2 weeks of treatment (around 30% in patients taking immediate-release metformin) but fewer than 5% of patients are intolerant at any dose. Side effects are much more common than with modified-release preparations, for example diarrhoea, nausea and vomiting (four times more common, 8–13%) and abdominal pain (twice as common, 5%). Nausea/vomiting and diarrhoea clearly increase with dose. Metformin is now so widely used that there is a risk that clinicians will omit to discuss these common side effects with patients.

Practice point

Metformin is likely to cause early gastrointestinal side effects, especially diarrhoea, nausea and vomiting. Side effects are dose-related.

There is an uncommon but characteristic syndrome in older people, comprising:

- profound anorexia and sometimes marked weight loss, without prominent typical metformin side-effects
- gradual onset after many years of apparently trouble-free metformin treatment, possibly related to the normal weight loss in the elderly
- patients currently normal weight or thin
- low HbA$_{1c}$.

Patients usually undergo extensive gastrointestinal investigations but, in the meantime, rapidly reduce the dose of metformin while carefully monitoring glycaemic control. Symptomatic response can be dramatic and gratifying.

Metformin and renal impairment

Metformin is excreted renally and largely unchanged. It therefore accumulates in renal impairment, with an associated increased risk of lactic acidosis – though the risks are extremely low. There is a popular widespread misunderstanding that metformin itself is nephrotoxic. In comparison with sulfonylureas, for example, metformin may be mildly renoprotective and slow the decline in eGFR, but independent of cases of lactic acidosis all-cause mortality is increased in people with advanced renal impairment who take metformin (G5, serum creatinine >530 µmol/l) (Hung *et al.*, 2015). In 2016, the European Medicines Agency approved its use in people with eGFR between 30 and 59 ml/min (G3a and 3b). **Table 10.3** shows current guidance on metformin dosing in CKD.

It is important to have a glycaemic strategy in place in patients with renal impairment who have discontinued metformin in case there is unexpected deterioration in control. This is sometimes in the setting of an acute illness requiring hospitalization, but even in ambulatory care abruptly discontinuing metformin – sometimes when there has been only a slight deterioration in renal function – is usually unnecessary and can result in severe hyperglycaemia. Medication to replace metformin or supplement it in reduced doses will depend on co-existing medications and the degree of renal impairment, but therapeutic options are often limited, since GLP-1-receptor agonists and SGLT2 inhibitor agents cannot be

Table 10.3 Metformin dosing in CKD.

eGFR level (ml/min)	GFR category	Action
≥60	G1-G2	No renal contraindication
45–59	G3a	Continue metformin
30–44	G3b	Lower metformin dose, e.g. halve, or half-maximal dose (no more than 1 g/day)
<30	G4-G5	Discontinue

Source: Lipska et al., 2011. Reproduced with permission of American Diabetes Association.

used, and although several DPP4-inhibitor drugs can be used even in advanced renal impairment, they are less effective in controlling glycaemia than metformin (see later). In many cases introducing or intensifying insulin treatment is the best option.

Practice point

Make a plan with patients who have eGFR <45 for the staged withdrawal of metformin if renal function continues to deteriorate, and for re-establishing glycaemic control with other agents. But metformin is safe in patients with eGFR above 30.

Metformin in liver disease

The mildly abnormal liver function tests frequently encountered in people with non-alcoholic fatty liver disease are not a contraindication to metformin, and metformin treatment (as with statins and the glitazones) may well cause a drop in transaminase levels – though this probably does not indicate an improvement in hepatic structure. Severe hepatic impairment is considered a contraindication to metformin, though the evidence is historical, and metformin is probably safe even in people with cirrhosis (Bhat et al., 2015). Uncontrolled heart failure would require a major rethink of glycaemic treatment in any case, and in one study nearly one-half of patients with heart failure were being treated with metformin alone. It may carry a long-term mortality benefit even in patients acutely admitted with heart failure (Fácila et al., 2017). Stable ischaemic heart disease, including coronary bypass patients and those with stents, is not a contraindication, but metformin is frequently discontinued (often unnecessarily) during an inpatient stay and clear advice to primary care teams to reinstate treatment is often omitted.

Lactic acidosis

Lactic acidosis is a feared complication of metformin treatment, though it is vanishingly rare, and a Cochrane review in 2006 concluded that there was no increased risk in metformin-treated patients. Metformin-associated lactic acidosis is Type B (non-hypoxic), and is characterized by:

- blood pH <7.0 (i.e. severe acidosis)
- very high lactate (>15 mmol/l)
- large anion gap (>20 mmol/l)
- renal insufficiency (eGFR <45 ml/min or serum creatinine >180 μmol/l).

Despite the often very severe metabolic derangement, the prognosis compared with other causes of lactic acidosis is good (Kalanter-Zadeh *et al.*, 2013). Patients need early intensive care input and often respond well to veno-venous haemofiltration which simultaneously corrects the acidosis and acute kidney injury and removes metformin.

Contrast-induced nephropathy and lactic acidosis

A murky area lacking in evidence compensated for by a huge proliferation in guidance. Lactic acidosis secondary to renal impairment caused by iodinated contrast media is extremely rare but preventive measures must be in place. Patients with normal renal function can continue to take metformin normally, but those with eGFR between 30 and 60 ml/min and those with normal renal function but multiple comorbidities should discontinue it at the time of the procedure; it should be reinstated after 48 hours if renal function is stable. Avoid contrast if eGFR <30. The tendency not to reinstate treatment, especially after short hospital admissions, needs active correction.

Practice point

Discontinue metformin at the time of contrast investigations in those with eGFR 30–60 and in people with normal renal function but multiple comorbidities. Reinstate after 48 hours once renal function is stable.

Vitamin B$_{12}$ deficiency

Much research time has gone into investigating this known side effect of prolonged metformin treatment. The prevalence of simple serum vitamin B12 deficiency is between 10 and 20% in different studies, up to twice as frequent as in non-metformin users. However, there is no evidence that these low levels are associated with anaemia or an increased risk of peripheral neuropathy. Multiple abnormalities of vitamin B12 metabolites have been described, but the clinical correlates are even less clear. Though frequently urged, routine, and even occasional, serum B12 measurements are not required outside their non-diabetic indications. But aside from diabetes, nutritional B12 deficiency seems to be on the rise, and the additional impact of long-term metformin treatment on serum B12 levels (mean fall from meta-analysis of approximately 60 pmol/l) may cause people with borderline dietary intake to slip into at least biochemical deficiency (Chapman *et al.*, 2016).

AGENTS TO BE USED AFTER METFORMIN

If glycaemic guidelines agree on anything, it is that metformin is the default first-line glycaemic treatment for Type 2 diabetes; but even this may not have a watertight evidence base. The evidence for its cardiovascular benefit is weak and although durability of effect is better than for other agents it is unimpressive in a long-term condition. But it is cheap, effective and generally well tolerated with a low risk of hypoglycaemia, and there will be no emerging long-term adverse effects after 40 years of use worldwide. It is likely to retain its priority status for a long time, especially if a group of well-designed cardiovascular endpoint trials in progress give positive results (Lexis and van der Horst, 2014); but there is no need to use it early if glycaemic control can be maintained with lifestyle measures. Its contribution to vascular risk reduction is small compared with that of angiotensin blocking agents and statins

(Boussageon *et al.*, 2016). Metformin was in danger of becoming 'the new aspirin', and aspirin is no longer recommended in primary prevention.

SULFONYLUREAS AND PRANDIAL GLUCOSE REGULATORS (MEGLITINIDES)

Key practice points

- Sulfonylureas are safe, effective and cost effective if used with care; expect HbA$_{1c}$ reduction of approximately 0.7%
- They have better durability than DPP-4 inhibitors
- Do not start them in people over 70
- Because of the risk of severe hypoglycaemia, avoid sulfonylureas in elderly people who may already be in satisfactory glycaemic control, and in patients with multiple comorbidities and taking polypharmacy. Avoid ultra-low HbA$_{1c}$ targets, for example <7.0% (53)
- Hypoglycaemia is mostly avoidable by using gliclazide as the preferred agent

Metformin has led a relatively untroubled existence. The same cannot be said for sulfonylureas. Although they have been used for more than 40 years, they have been subjected to continuous scrutiny over their efficacy and safety, especially hypoglycaemia. Like metformin, there are not likely to be any further safety concerns emerging in the foreseeable future, but since the demise of the glitazones, they have been thrust into the spotlight, as they again became the standard comparator drugs for new agents. UKPDS, which used the obsolete long-acting agents glibenclamide and chlorpropamide, has imprinted the label of hypoglycaemia on the sulfonylureas as a group.

Broadly, their efficacy is the same or possibly slightly greater, at least in the short- to medium-term, compared with other agents and they are metabolically neutral concerning lipids and inflammatory markers. There have been recurrent concerns expressed over their cardiovascular safety. This started in the early 1960s with the contested and still-unresolved UGDP (University Group Diabetes Program) and continued with studies of older agents that demonstrated reduction of cardiac ischaemic resistance, and the unexpected finding of increased mortality when sulfonylureas were used in combination with metformin in the UKPDS (a finding selectively and promptly ignored in clinical practice). The relative lack of long-term glycaemic efficiency has been noted in several studies. However, USA and UK guidelines still recommend their use after metformin and the World Health Organization includes gliclazide in its model list of essential medicines for older people. Fortunately, there are good-quality contemporary trials that allow us to consider the current role of these old and inexpensive workhorse medications.

Mechanism of action

Sulfonylureas are insulinotropic agents, causing β-cell stimulation by their action at specific cell-surface receptors. Early first-phase insulin secretion resulting from insulin release from preformed insulin-containing granules is followed by a prolonged second phase of insulin secretion insulin. Unlike the DPP-4 inhibitors, secretion of insulin continues regardless of ambient glucose levels, resulting in an increased risk of hypoglycaemia. Sulfonylureas have no meaningful extra-pancreatic actions and do not modulate peripheral insulin resistance. Effects on insulin-resistant characteristics, for example blood pressure, dyslipidaemia and inflammation, are negligible.

The sulfonylureas are usually classified by their pharmacological half-life but, in practice, the critical consideration is their propensity to cause hypoglycaemia. The only truly short-acting sulfonylurea, tolbutamide, is barely used these days (though apart from the need for dosing more than once-daily, its demise was dictated largely by fashion and in the United Kingdom an inflated generic price). Glibenclamide (USA: glyburide) should no longer be used because of the high risk of severe hypoglycaemia. Gliclazide is becoming the favoured sulfonylurea: it is as effective as other agents and the risk of hypoglycaemia is lower (see later). Its hypoglycaemia safety seems to reside in its molecular structure; there is no difference between the immediate and modified- release forms either in glycaemic potency or hypoglycaemia rates.

Glycaemic efficiency and durability

Sulfonylureas are effective glucose-reducing agents. As with metformin, there is a strong relationship between baseline HbA_{1c} and its subsequent fall; for example, when glipizide was added to metformin, HbA_{1c} fell by approximately 0.5% in patients with baseline HbA_{1c} of 7–8% (53–64), but by about 1.0% when baseline was between 8 and 9% (64 and 75) (Nauck et al., 2007). All sulfonylureas have approximately the same glycaemic effect, comparable to that of newer agents (e.g. ~0.5% improvement with both glimepiride and liraglutide) (Nauck et al., 2013).

Sulfonylurea doses are often pushed too high, with no improvement in glycaemia but an increased risk of hypoglycaemia. The maximum dose of standard gliclazide, for example, is stated in the British National Formulary as 320 mg daily, but the maximum practical dose is 240 mg daily, taken in two divided doses. Modified-release gliclazide 30 mg is similar in effect to 80 mg standard gliclazide.

The question of durability has dogged the sulfonylureas. In monotherapy studies they reach a lower nadir HbA_{1c} than other agents. Thereafter failure occurs more quickly than with metformin or glitazones, but DPP-4 inhibitors are less durable than sulfonylureas (Mamza et al., 2016). In the long-term ADVANCE trial, which used modified-release gliclazide as primary treatment in both the intensive and standard glucose control groups, HbA_{1c} remained stable up to six years in patients on gliclazide monotherapy, without evidence of an initial decline followed by 'rebound' (which may in part be related to the titration regimen dictated by trial design) (Zoungas et al., 2010) (**Figure 10.4**).

Sulfonylureas, like many other therapies, are promoted as being of greater value in the early stages of diagnosed diabetes; this may be the case, but that does not mean they cease to have any value later on. For example, near-maximum dose glimepiride (4 mg daily) was added to metformin and insulin in patients with a median age of 66 years and 16 years diabetes. Average HbA_{1c} fell by 0.6% and most patients needed a reduction in insulin dose – defined by either of these, about two-thirds of patients responded (Nybäck-Nakell et al., 2014). A brief and carefully monitored retrial of a sulfonylurea is therefore warranted if there were no clear reasons for discontinuing it the first time.

Effects on weight and hypoglycaemia

Weight gain with sulfonylureas is seen as a concern. Mean weight gain in the UKPDS over 10 years was about 5 kg, compared with 2.5 kg in the diet-controlled group. However, in the huge ADVANCE study, intensive control with insulin caused 2 kg weight gain over five years, while there was minor weight loss in those treated with gliclazide and metformin (Zoungas et al., 2010). In a modern two-year study, there was only 0.7 kg weight gain over two years with glimepiride, though the comparator drug liraglutide caused significant weight loss; see later (Nauck et al., 2013). Major sulfonylurea-induced weight gain may be historical in studies with perhaps more rapid dose escalation.

(a)

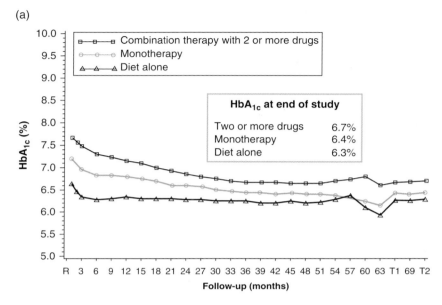

Figure 10.4 Glycaemic control in the patients in the ADVANCE trial. Glycaemia is stable throughout in all groups, with no evidence for glycaemic failure in those on gliclazide monotherapy. *Source*: Zoungas *et al.*, 2010. Reproduced with permission of Elsevier.

Practice point

With careful use, sulfonylureas cause only small weight gain compared with the several kilograms gain seen in older studies.

In clinical trials, hypoglycaemia is extremely uncommon. In the UKPDS, 1.2% of sulfonylurea-treated patients reported hypoglycaemia each year, compared with 4–5% with insulin and 0.3% treated with metformin (Wright *et al.*, 2006). Hypoglycaemia is demonstrably much less common with gliclazide than other sulfonylureas. In the ADVANCE study approximately 2% over the whole trial had an episode of severe hypoglycaemia, corresponding to an event rate of 0.07/1000 patient years) (Zoungas *et al.*, 2010). In a further meta-analysis, only one patient in 2500 had a severe hypoglycaemic event – and that patient was also using insulin. Patients at high risk of sulfonylurea-induced hypoglycaemia can be identified clinically (**Box 10.2**); these patients should have alternative medication that carries negligible risk. Reassess any patients over 70 taking a sulfonylurea.

Practice point

Severe hypoglycaemia with gliclazide is very uncommon in clinical trials. In clinical practice, regular supervision of patients with specific questioning about hypoglycaemia is needed. In hospital the peak time for hypoglycaemia in patients taking sulfonylureas and insulin is 6:00 a.m.

> **Box 10.2** Clinical characteristics of patients developing severe sulfonylurea-related hypoglycaemia.
>
> - Use of glibenclamide, glimepiride or gliquidone.
> - Over 70 years old.
> - Long known duration Type 2 diabetes, e.g. 15 years.
> - Multiple comorbidity; admission with infection.
> - Multiple medications.
> - Previous admission with hypoglycaemia.
> - Reduced eGFR.
> - Poor pre-admission nutrition (BMI around 26, laboratory markers of poor nutrition common).
> - Low HbA$_{1c}$ on admission, e.g. 6.5–7.0%, 48–53.
>
> *Source*: adapted from Scheiter *et al.*, 2012.

In outpatient practice, mild hypoglycaemia is commonly reported 2–3 hours after breakfast, usually while exercising, or before a delayed lunch. Some of these patients will already be in overtight glycaemic control. In hospital, patients taking sulfonylureas are – potentially hazardously – prone to their highest risk of hypoglycaemia around 6:00 a.m. (Rajendran *et al.*, 2014).

Non-glycaemic effects
Minor effects on lipids, inflammatory indices and indicators of oxidant status have been repeatedly reported. They are not meaningful. All sulfonylureas are available in generic form. No further agents will be introduced commercially but they should not be forgotten.

Drug interactions
Although hepatically metabolized, sulfonylureas are safe in liver disease unless severe; there is a risk of hypoglycaemia. They need to be used with caution in severe kidney disease, though gliclazide is safe, so long as glycaemia is monitored carefully. There is a possibility of haemolysis in patients with G6PD deficiency. Hypoglycaemia may occur with some antibiotics that are metabolized through the same CYP pathway. In order of decreasing likelihood:

- clarithromycin (nearly fourfold increased risk)
- levofloxacin
- co-trimoxazole
- metronidazole
- ciprofloxacin.

Meglitinides: repaglinide and nateglinide
These interesting agents – short-acting insulin secretagogues that operate at the sulfonylurea receptor – were introduced in the late 1990s at a time when there were no drugs for Type 2 diabetes other than the medications used in the UKPDS (sulfonylureas, metformin and human insulins), when clinical trial programmes for new agents were less extensive, and around the same time the glitazones were causing excitement. They are little used, in part because any benefits they have over the similar-acting sulfonylureas are difficult to discern from the evidence and because there is little confidence that they are less prone to causing hypoglycaemia despite their short action.

Nateglinide, a phenylalanine derivative, has a short action similar to that of repaglinide at the SUR1 receptor, closing potassium channels and causing insulin secretion. In the initial trials, repaglinide was as effective as glibenclamide and possibly more than glip-izide; hypoglycaemia in both studies was uncommon. There is no clear demonstration of a clinical dose-response relationship over its licensed range (0.5–4 mg before each meal, maximum dose 12 mg daily). While the idea of a 'prandial glucose regulator' is appealing, and some patients vary the dose according to meal size, there is no evidence that precision use in this way improves glycaemia or reduces the risks of hypoglycaemia. It has never been trialled against gliclazide, and like nateglinide is formally licensed only in combination with metformin.

Practice point

20 years after its introduction there is no evidence that repaglinide is safer or more effective than sulfonylureas in current use.

DRUGS ACTING ON THE INCRETIN SYSTEM

These important groups of drugs, introduced from the mid-2000s onwards, have focused physiological and clinical attention on the previously neglected endocrine role of the gastrointestinal tract in modifying appetite, gut motility, insulin secretion and weight control. Their development was based on the physiological understanding of the incretin system. Gut-derived substances affecting carbohydrate metabolism were first mooted in classically epic animal studies by the great physiologists William Bayliss (1860–1924) and Ernest Starling (1866–1927), but the incretin effect was not described until 1969: the observation that for a given achieved blood glucose level, orally-administered glucose generated a higher systemic insulin level than intravenous glucose. In the same year, the term 'entero-insular axis' was coined – an important concept linking gut-derived stimuli and pancreatic islet function. GIP (now named glucose-dependent insulinotropic hormone) was the first incretin to be sequenced in 1970, and the major current therapeutic target, GLP-1, in 1983.

The incretin effect is reduced in Type 2 diabetes through a combination of GLP-1 deficiency and defective GLP-1 signalling, though incretin abnormalities are not a primary cause of Type 2 diabetes. GLP-1 is released from gut L-cells within 10–15 minutes of starting to eat and levels are elevated for several hours as a result of different populations of L-cells being sequentially stimulated (Gribble, 2008).

The effect of GLP-1 is predominantly in the postprandial phase. In addition to insulin secretion, two additional effects are important: decreasing postprandial glucagon levels (an important factor in the hyperglycaemia of Type 2 diabetes) and slowing gastric emptying. There is also a direct effect on satiety via the hypothalamus.

Two pharmacological strategies are now familiar: the development of injected long-acting GLP-1-receptor agonists and of inhibitors of the enzyme dipeptidyl peptidase IV (DPP-4), the major plasma factor that degrades endogenous GLP-1, prolonging its action.

These drugs therefore have fascinating properties that have captivated clinicians. However in clinical practice the DPP-4 inhibitors have generally unremarkable glycaemic effects, and weight loss is seen only with the GLP-1-receptor agonists. But they undoubtedly represent the beginning of a new phase in the understanding and treatment of Type 2 diabetes.

DPP-4 INHIBITORS (GLIPTINS)

Key practice points

- Weaker glycaemic effect (e.g. HbA_{1c} fall approximately 0.3–0.5%) than other drugs in widespread use
- Cardiovascular safety confirmed in large follow-up studies
- No or very low risk of hypoglycaemia
- Very slight increase in risk of acute pancreatitis
- Expensive: monitor response carefully and discontinue if glycaemic response is minimal or the effect wanes

Glycaemic efficiency and durability

The first agent, sitagliptin, was introduced in 2006–2007. Taking sitagliptin 100 mg daily as representative of this large group now consisting of around six compounds, and the relationship between baseline HbA_{1c} and subsequent glycaemic improvement, expect a fall of around 0.5% with baseline HbA_{1c} between 7 and 8% (53–64), and 0.8–1.0% in patients with values >8.5% (69). The approximately 0.5–0.6% reduction is also seen in meta-analysis and confirms that this group of drugs has less glycaemic potency than other agents (for example, in a direct 18-month comparison from a baseline HbA_{1c} of 8.0% (64), mean HbA_{1c} reduction was 0.9% with empagliflozin 25 g daily and 0.7% with sitagliptin 100 mg daily; Roden et al., 2015). However, there is naturally wide interindividual variation, so individuals may have meaningful responses. Careful monitoring of HbA_{1c} is needed. In a meta-analysis, glycaemic control with DPP4-inhibitors deteriorated in the second year of treatment. Overall HbA_{1c} difference from placebo in the placebo-controlled but not target-driven three-year TECOS study using sitaglitpin was only 0.3% (Green et al., 2015).

Dose-response relationships are flat. Lower doses are available for use in patients with renal impairment but in most cases there is no need for dosage titration. Many also come in fixed-dose combinations with metformin, either 850 mg or 1000 mg, and are taken twice daily. They may be helpful for patients not achieving glycaemic target on maximum metformin.

Most can be used in varying degrees of renal impairment (**Table 10.4**). In clinical practice, there may not be much benefit of around 0.5% HbA_{1c} reduction in patients with CKD, ESRD or those on dialysis (see **Chapter 4** for a broader discussion of diabetes management in renal impairment). With a few exceptions they are licensed with insulin where they have the same glycaemic effects as in combination oral therapy (HbA_{1c} fall ~0.4%). They should not be trialled in patients in poor control on insulin.

Practice point

DPP-4 inhibitors are relatively weak drugs. Monitor carefully to identify patients who have a consistent beneficial effect. They are of little practical value for insulin-treated patients in poor control.

Table 10.4 Dosing of DPP-4 inhibitors (gliptins) in renal impairment.

DPP-4 inhibitor	Full dose	Dose reductions in renal impairment
Sitagliptin (Januvia)	100 mg morning	eGFR 30–50 ml/min – 50 mg eGFR <30, ESRD (dialysis) – 25 mg
Saxagliptin (Onglyza)	5 mg morning	Moderate/severe renal disease – 2.5 mg ESRD – do not use
Linagliptin (Trajenta)	5 mg morning	Dose unchanged in all degrees of renal impairment, including (with caution) in dialysis
Vildagliptin (Galvus)	50 mg bd	All degrees of renal impairment and ESRD – 50 mg
Alogliptin (Vipidia)	25 mg morning	eGFR 30–60 ml/min – 12.5 mg eGFR 15–30, dialysis – 6.25 mg

Effects on weight and risk of hypoglycaemia

All compounds are weight neutral and do not by themselves cause hypoglycaemia, but in a cardiovascular outcome study in high-risk patients (SAVOR-TIMI 53) those treated with saxagliptin or a sulfonylurea (especially glibenclamide) had higher hypoglycaemia rates than the placebo group; higher rates were identified in diabetic kidney disease, old age and long duration of diabetes, and baseline HbA_{1c} ≤7.0% (53). Overall, however, only 2% of patents reported a severe hypoglycaemic event over two years. Since most patients will be using multiple diabetes therapies, they should be warned about hypoglycaemia when a DPP-4 inhibitor is added (Cahn et al., 2016).

Non-glycaemic effects and adverse effects

DPP-4 inhibitors have no significant non-glycaemic effects. Like the injected GLP-1-receptor agonists both the USA and European drug agencies consider that acute pancreatitis might be increased, but any absolute increase in risk is very small (e.g. 0.13% in a combined analysis) (Tkáč and Raz, 2017). In the huge TECOS cardiovascular follow-up study (14 500 patients for three years) the incidence of both acute pancreatitis and pancreatic cancer was no higher in patients treated with sitagliptin. Heart failure was raised as a possible risk in early studies but the long-term follow-up studies have not confirmed this and overall they do not increase cardiovascular risk. In the SAVOR-TIMI 53 cardiovascular safety trial, saxagliptin reduced albumin creatinine ratios independently of improvement in glycaemia, but there were no concomitant improvements either in eGFR or hard renal endpoints; likewise, sitagliptin in TECOS did not have any impact on CKD outcomes, though it confirmed again the serious adverse cardiovascular outcomes in CKD, with event rates increased by about 40% in patients with G3b compared with G1 (Cornel et al., 2016).

GLP-1-RECEPTOR AGONISTS

The biology and physiology of GLP-1-receptor agonists have been rehearsed in detail and they are in widespread use more than 10 years after the introduction of the prototype agent exenatide (**Table 10.5**). However, their portfolio of desirable features – moderate but sometimes marked weight loss and glycaemic impact, and low risk of hypoglycaemia – must be balanced against the need for injection (rarely, though, a major problem for patients), occasional marked adverse effects, especially gastrointestinal, variable durability and expense. In non-human species they are potent growth agents for the gut and, although careful analysis cannot confirm a meaningful risk of acute and chronic

Table 10.5 GLP-1-receptor agonist drugs.

Drug	Approval date (Europe/USA)	Usual maintenance dose	Notes	Titles of clinical trial program/notes
*Exenatide	2006/2005	5–10 µg twice daily. Take within an hour of two main meals at least 6 h apart 2 mg weekly	Prototype clinical agent. EXSCEL (2017; 2mg preparation). Neutral CV outcomes in patients with or without known CV disease.	
Liraglutide	2009/2010	1.2 mg once daily (1.8 mg available but not recommended)	Positive CV outcome study (LEADER, 2016). Effective in moderate renal impairment (eGFR 30–59) and in ESRD but higher rate of gastrointestinal side effects leading to stopping treatment	LEAD, LEADER, BEGIN. Titratable fixed-ratio combination of liraglutide and insulin degludec (iDegLira) is available
Lixisenatide	2013/2016	20 µg once daily. Take within an hour of the morning or evening meal	Neutral CV outcome study (ELIXA, 2015)	GetGoal. Titratable fixed-ratio combination of lixisenatide and insulin glargine (iGlarLixi) is available
*Dulaglutide	2015/2014	0.75 mg or 1.5 mg weekly	Glycaemic impact of 1.5 mg dose is similar to that of liraglutide 1.8 mg daily. Modest weight reducing properties. Glycaemic reduction in Japanese subjects is greater than with daily insulin glargine	AWARD. Long-term CV safety trial (REWIND). Neutral CV outcomes across phase 3 trials
*Albiglutide	2014/2014	30 mg or 50 mg weekly		HARMONY. Licensed for renal impairment with eGFR >30. 30 mg dose is more effective than 50 mg short term in Japanese patients
*Semaglutide	2017/2017	0.5 or 1.0 mg weekly	Although no head-to-head data, seems especially effective in improving glycaemia and reducing weight	Neutral CV outcomes across phase 3 trials. Oral (daily) formulation in clinical trials. Signal of increased retinopathy, possibly related to high glycaemic effectiveness

Cardiovascular studies are undertaken in high or very high risk patients.
CV: cardiovascular
*Weekly injection

pancreatic complications, signals persist. Importantly, different agents in this class have meaningful differences in glycaemic and weight responses and in side-effect profiles and one agent, the weekly taspoglutide, was withdrawn in late clinical trial development because of high rates of side effects, including injection-site problems.

They have multiple modes of action, which may account for some of the variation seen in clinical trials and the variability in individual responses. Because they augment postprandial insulin secretion, they have a predominant effect on postprandial rather than fasting glucose levels. There was a good deal of interest in this difference in the 2000s, when it was proposed that atherosclerosis might be promoted by postprandial changes in glucose, reactive oxygen species and lipids. A definitive trial of non-incretin drugs in postmyocardial infarction patients (HEART2D) was negative (Raz et al., 2009). Differences between agents in achieved postprandial glucose levels are statistical and not of clinical significance. Much of the heat of this discussion has fortunately dissipated; but the light has largely gone out too, much as did the once fierce controversy about the atherogenicity of injected insulin.

Glycaemic efficiency and durability

Phase 3 clinical trial programmes of new glycaemic agents are now of great complexity, often performed under an upbeat banner acronym, and largely undertaken to ensure there is regulatory information on coprescribing with other glycaemic agents. Analysing the effects of various combinations is formidably difficult and isolated comparisons of limited significance to patients or doctors. Durability of an expensive injected agent is as important as its absolute glycaemic benefit and trials with the longest randomized phases in practical combinations should be the focus. Valuable data are emerging from the long-term cardiovascular safety trials, which have the major advantage of being placebo-controlled. In addition, they are analysed by intention-to-treat rather than the less reliable 'completer' data of the many open-label extension studies. Finally, although they are not treat-to-target studies, their protocols require optimum glycaemic control in all patients and the trial data show this is achieved in both placebo and active-treatment groups.

Broadly, when added to any standard existing agent – that is, in dual therapy – GLP-1-receptor agonists are as effective as other agents. For example, liraglutide and glimepiride each reduced HbA_{1c} by about 0.5–0.6% when added to metformin in a two-year study (Nauck et al., 2013). The effect was slightly smaller, −0.3%, compared with placebo in an 18-month trial of lixisenatide (**Figure 10.5**) (Bolli et al., 2014); it looks as if there is greater variability in glycaemic response with different GLP-1 agents than with other classes of medication, and in some well-conducted longer-term studies HbA_{1c} fell by up to 0.8–1.0%. In addition to possibly superior glycaemic effects, six months' treatment with semaglutide 1 mg weekly resulted in mean weight loss of 5 kg compared with a gain of 1 kg with basal glargine (see later) (Aroda et al., 2017). Limited data suggests that these agents are equally effective in other ethnic groups (data exist for lixisenatide in South-East Asian people and for liraglutide in Latino/Hispanics).

GLP-1-receptor agonists in long-duration trials

Valuable clinical data are emerging from long-term studies of GLP-1-receptor agonists, especially the cardiovascular safety studies, which include large numbers of patients. In addition, they are placebo-controlled and analysed by intention-to-treat, both important features of a clinical trial landscape populated by intrinsically problematical open-label

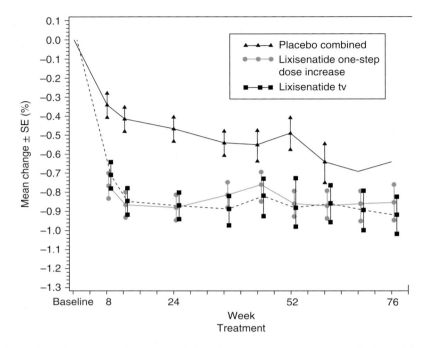

Figure 10.5 Double-blind placebo-controlled randomized trial of lixisenatide in patients poorly controlled on metformin. Baseline HbA$_{1c}$ was ~8.2% (66) *Source*: Bolli *et al.*, 2014. Reproduced with permission of John Wiley & Sons. Note the prompt and significant placebo reduction of ~0.6%, resulting in a placebo-corrected HbA$_{1c}$ decrease of only ~0.3% and the sustained decrease in HbA$_{1c}$ with lixisenatide.

'completer'-type studies. All the agents will eventually complete their mandated cardiovascular safety studies and they will be a major resource for informing rational practice. Examples include:

> *Exenatide (weekly) vs basal glargine* (three-year study; Diamant *et al.*, 2014). Although not placebo-controlled, this trial showed that, long-term, exenatide and glargine (titrated to a mean 37 units daily) gave similar and stable reductions in HbA$_{1c}$ to about 7.0% (53) with a similarly stable overall reduction in weight of 4.5 kg.
>
> *Liraglutide/lixisenatide/semaglutide vs placebo added to stable oral agents.* These are all longer-term cardiovascular studies (see below) lasting two or four years:
>
> - Liraglutide (LEADER, 4 years; Marso *et al.*, 2016a)
> - Lixisenatide (ELIXA, 2 years; Pfeffer *et al.*, 2015)
> - Semaglutide (SUSTAIN-6, 2 years; Marso *et al.*, 2016b)

Glycaemic control in all of these studies was reasonably stable, though it showed a mild upwards 'tick' pattern after reaching a nadir at 3–12 months with the GLP-1-receceptor agonists. Glycaemic control in the placebo-treated groups was remarkably stable, confirming the high standard of care in all patients included in these studies, though placebo-subtracted HbA$_{1c}$ differences were small, <0.5%, with both liraglutide and lixisenatide.

The apparently much more potent semaglutide maintained stable HbA_{1c} levels over two years with a difference of around 1.4% at the end of the trial. Durability, therefore, appears to vary with the agent used and is greater for exenatide and semaglutide than liraglutide or lixisenatide.

Practice point

Expect ~0.5% HbA_{1c} or greater reduction with GLP-1-receptor agonist treatment. In longer-term studies, exenatide and semaglutide appear to have greater durability of effect than liraglutide or lixisenatide.

NICE Guidance (2010/2015–2016)

In 2010, NICE (UK) proposed that GLP-1-receptor agonists could be used for an initial period of six months and continued if HbA_{1c} had fallen by 1% or more (and initial body weight had decreased by ≥3%). The advice remained unchanged in the 2015–2016 guidance. The glycaemic criterion was widely considered to be too stringent given the overall glycaemic efficacy of this group. It is stringent, but again importantly highlights the need for very close liaison with patients taking these expensive drugs, and for regular discussions about progress and alternative therapies.

GLP-1-receptor agonist treatment combined with basal insulin

These drugs are now widely used in combination with insulin (and there are titratable fixed-ratio mixtures of degludec and liraglutide, and of glargine and lixisenatide; see later) and clinical trials confirm the safety and efficacy of the combination. NICE suggests specialist supervision for this combination but a specialist contribution to the *discussion* about starting is important, though probably not as important as planning ahead for next steps if there is an inadequate response once maximum doses of both components have been reached.

Trial design is often of baroque complexity but broad approaches have been:

- *Adding GLP-1-receptor agonist to patients inadequately controlled on basal insulin.* Exenatide and liraglutide have been studied in this way and improvement in glycaemia (e.g. HbA_{1c} fall around 1.0% with baseline values of 7.5–8.5%, 58–69) can be more effective than adding mealtime bolus insulin (Thomsen et al., 2017). Improvements were less numerically impressive with lixisenatide, but carefully monitored this approach can be valuable, with possible benefits for patient satisfaction and adherence, compared to multiple daily insulin injections. The strategy is also valuable where high-dose basal insulin has failed: mean HbA_{1c} fell from 9.0% (75) to 7.9% (63) after liraglutide 1.8 mg daily was added to a mean daily insulin dose of about 250 units/day insulin. Weight did not change but insulin doses fell by 12%; during the first month hypoglycaemia was more frequent in liraglutide-treated patients but beyond that up to six months there were no differences (Vanderheiden et al., 2016).
- *Adding basal insulin to pre-existing GLP-1-receptor agonist treatment.* Despite this being a very common clinical scenario, there are (perhaps not surprisingly, but certainly disappointingly) few studies. A complex sequential trial found that gradual titration of insulin detemir to a mean dose of 40 units reduced HbA_{1c} by a further 0.5% from 7.6% (60) when added to metformin and liraglutide 1.8 mg daily; weight loss was just under 1 kg (DeVries et al., 2012).

- *Titratable fixed-ratio combinations of GLP-1-receptor agonists and insulin.* Two are available: iDegLira, a combination of degludec (dose range from 10–50 U daily) and liraglutide (0.6–1.8 mg daily); and iGlarLixi, glargine (15–60 U daily) and lixisenatide (5–20 µg daily). The logic of fixed-dose combinations, at least in hypertension, is impeccable (see **Chapter 11**), where they are likely to improve adherence and may enhance blood pressure response because of the inevitable variation in the responsiveness of individuals to each component. This is shown indirectly in the DURA-TION-3 study (Diamant et al., 2014; see previously), comparing insulin glargine and weekly exenatide over three years, and one of the very few studies to present data on non-responders. Stable control with either agent was achieved in about one-half the study population; equal numbers of the remaining one-half failed to achieve control with either agent (**Figure 10.6**). Durable control is likely to be achieved in a meaningful proportion of these patients with fixed-ratio combination treatment.

Oral diabetes agents are widely available in fixed-dose combinations with metformin, but these are used once the usual maximum dose of metformin (2 g daily) has been reached and further glucose lowering is required. The injectable, titratable fixed-ratio (rather than fixed-dose) combinations will usually be added on to maximum metformin with or without one or more oral agents. Both components of the combinations are relatively powerful, so it is not surprising that major reductions in HbA_{1c} are seen. For example, while degludec at a mean dose of 45 units daily reduced HbA_{1c} by approximately 0.8%, when combined with liraglutide (at a daily dose near 1.8 mg daily) there was a further 1.0% reduction (Buse et al., 2014). Optimum titration regimes have not been explored in detail but a single dosage step each week is effective. Their logic may be

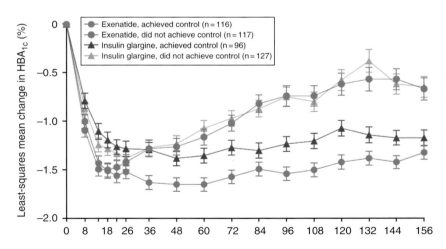

Figure 10.6 Responders and non-responders to weekly exenatide or basal glargine in the DURATION-3 study. One-half of the study patients failed to achieve stable control, divided approximately equally between those taking the two treatments. Interestingly, the mean achieved insulin dose was no different in responders and non-responders. This study boosts the case for the use of fixed-ratio combinations of basal insulin and GL1-receptor agonists. *Source*: Diamant et al., 2014. Reproduced with permission of Elsevier.

sound but physician resistance to using even generically-available fixed-dose combinations in hypertension is ingrained. Additional concerns about the fixed-ratio insulin/GLP-1-receptor agonist preparations include:

- expense
- lack of long-term data
- practical steps to take once maximum dosage steps have been reached in individuals.

> **Practice point**
>
> Consider adding a GLP-1-receptor agonist if HbA$_{1c}$ is not at target with basal insulin. HbA$_{1c}$ falls of 1% have been reported. The converse – adding basal insulin to a GLP-1-receptor agonist – may be as effective, but there are few trials of this common scenario.

Continuous subcutaneous exenatide

In an elegant dose-finding study exenatide delivered for a year by an osmotic pump implanted subcutaneously gave substantial and sustained reductions in HbA$_{1c}$ (e.g. 1.0–1.5% from a baseline of about 8.0%, 64) and meaningful weight loss (e.g. about 10% from a baseline of about 100 kg) in patients taking metformin; outcomes were best at a daily dose of 60 µg. Phase 3 clinical studies are underway (Henry et al., 2014). At the very least this demonstrates elegant pharmacology and technology in the therapy of Type 2 diabetes.

Effects on weight and risk of hypoglycaemia

GLP-1-receptor agonist drugs cause weight loss through several mechanisms that are yielding to careful analysis. In meta-analyses of trials averaging 31 weeks, placebo-adjusted weight loss was approximately 2 kg for liraglutide and exenatide. In the few double-blind trials longer than six months, weight continues to fall very slowly up to 72 weeks. There is a definite placebo weight response compared with placebo oral DPP-4-inhibitor and SGLT2 inhibitor agents, amounting to about −0.7 kg; this difference is strongly related to the degree of weight loss seen with the active drug. Reassuringly (or perhaps not) placebo GLP-1-receptor agonists do not have a similar effect on HbA$_{1c}$ (de Wit et al., 2016). In long-term studies up to four years (see previously) weight loss appears to be maintained.

The only agent to be formally studied in obesity is liraglutide, used at doses higher than in diabetes (up to 3 mg daily). Earlier studies had shown mean weight loss of approximately 5 kg in non-diabetic and prediabetic patients over a year, though there was high variability in individual response. Liraglutide reduced the rate of progression to diabetes. In the large year-long SCALE study of Type 2 patients with a mean baseline weight of 106 kg, mean placebo-subtracted weight loss was similar to that in non-diabetic subjects, 4%, at the 3 mg dose, and 2.7% at the 1.8 mg dose (Davies et al., 2015). Comparisons between the effects of the two doses should be made with caution, but in any case this was not a monotherapy trial: all patients were given a 500 kcal/day deficit diet and advised on increased physical activity (≥150 min/week). There were more gastrointestinal side effects at the higher dose.

In meta-analyses of GLP-1-receptor agonists, systolic blood pressure decreased by approximately 3 mm, partly accounted for by the weight loss, with little impact on diastolic pressure. Weight loss depends on baseline eating behaviour and is greatest in those exhibiting restrained eating behaviour (e.g. making a deliberate attempt at restricting eating at mealtimes), lowest in those with external eating behaviour (e.g. 'do you eat more than usual when food looks and smells good'?); others (e.g. emotional eating) were associated with intermediate weight loss (de Boer *et al.*, 2016). Although functional studies, including fMRI, are surprisingly limited in these important drugs, external eaters may have attenuated brain responses to GLP-1-receptor agonists. Meaningful weight loss, around 13 kg, was found in very obese patients with mean BMI 41 planned for bariatric surgery, though this potentially helpful manoeuvre requires about six months' treatment (Iglesias *et al.*, 2015).

Practice point

Weight loss with GLP-1-receptor agonists is associated with eating behaviour at baseline: those with restrained eating have the largest weight response. GLP-1-receptor agonists can help achieve meaningful weight loss in the six months before bariatric surgery.

Hypoglycaemia

Severe hypoglycaemia is very uncommon, even when are used with insulin. Symptomatic hypoglycaemia occurred in 2–3% of patients taking insulin, metformin and lixisenatide (Bolli and Owens, 2014). Trials often report hypoglycaemia, not surprisingly, when these agents are used in combination with sulfonylureas. Reassuringly, in the LEADER trial (see later), there were fewer episodes of hypoglycaemia in the liraglutide-treated group, probably because they required less additional glycaemic treatment (especially insulin, sulfonylureas and glinides).

Practice point

Hypoglycaemia risk is low in patients treated with a GLP-1-receptor agonist and insulin, but be aware of the risk when used in combination with a sulfonylurea.

Cardiovascular outcomes in long-term studies of patients with established vascular disease

The potential acute benefit of GLP-1-receptor agonist treatment on myocardial function and structure observed in small early studies was not apparent when exenatide was given to non-diabetic postmyocardial infarction patients immediately before percutaneous coronary intervention (Roos *et al.*, 2016), nor in long-term use in diabetic patients who had had an acute coronary syndrome in the previous six months (ELIXA study) (Pfeffer *et al.*, 2015). It was, therefore, a surprise that in the four-year LEADER follow-up using liraglutide there was an approximate 20% reduction in major cardiovascular outcomes and of all-cause mortality (Marso *et al.*, 2016a), and all types of myocardial infarction were just statistically lower in patients with known cardiovascular disease. Strangely, though, non-fatal myocardial infarction, non-fatal stroke and heart failure were not reduced. Without formal prospective studies there can be no mechanistic explanations for these inconsistent results – a situation analogous to the increased mortality seen with tight glycaemia control in the ACCORD study and equally resistant to explanation using the most inventive statistical machinations. However, there is formal confirmation of the lack of benefit in heart failure. A prospective study in patients previously hospitalized for heart failure and with reduced left ventricular ejection fraction was neutral for mortality, rehospitalization and changes in N-terminal pro-B-type natriuretic peptide. Liraglutide is safe in heart failure, but not beneficial (Margulies et al., 2016).

While still an investigational result, a weekly GLP-1-receptor agonist, semaglutide, was found to reduce a range of cardiovascular outcomes in a two-year placebo-controlled trial (SUSTAIN 6) (Marso et al., 2016b), including cardiovascular death, and non-fatal myocardial infarction and stroke, but there was an excess of significant retinopathy, attributed, implausibly, to the rapid reduction in blood glucose levels. The difference of 1.0% HbA_{1c} and 4.3 kg weight compared with the placebo group are unlikely to have contributed substantially to the cardiovascular benefit over such a short period, given the lack of cardiovascular benefit with approximately similar changes seen in the 'lifestyle' Look AHEAD study; but as in all cardiovascular safety studies very high-risk patients are targeted for inclusion (and the extremely high risk postmyocardial infarction patients recruited in the ELIXA study (lixisenatide) may explain the lack of benefit from drug treatment).

It is critically important for clinicians to appreciate the clinical profile of patients who have been found to benefit in these long-term studies (more will be reported over the next few years). Regrettably, the titles of the articles describing the results with liraglutide and semaglutide do not include any notion of the high risk patients included. **Table 10.6** compares the clinical characteristics of patients in LEADER, SUSTAIN-6 and ELIXA studies; the first two are rather similar. The potential for the results of the first two studies, comprising a very small proportion of general Type 2 patients, to 'bleed' into widespread but unjustified long-term prophylactic treatment in patients with more recent-onset diabetes – apart from the established clinical indications – must be resisted until larger studies in more heterogeneous groups have reported; the same applies to the cardiovascular outcome studies of SGLT2 inhibitors (see later) and to aspirin and angiotensin blockade in earlier eras.

Practice point

The GLP-1-receptor agonists liraglutide and semaglutide may have cardiovascular outcome benefits, but so far only in patients with established cardiovascular disease.

Side effects

The gastrointestinal side effects, especially mild to moderate nausea usually occurring in the first eight weeks of treatment and decreasing thereafter, are well known. Both nausea and vomiting leading to discontinuation of treatment are about twice as common with active drug as with placebo. Gastrointestinal side effects are generally lower with the long-acting agents and they have a tendency to statistically better glycaemic control.

Table 10.6 Clinical characteristics of patients recruited into long-term cardiovascular out-come studies with GLP-1-receptor agonists liraglutide (LEADER), semaglutide (SUSTAIN-6), and exenatide (ELIXA), and the SGLT2-inhibitor empagliflozin (EMPA REG OUTCOME).

	LEADER (liraglutide)	SUSTAIN-6 (semaglutide)	ELIXA (exenatide)	EMPA REG (empagliflozin)
Total number of patients	9340	3297	6068	7000
Male (%)	64	61	60	73
Duration diabetes, years	13	14	9	No pooled info
Baseline HbA$_{1c}$	8.7% (72)	8.7% (72)	7.6% (60)	8.1% (65)
Body weight, kg	92 (BMI 33)	92	85 (BMI 30)	86 (BMI 31)
Prior myocardial infarction, %	31	33	100 ACS	47
Prior stroke, %	16	15	5	23
Prior revascularization, %	39		8	25 (CABG)
Heart failure, %	14 (NYHA II-III)	24	22	10
Blood pressure, mm Hg	136/77	136/77	130	135/77
LDL cholesterol, mmol/l		2.1	2.0	2.2

Sources: Marso *et al.*, 2016a, 2016b; Pfeffer *et al.*, 2015; Zinman *et al.*, 2015).

Practice point

Ensure patients are not taking an oral gliptin and an injected GLP-1-receptor agonist at the same time. In practice it is best to avoid GLP-1-receptor agonists in patients with known gallstones or advanced neuropathy (risk of gastroparesis).

Pancreatic

Because of their pancreatic action, there has been careful scrutiny for acute pancreatitis and pancreatic cancer in patients treated with GLP-1-receptor agonists. About one-quarter of patients taking liraglutide develop raised pancreatic amylase or lipase, or both, and this proportion is much higher in patients with advanced renal impairment. In both the ELIXA and LEADER studies there was no increased risk of acute pancreatitis, but there was a higher rate of gallstone and severe gallstone disease with liraglutide in the LEADER study. It would be wise not to use these drugs in people with clinical or radiological evidence of gallstones, and although there will never be sufficient data to put it on a formal footing, they should not be used in people with advanced neuropathy and a consequent high risk of gastroparesis. There are no data on the effect of DPP-4 inhibitor drugs on pancreatic enzyme levels in humans, but there have been sporadic reports of acute pancreatitis. Inadvertently, patients may end up on both classes of agents. There is a case report of fatal necrotizing pancreatitis in a patient well-established on an injected GLP-1-receptor agonist after a DPP-4 inhibitor was added. There were concerns about thyroid C-cell tumours and hyperplasia in experimental animals treated with GLP-1-receptor agonists; these tumours are rare in humans and only very long-term pharma-covigilance will resolve this question, as it will with pancreatic cancers, which were numerically higher in liraglutide-treated patients in the LEADER study.

SGLT2 INHIBITORS ('FLOZINS')

Key practice points

- Glucose- and weight-lowering agents that act independently of β-cell function and insulin resistance
- Long-term glycaemic effectiveness is modest (approximately −0.5% HbA$_{1c}$ reduction at 2–4 years with empagliflozin)
- In patients with advanced atherosclerotic disease, empagliflozin reduced cardiovascular and renal endpoints and admissions with heart failure
- Use with caution in the elderly; canagliflozin carries a higher fracture rate

This fascinating group of glycosuric agents was introduced in 2012. Canagliflozin, dapagliflozin and empagliflozin are currently available, with several more compounds waiting in the wings. It is interesting that in the age of genomics, the mechanism of action of these drugs (transport blocker) is similar to that of many other very old and very successful drugs; but that should not blind us to the possibility of significant side effects. In contrast, however, the first definitive indication of cardiovascular benefit of any glycaemic drug has emerged with empagliflozin (see later). This group of drugs acts at the SGLT2 transporter in the proximal renal tubule, to inhibit reabsorption of about 90% of glucose; the small residual glucose is reabsorbed by SGLT1 situated slightly more distally. SGLT2 inhibitor drugs are less effective antihyperglycemic agents in impaired renal function. Their renal action means they are independent of insulin sensitivity and β-cell function and therefore do not cause weight gain or hypoglycaemia.

Glycaemic efficiency and durability

Dapagliflozin, canagliflozin and empagliflozin are currently licensed in the United Kingdom (**Table 10.7**). Several others are in development. Dosing is flat, once-daily and at any time of the day, and they are licensed in combination with all other drugs, including insulin. The formal advice is to start with the lower dose and increase as necessary, but there are no meaningful differences in achieved glycaemia between the two doses. They are effective drugs, with a clear baseline-related effect on glycaemic benefit. Over one year in metformin-treated patients with baseline HbA$_{1c}$ about 8.0% (64), canagliflozin 100 mg or 300 mg daily and glimepiride 6–8 mg daily were equally effective, reducing HbA$_{1c}$ by 0.8–0.9% (Cefalu et al., 2013). Falls of >1% occur in patients with baseline HbA$_{1c}$ >9% (75). In Type 2 patients on basal insulin, in a long 18-month double-blind placebo-controlled study, empagliflozin 25 mg daily reduced HbA$_{1c}$ by 0.6–0.7% from baseline 8% (64) (Rosenstock et al., 2015). In the single very long study, the placebo-controlled EMPA-REG OUTCOME study, glycaemic outcomes with empagliflozin were less impressive, with reductions of −0.5% at two years, and −0.4% at four years (Zinman et al., 2015). Because the flozins act independently of insulin they are of potential value in Type 1 diabetes, but because of concern about diabetic ketoacidosis (see below) they must be restricted to Type 2 patients with classic overweight phenotype until formal safety and efficacy trials are completed. The dosing in renal impairment is complex and differs for each agent, but the contraindications are largely due to supposed ineffectiveness in renal impairment, rather than increased risks of side effects.

Table 10.7 SGLT2 inhibitor drugs.

Drug	Dose	Adjustments in renal impairment	CV outcome studies; comments
Canagliflozin	100 mg daily, increasing to 300 mg daily	Do not start if eGFR <60 ml/min Reduce dose to 100 mg daily if eGFR falls to <60 ml/min Discontinue if eGFR <45 ml/min	CANVAS study (CANVAS-R, renal outcomes)
Dapagliflozin Empagliflozin	10 mg daily 10 mg daily, increasing to 25 mg daily	Use only if eGFR >60 ml/min Do not start if eGFR <60 ml/min Reduce dose to 10 mg if eGFR falls to <60 ml/min Discontinue if eGFR <45 ml/min	DECLARE-TIMI 58 (2019) Clear cardiovascular benefit in high risk patients (EMPA-REG OUTCOME) Benefits also in renal disease (**Chapter 4**), as well as heart failure (**Chapter 6**)

Effects on weight and risk of hypoglycaemia

This group of drugs causes consistent weight loss, around 1.5–3 kg which persists up to two years in trials. However, despite continuing glycosuria, weight loss levels off, so other compensatory mechanisms must be coming into play. Because of the consistent mechanism underlying weight loss, the occasional huge weight loss seen with GLP-1-receptor agonist drugs does not occur with the SGLT2 inhibitors, but both groups have overall similar effects on weight. In the EMPA-REG OUTCOME study, placebo-corrected weight loss of approximately 2 kg was maintained up to four years of follow-up. Hypoglycaemia is much the same as with the GLP-1-receptor agonist drugs; rates are not increased compared with placebo, but hypoglycaemia is more frequent in patients treated with sulfonylureas and insulin.

Practice point

Anticipate consistent weight loss of about 2 kg with the SGLT2 inhibitor drugs.

Non-glycaemic effects

SGLT2 inhibitors mildly benefit a portfolio of cardiovascular risk factors (for example, systolic blood pressure, HDL and serum urate) but similar effects have been excitedly reported with other glycaemic drugs in the past that have shown no overall cardiovascular benefit. Empagliflozin, however, in the cardiovascular safety study (EMPA-REG OUTCOME; Zinman et al., 2015) showed a striking and clinically meaningful reduction in cardiovascular outcomes in patients with established coronary, cerebrovascular or peripheral vascular disease, though the pattern of benefit is unusual and as with liraglutide in LEADER the mechanism(s) cannot be inferred from the clinical trials (**Table 10.6**). Major cardiovascular outcomes were reduced by 14% (1.6% absolute risk reduction), cardiovascular deaths fell by 2% and all-cause death by 2.5% (both absolute reductions). Notably, and against any haemodynamic explanation, stroke and transient ischaemic episodes were not reduced, but the risk of hospital admission for heart failure was reduced by 35%. Data for other SGLT2 inhibitors is awaited; a prospectively prespecified meta-analysis of clinical trials with dapagliflozin showed a benefit (approximately 20% risk reduction) both in the overall study population and those with cardiovascular disease (Sonesson et al., 2016). Reductions in heart failure hospitalization were again striking. In a post hoc analysis of a two-year trial in older patients between 55 and 80 years old taking canagliflozin 100 or 300 mg daily, cardiovascular biomarkers, including NT-proBNP, remained stable, while they increased in the placebo group, and although the reasons for these changes are not known, they may emerge as plausible mechanisms for cardiovascular event reduction, especially heart failure (Januzzi et al., 2017). The renal benefits are striking (see later and **Chapter 4**).

On the basis of these findings, this group of drugs is likely to be preferentially used in people with established cardiovascular disease, with again the risk of prescribing 'bleed' into much wider groups of Type 2 patients including those with any degree of diabetic renal disease. However, the drugs are expensive, and since patients without cardiovascular disease gain no specific benefits, proven strategies, such as careful blood pressure control and intensive LDL lowering, are likely to be just as valuable. Baseline characteristics in the EMPA REG OUTCOME study were suboptimal for these high-risk patients, for example total cholesterol 4.2 mmol/l, LDL 2.2 mmol/l and triglycerides 1.9 mmol/l, and systolic blood pressure perhaps a little high at 135 mm Hg. Only 78% of patients were taking a statin; mean baseline HbA_{1c} was 8.1% (65).

Practice point

Some important cardiovascular outcomes were reduced with empagliflozin treatment in high-risk vascular patients; heart failure events showed a particularly early reduction. Conventional cardiovascular risk factors were in poor control at baseline.

Side effects

Genito-urinary and bones

The persistent heavy glycosuria predisposes to fungal genital infections, especially in those who have had previous infections. In the EMPA REG OUTCOME study there was no excess of complicated urinary tract infection, but there is a higher risk in those with chronic or recurrent infection. Although the SGLT2 inhibitors are not classical diuretics, they are associated with urinary frequency. Volume depletion is seen more often in the over 75s and in those taking loop diuretics. Although renal outcomes are improved in patients taking empagliflozin, eGFR fell acutely by about 5% in the first 12 weeks of treatment in the EMPA REG OUTCOME study, remaining stable thereafter (Wanner et al., 2016).

There was a signal of increased risk of lower limb amputations in the long-term CANVAS study of canagliflozin, and increased upper- and lower-limb fracture risk in this older group with known cardiovascular disease. SGLT2 inhibitors alter calcium and

---

Practice point

Use SGLT2 inhibitor drugs with caution in the elderly and those with recurrent or chronic urinary infections or who are taking loop diuretics.

phosphate metabolism and increased phosphate reabsorption may lead to secondary hyperparathyroidism. These are further considerations in the use of these drugs in older and more frail people.

Normoglycaemic diabetic ketoacidosis

The US Food & Drug Administration (FDA) issued a warning on this side effect in 2015; it is still rare but potentially very hazardous as casual blood glucose levels are often low (e.g. <14 mmol/l) and may delay or prevent accurate diagnosis. The mechanisms are varied:

- insulin doses may be reduced because of improved glycaemia and become insufficient to suppress lipolysis and ketogenesis
- increased fat oxidation and ketone production (Daniele et al., 2016)
- increased glucagon secretion.

An additional clinical risk factor may be low carbohydrate diets, especially with further reduction in food intake because of an intercurrent illness (Farjo et al., 2016). American guidelines suggest discontinuing SGLT2 inhibitor treatment at least 24 hours before elective surgery, planned invasive procedures or severe stressful activity such as running a marathon (Handelsman et al., 2016). While physiologically sound, practical implementation, especially in the inpatient setting – as with metformin – will be difficult. In emergency departments, all patients using these agents should have a capillary ketone measurement regardless of the blood glucose level.

In a short, 18-week double-blind trial of canagliflozin in Type 1 patients with inadequately controlled glycaemia (HbA$_{1c}$ 7–9%, 53–75), nearly 10% had some form of ketone-associated adverse event and 6% of patients taking the higher dose developed actual ketoacidosis (Peters et al., 2016). SGLT2 inhibitors must not be used in Type 1 patients. While this is evident in those with 'classical' Type 1 (and it is unlikely they will be licensed in Type 1) it raises concerns about their use in patients with diagnosed Type 2 diabetes that is actually later-onset autoimmune diabetes, with a higher associated risk of insulin deficiency.

Practice point

SGLT2 inhibitors are not licensed for Type 1 diabetes; they should be used with caution in people with phenotypic features of later-onset autoimmune diabetes (see **Chapter 1**).

OTHER NON-INSULIN AGENTS

Thiazolidinediones (glitazones): hero to almost zero

No fewer than four pages were devoted to these insulin-sensitising drugs in the last edition of *Practical Diabetes Care*. The current short paragraph reflects their current minimal use. Increased cardiovascular risk resulted in effectively the worldwide withdrawal of rosiglitazone in 2010, but a portfolio of other side effects remain, the most problematic from the patient viewpoint being substantial weight gain and peripheral oedema. Pioglitazone survives, though mostly in guidelines. In the huge IRIS study in patients with stroke and transient cerebral ischaemia the risk of further stroke or myocardial infarction was significantly reduced (Kernan et al., 2016), echoing the more contested data of macrovascular event reduction in the PROActive study (Dormandy *et al.*, 2005), but this group of drugs is now irretrievably tainted for practitioners and patients alike, overtaken by the flozins and incretin-related therapies, and pioglitazone is almost never initiated in clinical practice.

Acarbose: α-glucosidase inhibitors

One of a family of agents (voglibose and miglitol are available outside the United Kingdom) that inhibits enzymes which break down polysaccharides and sucrose in the small intestine, delaying postmeal peaks of glucose. The STOP-NIDDM trial (2002) demonstrated a powerful effect in reducing progression of impaired glucose tolerance to diabetes, though with no legacy effect. There was also some contested evidence for a reduction in cardiovascular events and new-onset hypertension. In a UKPDS substudy, acarbose reduced HbA_{1c} by approximately 0.5%; although it is considered a weak agent, it is no less so than DPP-4 inhibitors. Their perceived weakness and the very real gastro-intestinal side effects, especially flatulence, have led to its near-complete erasure from the mental pharmacopeia of practicing physicians. However, in Chinese subjects it is as effective in initial therapy as metformin (HbA_{1c} reduction over 1 year about 1% from a baseline 7.5%, 58), with a low side-effect rate possibly due to the gradual titration regimen (50 mg once daily, increasing over 4 weeks to 100 mg three times daily) (Yang *et al.*, 2014). The good response has been attributed in part to the high carbohydrate diet of many Chinese people (in this study nearly two-thirds of energy intake was carbohydrate), though this would not explain the similar response to metformin. Acarbose treatment could, therefore, be effective in certain groups, though it did not reduce cardiovascular events in a large pre-diabetic Chinese population (Holman *et al.*, 2017).

Pramlintide and bromocriptine

These agents are not available in the United Kingdom. Pramlintide is synthetic amylin, a peptide of obscure function cosecreted with insulin. Taken together with prandial insulin in both Type 1 and 2 diabetes it improves some glycaemic measures, but even where available it is not widely used.

The dopamine agonist bromocriptine, usually used in hyperprolactinaemia, exerts its glucose-lowering effects via central dopaminergic and sympathetic pathways rather than peripheral action, and a quick-release preparation taken once daily is available in the USA. Modest falls around 0.5% HbA_{1c} are described, but its use is limited by nausea and vomiting.

Colesevelam

Similar to the long-obsolete bile acid sequestrant resins used to treat hypercholesterolaemia, colesevelam also has some glucose lowering properties (e.g. HbA_{1c} falls of about 0.3%). Although available in the United Kingdom, it is almost never prescribed on account of gastrointestinal side effects, the need for multiple daily dosing and its prohibitive cost.

INSULIN TREATMENT

The idea of insulin treatment is unpopular with patients and a proposal to start insulin is usually resisted. In the 4-T study – see later – recruited patients gave encouragingly positive feedback on the experience, but this may not accurately represent the everyday experience of often pressured clinicians – and patients – out of the clinical trial environment (Jenkins *et al.*, 2010). Patient-level resistance to insulin treatment contrasts with its ringing endorsement in guidelines, including an ADA recommendation for the use of

> **Box 10.3** Claims for the benefits of insulin treatment in Type 2 diabetes.
>
> - It is the most effective glucose-lowering agent.
> - It has 'unlimited' capacity to lower blood glucose.
> - It better preserves β-cell function.
> - It reduces endpoints meaningful for patients.

basal insulin after metformin, where it is described as having the 'highest' glycaemic efficacy compared with other available agents, but is qualified by high hypoglycaemia risk, weight gain and its variable cost (**Box 10.3**). There are sporadic references in the literature to the 'unlimited' ability of insulin to reduce blood glucose levels, but perhaps also the beginnings of a new movement questioning the supremacy of insulin treatment, based on increasing concerns about its safety, and advocating wherever possible combination treatment with non-insulin agents (Schwartz et al., 2016).

Is the claim for insulin's 'highest' glycaemic efficacy supported by evidence? There are very few monotherapy trials to guide us in this question, but in the UKPDS, the tick-shaped trajectory of HbA_{1c} in the insulin-treated group was identical over a decade to that of groups treated with sulfonylureas. However, there are good studies of insulin versus combination oral therapy that do indicate that two non-insulin agents may be needed to match its glycaemic efficiency. A randomized three-year study in newly-diagnosed patients, comparing insulin+metformin with metformin+pioglitazone+glibenclamide (after a run-in period of three months of metformin+insulin in all patients), found that glycaemia, weight and rate of hypoglycaemia were identical in the two groups; it concluded that insulin treatment was appropriate for early use in Type 2 diabetes. However, sequential testing showed that there were no differences in β-cell function between the two groups. An argument commonly used to promote early use of insulin treatment is that it better preserves insulin secretion, but the contention is not supported by this or other careful studies (Harrison et al., 2012).

Is insulin more effective in patients with established diabetes? Again, when compared in trials against judicious combination therapy, the answer is that it seems to be as effective as approximately two non-insulin agents. For example, patients poorly controlled (mean HbA_{1c} 9.7%, 83) on two oral agents were treated either with triple oral therapy by adding rosiglitazone, or were maintained on metformin treatment with additional twice-daily biphasic 30/70 insulin. Over six months, HbA_{1c} fell by 2.1% to 7.6% (60) in both groups, though initially the fall was more rapid in the insulin treated patients (Schwartz et al., 2003). Given the approximate glycaemic equivalence of most non-insulin agents (see previously), the fact that these studies used agents that are now either obsolete (glibenclamide) or have been withdrawn (rosiglitazone) is not relevant. On the basis of glycaemic advantage only the individual patient can properly decide whether insulin treatment is more troublesome than two additional oral agents.

The critical question is whether insulin improves outcomes that matter to patients. The concern that exogenous insulin may be pro-atherogenic was exhaustively aired several years ago and the conclusion was that there was no evidence for such an adverse effect, though the concern was based on sound biochemistry. In the end the debate was terminated in part by the more pressing concerns of potential harm of the glitazones and other non-insulin agents. In short, there is no conclusive evidence that insulin treatment improves all-cause mortality of cardiovascular outcomes in Type 2 patients compared with oral hypoglycaemic treatment (Li et al., 2016).

The complex ORIGIN trial failed to show that long-term treatment (approximately seven years) with basal insulin glargine had any benefit on cardiovascular endpoints in a mixed group of subjects with early Type 2 diabetes and prediabetes, and a baseline HbA$_{1c}$ (6.4%, 46) that was just short of the diagnostic level for diabetes. All patients remained in excellent stable control both during the randomized phase of the trial with only tiny differences between the groups and also in follow-up of more than 2½ years (HbA$_{1c}$ 6.7%, 50) with no differences between the previous treatment groups) (ORIGIN Trial Investigators, 2016). Hypoglycaemia of all grades was more common in the glargine-treated group, and at the end of the trial the glargine-treated patients were on average 2 kg heavier than the control group. The positive conclusion from this huge study is that insulin and non-insulin treatments can both maintain excellent glycaemia over a very long period when instituted early, but it cannot be used to sustain arguments for prioritizing insulin over any other approved agents, other than on the grounds of interesting pathophysiology (e.g. glucotoxicity or lipotoxicity) that is not supported by clinical outcome data.

Nevertheless, valuable strategies have emerged that allow patients to remain in good and stable glycaemic control with insulin, usually in combination with other agents

INSULIN TREATMENT IN TYPE 2 DIABETES

Mandatory insulin treatment
There is a small heterogeneous group of patients who must start insulin treatment soon:

- Patients with features of latent autoimmune diabetes of adults (LADA) in poor control (see **Chapter 1**).
- Normal weight or thin patients, and those with progressive weight loss and persistent poor control (e.g. HbA$_{1c}$ >8.0%, 64) despite good adherence to several non-insulin agents, or who have had a poor response to them.
- The unusual patients with proximal femoral neuropathy (neuropathic cachexia; see **Chapter 5**).
- Patients already in poor control who are likely to need long-term or frequent intermittent courses of steroids.

> **Practice point**
>
> Very poor control in someone losing weight or not obese to begin with? They may have autoimmune diabetes – and are likely to need 'full' insulin replacement.

Metformin should be stopped in patients with normal body mass index or who have lost weight; other agents should also be stopped except in overweight patients starting steroids. Patients should in general start full insulin treatment with basal-bolus insulin or biphasic insulin.

Elective insulin treatment
The usual scenario is a patient with diabetes of known 5–10 years' duration. Glycaemic control has been slipping over a few years with HbA$_{1c}$ climbing towards and beyond about 8% (64). Most patients will be taking full dose or maximum tolerated metformin, and usually two other non-insulin agents. The possible combinations of non-insulin agents are legion but in current practice will usually be a sulfonylurea in combination with either a GLP-1-receptor agonist, oral DPP-4 inhibitor, SGLT2 inhibitor,

Table 10.8 Characteristics of patients starting insulin in the 4-T study (2007) and the DURABLE trial (2011).

	4-T (12 months)	DURABLE (6 months)
White ethnic groups, %	92	70–80
Mean age, yr	62	57–59
Mean duration of diabetes, yr	9	8.5–10
HbA$_{1c}$, % (mmol/mol)	8.6 (70)	9.0–9.1 (75–76)
Fasting glucose, mmol/l	9.7	10–11
Weight, kg	86	90–92
BMI	30	32
BP	138/80	
Macrovascular disease/retinopathy/ nephropathy, %	22/15/9	

Sources: Holman *et al.*, 2007, Buse *et al.*, 2011.

or – rarely – pioglitazone. The characteristics of patients starting insulin in the UK randomized 4-T study (Holman *et al.*, 2007) and in the international DURABLE study (Buse *et al.*, 2011) are shown in **Table 10.8**. Baseline HbA$_{1c}$ in most insulin initiation trials remains stubbornly higher than the guideline recommendations, usually 8.5–9.0% (69–75). The decision to start insulin remains very difficult, but at least there are good clinical trials that help the decision which insulin regimen to start.

In view of the recent long-term trials that have confirmed the broadly equal glycaemic efficacy of basal insulin and a GLP-1-receptor agonist, it is always worth considering the latter, or conceivably a fixed-ratio combination of basal analogue insulin and GLP-1-receptor agonist in someone taking neither agent (see previously).

Which insulin regimen?
The widely quoted study of Monnier *et al.* (2007) proposed that in Type 2 diabetes loss of postprandial glucose control preceded fasting hyperglycaemia as overall glycaemic worsened. Monnier's thesis was supported in a DURABLE substudy using seven-point glucose profiles (Scheen *et al.*, 2015). As HbA$_{1c}$ increased, the relative contribution of postprandial hyperglycaemia to total glycaemia decreased from 41% to 27%, while that of fasting hyperglycaemia increased from 59% to 73%. In Asians (in this study, people of South-East Asian, rather than South Asian origin), postprandial hyperglycaemia at all HbA$_{1c}$ levels contributed about 10% more to overall hyperglycaemia than in the white population. There has always been a hope that patients with predominant fasting hyperglycaemia could be prioritized for a trial of basal insulin, while those with postprandial hyperglycaemia might respond better to prandial or biphasic insulin, but there is no evidence yet for this approach. In motivated people, and where there are resources, there may be a case for an initial diagnostic continuous glucose monitoring to help target alternative regimens to standard basal insulin (e.g. twice-daily biphasic insulin), especially in South-East Asian people.

In practice, though, by 10 years of diagnosed diabetes there is severe clinical hyperglycaemia. In both the 4-T and DURABLE studies, elevated HbA$_{1c}$ (e.g. 8.5–9.0%, 69–75) was consistently associated with severe fasting hyperglycaemia (e.g. 10–11 mmol/l); in addition, in the 4-T study there was, not surprisingly, marked postprandial hyperglycaemia (mean 12.5 mmol/l). Relevant to the practical titration of insulin doses

Table 10.9 Expectations of basal insulin treatment in Type 2 diabetes: 4-T and DURABLE trials.

Outcome	4-T	DURABLE
Reduction in HbA$_{1c}$, %	1.4	1.7
Final HbA$_{1c}$, % (mmol/mol)	7.6 (60)	7.3 (56)
Weight gain, kg	1.9	2.5
Hypoglycaemia compared with twice-daily biphasic insulin	Doubled	Higher overall hypoglycaemia, lower nocturnal hypoglycaemia, no differences in severe hypoglycaemia
Total final basal insulin dose, U	42	~36
Insulin dose, U/kg/day	0.50	0.40

and the overall low risks of nocturnal hypoglycaemia with basal insulin, there was sustained nocturnal hyperglycaemia (3:00 a.m. values were very similar, 9.5 mmo/l, to fasting levels).

We will set aside the group in the 4-T study treated with three-times daily rapid-acting analogue (without basal insulin), as this was and remains an unconventional regimen, and gave similar results to the group managed with twice-daily biphasic insulin. In both studies biphasic insulin was statistically marginally better than basal insulin, both in HbA$_{1c}$ reduction (7.3% vs 7.6%, 56 vs 60, in 4-T) and durability of maintaining target HbA$_{1c}$ <7.0% (53). However, these marginal advantages will not be apparent in individuals and were outweighed by greater weight gain with biphasic insulin and, in the 4-T study, increased hypoglycaemia. Outline results of these trials are shown in **Table 10.9**.

> **Practice point**
>
> Overnight basal insulin is the best starting regimen for most Type 2 patients who need insulin, but consider a GLP-1- receptor agonist in someone not already taking one.

Starting basal insulin

This takes time and even experienced specialist nurses will need about an hour to fully educate and involve the patient and carers. The whole process is intensive for healthcare professionals and patients alike, and it must not be embarked on lightly, and without a clear plan for follow-up. Although self-titration is critical for engagement and optimum results, insulin initiation cannot be delegated solely to the patient, and the more frequent the contact with specialist nurses, the better the glycaemic outcome (Swinnen and Devries, 2009). Telephone contact is preferable, as it helps maintain a focus on the key tasks of dosage adjustment and glycaemic targets.

Insulin titration regimen: 'aggressive' or pragmatic? Desirable fasting glucose level

Clinical trials in general adopt a highly structured basal insulin titration regimen, often targeting low or very low fasting glucose levels. Many trials last only for six months, so there is a practical need to achieve stable low levels as quickly as possible; this is not a priority in general clinical practice where hyperglycaemia has often been slowly progressing

Table 10.10 Examples of basal insulin titration regimens in clinical trials compared with a pragmatic example for clinical practice.

Fasting glucose (mmol/l)	Degludec vs glargine (2012)	NPH vs glargine (2003)	Example in general clinical practice
>15			**+2 units every few days or**
>10	+8 units	+8 units	**increase by 10% at higher**
9	+6 units	+6 units	**insulin doses**
8			
7	+4	+4	**Don't increase insulin dose**
6	+2	+2	
5	Dose unchanged		**Decrease if hypoglycaemia**
4	−2 units		
3	−4 units		

Sources: Zinman *et al.*, 2012, Riddle *et al.*, 2003.

for years. With the advent of long-acting analogues with pharmacokinetic evidence of smooth action, several trials have justified targeting fasting values indistinguishable from non-diabetic levels (e.g. 4–5 mmol/l) (Zinman *et al.*, 2012). Not surprisingly, very few trials have achieved these and the usual final fasting level is about 7–8 mmol/l, though occasionally 6 mmol/l.

The regimen adopted in trials often requires uptitration of insulin doses by two or even four units once fasting levels of 6–7 mmol/l have been reached; in routine clinical practice these levels would be considered quite satisfactory and most practitioners will not recommend further increases in insulin doses. The 'aggressive' dose titration (a descriptor commonly used in clinical trial reports) may have consequences for accentuating differences in nocturnal hypoglycaemia rates between different long-acting analogues (**Table 10.10**; see later).

Further confirmation of satisfactory fasting glucose targets comes from the ADAG study (Wei *et al.*, 2014). For example, in order to target HbA$_{1c}$ between 7.0% and 7.5% (53–58) mean fasting glucose should be about 8 mmol/l (range 7.4-8.9) and between 6.5% and 7.0% mean fasting glucose should be 7.7 mmol/l (range 7.7–8.2). These values are higher than the wide preprandial range proposed by the American Diabetes Association, that is 4.4–7.2 mmol/l (desirable fasting range not stated), but are well away from the hypogly-caemia hazard zone.

Dose titration

The labour-intensive regimens (for patients and professionals alike) in clinical trials are not practical for everyday use. Median starting insulin dose in the 4-T study was 16 units (interquartile range 10–24); this was effective and safe but in practice a lower dose is usually used, for example 10 units, or, wholly arbitrarily, at the same number of units as the baseline fasting glucose in mmol/l. Many trials aim for dosage titration about twice a week, based on the previous few days' glucose measurements, and this is reasonable, as long as dose increments are small and consistent. Since most modern trials find that target fasting glucose levels are reached with 40–50 units basal insulin, twice-weekly upwards titration by two units each time will allow most patients to achieve reasonable control within 2–3 months (actually a shorter time than in many clinical trials, where insulin doses do not start to plateau until 4–5 months). Slow and steady may in this instance achieve at least a safe arrival.

However, reliable and safe outcomes can only be achieved with carefully documented suggestions for patients to self-titrate, frequent communication with their diabetes practice team and reassurance that the final dose of insulin, although perhaps three or four times the starting dose, is generally needed.

Maintain metformin and perhaps optimize the dose at 2 g daily. Tail off or stop any non-insulin agents that have not been of meaningful glycaemic benefit to the patient, and reduce any sulfonylurea to the maximum effective dose (see previously). Do not discontinue sulfonylureas, even in long-duration Type 2 diabetes, as it may result in gly-caemic deterioration, though studies showing this interesting phenomenon have been carried out in South-East Asian patients (Srivanichakorn et al., 2015). If a sulfonylurea is continued, then it is worthwhile ensuring that patients carry out prelunch glucose meas-urements to confirm that now they have achieved lower fasting levels, they are not slip-ping into hypoglycaemia on their old sulfonylurea dose.

Practice point

A practical basal insulin regimen could start with 10 units at bedtime, increasing by two units twice a week with daily fasting home glucose monitoring until target fasting glucose is reached (e.g. 7 mmol/l).

Although the full 24-month DURABLE study found some evidence that in older people (mean age 69 years) biphasic insulin had greater durability and better effects on glycae-mic control than basal glargine, it was not generalizable, as it excluded patients not achieving an HbA_{1c} target <7.0% (53) at six months. However, those with HbA_{1c} >7.0% were entered into a large and important substudy (see later).

Practice point

Although there are no agreed fasting glucose targets for patients starting basal insulin treat-ment, a reasonable and achievable range would be 7–8 mmol/l.

Which insulin?

Prodigious research and marketing energy has been devoted to the minutiae of discuss-ing whether human isophane (NPH) or one of the long-acting analogue insulins, which continue to proliferate, is preferable for basal use in Type 2 diabetes. They are identical in glucose-lowering effect and trials lasting up to six months show superimposable trajectories of both fasting glucose and HbA_{1c} (for example, NPH compared with glar-gine) (Riddle et al., 2003). The argument has therefore shifted to considerations of dif-ferences in rates of hypoglycaemia between NPH and long-acting analogues, and with the introduction of a new long-acting analogue to comparing hypoglycaemia rates against those of an older analogue, usually the prototype glargine. These arguments have rarely enlightened the practitioner. The evidence for NPH compared with glargine and detemir is summarized in a Cochrane meta-analysis (Horvath et al., 2007):

- there is no difference in rates of severe hypoglycaemia between NPH and either insulin detemir or glargine;
- statistically there is a lower risk of symptomatic, overall and nocturnal hypoglycaemia.

Likewise there are only small differences between long-acting analogues (**Figure 10.7**). Another Cochrane review comparing insulin glargine and detemir found similar glycaemic control, and no differences in any type of hypoglycaemia, though by the end of the trials 14–57% of patients were injecting detemir twice-daily, and they needed higher doses than glargine for equivalent glycaemic effect (a consistent finding in clinical trials

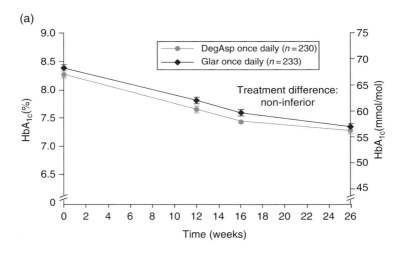

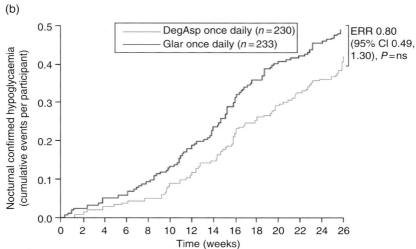

Figure 10.7 Characteristic effects of basal insulin treatment on glycaemic control and hypoglycaemia rates in Type 2 diabetes. In this case the preparations were a 30/70 mixture degludec/aspart and the standard for comparative trials, glargine. (a) HbA$_{1c}$, (b) rates of nocturnal hypoglycaemia, showing a numerically lower incidence with the biphasic mixture, though in this case the difference was not statistically significant, (c) fasting glucose. See text for further discussion of this phenomenon. *Source*: Kumar *et al.*, 2017. Reproduced with permission of John Wiley & Sons.

(c)

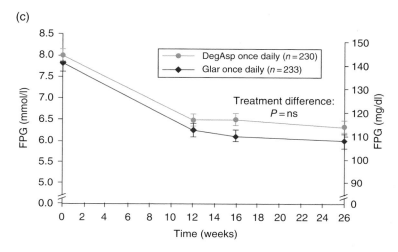

Figure 10.7 (Continued)

that increases the effective cost of this insulin preparation). Weight gain was statistically slightly less with detemir (for example in one trial 0.6 kg compared with 1.4 kg for glargine). Swinnen *et al.* (2011) concluded there were no meaningful differences between the two preparations.

It was hoped that the 'ultra-long' acting insulin degludec would permit alternate three times weekly dosing, but used in this way glycaemia was inferior to that of daily glargine with no differences in hypoglycaemia (Zinman *et al.*, 2013). In once-daily usage it has the same glycaemic effect as glargine; confirmed and severe hypoglycaemia rates were similar, but nocturnal hypoglycaemia was marginally less frequent.

Basal insulin is effective in Chinese and Japanese patients poorly controlled on metformin and a sulfonylurea, but a single dose of biphasic insulin gave the same HbA_{1c} reduction with no differences in hypoglycaemia (Yang *et al.*, 2013).

Despite these extensive trials that aimed to establish clear superiority of one long-acting analogue preparation over another, human NPH (isophane) insulin remains the most appropriate insulin for overnight basal insulin treatment in overweight Type 2 patients not achieving glycaemic targets using maximum appropriate non-insulin treatment. Patients with a more 'Type 1-LADA' phenotype may prefer glargine, which in many countries has become the standard basal insulin treatment for all Type 2 patients, but there is no convincing evidence for its superiority, and it is likely that practitioners have generally become more adept at using basal insulin treatment in the two decades since the introduction of glargine. As in all aspects of insulin treatment, professional engagement with an educated patient is more important in ensuring good therapeutic outcomes than minute differences in overnight hypoglycaemia rates between competing products. Practical points are very important, especially those that ease the burden of injections, and inevitably there will be local variations, but, for example, UK patients should be offered insulin preparations available in disposable pens:

- *Isophane insulin (NPH)*: Humulin I, Insuman Basal SoloStar, Insulatard InnoLet.
- *Long-acting analogues*: Glargine (Lantus SoloStar, Toujeo [300 U/ml] SoloStar, Abasaglar KwikPen); detemir (Levemir FlexTouch); degludec (Tresiba [100 U/ml and 200 U/ml] FlexTouch.

Practice point

Human NPH (isophane) insulin is first-choice for basal insulin treatment in Type 2 diabetes; insulin glargine is a suitable alternative. There is no meaningful advantage using any of the more recent long-acting insulin analogues.

How long should we persist with basal overnight insulin treatment?

It was a widespread view not so long ago, and very much of the technocratic era where insulin was considered to have unlimited power to reduce blood glucose level, that there was no degree of insulin resistance that could not be overcome if sufficiently high doses were given. In occasional cases, this may have been the case, but in most patients diminishing returns seemed to set in: weight continued to increase without commensurate further reductions in HbA_{1c} and, equally important, patients became demotivated because of little apparent progress, while they still often faced multiple injections. Although high-concentration analogues have been introduced as patent expiry looms, until recently no pen devices could deliver more than 80 units in one shot. Very high doses can now be more conveniently delivered, but trial data and not the availability of devices must guide clinical practice.

However, there is some evidence for cautiously persisting with basal insulin beyond the 40–50 units daily used in most conventional trials. Although the EDITION 2 study (Yki-Järvinen *et al.*, 2014) was primarily concerned with the safety and efficiency of high-concentration (U300) insulin glargine, it studied a large and clinically-relevant group of relatively young patients (mean 58 years), with long diabetes duration (mean 12 years), severely overweight (mean BMI 35) and in poor control (mean HbA_{1c} 8.2%, 66), despite oral hypoglycaemics and basal insulin at a mean dose of 65 units (the protocol required patients to be taking 42 units or more a day). Although only a six-month trial, by increasing insulin glargine to a mean of 90 units (0.85–0.90 units/kg/day), HbA_{1c} fell by approximately 0.6% to 7.6% (59), with almost no weight gain. (There were no meaningful differences between the groups taking U100 and U300 glargine.) Durability is, though, critical and as with so many agents there is no useful data beyond the short reach of randomisation (see later).

However, this is an intensive process for patients and professionals, and although there are no studies comparing progression to higher-dose basal insulin with the addition of a GLP1-receptor agonist (see previously), the latter manoeuvre is likely to be equally effective and may be less troublesome for patients. A large population-based study in Denmark found that when a GLP-1-receptor agonist was added around a year after starting basal insulin treatment it was more effective in achieving HbA_{1c} values <7.0% or <7.5% (53 or 58) than insulin intensification using either premixed insulin or bolus insulin (Thomsen *et al.*, 2017).

Practice point

In patients still not at target HbA$_{1c}$ taking 40–60 units of basal insulin, consider either further increasing the dose or adding a GLP-1-receptor agonist.

Durability of basal insulin treatment

The data are very sparse. However, there is no reason to expect that basal insulin maintains glycaemic targets with more persistence than any other glucose-lowering agents. In the DURABLE study, around 50% of patients failed to maintain the admittedly very stringent HbA$_{1c}$ target of 7% (53) or lower up to two years, and this was in a study cohort where those not achieving that same target in the first six months of the study had been excluded. Because responses to insulin treatment are idiosyncratic, patients must have frequent reviews until stable glycaemia is established. Flexibly providing the services needed for individuals is much more important than the locus of care.

PROGRESSING INSULIN TREATMENT

This very difficult clinical situation – how to advance insulin treatment in patients not achieving adequate glycaemic control and usually taking basal insulin together with one or more non-insulin agents – is poorly illuminated by the clinical trial repertoire, and not just from the point of view of glycaemia. Patients have disparate needs and expectations at this stage of their diabetes – often many years after diagnosis, with a substantial burden of vascular complications – and may already be somewhat jaded by the experience of initiating insulin. However, there has been a major change in approach over the past decade: previously patients requiring more than basal insulin would have been encouraged to move immediately to the basal-bolus regimen that is the norm in Type 1 diabetes. This failed to recognize that Type 2 patients are very rarely so insulin deficient that they require the 24-hour insulin coverage needed in Type 1 diabetes.

The 4-T study ran on for another two years after the initial randomization to complete three years (Holman *et al.*, 2009). It was published in 2009, around the same time as the major vascular trials (ADVANCE, ACCORD and VADT); ultra-tight glycaemia was still the accepted strategy and in the 4-T study additional insulin was added when HbA$_{1c}$ exceeded 6.5% (48). Additional insulin was needed in 70–80% of patients, and at that point the sulfonylurea was discontinued. The biphasic insulin regimen was advanced by adding in prandial lunchtime insulin at a starting dose of 10% of the total daily insulin dose. In the basal group, 10% of the total daily insulin dose was added before each meal (this approach has probably been superseded by the 'basal-plus' regimen: see later).

The conclusions were clear:

- Under study conditions, it is possible to maintain good glycaemic control (HbA$_{1c}$ 6.8–7.1%, 51–54) with basal, twice-daily biphasic or prandial insulin.
- Hypoglycaemia and weight gain were lowest in the basal group.
- At trial end patients were taking 1.2 U/kg/day insulin (of which 60% was prandial); they had effectively converted to a standard basal-bolus regimen; this probably accounts for most of the mean 3.6 kg weight gain.

Practical insulin regimens after basal insulin

'Basal plus' regimen

'Basal plus' is the sound concept of incremental addition of prandial insulin doses where glycaemia has not been optimized with basal insulin alone; daytime non-insulin agents are continued. The first insulin dose is added before the meal with the highest carbohydrate content – for most patients this will be dinner. Postprandial fingerprick measurements will direct gradual dose titration to achieve values <10 mmol/l, though in principle it could be achieved more precisely using short-term continuous glucose monitoring. A six-month trial compared 'basal plus' with twice-daily biphasic insulin in patients with likely postprandial hyperglycaemia, that is fasting glucose levels <7 mmol/l but HbA_{1c} >7.0% (53) (Vora et al., 2015). There were no differences in achieved glycaemia, weight (2 kg mean gain in each) or rates of overall hypoglycaemia, but there was more nocturnal hypoglycaemia in the basal plus group, hinting at the possibility of insulin 'stacking' from a late evening meal and early bedtime basal insulin (this is also a problem in working-age Type 1 patients). Treatment satisfaction was higher with basal plus than with twice-daily biphasic insulin, but overall quality of life was the same.

The ADA/EASD guideline for introducing basal-plus insulin is sound and conservative:

- start with four units (or 0.1 units/kg, or 10% of basal dose) before the main carbohydrate-containing meal
- titrate by one or two units or 10–15% twice-weekly until postprandial target is reached
- decrease by two or four units if there is hypoglycaemia.

As with all insulin regimens, supported self-titration is best (though it may not be suitable for all patients) and, as in patients starting basal insulin, remind them that although the starting insulin dose is deliberately low, some people may need 20 U or more if they have a substantial carbohydrate-containing meal (e.g. 100 g pasta – a medium-sized portion for an adult male) and also have a tendency to insulin resistance. Technique and detail are important: wherever possible – and it is more likely to be possible with the evening meal than any other meal in working-age patients – insulin should be taken 15–20 minutes before meals or, failing that, immediately before (but certainly not after). Although the tendency will normally be to suggest a rapid-acting analogue, there is no evidence for their superiority in this situation compared with the slower and more gentle action of human soluble insulin, which may be more suitable in patients who eat early (e.g. 6–7 p.m.) and have high-carbohydrate meals.

There are no trials of regimens that test the efficacy of adding further prandial doses beyond the one taken with the largest meal in the basal plus regimen. Intuitively the effect might be limited. There is no study comparing the outcomes of a basal-bolus regimen gradually implemented compared with instituting it all at once (but see later).

Practice point

Basal plus insulin is as effective as twice-daily biphasic insulin and it is easy to implement if needed after basal insulin.

Basal bolus regimen

Intensifying insulin treatment in Type 2 diabetes has not until recently been informed by much evidence and in many cases patients ended up using a basal bolus regimen comprising up to five injections a day. Trials of insulin intensification beyond basal-plus or twice-daily biphasic insulin vary in quality, but there are studies that can inform everyday practice.

The DURABLE follow-on study randomized patients with HbA_{1c} >7.0% (53) on basal or twice-daily biphasic insulin and attempted to intensify treatment from their actual baseline HbA_{1c} of approximately 8.0% (64) using various regimens: basal bolus insulin, twice-daily 25/75 biphasic insulin or prandial three times daily 50/50 biphasic mixture (Miser et al., 2010). Sulfonylureas were discontinued but metformin and glitazones continued. This was a commendably realistic six-month trial. Clinicians were allowed to titrate as they felt appropriate, with a preprandial target of 6.1 mmol/l. The baseline insulin dose of 40–50 units/day increased by about 60% to a final dose of 70–74 units/day. Regardless of the new regimen, HbA_{1c} did not improve and remained solidly at approximately 8% (64). Positively, patients gained little weight (0.6–1.4 kg) and hypoglycaemia rates did not differ between the different regimens.

Patients in the DURABLE study were not typical of participants in other trials, or indeed of many patients in clinical practice, where baseline HbA_{1c} values are often much higher (e.g. 9.0–9.5%, 75–80). But even in these patients, basal bolus insulin was not meaningfully better than simpler regimens, another reminder that Type 1 and 2 diabetes are fundamentally different. Basal-bolus insulin should not be a desired target regimen in Type 2 diabetes. For example, Rosenstock et al. (2008) randomized patients in poor control on glargine and oral agents (mean HbA_{1c} 8.8, 73) to basal bolus or three-times daily 50% biphasic mixture. HbA_{1c} at the end of the six-month study was numerically lower but clinically no different in the basal-bolus group (6.8%, vs 7.0%, 51 vs 53).

Practice point

Standard insulin intensification, for example conversion of a basal-plus regimen to basal-bolus or to three times daily prandial biphasic insulin, does not improve control.

Biphasic insulin

Broad conclusions from studies previously discussed are:

- Basal insulin, carefully implemented, is often as good as any other, more complex regimen.
- Thereafter, basal plus insulin is as effective as twice-daily biphasic insulin. Targeting one or other regimen to different groups of patients is likely to be based on pragmatic considerations such as meal planning. For example, twice-daily biphasic insulin might suit patients regularly eating breakfast and evening meals approximately 12 hours apart; basal plus might be better for working-age patients rushing out to work after a small (or no) breakfast and eating dinner at varying times.
- It is not known whether progressive addition of mealtime insulin beyond the single injection in basal plus carries additional glycaemic benefit.
- Patients in poor control on basal (or possibly basal plus) should be considered for twice- or three-times daily prandial biphasic insulin.
- Basal-bolus regimens are generally not more effective than biphasic insulin. This important conclusion is supported by a meta-analysis of trials up to 2015 (Giugliano et al., 2016).

Table 10.11 Biphasic insulin preparations appropriate for use in Type 2 diabetes in the United Kingdom.

Brand name (UK)	Formal designation	Components	Presentations/ comment
Biphasic human insulin preparations			
Humulin M3	Biphasic isophane insulin	Soluble 30% Isophane 70%	Available in 3 ml cartridges and disposable pen (Humulin M3 KwikPen)
Insuman Comb 15/25/50	Biphasic isophane insulin	Soluble 15%/25%/50% Isophane 85%/75%/50%	Available in 3 ml cartridges Insuman Comb 25 available as disposable pen (Insuman Comb 25 SoloStar)
Biphasic analogue insulin preparations			
NovoMix 30	Biphasic insulin aspart BIAsp 30	Insulin aspart 30% Insulin aspart protamine 70%	Available in 3 ml cartridges (Penfill) and disposable pens (FlexPen, FlexTouch)
Humalog Mix25 Humalog Mix50	Biphasic insulin lispro	Insulin lispro 25%/50% Insulin lispro protamine 75%/50%	Available in 3ml cartridges and disposable pens (Humalog Mix25 KwikPen, Humalog Mix50 KwikPen) State the name of the insulin preparation in full (remember there is the rapid-acting 'Humalog')
Ryzodeg	Insulin degludec/ insulin aspart IDegAsp	Insulin aspart 30% Insulin degludec 70%	Available in 3ml disposable pens (FlexTouch)

One pork biphasic insulin preparation is available in the UK (Hypurin Porcine 30/70, soluble 30%, 70% isophane) in cartridges.

Any residual concerns about using premixed insulins in Type 2 diabetes can no longer be sustained when the evidence is considered. Again, the contrast with Type 1 diabetes could not be clearer. Practitioners must be confident using them (**Table 10.11**), but importantly, outcomes are not meaningfully different with any of the available preparations.

Practice point

There are no meaningful differences between biphasic insulin preparations. It is entirely reasonable to use human biphasic isophane insulin twice daily.

Implementing biphasic insulin treatment

The intensity of insulin titration will differ according to the individual patient's needs and preferences, bearing in mind the priority of avoiding severe hypoglycaemia. The regimens used in clinical trials, especially those in the 2000s, tended towards the vigorous, with the aim of achieving low target HbA$_{1c}$ values, for example 6.5% (48) or lower. A gentler approach is usually sound, though there are countless ways of doing this. For example:

- If patients are transferring from basal or basal plus, divide the current basal dose, giving either 50% before breakfast and evening meal or, more traditionally 2/3 before breakfast, 1/3 before evening meal.
- Titrate every 3–4 days by two units, targeting postprandial glucose levels <10 mmol/l.
- In patients at work, this is difficult to do in practice – especially postbreakfast measurements; a prelunch target could be similar to the general ADA target of >4–7 mmol/l.
- Advise patients to watch for mid- to late-morning hypoglycaemia, especially if they have a particularly busy physical schedule in the morning.

In most trials of biphasic insulin, patients eventually require about 0.5 units/kg/day, that is about 40-60 units.

Beyond complex regimens: the patient in persistent poor control (e.g. HbA$_{1c}$ >9%, 75) on multiple daily insulin doses and non-insulin agents

We may be getting better at implementing structured and more or less evidence-based insulin treatment in patients newly requiring insulin, but a common pre-existing problem, and one that is especially distressing for patients is consistent poor control while using high-dose multiple daily insulin injections with a variable number of non-insulin agents. There is no large-scale trial evidence to guide managing this situation. However, we know the characteristics of patients with persistent poor control for more than a year (HbA$_{1c}$ >8.0% [64]) (Crowley et al., 2014), the majority taking insulin. They comprised about 12% of Type 2 patients, were younger at onset – mean 47 years – than those in better control and had a long duration (mean 14 years). Actual mean HbA$_{1c}$ was nearly 10% (86). There was evidence of poor adherence to oral hypoglycaemic agents and statins, suggesting again the importance of focusing on rationalizing medication. The authors proposed largely behavioural approaches, but these have not been tested.

How in practice to manage this difficult situation elicits much opinion and strikingly little evidence. However, consider the following:

- Change from complex basal-bolus regimens to biphasic insulin, which at least will reduce the injection burden and is likely not to cause further deterioration in control (remember that at these high absolute levels, the variability of HbA$_{1c}$ measurements will appear to be high, so it is especially important not to over-interpret changes of 1.0–1.5%). We must acknowledge that further 'intensification' of multiple daily dose insulin will not work. For example in the OpT2mise study – see later – intensification if HbA$_{1c}$ >8.4% (68) failed in more than 90% of patients (Schütz-Fuhrmann et al., 2017).
- Introduce non-insulin agents that might help:
  - GLP-1-receptor agonist,
  - SGLT2 inhibitor,
  - Possibly low-dose pioglitazone.
- Reintroduce a sulfonylurea, even in long-duration diabetes when these drugs have often been discontinued years ago (Nybäck-Nakell et al., 2014).
- Optimise metformin.
- Start a conversation about bariatric surgery (see later).
- Although not yet currently available in Type 2 diabetes, insulin pump treatment may be a future option (see later).

Practice point

Around 10% of patients, often young with long duration, have persistent poor control (HbA$_{1c}$ >8.0%, 64) taking insulin with or without multiple non-insulin agents. Further intensification of multiple daily dose insulin if HbA$_{1c}$ >8.4% (68) is futile.

Increasingly familiar with developments in transplant options for Type 1 diabetes, Type 2 patients sometimes enquire about the possibility of islet or pancreas transplants. Although occasionally mentioned in the literature, leaving aside all other considerations, it should be pointed out that there are insufficient organs available even for the priority group, complicated Type 1 patients but there is a much wider range of options for glycaemic control in Type 2 diabetes.

Resistant hyperglycaemia

Constraints on prescribing combination therapies are much less stringent than before but it is worthwhile requesting an independent clinical opinion once patients have persistent poor control on a wide variety of agents. It is widely appreciated by patients, may be of some value by allowing a fresh pair of eyes to spot immediately fixable points and new combinations, and may reduce the patient's medication burden. But we must recognize limitations. The phenomenon of glycaemic 'tracking' is well known in Type 1 diabetes and describes the persistence of glycaemia over many years in spite of consistent thoughtful clinical input, and although it has not been formally been described in Type 2 diabetes, the group of patients in persistent poor control described by Crowley et al. (2014) probably mostly comprises these patients. When all reasonable attempts have been made, after careful review and discussion, agreeing to a form of pharmacological ceasefire should not be considered a failure either on the part of practitioners or patients. Focus attention on more remediable elements, especially proteinuria, blood pressure and lipids. It is striking that while resistant hypertension is described and strategies understood, many practitioners do not acknowledge the presence of resistant hyperglycaemia. Some of the reasons for this have been discussed already, especially the notion that diabetes has the perfect pharmacopoeia for correction of hyperglycaemia in everyone. If this were the case, then the current chapter would have been considerably shorter.

Practice point

Resistant hyperglycaemia, like resistant hypertension, exists. Rationalize, simplify and carefully optimize all agents, not forgetting that drug classes abandoned many years ago, often for forgotten reasons, may be worthwhile reintroducing. Thereafter, focus on other risk factors, especially blood pressure, proteinuria and LDL.

INSULIN PUMP TREATMENT IN TYPE 2 DIABETES

Can insulin pump treatment in Type 2 patients replicate the undoubted glycaemic benefits seen in Type 1 diabetes? It has been trialled in small uncontrolled studies, but the inelegantly named OpT2mise trial (2014) soundly studied patients in poor control (mean HbA$_{1c}$ 9.0%, 75) despite multiple daily insulin injections (mean total dose approximately

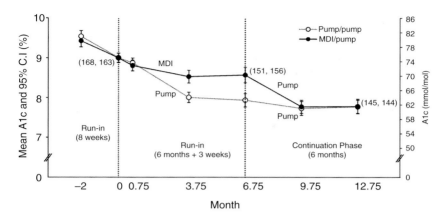

Figure 10.8 Effectiveness of up to one year of insulin pump treatment in the OpT2mise study showing a consistent ~0.7% HbA$_{1c}$ reduction in patients previously in very poor control while taking basal-bolus insulin. Source: Aronson *et al.*, 2016. Reproduced with permission of John Wiley & Sons.

110 units/day, 1.1 units/kg/day). During a two month run-in period to optimize multiple daily insulin treatment, HbA$_{1c}$ in all patients fell by about 0.5%. In the subsequent active six-month treatment phase, it fell by a further 0.4% to 8.6% (70), but by 1.1% to 7.9% (63) in the pump group, yielding an overall difference between the two groups of 0.7%. At the six-month point the multiple daily insulin group was then changed to pump treatment. At both six and twelve months all patients, by then pump treated, had the same mean HbA$_{1c}$, 7.9% (63) (**Figure 10.8**). There was only one episode of severe hypoglycaemia in each group. In the group changed from multiple daily insulin to pump treatment, total insulin dose fell by nearly 20%, but disappointingly there was no associated weight loss: both groups gained about 2 kg.

HYPOGLYCAEMIA IN INSULIN-TREATED TYPE 2 PATIENTS

There are few prospective studies. In the old UKPDS, annually between 1% and 4% of insulin-treated patients had an episode of severe hypoglycaemia, with a hint that the rate increased with longer follow-up. This was about a two- to fourfold increased rate compared with the group treated with sulfonylureas. More recently, and probably with the benefit of greater experience of insulin treatment in Type 2 diabetes, the UK Hypoglycaemia Study Group (2007) found that in patients treated for less than two years, the rate of severe hypoglycaemia – 7% – was the same in insulin- and sulfonylurea-treated patients.

The results of the ACCORD glycaemia study, indicating increased mortality in intensively treated patients, usually taking insulin, properly heightened concerns. Prospective data are hard to find, but a careful retrospective UK study echoed some of these anxieties in finding a 50–60% increased risk of cardiovascular death and a near twofold increase in all-cause mortality in insulin-treated Type 2 patients after a recorded hypoglycaemic event of any severity (Khunti *et al.*, 2015). The median latent period between hypoglycaemia and death was 1½ years in both Type 1 and Type 2 patients. In the

ORIGIN trial of glargine or standard glycaemic care in people with dysglycaemia and high cardiovascular risk, severe hypoglycaemia (requiring help or blood glucose ≤2.0 mmol/l) was associated with a 60–80% increased risk of cardiovascular outcomes, including death and arrhythmic death. Although insulin was not associated with an increased relative risk of adverse outcomes, severe hypoglycaemia was – inevitably – around three times more frequent in insulin-treated patients (ORIGIN Trial Investigators, 2013). Interpreting causality is troubled, but the consistency of the association with different study designs and across both types of diabetes makes it imperative to avoid hypoglycaemia in insulin-treated patients, and to take vigorous remedial action to minimise further risk in anyone reporting or recording hypoglycaemia. It is important to recall that it is not just patients with low HbA_{1c} values who are at risk of hypoglycaemia; patients in very poor control also have severe hypoglycaemic events. Where available, diagnostic continuous glucose monitoring is valuable in diagnosis and management. Regardless, this repeated signal of concern should be a major factor in cooling persistent ardent calls for early insulin treatment in Type 2 diabetes which, as we have seen, carries no discernible benefit compared with non-insulin treatment. Since there are no differences in severe hypoglycaemia rates between different long-acting insulin analogues, switching insulin preparations in the hope of reducing this risk does not accord with the evidence.

Practice point

Hypoglycaemia in insulin-treated Type 2 patients may be associated with cardiovascular mortality. This is another reason for deferring insulin treatment where other non-insulin strategies are available, especially in people with known cardiovascular disease.

BARIATRIC/METABOLIC SURGERY

Sustained weight loss of 5–10% has important metabolic benefits (though does not – see Look AHEAD – reduce the risk of premature death or of cardiovascular disease). However, the 20–30% body weight loss often seen with bariatric surgery has profound and widespread effects, including a high probability of permanent remission ('cure') of Type 2 diabetes and reduction in associated cardiovascular risk factors, cardiovascular endpoints, premature death and, possibly, cancer risk. The interest in bariatric surgery is not surprising; less expected was the time it took to establish it in the hierarchy of recognized treatments for diabetes (Rubino *et al.*, 2016). In common with many innovations in medicine, the surgical techniques were developed well in advance of proper clinical trials assessing their effect. This has been rectified, though not fully, and long-term studies in Type 2 patients have been delayed in comparison with those involving non-diabetic obesity, where there are valuable observational studies, especially the Swedish Obese Subjects (SOS) study (**Figure 10.9**). Most studies of surgery in Type 2 diabetes have focused on glycaemia remission rates.

Advances in the understanding and practical implementation of what, in the context of Type 2 diabetes, is more appropriately termed 'metabolic surgery' have been reported in the past five years. However, there is a long history of surgical approaches to obesity, starting in the late 1960s in the USA with intestinal bypass procedures from jejunum to ileum or colon that induced weight loss through malabsorption, with generally poor medical results, and what seems to have been no central effects on appetite. The now-standard operation, Roux-en-Y gastric bypass, was introduced in 1993. There was a

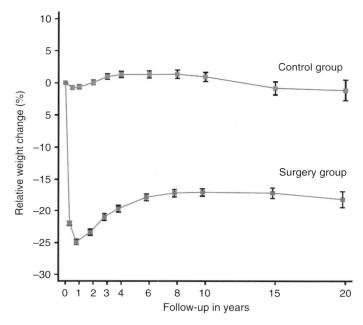

Figure 10.9 Long-term weight loss in the Swedish Obese Subjects study. After 20 years, surgical subjects maintained an approximate 20% weight loss, while the medically-treated control group showed no significant weight changes. Approximately 15% each of the subjects had prediabetes and diabetes. In the STAMPEDE study in diabetic subjects (see text) weight loss at three years was similar to SOS. *Source*: Jamaly *et al.*, 2016.

vogue for reversible gastric banding, but it has less profound effects on weight and diabetes remission (see later), complication rates are no lower than for more substantial interventions and high reoperation rates are reported. In recent years, sleeve gastrectomy, a simple subtotal gastrectomy procedure, has become popular and in some centres has become the most commonly used operation (**Figure 10.10**). More radical procedures, for example biliopancreatic diversion, are only used occasionally.

How does bariatric surgery improve glycaemia in Type 2 diabetes?

The reasons for the effectiveness of metabolic surgery and the remarkable stability of the resulting glucose levels in many patients are still debated. Glucose levels fall very rapidly after surgery, before weight loss can be detected. Calorie restriction is still, however, an important factor, causing the expected reduction in postprandial glucose and insulin concentrations due to increased hepatic insulin sensitivity – similar to the effects of very low calorie diets (see **Chapter 9**). Changes in gut hormones have been extensively studied. For example, circulating GLP-1 levels increase substantially after the two common procedures that exclude substantial parts of the stomach, Roux-en-Y gastric bypass and vertical sleeve gastrectomy – but not laparoscopic adjustable gastric banding. The two former procedures increase ileal transit of food, which probably increases GLP-1 secretion, with associated improvement in β-cell function. Other gut factors may contribute, for example changes in bile acids – which may themselves increase GLP-1 secretion – and

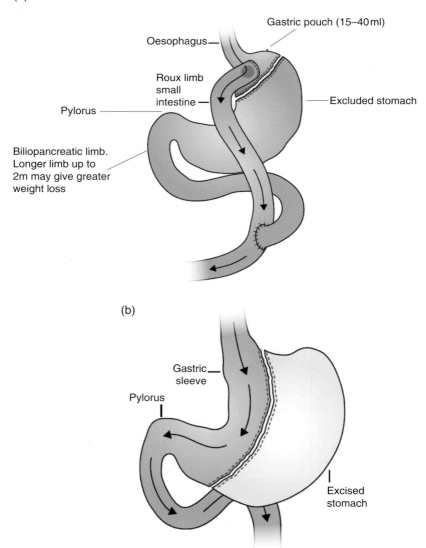

Figure 10.10 (a) Roux-en-Y gastric bypass and (b) sleeve gastrectomy: 70–80% of the stomach is excised.

the intestinal microbiota, though at present there is more experimental than clinical evidence to support them (Madsbad *et al.*, 2014).

'Remission' of Type 2 diabetes

'Remission' of Type 2 diabetes has been seen as a major goal of bariatric procedures and there has inevitably been a vigorous numerological debate about its definition (including HbA_{1c} levels and associated medication needed to maintain those levels). It is, of course important, as bariatric surgery is a valuable means of restoring good blood glucose control in patients with resistant hyperglycaemia, discussed previously. But there is a strong case for moving the focus – as in bariatric surgery in non-diabetic people – from glycaemic measures and weight loss towards meaningful event outcomes. In the meantime, the International Diabetes Federation (IDF) uses a portfolio of measures to judge intermediate outcomes – improvement or optimization of the overall metabolic state – while the American Diabetes Association currently still uses only glycaemic measures (**Box 10.4**). All these are arbitrary.

The STAMPEDE trial (Schauer *et al.*, 2014) is the only trial in diabetes where patients were strictly randomized to intensive medical therapy, Roux-en-Y bypass or vertical sleeve gastrectomy. These clinically representative younger patients, mean age 48 years, were followed up for three years. Key results in the surgical groups are shown in **Table 10.12**. Importantly, blood pressure did not fall and although mean triglycerides fell by 30–46% and HDL-cholesterol increased by 35%, LDL-cholesterol was overall unchanged.

Box 10.4 Definitions of metabolic outcomes of bariatric surgery. Modified after Miras and le Roux, 2014).

International Diabetes Federation (IDF)
Optimization of the metabolic state:
- Weight loss >15%.
- HbA_{1c} ≤6.0% (42) without hypoglycaemia.
- Blood pressure <135/85 mm Hg.
- Lipids: total cholesterol <4.0 mmol/l, triglycerides <2.2 mmol/l, LDL-cholesterol <2.0 mmol/l.
- Reduced drug treatment or no drug treatment (where drug treatment is still required, reduced doses compared with the preoperative state).

Substantial improvement in the metabolic state:
- HbA_{1c} lowered by >20%.
- LDL <2.3 mmol/l.
- BP <135/85.
- Reduced drug treatment.

American Diabetes Association
HbA_{1c}
- Complete remission: <6.0% (42).
- Partial remission: <6.5% (48).

Fasting glucose
- Complete remission: <5.6 mmol/l for at least one year without drug treatment or ongoing procedures.
- Partial remission: 5.6–6.9 mmol/l for at least one year without drug treatment or continuing procedures.

Table 10.12 Impact of bariatric surgery in Type 2 diabetes (STAMPEDE, 2014).

	Baseline	3 years after surgery
Weight, kg	105	80
HbA$_{1c}$, % (mmol/mol)	9.3 (78)	6.7–7.0 (50–53)
Change in weight from baseline, %		−21–25
Insulin use, %	45	7
Mean number of diabetes medications	2.5	0.5–1.0
Mean number of all medications	4.6–5.2	1.4–2.3

Source: Schauer *et al.*, 2014. Reproduced with permission of Massachusetts Medical Society.

After 10 years, 30% of the diabetic patients, compared with 6% of the medical control patients entered into the Swedish Obese Subjects study were still taking no diabetes medication with fasting glucose <6.1 mmol/l (Sjöstrom *et al.*, 2014). This is an impressive finding; the hope is that in subjects who did not remit, surgery in some way 'reset' the glycaemic clock, allowing them to be on substantially less medication than the medically managed patients.

After 15 years follow up in the SOS study, the risk of non-diabetic participants remaining free of diabetes was about 85% lower than in the medically-treated group. The risk reduction did not differ with the level of obesity (though entry to the study was restricted to men with BMI ≥34 and females ≥38) (Carlsson *et al.*, 2012). Although this important finding has not been incorporated into formal guidance, it may be a persuasive additional factor in discussing the options for bariatric surgery in people with a very strong first-degree family history of Type 2 diabetes.

Long-term health outcomes

Very few data are available for diabetic people apart from the microvascular and macrovascular outcomes in the SOS study (see later). However, the same study has carefully followed up non-diabetic subjects for a very long time and outcomes are likely to be similar, as they are for other interventions in diabetic compared with nondiabetic people.

After a median follow-up of nearly 15 years, the SOS study reported a near-50% reduction in the risk of cardiovascular deaths in the surgical compared with the medical control group; the risk of first-time cardiovascular deaths (myocardial infarction or stroke, fatal or not) was reduced by about 30%. These are compelling data, albeit not from a strictly randomized trial (Sjöstrom *et al.*, 2012). Cancer risk was reduced in women by about 40% but there was no effect in men, reinforcing the role of obesity in some cancer types in women, notably cancers of the breast and endometrium.

Microvascular and macrovascular complications

Diabetic complications in the nearly 350 SOS subjects at baseline were reported in 2014 after an average follow-up of almost 18 years (Sjöstrom *et al.*, 2014). A basket of significant microvascular complications was reduced by 55%, and macrovascular events by 30%, but the data on complications was derived from a national Swedish database, which while complete, was less likely to capture details of, for example, retinopathy status. In the STAMPEDE study (Schauer *et al.*, 2014) in the surgical groups the low baseline levels of microalbuminuria fell further. Only a small number of patients had albuminuria, but there was a significant tendency to resolution at three years in both surgical groups; this was statistically significant in the bypass group (60%, 8 out of 13).

The critical question, awaiting a large trial, is whether persistent, very long-term reductions in glycaemia and improvements in other cardiovascular risk factors seen after bariatric surgery will have a greater impact on diabetic complications than the generally negative effects seen in the glycaemic studies of the 2000s. Specifically, do retinopathy and neuropathy, which seem most resistant to the effects of good glycaemia in Type 2 diabetes, respond to the dramatic glycaemic effects of bariatric surgery? Conversely, since glycaemic control seems to be a meaningful factor in progression of diabetic kidney disease in Type 2 diabetes, will this complication respond to bariatric surgery in a way that is beneficial to patients? A meta-analysis of poor-quality studies predictably found no benefit (Zhou et al., 2016) but, more promisingly, a large retrospective study of non-diabetic people found a lower rate of decline in eGFR and a substantial reduction in the risk of a doubling in serum creatinine or ESRD about four years after bariatric intervention (Chang et al., 2016), though even this is a far cry from improving the outlook in established diabetic renal disease, which was seen so spectacularly within 5–10 years of pancreatic transplantation in Type 1 patients (see **Chapter 4**). Finally, and most importantly, can bariatric intervention reduce the long timescale needed for the (modest) cardiovascular benefits seen in follow-up studies of ADVANCE, ACCORD and VADT?

Indications for bariatric surgery

Metabolic surgery is increasingly recommended in countries with advanced healthcare systems and with increasingly liberal indications according to simple criteria of body mass index. However, because it is still considered a treatment for obesity and not for an abnormal metabolic state, it is often considered late. The recommendations of International Diabetes Organizations (Rubino et al., 2016) seek to re-orientate the mental framework of practitioners towards the metabolic rather than the weight aspects. Their recommendations, together with the more traditional ones favoured by NICE in the United Kingdom, are shown in **Box 10.5**. In many healthcare systems, and in spite of guidance, there are often significant barriers to patients gaining access to metabolic surgery. In constrained systems, considerations of lifelong savings on medication, possible avoidance of complications and improved quality of life do not always carry the weight they should. Hopefully the laudable aspirations of the guidelines to move procedures away from bariatric to metabolic will pay off in time, though there is a long way to go: the UK National Bariatric Surgery Registry (2011–2013) found that only about 10% of procedures in men and about 15% in women were performed in people with BMI <40 (www.nbsr.co.uk).

Complications of bariatric surgery

Operative complications

Between 2009 and 2013 overall operative mortality in the UK was 0.11%, comparable with the best outcomes worldwide. The recorded surgical complication rate for primary operations was 2.9%. The evidence for thromboembolic events is weak, but they occur at about 1%, with a very low mortality (<0.05%). Reoperation rates are significant, but lower for bypass than sleeve gastrectomy (3% vs 7%) (Chang et al., 2014). Incisional hernia occurs in about 2% of patients followed up for two years. Repair is time-consuming and costly.

Box 10.5 Patient selection for bariatric/metabolic surgery.

Reduce BMI cut-off levels appropriately (i.e. by about 2.5 BMI points) for people of South Asian family origin.

NICE (UK, 2014)
Consider bariatric surgery if all the following are fulfilled:
- BMI 35–40 in the presence of Type 2 diabetes.
- Adequate unsuccessful trial of non-surgical approaches to weight loss in a specialist [Tier 3] service.
- Fit for anaesthesia and willing to commit to long-term follow-up.

Exceptionally it can be considered in young people who have completed or nearly completed physiological maturation.

Recommendations in people with recent onset diabetes
- Expedited assessment if BMI ≥35 and being managed in a specialist [Tier 3] service.
- Assessment if BMI 30–34.9.

International Diabetes Organizations (2016)
Metabolic surgery is *recommended* as a treatment option in people with Type 2 diabetes with:
- Class III obesity (BMI ≥40) regardless of glycaemic control or complexity of glucose-management regimen.
- Class II obesity (BMI 35-39.9) with inadequately controlled glycaemia despite optimal lifestyle and medical therapy.

Consider metabolic surgery as a treatment option in people with Type 2 diabetes people with:
- Class 1 obesity (BMI 30.0–34.9) and inadequately controlled hyperglycaemia despite optimal medical treatment with oral or injected agents.

Gastrointestinal side-effects

Dumping
Common many years ago when similar procedures used to be done for peptic ulcer, but still encountered, and awareness of occasional severe and refractory cases is increasing (Tack and Deloose, 2014). *Early dumping* is characterized by prominent gastrointestinal symptoms – abdominal pain, diarrhoea, borborygmi, bloating and nausea. There can be vasomotor symptoms (flushing, palpitation, perspiration, tachycardia, hypotension, syncope). These are caused by rapid passage of hyperosmolar nutrients into the small bowel, causing release of gut hormones and fluid shifts into the gut. *Late dumping* refers to hypoglycaemia occurring about three hours after eating, resulting from rapid gastric emptying leading to high intestinal glucose concentrations with associated hyperinsulinaemia and hypoglycaemia, though fortunately not usually severe enough to cause neuroglycopenic symptoms. Purely restrictive procedures might not be expected to cause dumping, and although it is less common after sleeve gastrectomy than Roux-en-Y bypass, it does occur. Glucose tolerance tests for gestational diabetes and in postpartum monitoring may be unreliable where there is dumping.

Gastrooesophageal reflux disease (GORD)
Reflux disease is common in obesity and most studies see an improvement after bypass. There are less consistent improvements after sleeve gastrectomy and it may not be the preferred procedure in patients with severe pre-existing reflux. Hiatus hernia is a

contraindication unless it can be repaired. New-onset reflux, both acid- and non-acid induced, is described after sleeve gastrectomy.

Other long-term metabolic side-effects

Beta-cell hypertrophy or proliferation, leading to the much-debated nesidioblastosis, can rarely result in severe hyperinsulinaemic hypoglycaemia. Very rarely a bariatric procedure may uncover a pre-existing islet tumour. Awareness is critical. Vitamin D deficiency in obesity is common, is described in 25–75% of patients undergoing bariatric surgery and is probably as common postoperatively (Tack and Deloose, 2014). There is continuing concern about increased fracture risk after bariatric surgery. The SOS study did not report fracture incidence, but in the careful STAMPEDE study total bone mineral content in the surgical groups fell by approximately 8% at two years, and hip bone mineral density by a similar amount, with a strong correlation between this measurement and the degree of weight loss. These changes occurred despite full calcium and vitamin D replacement (Maghrabi et al., 2015).

Practice point

After bariatric surgery total bone mineral content and hip bone density both fall within two years. Changes are more marked in people with greater weight loss.

Renal stone disease was a frequent complication of the very early, abandoned, procedure of jejunoileal bypass for weight loss. This was due to oxalate hyperabsorption and stone formation. Although the complication is less frequent after bypass, it still occurs twice as commonly as in obese non-surgical patients. There appears to be a substantially lower risk in people who have restrictive procedures. One study has uncovered a doubled risk of chronic kidney disease after bypass and the more radical malabsorptive procedures (Lieske et al., 2015).

Non-metabolic benefits of bariatric surgery

Quality of life, genito-urinary function, sleep

A meta-analysis (Jumbe et al., 2016) moderated the intuitive view that broad quality of life indicators improve after surgery: physical, but not psychological quality of life improved. This is borne out by the STAMPEDE study, which used the RAND 36-Item Health Survey. While there was evidence of global improvement that reached statistical significance for bodily pain, general health and energy/fatigue, social functioning, and role limitations due to both physical and emotional problems showed non-significant improvements. Bariatric surgery is not a cure-all: poor psychological function can persist and a large retrospective study, while confirming overall improved mortality, found a substantial increase in non-disease deaths, for example accidents and suicide (Adams et al., 2007).

Both male and female sexual function improve, especially in the six months after surgery. Lower urinary tract symptoms in men improve. In one study urinary incontinence resolved in around half of women, together with an improvement in other pelvic floor symptoms (Shimonov et al., 2017).

While hospitalization in the 30 days after surgery (mostly for nausea, vomiting and abdominal pain) is common (2–4%), overall hospitalization for any reason and for diabetes-related problems fall by about 30%. Emergency department attendances and hospital admissions for people with pre-existing heart failure fell significantly in the second postoperative year.

Sleep apnoea is usually asserted to improve after surgery, but the quality of most studies is poor, perhaps because it is over-readily assumed that sleep quality is bound to get better. Neither the SOS nor STAMPEDE studies has reported the effect of surgery on sleep.

Postbariatric surgery monitoring

NICE (CG189) stressed the importance of at least two years' follow-up in the surgical service, and thereafter annual monitoring under a shared care arrangement.

While some patients will be under long-term follow-up from their specialist bariatric centre, some will move away from their original centre and some, inevitably, will be lost to hospital follow-up.

Nutritional support is critical (Marcotte and Chand, 2016). Wernicke's encephalopathy and Korsakoff's psychosis due to Vitamin B1 deficiency (B1 is absorbed in the duodenum and proximal jejunum) is uncommon but can be fatal. The usual clinical scenario is prolonged vomiting and consequent failure to take vitamin supplements. It is more common after malabsorptive procedures but has been reported after all bariatric interventions.

UK guidance on long-term follow up was published in 2014 by the British Obesity and Bariatric Surgery Society; it is summarized in **Tables 10.13 and 10.14**.

Practice point

Encourage adherence to mineral and vitamin supplements in all postbariatric patients, but especially in women of child-bearing age.

Table 10.13 Indications for requesting specific blood tests following Roux-en-Y bypass or sleeve gastrectomy (BOMMS, 2014).

Laboratory test/procedure	Frequency
Thiamine (vitamin B1)	Not routinely tested, but thiamine deficiency can result from prolonged vomiting; admit and treat with intravenous thiamine
Vitamin B12	6 and 12 months, then annually
Zinc, copper	Annually Check zinc if unexplained anaemia, hair loss or changes in taste acuity Check copper if unexplained anaemia or poor wound healing. Zinc and copper levels affect each other
Vitamin A	Measure only if there is steatorrhoea or symptoms of vitamin A deficiency, e.g. night blindness
INR	If excessive bruising; may indicate vitamin K deficiency
Selenium	Check if unexplained fatigue, anaemia, metabolic bone disease, chronic diarrhoea or heart failure

Table 10.14 Vitamin supplements following Roux-en-Y bypass or sleeve gastrectomy.

Vitamins and minerals recommended	Preparations (UK)
Multivitamin and mineral supplement should contain: Iron Selenium Copper (minimum 2 mg) Zinc (ratio of 8–15 mg zinc for each 1 mg copper)	Once daily Forceval (soluble and capsule) Over the counter preparations, e.g. Sanatogen A-Z Complete (2 daily)
Iron 45–60 mg daily (increase to 100 mg daily in menstruating women)	Contained in Ferrous sulfate 200 mg Ferrous fumarate 210 mg Ferrous gluconate 300 mg
Folic acid	Sufficient in multivitamin and mineral supplement Encourage consumption of folate-rich foods
Vitamin B12	Intramuscular vitamin B12 1 mg every three months
Calcium and vitamin D	Ensure good intake through nutrition Most patients will need 800 mg calcium daily and vitamin D 20 mcg daily

Pregnancy

About 80% of bariatric procedures are performed in women, many of child-bearing age. There are little data on pregnancy outcomes in women who have had surgery, but a study from Sweden found, not surprisingly, that gestational diabetes was much less common in postsurgical women than preoperative BMI-matched control women. Likewise, excessive foetal growth was less common and congenital abnormalities no higher, but there was a higher risk of small-for-gestational age infants, and a hint that stillbirth or neonatal death rates could be higher (Johansson et al., 2015). Other, smaller, studies have found a higher rate of spontaneous preterm birth. In the Swedish study median interval between surgery and conception was just over a year, during a period of continuing weight loss, which may affect foetal nutrition. Poor adherence to micronutrient supplementation and vitamin D deficiency may contribute to poor maternal nutrition. Education about the need for supplementation with folic acid is especially critical in this group (Dolin et al., 2016), but perhaps the most important thing is to remember to discuss pregnancy in these subjects as early as possible, preferably in the preoperative phase.

Endoscopic duodenal–jejunal bypass liner

A bariatric procedure, this device, first described in 2008, is an impermeable 80-cm-long tube placed endoscopically in the proximal jejunum and tethered to the duodenal bulb. Biliary and pancreatic fluids do not mix with food proximally, and it is therefore a malabsorptive procedure, similar to Roux-en-Y, with no restriction. Studies are small. Where available it is licensed only for 12 months use, after which it is removed. The technology of the device is more celebrated than its clinical outcomes. Procedural complications are frequent, including failure to implant, device migration and local effects, including minor trauma and haematemesis. A novel procedure of duodenal resurfacing with hydrothermal ablation has been reported in a small number of poorly-controlled obese patients.

Over six months, HbA$_{1c}$ improved by 1.2–2.5% depending on the length of duodenum ablated. While glucose levels tended to rebound by the end of the study, some patients had stable glycaemia (Rajagopalan *et al.*, 2016). Like the bypass liner, this procedure has a long investigational path to traverse before it comes into widespread use.

References

ACCORD Study Group; Gerstein HC, Miller HE *et al*. Long-term effects of intensive glucose lowering on cardiovascular outcomes. *N Engl J Med* 2011;364:818–28 [PMID: 21366473] PMC4083508.

ACCORDION (Action to Control Cardiovascular Risk in Diabetes Follow-On) Eye Study Group and the Action to Control Cardiovascular Risk in Diabetes Follow-On (ACCORDION) Study Group. Persistent effects of intensive glycaemic control on retinopathy in type 2 diabetes in the Action to Control Cardiovascular Risk in Diabetes (ACCORD) Follow-On Study. *Diabetes Care* 2016; 39:1089–100 [PMID: 27289122] PMC4915557.

Adams TD, Gress RE, Smith SC *et al*. Long-term mortality after gastric bypass surgery. *N Engl J Med* 2007;357:753–61 [PMID: 17715409] Free full text.

Anagnostou E. Aman MG, Handen BL *et al*. Metformin for treatment of overweight induced by atypical antipsychotic medication in young people with autism spectrum disorder: a randomized clinical trial. *JAMA Psychiatry* 2016;73:928–37 [PMID: 2755593].

Aroda VR, Bain SC, Cariou B *et al*. Efficacy and safety of once-weekly semaglutide versus once-daily insulin glargine as add-on to metformin (with or without sulfonylureas) in insulin-naive patients with type 2 diabetes (SUSTAIN 4): a randomised, open-label, parallel-group, multicentre, multinational, phase 3a trial. *Lancet Diabetes Endocrinol* 2017;5:355–66 [PMID: 28344112].

Aronson R, Reznik Y, Conget I *et al*. OpT2mise Study Group. Sustained efficacy of insulin pump therapy compared with multiple daily injections in type 2 diabetes: 12-month data from the OpT2mise randomized trial. *Diabetes Obes Metab* 2016;18:500–7 [PMID: 26854123].

Best JD, Drury PL, Davis TM *et al*. Fenofibrate Intervention and Event Lowering in Diabetes Study Investigators. Glycemic control over 5 years in 4,900 people with type 2 diabetes: real-world diabetes therapy in a clinical trial cohort. *Diabetes Care* 2012;35:1165–70 [PMID: 22432105] PMC3329812.

Bhat A, Sebastiani G, Bhat M. Systematic review: preventive and therapeutic applications of metformin in liver disease. *World J Hepatol* 2015;7:1652–9 [PMID: 26140084] PMC4483546.

de Boer SA, Lefrandt JD, Petersen JK *et al*. The effects of GLP-1 analogues in obese, insulin-using type 2 diabetes in relation to eating behaviour. *Int J Clin Pharm* 2016; 38: 144–151 [PMID: 26597956] PMC4733138.

Bolli GB, Owens DR. Lixisenatide, a novel GLP-1 receptor agonist: efficacy, safety and clinical implications for type 2 diabetes mellitus. *Diabetes Obes Metab* 2014;16:588–601 [PMID: 24373190].

Bolli GB, Munteanu M, Dotsenko S *et al*. Efficacy and safety of lixisenatide once daily vs. placebo in people with Type 2 diabetes insufficiently controlled on metformin (GetGoal-F1). *Diabet Med* 2014;31:176–84 [PMID: 24116597] Free full text.

Boussageon R, Gueyffier F, Cornu C. Metformin as firstline treatment for type 2 diabetes: are we sure? *BMJ* 2016;352:h6748 [PMID: 26747716] Free full text.

Buse JB, Wolfenbuttel BH, Herman WH *et al*. The DURability of Basal versus Lispro mix 75/25 insulin Efficacy (DURABLE) trial: comparing the durability of lispro mix 75/25 and glargine. *Diabetes Care* 2011;34:249–55 [PMID: 21270182] PMC3024329.

Buse JB, Visbøll T, Thurman J *et al*.; NN9068-3912 (DUAL-II) Trial Investigators. Contribution of liraglutide in the fixed-ratio combination of insulin degludec and liraglutide (IDegLira). *Diabetes Care* 2014;37:2926–33 [PMID: 25114296].

Buse JB, DeFronzo RA, Rosenstock J *et al*. The primary glucose-lowering effect of metformin resides in the gut, not the circulation: results from short-term pharmacokinetic and 12-week dose-ranging studies. *Diabetes* 2016;39:198–205 [PMID: 26285584].

Cahn A, Raz I, Mosenzon O *et al*. Predisposing factors for any and major hypoglycaemia with saxagliptin versus placebo and overall: analysis from the SAVOR-TIMI 53 Trial. *Diabetes Care* 2016;39:1329–37 [PMID: 27222508].

Carlsson LM, Peltonen M, Ahlin S et al. Bariatric surgery and prevention of type 2 diabetes in Swedish obese subjects. *NEJM* 2012;367:695–704 [PMID: 22913680] Free full text.

Cefalu WT, Leiter LA, Yoon K et al. Efficacy and safety of canagliflozin versus glimepiride in patients with type 2 diabetes inadequately controlled with metformin (CANTATA-SU): 52 week results from a randomised, double-blind, phase 3 non-inferiority trial. *Lancet* 2013;382:941–50 [PMID: 23850055].

Chang SH, Stoll R, Song J et al. The effectiveness and risks of bariatric surgery: an updated systematic review and meta-analysis, 2003–2012. *JAMA Surg* 2014;149:275–87 [PMID: 24352617] PMC3962512.

Chang AR, Chen Y, Still C et al. Bariatric surgery is associated with improvement in kidney outcomes. *Kidney Int* 2016;90:164–71 [PMID: 2718199] PMC4912457.

Chapman LE, Darling AL, Brown JE. Association between metformin and vitamin B12 deficiency in patients with type 2 diabetes: a systematic review and meta-analysis. *Diabetes Metab* 2016;42:316–27 [PMID: 27130885].

Cornel JH, Bakris GL, Stevens SR et al. TECOS Study Group. Effect of sitagliptin on kidney function and respective cardiovascular outcomes in type 2 diabetes: outcomes from TECOS. *Diabetes Care* 2016;39:2304–10 [PMID: 27742728].

Crowley MJ, Holleman R, Klamerus ML et al. Factors associated with persistent poorly controlled diabetes mellitus: clues to improving management in patients with resistant poor control. *Chronic Illn* 2014;10:291–302 [PMID: 24567193] PMC4317345.

Daniele G, Xiong J, Solis-Herrera C et al. Dapagliflozin enhances fat oxidation and ketone production I patients with type 2 diabetes. *Diabetes Care* 2016;39:2036–41 [PMID: 27561923] PMC5079607.

Davies MJ, Bergenstal R, Bode B et al. NN8022-1922 Study Group. Efficacy of liraglutide for weight loss among patients with type 2 diabetes: the SCALE diabetes randomized clinical trial. *JAMA* 2015;314:687–99 [PMID: 26284720].

DeVries JH, Bain SC, Rodbard HW et al. Liraglutide-Detemir Study Group. Sequential intensification of metformin treatment in type 2 diabetes with liraglutide followed by randomized addition of basal insulin prompted by A1C targets. *Diabetes Care* 2012;35:1446–54 [PMID: 22584132] PMC3379583.

Diamant M, Van Gaal L, Guerci B et al. Exenatide once weekly versus insulin glargine for type 2 diabetes (DURATION-3): 3-year results of an open-label randomised trial. *Lancet Diabetes Endocrinol* 2014;2:464–73 [PMID: 24731672].

Dolin C, Ude Welcome AO, Caughey AB. Management of pregnancy in women who have undergone bariatric surgery. *Obstet Gynecol Surv* 2016;71:734–40 [PMID: 28005136].

Dormandy JA, Charbonnel B, Eckland DJ et al. PROactive Investigators. Secondary prevention of macrovascular events in patients with type 2 diabetes in the PROactive Study (PROspective pioglitAzone Clinical Trial In macrovascular Events): a randomised clinical trial. *Lancet* 2005;366:1279–89 [PMID: 16214598].

Ekström N, Svensson AM, Miftaraj M et al. Durability of oral hypoglycemic agents in drug naive patients with type 2 diabetes: report from the Swedish National Diabetes Register (NDR). *BMJ Open Diabetes Res Care* 2015;3:e000059 [PMID: 25815205] PMC4368982.

Fácila L, Fabregat-Andrés Ó, Bertemeu V et al. Metformin and risk of long-term mortality following an admission for acute heart failure. *J Cardiovasc Med (Hagerstown)* 2017;18:69–73 [PMID: 27341193].

Farjo PD, Kidd KM, Reece JL. A case of euglycemic diabetic ketoacidosis following long-term empagliflozin therapy. *Diabetes Care* 2016;39:e165–6 [PMID: 27436273].

Fujioka K, Brazg RL, Raz I et al. Efficacy, dose-response relationship and safety of once-daily extended-release metformin (Glucophage XR) in type 2 diabetic patients with inadequate glycaemic control despite prior treatment with diet and exercise: results from two double-blind, placebo-controlled studies. *Diab Obes Metab* 2005;7:28–39 [PMID: 15642073].

Gæde P, Lund-Andersen H, Parving HH, Pedersen O. Effect of a multifactorial intervention on mortality in type 2 diabetes. *N Engl J Med* 2008;358:580–91 [PMID: 18256393] Free full text.

Gæde P, Oellgaard J, Carstensen B et al. Years of life gained by multifactorial intervention in patients with type 2 diabetes and microalbuminuria: 21 years follow-up of the Steno-2 randomised trial. *Diabetologia* 2016;59:2298–307 [PMID: 27531506].

Garber AJ, Duncan TG, Goodman AM et al. Efficacy of metformin in type II diabetes: results of a double-bind, placebo-controlled, dose-response trial. Am J Med 1997;103:491–7 [PMID: 9428832].

Giugliano D, Chiodini P, Maiorino MI et al. Intensification of insulin therapy with basal-bolus or premixed insulin regimens in type 2 diabetes: a systematic review and meta-analysis of randomized controlled trials. Endocrine 2016;51;417–28 [PMID: 26281001].

Green JB, Bethel MA, Armstrong PW et al. TECOS Study Group. Effect of sitagliptin on cardiovascular outcomes in type 2 diabetes. N Engl J Med 2015;373:232–42 [PMID: 26052984] Free full text.

Gribble FM. Targeting GLP-1 release as a potential strategy for the therapy of Type 2 diabetes (RD Lawrence Lecture 2008). Diabetic Med 2008;25:889–94 [PMID: 18959599].

Handelsman Y, Henry RR, Bloomgarden ZT et al. American Association of Clinical Endocrinologists and American College of Endocrinology position statement on the association of SGLT-2 inhibitors and diabetic ketoacidosis. Endocr Pract 2016;22:753–62 [PMID: 27082665].

Harrison LB, Adams-Huet B, Raskin P, Lingvay I. β-cell function preservation after 3.5 years of intensive diabetes therapy. Diabetes Care 2012;35:1406–12 [PMID: 22723578] PMC3379585.

Hayward RA, Reaven PD, Witala WL et al. VADT Investigators. Follow-up of glycemic control and cardiovascular outcomes in type 2 diabetes. N Engl J Med 2015;372:2197–206 [PMID: 26039600] Free full text.

Henry RR, Rosenstock J, Logan D et al. Continuous subcutaneous delivery of exenatide via ITCA 650 leads to sustained glycemic control and weight loss for 48 weeks in metformin-treated subjects with type 2 diabetes. J Diabetes Complications 2014;28:393–8 [PMID: 24631129] Free full text.

Holman RR, Thorne KI, Farmer AJ et al. 4-T Study Group. Addition of biphasic, prandial, or basal insulin to oral therapy in type 2 diabetes. N Engl J Med 2007;357:1716–30 [PMID: 17890232] Free full text.

Holman RR, Paul SK, Bethel MA et al. 10-year follow-up of intensive glucose control in type 2 diabetes. N Engl J Med 2008;359:1577–89 [PMID: 18784090] Free full text.

Holman RR, Farmer AJ, Davies MJ et al. 4-T Study Group. Three-year efficacy of complex insulin regimens in type 2 diabetes. N Engl J Med 2009;361:1736–47 [PMID: 19850703].

Holman RR, Coleman RL, Chan JCN et al. ACE Study Group. Effects of acarbose on cardiovascular and diabetes outcomes in patients with coronary heart disease and impaired glucose tolerance (ACE): a randomised, double-blind, placebo-controlled trial. Lancet Diabetes Endocrinol 2017. [Epub ahead of print] [PMID: 28917545]

Horvath K, Jeitler K Berghold A et al. Long-acting insulin analogues versus NPH insulin (human isophane insulin) for type 2 diabetes mellitus. Cochrane Database Syst Rev 2007 18;(2):CD005613 [PMID: 17443605].

Hung SC, Chang YK, Liu JS et al. Metformin use and mortality in patients with advanced chronic kidney disease: national, retrospective, observational cohort study. Lancet Diabetes Endocrinol 2015;3:605–14 [PMID: 26094107].

Iglesias P, Civantos S, Vega B et al. Clinical effectiveness of exenatide in diabetic patients waiting for bariatric surgery. Obes Surg 2015;25:575–8 [PMID: 26589020].

Jamaly S, Carlsson L, Peltonen M et al. Bariatric surgery and the risk of new-onset atrial fibrillation in Swedish Obese Subjects. J Am Coll Cardiol 2016;68:2497–504 [PMID: 27931605] PMC5157934.

Januzzi JL, Butler J, Jarolim P et al. Effects of canagliflozin on cardiovascular biomarkers in older adults with type 2 diabetes. J Am Coll Cardiol 2017;70:704–12 [PMID: 28619659] Free full text.

Jenkins N, Hallowell N, Farmer AJ et al. Initiating insulin as part of the Treating to Target in Type 2 Diabetes (4-T) trial: an interview study of patients' and health professionals' experiences. Diabetes Care 2010;33:2178–80 [PMID: 20592050] PMC2945156.

Johansson K, Cnattingius S, Näslund I et al. Outcomes of pregnancy after bariatric surgery. N Engl J Med 2015;372:814–24 [PMID: 25714159] Free full text.

Jumbe S, Bartlett C, Jumbe SL, Meyrick J. The effectiveness of bariatric surgery on long term psychological quality of a life – a systematic review. Obes Res Clin Pract 2016;10:225–42 [PMID: 26774500].

Kalanter-Zadeh K, Uppot RN, Lewandrowski KB. Case records of the Massachusetts General Hospital. Case 23-2-13. A 54-year-old woman with abdominal pain, vomiting, and confusion. [Metformin toxicity and its management]. N Engl J Med 2013;369:374–82 [PMID: 23841704].

Kernan WN, Viscoli CM, Furie KL et al. IRIS Trial Investigators. Pioglitazone after ischemic stroke or transient ischemic attack. N Engl J Med 2016;374;1321–31 [PMID: 26886418] PMC4887756.

Khunti K, Davies M, Majeed A et al. Hypoglycemia and risk of cardiovascular disease and all-cause mortality in insulin-treated people with type 1 and type 2 diabetes: a cohort study. Diabetes Care 2015;38:316–22 [PMID: 25492401].

Kumar S, Jang HC, Demirag NG et al. Efficacy and safety of once-daily insulin degludec/insulin aspart compared with once-daily insulin glargine in participants with Type 2 diabetes: a randomized, treat-to-target study. Diabet Med 2017;34:180–8 [PMID: 27027878] PMC5248644.

Lexis CP, van der Horst IC. Metformin for cardiovascular disease: promise still unproven. Lancet Diabetes Endocrinology 2014;2:94–5 [PMID: 24622700] Free full text.

Li J, Tong Y, Zhang Y et al. Effects on all-cause mortality and cardiovascular outcomes in patients with type 2 diabetes by comparing insulin with oral hypoglycemic agent therapy: a meta-analysis of randomized controlled trials. Clin Ther 2016;38:372–86 [PMID: 26774276].

Lieske JC, Mehta RA, Milliner DS et al. Kidney stones are common after bariatric surgery. Kidney Int 2015;87:839–45 [PMID: 25354237] PMC4382441.

Lipska KJ, Bailey CJ, Inzucchi SE. Use of metformin in the setting of mild-to-moderate renal insufficiency. Diabetes Care 2011;34:1431–7 [PMID: 21617112].

Lipska KJ, Yao X, Herrin J et al. Trends in drug utilization, glycemic control, and rates of severe hypoglycemia, 2006–2013. Diabetes Care 2017;40:468–75 [PMID: 27659408].

Madsbad S, Dirksen C, Holst JJ. Mechanisms of changes in glucose metabolism and bodyweight after bariatric surgery. Lancet Diabetes Endocrinol 2014;2:152–64 [PMID: 24622719].

Maghrabi AH, Wolski K, Abood B et al. Two-year outcomes on bone density and fracture incidence in patients with T2DM randomized to bariatric surgery versus intensive medical therapy. Obesity (Silver Springs) 2015;23:2344–8 [PMID: 26193177] PMC4701611.

Malanda UL, Welschen LM, Riphagen II et al. Self-monitoring of blood glucose in patients with type 2 diabetes mellitus who are not using insulin. Cochrane Database Syst Rev 2012;1:CD005060 [PMID: 22258959].

Mamza J, Mehta R, Donnelly R, Idris I. Important differences in the durability of glycaemic response among second-line treatment options when added to metformin in type 2 diabetes: a retrospective cohort study. Ann Med 2016;48:224–34 [PMID: 26982210].

Marcotte E, Chand B. Management and prevention of surgical and nutritional complications after bariatric surgery. Surg Clin North Am 2016;96:843–56 [PMID: 27473805].

Margulies KB, Hernandez AF, Redfield MM et al. NHLBI Heart Failure Clinical Research Network. Effects of liraglutide on clinical stability among patients with advanced heart failure and reduced ejection fraction: a randomized clinical trial. JAMA 2016;316:500–8 [PMID: 27483064] PMC5021525.

Marso SP, Daniels GH, Brown-Frandsen K et al. LEADER Steering Committee; LEADER Trial Investigators. Liraglutide and cardiovascular outcomes in type 2 diabetes. N Engl J Med 2016a;375:311–22 [PMID: 27295427] PMC4985288.

Marso SP, Bain SC, Consoli A et al.; SUSTAIN-6 Investigators. Semaglutide and cardiovascular outcomes in patients with Type 2 diabetes. N Engl J Med 2016b;375:1834–44 [PMID: 27633186] Free full text.

McCormack J, Greenhalgh T. Seeing what you want to see in randomised controlled trials: versions and perversions of UKPDS data. United Kingdom Prospective Diabetes Study. BMJ 2000;320:1720–3 [PMID: 10864554] PMC1127485.

McCreight LJ, Bailey CJ, Pearson ER. Metformin and the gastrointestinal tract. Diabetologia 2016;59:426–35 [PMID: 26780750] PMC4742508.

Miras AD, le Roux CW. Metabolic surgery: shifting the focus from glycaemia and weight to end-organ health. Lancet Diabetes Endocrinol 2014;2:141–51 [PMID: 24622718].

Miser WF, Arakaki R, Jiang H et al. Randomized, open-label, parallel-group evaluations of basal-bolus therapy versus insulin lispro premixed therapy in patients with type 2 diabetes mellitus failing to achieve control with starter insulin treatment and continuing oral antihyperglycemic drugs: a noninferiority intensification substudy of the DURABLE trial. Clin Ther 2010;32:896–908 [PMID: 20685497].

Monnier L, Colette C, Dunseath GJ, Owens DR. The loss of postprandial glycemic control precedes stepwise deterioration of fasting with worsening diabetes. *Diabetes Care* 2007;30:263–9 [PMID: 17259492].

Nauck MA, Meininger G, Shen D *et al*. Sitagliptin Study 024 Group. Efficacy and safety of the dipeptidyl peptidase-4 inhibitor, sitagliptin, compared with the sulfonylurea, glipizide, in patients with type 2 diabetes inadequately controlled on metformin alone: a randomized, double-blind, non-inferiority study. *Diabetes Obese Metab* 2007;9:194–205 [PMID: 17300595].

Nauck M, Frid A, Hermansen K *et al*. Long-term efficacy and safety comparison of liralgutide, glimepiride and placebo, all in combination with metformin in type 2 diabetes: 2-year results from the LEAD-2 study. *Diabetes Obes Metab* 2013;15:204–12 [PMID: 22985213].

Nybäck-Nakell Å, Adamson U, Lins PE, Landstedt-Hallin L. Adding glimepiride to insulin+metformin in type 2 diabetes of more than 10 years duration – a randomised, double-blind, placebo-controlled, cross-over study. *Diabetes Res Clin Pract* 2014;103:286–91 [PMID: 24485398].

ORIGIN Trial Investigators; Mellbin LG, Rydén L, Riddle MC *et al*. Does hypoglycaemia increase the risk of cardiovascular events? A report from the ORIGIN trial. *Eur Heart J* 2013;34:3137–44 [PMID: 23999452].

ORIGIN Trial Investigators. Cardiovascular and other outcomes postintervention with insulin glargine and omega-3 fatty acids (ORIGINALE). *Diabetes Care* 2016;39:709–16 [PMID: 26681720].

Paul SK, Klein K, Thorsted BL *et al*. Delay in treatment intensification increases the risks of cardiovascular events in patients with type 2 diabetes. *Cardiovasc Diabetol* 2015;14:100 [PMID: 26249018] Free full text.

Peters AL, Henry RR, Thakkar P *et al*. Diabetic ketoacidosis with canagliflozin, a sodium-glucose cotransporter 2 inhibitor, in patients with type 1 diabetes. *Diabetes Care* 2016;39:532–8 [PMID: 26989182].

Pfeffer MA, Claggett B Diaz R *et al*. ELIXA Investigators. Lixisenatide in patients with type 2 diabetes and acute coronary syndrome. *N Engl J Med* 2015;373:2247–57 [PMID: 26630143].

Rajagopalan H, Cherrington AD, Thomspon CC *et al*. Endoscopic duodenal mucosal resurfacing for the treatment of type 2 diabetes: 6-month interim analysis from the first-in-human proof-of-concept study, *Diabetes Care* 2016;39:2254–61 [PMID: 27519448].

Rajendran R, Kerry C, Rayman G; MaGIC Study Group. Temporal patterns of hypoglycaemia and burden of sulfonylurea-related hypoglycaemia: a retrospective multicentre audit of hospitalised patients with diabetes. *BMJ Open* 2014;4:e005165 [PMID: 25009134] Free full text.

Raz I, Wilson PW, Strojek K *et al*. Effects of prandial versus fasting glycemia on cardiovascular outcomes in type 2 diabetes: the HEART2D study. *Diabetes Care* 2009;32:381–6 [PMID: 19246588] PMC264013.

Reaven G. HOMA-beta in the UKPDS and ADOPT. Is the natural history of type 2 diabetes characterised by a progressive and inexorable loss of insulin secretary function? Maybe? Maybe not? *Diab Vasc Dis Res* 2009;6:133–8 [PMID: 20368203].

Riddle MC, Rosenstock J, Gerich J; Insulin Glargine 4002 Study Investigators. The treat-to-target trial: randomized addition of glargine or human NPH insulin to oral therapy of type 2 diabetic patients. *Diabetes Care* 2003;26:3080–6 [PMID: 14578243].

Roden M, Merker L, Chistiansen AV *et al*. EMPA-REG™ EXTEND MONO investigators. Safety, tolerability and effects on cardiometabolic risk factors of empagliflozin monotherapy in drug-naïve patients with type 2 diabetes: a double-blind extension of a phase III randomized controlled trial. *Cardiovasc Diabetol* 2015;14:154 [PMID: 26701110] PMC4690334.

Roos ST, Timmers L, Biesbroek PS *et al*. No benefit of additional treatment with exenatide in patients with an acute myocardial infarction. *Int J Cardiol* 2016;220:809–14 [PMID: 27394978].

Rosenstock J, Ahmann AJ, Colon G *et al*. Advancing insulin therapy in type 2 diabetes previously treated with glargine plus oral agents: prandial premixed (insulin lispro protamine suspension/lispro) versus basal/bolus (glargine/lispro) therapy *Diabetes Care* 2008;31:20–5 [PMID: 17934150].

Rosenstock J, Jelaska A, Zeller C *et al*. EMPA-REG BASAL™ trial investigators. Impact of emapgliflozin added on to basal insulin in type 2 diabetes inadequately controlled on basal insulin: a 78-week randomized, double-blind, placebo-controlled trial. *Diabetes Obes Metab* 2015;17:936–48 [PMID: 26040302].

Rubino F, Nathan DM, Eckel RG *et al*. Delegates of the 2nd Diabetes Surgery Summit. Metabolic surgery in the treatment algorithm for type 2 diabetes: a joint statement by International Diabetes Organizations. *Diabetes Care* 2016;39:861–77 [PMID: 27222544].

Schauer PR, Bhatt DL, Kirwan JP *et al*. STAMPEDE Investigators. Bariatric surgery versus intensive medical therapy for diabetes – 3-year outcomes. *N Engl J Med* 2014;370:2002–13 [PMID: 24679060] Free full text.

Scheen AJ, Tan MH, Betteridge DJ *et al*. PROactive investigators. Long-term glycaemic effects of pioglitazone compared with placebo as add-on treatment to metformin or sulphonylurea monotherapy in PROactive (PROactive 18). *Diabet Med* 2009;26:1242–9 [PMID: 20002476].

Scheen AJ, Schmitt H, Jiang HH, Ivanyi T. Individualizing treatment of type 2 diabetes by targeting postprandial or fasting hyperglycaemia: Response to a basal vs a premixed insulin regimen by HbA$_{1c}$ quartiles and ethnicity. *Diabetes Metab* 2015;41:216–22 [PMID: 25881510].

Scheiter YD, Turvall E, Ackerman Z. Characteristics of patients with sulphonylurea-induced hypoglycaemia. *J Am Med Dir Assoc* 2012;13;234–8 [PMID: 21450199].

Schütz-Fuhrmann I, Castañeda J, Reznik Y *et al*. Factors affecting the benefit of insulin dose intensification in people with Type 2 diabetes: an analysis from the OpT2mise randomized trial. *Diabet Med* 2017;34:291–2 [PMID: 27770589].

Schwartz S, Sievers R, Strange P *et al*. INS-2061 Study Team. Insulin 70/30 mix plus metformin versus triple oral therapy in the treatment of type 2 diabetes after failure of two oral drugs: efficacy, safety, and cost analysis. *Diabetes Care* 2003;26:2238–43 [PMID: 12882842].

Schwartz SS, Jellinger PS, Herman ME. Obviating much of the need for insulin therapy in type 2 diabetes mellitus: a re-assessment of insulin therapy's safety profile. *Postgrad Med* 2016;128:609–19 [PMID: 27210018].

Shimonov M, Groutz A, Schachter P, Gordon D. Is bariatric surgery the answer to urinary incontinence in obese women? *Neurourol Urodyn* 2017;36:184–7 [PMID: 26473507].

Sjöstrom L, Peltonen M, Jacobson P *et al*. Bariatric surgery and long-term cardiovascular events. *JAMA* 2012;307:56–65 [PMID: 22215166].

Sjöstrom L, Peltonen M, Jacobsen P *et al*. Association of bariatric surgery with long-term remission of type 2 diabetes and with microvascular and macrovascular complications. *JAMA* 2014;311;2297–304 [PMID: 24915261].

Sonesson C, Johansson PA, Johansson E, Gause-Nilsson I. Cardiovascular effects of dapagliflozin in patients with type 2 diabetes and different risk categories: a meta-analysis. *Cardiovasc Diabetol* 2016;15:37 [PMID: 26895767] PMC4761166.

Srivanichakorn W, Sriwijitkamol A. Kongchoo A *et al*. Withdrawal of sulfonylureas from patients with type 2 diabetes receiving long-term sulfonylurea and insulin combination therapy results in deterioration of glycemic control: a randomized controlled trial. *Diabetes Metab Syndr Obes* 2015;8:137–45 [PMID: 25767401] PMC4354396.

Swinnen SG, Devries JH. Contact frequency determines outcome of basal insulin initiation trials in type 2 diabetes. *Diabetologia* 2009;52:2324–7 [PMID: 19756479] PMC2759009.

Swinnen SG, Simon AC, Holleman F *et al*. Insulin detemir versus insulin glargine for type 2 diabetes mellitus. *Cochrane Database Syst Rev* 2011;(7):CD006383 [PMID: 21735405].

Tack J, Deloose E. Complications of bariatric surgery: dumping syndrome, reflux and vitamin deficiencies. *Best Pract Clin Gastroenterol* 2014;28:741–9 [PMID: 25194187].

Tattersall R. Adult onset diabetes and the long awaited oral treatment, in Tattersall R: *Diabetes: The Biography (Biographies of Disease)*. Oxford: Oxford University Press, 2009, Chapter 6.

Thomsen RW, Baggesen LM, Søgaard M *et al*. Effectiveness of intensification therapies in Danes with Type 2 diabetes who use basal insulin: a population-based study. *Diabet Med* 2017;34:213–22 [PMID: 27279380].

Tkáč I, Raz I. Combined analysis of three large interventional trials with gliptins indicates increased incidence of acute pancreatitis in patients with type 2 diabetes. *Diabetes Care* 2017;40:284–6 [PMID: 27659407}.

UK Hypoglycaemia Study Group. Risk of hypoglycaemia in types 1 and 2 diabetes: effects of treatment modalities and their duration. *Diabetologia* 2007;50:1140–7 [PMID: 17415551].

UK Prospective Diabetes Study (UKPDS) Group. Intensive blood-glucose control with sulphonylureas or insulin compared with conventional treatment and risk of complications in patients with type 2 diabetes (UKPDS 33). *Lancet* 1998;352:837–53 [PMID: 9742976].

Vanderheiden A, Harrison L, Warshauer J et al. Effect of adding liraglutide vs placebo to a high-dose insulin regimen in patients with type 2 diabetes: a randomized clinical trial. *JAMA Intern Med* 2016;176:939–47 [PMID: 27273731].

Vora J, Cohen N, Evans M et al. Intensifying insulin regimen after basal insulin optimization in adults with type 2 diabetes: a 24-week, randomized, open-label trial comparing insulin glargine plus insulin glulisine with biphasic insulin aspart (LanScape). *Diabetes Obes Metab* 2015;17:1133–41 [PMID: 26085028].

Wanner C, Inzucchi SE, Lachin JM et al. EMPA-REG OUTCOME Investigators. Empagliflozin and progression of kidney disease in type 2 diabetes. *N Engl J Med* 2016;375:323–34 [PMID: 27299675] Free full text.

Wei N, Zheng H, Nathan DM. Empirically establishing blood glucose targets to achieve HbA1c goals. *Diabetes Care* 2014;37:1048–51 [PMID: 24513588] PMC3964488.

de Wit HM, Te Groen M, Rovers MM, Tack CJ. The placebo response of injectable GLP-1 receptor agonists vs. oral DPP4 inhibitors and SGLT-2 inhibitors: a systematic review and meta-analysis. *Br J Clin Pharmacol* 2016;82:301–14 [PMID: 26935973] PMC4917794.

Wright AD, Cull CA, Macleod KM, Holman RR; UKPDS Group. Hypoglycemia in type 2 diabetic patients randomized to and maintained on monotherapy with diet, sulfonylurea, metformin, or insulin for 6 years from diagnosis: UKPDS 73. *J Diabetes Complications* 2006;20:395–401 [PMID: 17070446].

Yang W, Xu X, Liu X et al. Treat-to-target comparison between once daily biphasic insulin aspart 30 and insulin glargine in Chinese and Japanese insulin-naïve subjects with type 2 diabetes. *Curr Med Res Opin* 2013;29:1599–608 [PMID: 23998560].

Yang W, Liu J, Sha Z et al. Acarbose compared with metformin as initial therapy in patients with newly diagnosed type 2 diabetes: an open-label, non-inferiority randomised trial. *Lancet Diabetes Endocrinol* 2014;2:46–55 [PMID: 24622668].

Yki-Järvinen H, Bergenstal R, Zieman M et al. EDITION 2 Study Investigators. New insulin glargine 300 units/mL versus glargine 100 units/mL in people with type 2 diabetes using oral agents and basal insulin: glucose control and hypoglycaemia in a 6-month randomized controlled trial (EDITION 2). *Diabetes Care* 2014;37:3235–43 [PMID: 25193531].

Zhou X, Li L, Kwong JS et al. Impact of bariatric surgery on renal functions in patients with type 2 diabetes: a systematic review of randomized trials and observational studies. *Surg Obes Relat Dis* 2016;12:1873–82 [PMID: 27421689].

Zhu H, Zhu Y, Leung SW. Is self-monitoring of blood glucose levels effective in improving glycaemic control in type 2 diabetes without insulin treatment: a meta-analysis of randomised controlled trials. *BMJ Open* 2016;6:e010524 [PMID: 27591016] PMC5020874.

Zinman B, Philis-Tsimikas A, Cariou B et al. NN1250-3579 (BEGIN Once Long) Trial Investigators. Insulin degludec versus insulin glargine in insulin-naive patients with type 2 diabetes: a 1-year, randomized, treat-to-target trial (BEGIN Once Long). *Diabetes Care* 2012;35:2464–71 [PMID: 23043166] PMC3507614.

Zinman B, DeVries JH, Bode B et al. NN1250-3724 (BEGIN:EASY AM) and NN1250-3718 (BEGIN:EASY PM) Trial Investigators. Efficacy and safety of insulin degludec three times a week versus insulin glargine once a day in insulin-naive patients with type 2 diabetes: results of two phase 3, 26 week, randomised, open-label, treat-to-target, non-inferiority trials. *Lancet Diabetes Endocrinol* 2013;1:123–31 [PMID: 24622318].

Zinman B, Wanner C, Lachin JM et al. EMPA-REG OUTCOME Investigators. Empagliflozin, outcomes, and mortality in type 1 diabetes. *N Engl J Med* 2015;373:2117–28 [PMID: 26378978].

Zoungas S, Chalmers J, Kengne AP et al. The efficacy of lowering glycated haemoglobin with a gliclazide modified release-based intensive glucose lowering regimen in the ADVANCE trial. *Diabetes Res Clin Pract* 2010:89:126–33 [PMID: 20541825].

Zoungas S, Chalmers J, Neal B *et al*. ADVANCE-ON Collaborative Group. Follow-up of blood-pressure lowering and glucose control in type 2 diabetes. *N Engl J Med* 2014;371:1392–406 [PMID: 25234206] Free full text.

Guidance

UK (NICE) *December 2015*
Type 2 diabetes in adults management (NG28). www.nice.org.uk/guidance/ng28 (last accessed 25 August 2017)

USA (ADA)
Diabetes Care 2016;39(suppl 1):S1–S106

Bariatric surgery
UK (NICE) *November 2014*
Obesity: identification, assessment and management (CG189). www.nice.org.uk/guidance/cg189 (last accessed 25 August 2017)

International Diabetes Organizations
Rubino F Nathan DM, Eckel RH *et al*. Delegates of the 2nd Diabetes Surgery Summit. Metabolic surgery in the treatment algorithm for type 2 diabetes: a joint statement by international diabetes organisations. *Obes Surg* 2016;27:2–21 [PMID: 27957699].

BOMSS (British Obesity and Metabolic Surgery Society) Guidelines on perioperative and postoperative biochemical monitoring and micronutrient replacement for patients undergoing bariatric surgery (September 2014). http://www.bomss.org.uk/bomss-nutritional-guidance/ (last accessed 25 August 2017).

11 Hypertension

Key points
- Focusing on cut-points and targets fails to emphasize the continuous change in risk of renal disease and macrovascular events across a wide range of systolic BP values
- All patients with Type 2 diabetes should aim for BP <130–140/80 mm Hg. In higher-risk patients, especially those with proteinuria and reduced eGFR, there may be further advantage in lower values
- At systolic levels <120 mm Hg there is no consistent benefit even in stroke reduction but renal events increase
- Ambulatory and home BP monitoring is central to effective management of hypertension
- Combined angiotensin blockade treatment is hazardous, and there are significant cardiovascular risks associated with postural hypotension (≥20 systolic or ≥10 mm Hg diastolic fall 3 minutes after standing from sitting independent of baseline blood pressure)
- Unlike glycaemia, there is no consistent legacy effect of prior good control of hypertension. Continuous treatment is needed. Adherence is central
- Type 1 patients have 'essential' hypertension exacerbated in long duration by premature arterial stiffening
- Recognize resistant and refractory hypertension, their poor cardiovascular prognosis and complexity

INTRODUCTION

Hypertension, however defined, is present in nearly all Type 2 patients. It is a powerful risk factor in non-diabetic people, but significantly more so in diabetes: epidemiological studies suggest a two- to fivefold increased risk just from coronary heart disease at any systolic blood pressure value. In the era of intervention studies, more positive converse data have emerged: although relative risk reduction is similar in diabetic and non-diabetic people, the increased absolute risk in diabetes results in dramatically lower cardiovascular event rates with focused BP control.

A unitary cause for hypertension has eluded researchers for a century and there clearly is not one; it will remain multifactorial in the majority of patients. Common, eminently treatable with clinically meaningful cardiovascular outcomes, it is unequivocally more important in diabetes management than glycaemia, yet blood pressure and its management, like lipids, is nearly always shoe-horned into the consultation after extensive consideration of blood glucose levels. Yudkin *et al.* (2010) estimated the numbers of people who needed to be treated in order to avoid a vascular event (**Figure 11.1**), using data from the United Kingdom Prospective Diabetes Study (UKPDS) and the large studies reporting in the 2000s. Reducing blood pressure by 10/5 mm Hg is more valuable than reducing HbA_{1c} by nearly 1% and has a similar effect to reducing LDL-cholesterol by 1 mmol/l.

Practical Diabetes Care, Fourth Edition. David Levy.
© 2018 John Wiley & Sons Ltd. Published 2018 by John Wiley & Sons Ltd.

Number of
patients

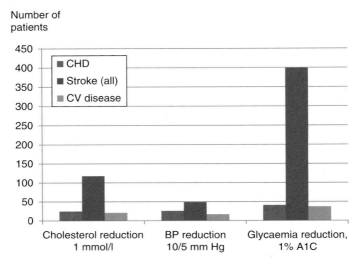

Figure 11.1 Numbers of patients needed to treat in order to prevent cardiovascular events in Type 2 diabetes. Improving glycaemia by 1% HbA$_{1c}$ is markedly less effective – and nearly always more difficult to achieve – than either reducing blood pressure by 10/5 mm Hg or LDL by 1 mmol/l. *Source*: Modified after Yudkin *et al.*, 2010.

In Type 1 diabetes hypertension has not been seen as a problem until mildly elevated albuminuria (microalbuminuria) is established, but there is increasing concern about 'essential' hypertension, especially systolic, in longer-established Type 1 diabetes, even when all measures of renal function are normal. In short, hypertension is an ever-present hazard in all forms of diabetes and the evidence for effective long-term treatment is unequivocal.

As with glycaemia and LDL, the practical management of hypertension is hindered by the guidelines focusing, necessarily, on cut-points and numerical targets. Nevertheless, in contrast with the lipid trials, which are drug and dose based (see **Chapter 12**), from UKPDS onwards there are substantial blood pressure trials that have randomized subjects to two numerical targets.

TYPE 1 DIABETES

Hypertension is intimately related to diabetic kidney disease in Type 1 diabetes and blood pressure is measurably higher (though still 'normal') when there is still only just-measurable albuminuria. Up to 30 or 40 years ago, established hypertension in Type 1 diabetes was usually seen in patients with renal disease. As advanced diabetic kidney disease has become less common, and the incidence of diabetes in the young has increased, hypertension without proteinuria or impaired renal function is the commonest scenario in Type 1 patients (Levy, 2016).

Practice point

Arteries stiffen early on in Type 1 diabetes, even when there is no proteinuria. One in four young adults between 25 and 40 years old will have definite hypertension (BP ≥140/≥90 mm Hg).

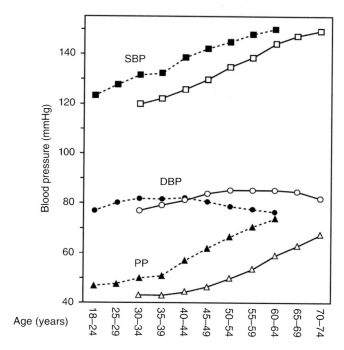

Figure 11.2 Age-related blood pressure changes in Finnish Type 1 patients. Filled symbols: normoalbuminuric subjects; open symbols: non-diabetic controls. Systolic blood pressure is elevated early on in Type 1 diabetes, diastolic blood pressure falls at an earlier age than in non-diabetic subjects, and pulse pressure rises rapidly with age. SBP: systolic blood pressure; DBP: diastolic blood pressure; PP: pulse pressure. *Source:* Rönnback *et al.*, 2008. Reproduced with permission of Wolters Kluwer Health, Inc.

Systolic blood pressure (SBP) rises with age in the non-diabetic population, as does diastolic blood pressure (DBP), until around age 60 years when it begins to fall. The slow rise in pulse pressure (SBP minus DBP) therefore accelerates after 60, Pulse pressure is the simplest clinical indicator of arterial stiffness and is a powerful risk factor for cardiovascular disease. Because the diastolic fall starts around 10–15 years earlier in Type 1 patients, pulse pressure becomes an even more important factor in arterial disease (**Figure 11.2**). The longitudinal FinnDiane study describes blood pressure in detail from 18 years onwards in Type 1 patients, its value enhanced by having a non-diabetic control group (**Box 11.1**) (Rönnback *et al.*, 2008).

Practicalities

There is little guidance on the management of hypertension in Type 1 diabetes in the absence of proteinuria. Diagnostic 24-hour ambulatory BP testing should be used widely and can help these often young people to engage with what they may consider another numerical exercise. Diagnostic criteria are the same as in non-diabetic people: clinic BP consistently ≥140/≥90 mm Hg requires treatment. Although an angiotensin-blocking agent will almost invariably be given first (ACE inhibitor, replaced by an angiotensin

> **Box 11.1** Hypertension in Type 1 patients >18 years in the FinnDiane Study.
>
> - Age-related changes are similar to those in non-diabetic people, but occur 10–15 years earlier. This phenomenon occurs in all age groups.
> - Diastolic blood pressure begins to fall in Type 1 patients in their 40s.
> - Pulse pressure is progressively higher in people with diabetes at all levels of albuminuria.
> - Glycaemia was not related to single HbA$_{1c}$ measurements in FinnDiane, but the risk of developing hypertension was lower in DCCT (Diabetes Control and Complications Trial) participants with better glycaemic control (multiple HbA$_{1c}$ measurements were made).
> - Discernible differences between people with and without diabetes are apparent by the early 30s onwards.
> - Diagnosed hypertension (≥140/≥90 mm Hg) is common and occurs in 20–25% of Type 1 patients aged 25–40.
> - By the time Type 1 patients are in their late 40s, the majority have either essential hypertension or isolated systolic hypertension.
>
> *Source*: Modified after Rönnback *et al.*, 2008.

receptor blocker if there is a cough or allergic reaction), this group of drugs is not mandatory if there are no microvascular complications (angiotensin blockers do not prevent retinopathy or albuminuria; see **Chapter 4**). A calcium-channel blocker might be more appropriate in these subjects and is safer in women of child-bearing age. Non-pharmacological interventions are important in young people, for example recommended activity levels, decreased salt intake and evidence-based dietary interventions, based on the DASH (Dietary Approaches to Stop Hypertension) recommendations (see later). These include increased fruit intake in moderation in diabetes, vegetables, beans, legumes, nuts, wholegrains and soy. Alcohol excess must be tackled (see later).

There are no prospective interventional studies of antihypertensive treatment in Type 1 subjects without baseline renal disease, but the relationship between outcomes and achieved blood pressure may not be the same as in Type 2 patients. For example, in long-term follow-up of the DCCT, mean blood pressure <120/70 mm Hg was associated with substantially reduced risks of developing macroalbuminuria or reaching chronic kidney disease G3. There are no reports of vascular events and blood pressure but event numbers were presumably too small to meaningfully analyse (Ku *et al.*, 2016).

TYPE 2 DIABETES

Gratifyingly, there has been no slow-down in major clinical trials in hypertension but headlines from the highest-profile studies, some in diabetes, some in general hypertension, have resulted in confusion for the practitioner. The widely-held 'lower [systolic blood pressure] is better' view was interrupted in the mid-2000s by the unexpected results of both the ADVANCE and ACCORD studies, which found no meaningful benefits of targeting lower systolic BP values on macro- or microvascular complications. More recently, however, intensive post hoc analyses, observational studies and meta-analyses, and the results of the meticulous SPRINT study in non-diabetic people, are likely to result in another re-think of BP targets in diabetes, broadly to significantly lower than the systolic BP level of <140 mm Hg that was established after the ACCORD study. However, the SPRINT study excluded people with diabetes and data on emergent diabetes during the trial and its outcomes will be needed before its important data can be meaningfully incorporated into guidance for diabetes (Nilsson and Kjeldsen, 2017). Inevitably we will – properly – be asked to individualize targets according to the risk profile of our patients, just as in glycaemic control, but there is still insufficient modern-era longitudinal data that will allow us to do this in anything but the most general fashion.

U- or J-shaped curves?

While there is no doubt that higher blood pressure is associated with continuously increasing risks of adverse cardiovascular effects, there is a long-standing debate whether there are similar effects at low levels – a J-shaped curve if less harmful than high blood pressure levels, U-shaped if similar. There are specific concerns from trials that people with diastolic blood pressure <70–75 mm Hg may be at particular risk. Academic considerations apart, the efficacy of modern antihypertensive treatments, especially in the elderly taking multiple medications may put vulnerable groups at risk of events both cardiovascular and non-cardiovascular, for example falls.

In the VALUE study, for example, hypertensive people at high cardiovascular risk were treated with a combination of the angiotensin receptor blocking agent valsartan, amlodipine, and hydrochlorothiazide. Although in non-adjusted statistical models there was a hint of a J-shape for cardiovascular events, it disappeared after full adjustments. It is possible that the J-shape seen in other studies is an artefact of confounding variables (Kjeldsen et al., 2016). However, while this may not be a consideration in the general high-risk population, there is still concern about an increase in other serious outcomes, especially renal, in patients with additional risk factors, especially proteinuria and impaired renal function (see later). Uncommon but important, such adverse outcomes are unlikely to influence the shape of the curve at the lower end of blood pressure measurements.

Postural hypotension (e.g. systolic fall 20 mm Hg or more, or diastolic fall 10 mm Hg or more) is consistently identified as a risk factor for major cardiovascular events, including heart failure. However in the ACCORD study postural hypotension was no more frequent in those treated to the intensive systolic BP goal (<120 mm) (Fleg et al., 2016). In the light of these concerns, postural BP changes should be more assiduously measured in people with Type 2 diabetes, who are likely to have the additional risk factor of autonomic neuropathy (see **Chapter 5**). In the ACCORD study, BP was measured up to three minutes after standing from the seated position.

Practice point

Postural hypotension (SBP fall ≥20 mm Hg, DBP ≥10 mm Hg) is a risk factor for mortality and heart failure, and is not limited to those with low blood pressure. Measure BP three minutes after standing up from seated.

TARGETS FOR BP IN TYPE 2 DIABETES

There is no disagreement that BP >160/90 mm Hg requires urgent treatment with two initial agents, or that >140/90 mm Hg requires treatment in Type 2 diabetes. The discussion focuses on optimum systolic blood pressure to minimize adverse cardiovascular and renal outcomes and adverse effects either of treatment or of excessively low blood pressure. It is also clear that coronary and cerebrovascular outcomes have a different relationship with blood pressure. Coronary vessels, unlike other vascular beds, fill during diastole, and low diastolic levels may be associated with an increased risk of cardiovascular events; low diastolic blood pressure also occurs in elderly people with stiff arteries and high pulse pressures, and this again is associated with increased cardiovascular events. For stroke risk, however, there is no limit below which there is no benefit. Large-scale trials are beginning to give more definitive guides to clinicians, but the differential impact of lowering blood pressure on different clinical outcomes means that clinical decisions are not simple.

CLINICAL TRIALS IN TYPE 2 DIABETES

The small hypertension arm of the UKPDS (approximately 1200 patients), published in 1998, is no longer relevant to clinical practice; achieved blood pressure in the intensively treated group (target <150/85 mm Hg) was 144/82 mm Hg, not far off the current threshold to start treatment. However the difference between the intensive and routinely-treated arms (10/3 mm Hg) significantly reduced stroke and heart failure (and measures of retinopathy and proteinuria) though there was no effect on myocardial infarction. Importantly, however, after long-term follow-up there was no legacy effect of prior lower blood pressure once randomisation had finished (Holman et al., 2008).

The ADVANCE (Patel et al., 2007) and ACCORD blood pressure studies (ACCORD Study Group, 2010) are more contemporary studies involving very large numbers of patients, but using different designs.

ADVANCE and ADVANCE-ON

The ADVANCE study was a trial of a fixed drug combination (the ACE inhibitor perindopril 4 mg and thiazide-like diuretic indapamide 1.25 mg daily) compared with placebo (therefore not a treat-to-target study). Over four years the difference between the two groups was 5.6/2.2 mm Hg from a baseline of 145/81 mm Hg. The risk of macro- and microvascular events, separately and combined, was reduced by approximately 9%, though this became statistically significant only when the two groups of outcomes were considered together. Risk reductions were similar regardless of baseline blood pressure and medications. Clinical benefits were in line with those of other studies of ACE inhibitor treatment, but less than expected from epidemiological studies. The non-significant reduction in stroke is striking given the high sensitivity of stroke events to even small reductions in blood pressure and has not been explained. The authors' view is that it is due to the play of chance, as a result of the relatively small difference in achieved systolic pressure. In four years of post-trial follow-up in the ADVANCE-ON study (Zoungas et al., 2014) blood pressure values harmonized at 145/80 mm Hg within six months of the end of the randomized trial period. All-cause and cardiovascular deaths continued to be lower in the previously treated group, but it was not a 'legacy' effect, as most of the events occurred during the randomized part of the trial.

> **Practice point**
>
> There is no blood pressure 'legacy' effect for major cardiovascular events in most clinical trials, but there may be some long-term advantage in reducing microvascular complications and heart failure even if blood pressure rises after the randomized period has finished.

ACCORD

The ACCORD study was the first major trial to randomize high cardiovascular risk patients to two systolic blood pressure strategies: standard (targeting systolic blood pressure <140 mm Hg) and intensive (<120 mm Hg). Baseline blood pressure was already fairly good (139/76 mm Hg). The maintained difference was substantial, approximately

14 mm (mean achieved systolic values 119 vs 134 mm Hg), but, despite this, there was no difference in the number of combined cardiovascular events, though the 40% stroke risk reduction was in line with expectations from other trials and epidemiological studies. However, although a large trial, it was not adequately powered, given the lower than expected rate of cardiovascular events during the trial (a persistent problem in modern clinical trials that are planned and executed over a very long period, during which major population changes in outcomes are seen epidemiologically).

ACCORD substudies suggest benefits of tight blood pressure control on an important range of outcomes, for example atrial fibrillation/P-wave indices (see **Chapter 6**), and ECG evidence of left ventricular hypertrophy (Soliman *et al.*, 2015). Perhaps there has been too much focus on the standard trial outcome of 'major adverse cardiovascular events' and insufficient on other, though clinically important, cardiovascular outcomes. Other trials have investigated alternative but important outcomes. The ROADMAP study of the angiotensin receptor blocker olmesartan found that after the end of the double-blind trial period, systolic blood pressure rose in the olmesartan treated group from 124 to 135 mm Hg during follow-up. However, patients previously treated with olmesartan had subsequently lower risks of developing microalbuminuria, retinopathy and heart failure, and in this trial there was a trend to lower major cardiovascular events (Menne *et al.*, 2014).

ACCOMPLISH

The important ACCOMPLISH study (Jamerson *et al.*, 2008) goes some way to explain the results of these other trials. It included large numbers of high-risk older people (mean age 67–70 years) both with and without diabetes. It gave valuable information on optimum combination drug therapy (see later) but, for the purposes of the current discussion on systolic blood pressure targets, the prospectively defined analysis of outcomes by 10 mm categories is unique and important (Weber *et al.*, 2016). In this analysis there were clear differences in patterns of cardiovascular and renal outcomes (**Figure 11.3**).

- *Composite cardiovascular endpoints* (cardiovascular death, non-fatal myocardial infarction, non-fatal stroke) were lower in the <140 mm Hg category compared with ≥140 mm Hg (uncontrolled) category. There was no difference at <130 mm Hg but there was loss of benefit at <120 mm Hg, again suggesting a J-shape, which was not present in the non-diabetic patients. This tended towards a U-shape for myocardial infarction with a striking increase in events at <120 compared with <130 mm Hg.
- *Stroke*: there was a linear decrease in events down to <120 mm Hg.
- *Renal endpoint* (increase >50% from baseline serum creatinine): the pattern of events was clearly a 'reverse-tick' in both diabetic and non-diabetic subjects, with the lowest event rate at 130–139 mm Hg. There was a progressive rise in events at lower values.

Practice point

For most older diabetic people with hypertension, optimum systolic blood pressure is 130–140 mm Hg, although stroke continues to decrease down to 110–120 mm Hg. Renal events increase when systolic pressure is lower than 130 mm Hg.

It is unlikely that further trials and meta-analyses will help the clinician and patients decide on specific numerical targets for treatment. Type 2 diabetes is a clinically heterogeneous disease and simple inclusion criteria, for example known duration of diabetes, will

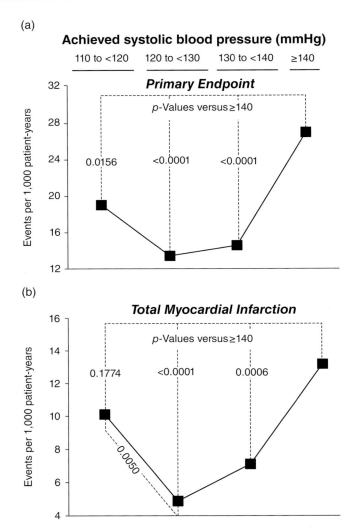

Figure 11.3 Cardiovascular and renal outcomes in diabetic participants in the ACCOMPLISH study plotted by achieved 10-mm systolic BP categories. (a) Primary endpoint (cardiovascular death, nonfatal myocardial infarction or stroke); (b) myocardial infarction; (c) stroke; (d) renal endpoint (50% rise in serum creatinine) in diabetic participants (results in people without diabetes are shown in (d)). The J-shaped curves were not seen in the non-diabetic participants, where there were straight-line relationships. The 'reverse tick' pattern for the renal endpoint was similar in diabetic and non-diabetic groups, but in all strata of blood pressure diabetic patients had approximately 50% more events. *Source*: Weber *et al.*, 2016. Reproduced with permission of John Wiley & Sons.

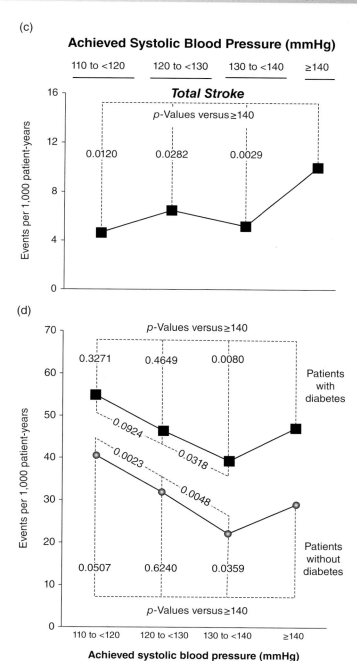

Figure 11.3 (Continued)

define very different populations of patients. As time goes on, more patients, regardless of allocation within trials, are taking powerful agents known to have meaningful effects on outcomes, especially aspirin and statins, and these will modify clinical risk at trial entry, resulting in many more trials underestimating the numbers needed to show clinical benefit. There are also powerful factors that are not usually taken into account, especially blood pressure variability in clinical practice; for example, detailed analysis of individual measurements during the VALUE trial showed that outcomes were strongly influenced by the proportion of recorded measurements within different ranges (Mancia *et al.*, 2016). In the ADVANCE study, the risk of macrovascular events was increased by 50% and of microvascular events (new or worsening nephropathy or retinopathy) by 85% in patients with the highest systolic pressure variability (that is, standard deviation) during the first two years of the trial (Hata *et al.*, 2013). While clinically this variable cannot so far be exploited therapeutically, it should help place rigid numerical targets in context.

For general cardiovascular risk reduction in Type 2 diabetes, systolic blood pressure should be consistently <140 mm Hg, with likely increased benefits down to 130 mm Hg. Systolic blood pressure <120, as in the tightly controlled ACCORD group, is not of definitive value and may harm. For patients with known cerebrovascular disease or at high risk of it benefits continue down to systolic values110–120 mm Hg.

BLOOD PRESSURE CONTROL IN TYPE 2 DIABETES – REAL LIFE

In real life, blood pressure control in Type 2 diabetes is not nearly as good as the guideline writers and target setters tell us it ought to be, though there is encouraging evidence from different countries and healthcare economies that it is improving over time – much as, for example mean HbA$_{1c}$ has improved in Type 2 diabetes in many countries.

Comparison of two NHANES studies in the USA found that while only 16% were controlled to <130/80 mm Hg in the earlier study from 1988 to 1994, nearly 30% were in this category during 1999–2004 (Suh *et al.*, 2009). Sweden has seen broadly similar trends, with discernible changes over the five-year period between 2005 and 2009: for example mean blood pressure fell from 141/77 to 136/76 mm Hg and, importantly, the proportion of patients with uncontrolled blood pressure (>140/90 mm Hg) decreased from 58 to 46%. These group trends were paralleled in individual patients. In the same study, the proportion of nephropathy patients with well-controlled hypertension increased from 12 to 21%, an especially impressive finding over a relatively short period in patients who frequently have difficult BP (Nilsson *et al.*, 2011). However, there remains the obvious concern that between 50 and 70% of all Type 2 patients still have uncontrolled hypertension.

Practice point

BP control in Type 2 patients is improving in many countries, but between 50 and 70% of patients still have uncontrolled BP (>140/90 mm Hg).

Blood pressure tracking

'Tracking' – the persistence of a measurement over a long period in spite of good clinical follow up and changes of treatment – is now emerging as an important phenomenon in blood pressure as it is in glycaemic control. In a large six-year study Walraven *et al.* (2015) found that about 85% of a cohort of Type 2 patients had adequate control over the whole period, that is systolic values about 140 mm Hg. About 6% eventually reached target, although slowly. An important group of nearly 10% of patients had difficult-to-control blood pressure: they either had worsening initial control followed by a poor treatment response or persistently worsening control. The last three groups contained more women, and people with a higher rate of micro- and macrovascular complications and who were taking more antihypertensive medication. Many will have resistant hypertension (see later).

Many patients hope that adherence to hypertension and diabetes treatment will improve once they retire. The evidence is it will not. Public sector workers in Finland were followed for three years before and four years after retirement for medication adherence (defined as <40% of days covered by treatment, though other measures gave similar results) (Kivimäki et al., 2013). The risk of poor adherence to antihypertensive medication in both men and women increased after retirement by 25–30% (in addition, men were twice as likely not to adhere to their antidiabetic medication, though there was no effect in women).

Practice point

Watch for *decreased* adherence to antihypertensive treatment once a patient has retired.

COMPLIANCE/ADHERENCE

The inconsistent legacy effects of antihypertensive treatment mean that treatment must be continuous. Poor adherence to treatment is associated with uncontrolled blood pressure (Krousel-Wood et al., 2011) and in a study of Korean patients admitted with ischaemic heart disease or stroke (infarction or haemorrhage), mortality of all three was higher in those with poor prior adherence (<50%) to antihypertensive medication (Kim et al., 2016). Although there are no longitudinal cohort studies, overall persistence with antihypertensive medication is about 80%. Structured pharmacist-based intervention may help. Over a year non-adherence to lipid-lowering and antihypertensive treatment (medication possession ratio <0.80) in Danish diabetic outpatients was 30% in a control group compared with 20% in the intervention group, and median measures of medication possession ratio slightly increased throughout the study year. The study was too small and short to demonstrate any benefits in blood pressure levels or cardiovascular outcomes, though there was a positive trend in the latter. In the usual-care group non-adherence to lipid-lowering medication and renin-angiotensin blocking agents was particularly high in this study, but there were no differences in adherence to β-blockers, diuretics or calcium channel blockers (Hedegaard et al., 2015), a timely reminder that expected adherence based on intuitive ideas of side-effect profiles may not be seen in practice.

Practice point

Perhaps one-third of people with diabetes take less than 80% of their medication. Adherence is not the same for all classes of medication.

NON-PHARMACOLOGICAL ('LIFESTYLE') APPROACHES TO HYPERTENSION IN TYPE 2 DIABETES

Intensive lifestyle intervention for blood pressure management is at least as effective as it is for blood glucose control, and there is a compelling evidence base, but in practice it is much less emphasized. One reason is that the wide availability of several valuable classes of drugs, now all generic, means that physicians tend to issue a prescription than consult the literature on lifestyle, and we do not have the hypertension equivalent of dieticians or diabetes specialist nurses. An elegant comparison between the pharmacological intervention used in the ACCORD blood pressure study and the intensive lifestyle intervention arm of Look AHEAD found they were equally effective in reducing systolic blood pressure to <140 mm Hg over four years. There was statistical support for greater efficacy of lifestyle measures in the obese (BMI >30) and of pharmacological intervention in the less obese; however, both are usually needed (Espeland *et al.*, 2015).

Practice point

Intensive lifestyle intervention for hypertension is as effective as drug treatment. A judicious combination of the two would significantly reduce drug usage and side effects.

Salt intake

Most Westerners consume a lot of salt – the average daily intake in the USA is 3400 mg/day. The recommendation in 2010 was <2300 mg (<1 teaspoon/day), decreasing to 1500 mg/day above the age of 50 years and in people with hypertension, diabetes or chronic kidney disease, and in those of African ethnicity. Patients with diabetes, hypertensive chronic kidney disease, women and older people are thought to be particularly salt-sensitive.

There is ample evidence for cardiovascular disease reduction in populations if overall salt intake is reduced and the linear relationship between reducing salt intake and fall in urinary salt excretion means that the benefit would continue at levels lower than current recommendations. Clinical studies inform clinical practice in individuals. For example, in the important five-year PREDIMED diet study (see **Chapter 9**) all-cause mortality was lower in subjects taking the recommended USA salt intake, while cardiovascular disease was higher in those taking more (Merino *et al.*, 2015). Therapeutically, salt reduction is clinically effective: reducing salt intake from an estimated 4500 mg/day to 2500 mg/day was more effective in proteinuria reduction than adding a second angiotensin blocking agent in patients with a variety of non-diabetic renal diagnoses. Mean systolic BP did not change with the additional angiotensin blocking agent but fell by 10 mm Hg after sodium restriction (Slagman *et al.*, 2011).

Practice point

Halving salt intake (added and included in snacks etc.) has the same effect on systolic blood pressure as one or two additional antihypertensive drugs.

Dietary Approaches to Stop Hypertension (DASH) diet

DASH is a portfolio approach to dietary management of hypertension that emphasizes fruits, vegetables and low-fat dairy products, and encourages low saturated and total fat intake (**Box 11.2**). The original short-duration randomized study is now 20 years old (Appel *et al.*, 1997) but there were dramatic benefits in hypertensive people (reduction 11/6 mm Hg) and population-relevant reductions in non-hypertensive people (4/2 mm Hg). The little long-term information is less consistent – there was no long-term impact on blood pressure levels in the Framingham Cohort Study, but a 30% reduction in

> **Box 11.2** Components of the DASH (Dietary Approaches to Stop Hypertension) diet (2000 kcal version).
>
> *Sodium*: standard up to 2300 mg/day; lower sodium diet, 1500 mg/day.
>
> *Grains*: 6–8 servings a day (bread [1 slice], cereal [1 oz dry], rice, pasta [½ cup cooked]); emphasize wholegrains over refined grains.
>
> *Vegetables*: 4–5 servings a day (1 serving = 1 cup raw leafy green vegetables or ½ cup cut-up raw or cooked vegetables).
>
> *Fruits*: 4–5 servings a day (1 serving = 1 medium fruit or ½ cup fresh, frozen or canned fruit without added sugar).
>
> *Low-fat dairy products*: 2–3 servings a day.
>
> *Lean meat, poultry and fish*: <6 servings (6 oz) a day.
>
> *Nuts, seeds and legumes*: 4–5 servings a week (⅓ cup (1½ oz) nuts, 2 tablespoons seeds or ½ cup cooked beans or peas).
>
> *Fats and oils*: 2–3 servings a day (total fat ≤27% of daily calories, emphasizing monounsaturated fats).
>
> *Sweets*: limit.

all-cause mortality in hypertensive participants in the NHANES study (Parikh *et al.*, 2009) – and heart failure was less common in people who adhered to the DASH diet. The intentions in the original concept may be yielding to considering broader and longer-term outcomes, but DASH invigorated research into lifestyle interventions for cardiovascular disease and cancer, and it shares many components with the Mediterranean diet (see **Chapter 9**).

Alcohol

In population studies, moderate alcohol intake, for example 21 or fewer standard drinks weekly in men and 14 or fewer in women, is consistently associated with a lower risk of cardiovascular events and all-cause mortality, giving rise to the shorthand U-shaped descriptor. In addition, the ADVANCE study found that moderate consumption was, as in some other studies in both Type 1 and 2 diabetes, associated with a lower risk of microvascular complications, but all macrovascular outcomes increased in heavy drinkers (Blomster *et al.*, 2014).

An elegant controlled study in Type 2 diabetes found that moderate red wine intake (about ⅓ bottle a day in women, slightly less than ½ bottle in men) caused slight increases in daytime but equal falls in nocturnal blood pressure, resulting in neutral 24-hour BP averages, though pulse rate increased throughout. Measures of glucose, inflammation, lipids and insulin sensitivity did not change (Mori *et al.*, 2016). This study confirmed that moderate alcohol intake up to the previous UK weekly limits is neutral for cardiovascular risk in Type 2 diabetes patients with reasonable 24-hour mean values (133/77 mm Hg). Heavy alcohol intake is not usually included in lists of factors associated with resistant hypertension (see later), but a study of ambulatory profiles in alcohol-dependent people found that 80% of hypertensive and 50% of normotensive individuals showed a significant fall in mean systolic pressure (13 and 8 mm Hg respectively) during 24-hours abstinence (Estruch *et al.*, 2003). Inevitably, there will be major individual variation in response to alcohol and reduction in intake but it is well worth exploring.

Practice point

Blood pressure in heavy drinkers with hypertension can fall significantly and rapidly after reducing alcohol intake.

Exercise

Aerobic endurance training is of substantial benefit in hypertensive subjects (e.g. 7/5 mm Hg reduction in meta-analysis). In one trial, aerobic interval training (treadmill three times a week to >90% of maximal heart rate) reduced ambulatory BP over 12 weeks by 12/8 mm Hg in hypertensive subjects (Molmen-Hansen et al., 2012). There is some, but so far limited, evidence for the benefit of dynamic resistance training 2–3 times a week.

Sleep

The literature on disturbed sleep and its relationship with hypertension is huge but the chains of causation, as with hyperglycaemia and other insulin resistant characteristics, are still insufficiently understood that firm therapeutic recommendations cannot be offered yet. This is another area where speculation, particularly about the role of the sympathetic nervous system, outweighs clinical trial data. Patients with obstructive sleep apnoea have a wide phenotype and their characteristics vary according to whether they have been selected from a hypertension, respiratory, cardiology or metabolic setting. Even in patients with resistant hypertension (see later), RCT results are not impressive, though two recent studies have shown minor effects on nocturnal BP, and one showed an increase in the proportion of patients with a nocturnal dipping pattern (≥10% fall in mean night-time BP compared with mean daytime BP). Adherence to continuous positive airway pressure (CPAP) treatment can be poor and in the same study there was a weak correlation between duration of CPAP and decrease in 24-hour mean BP (Martinez-Garcia et al., 2013). As discussed in **Chapters 10** and **13**, there is a dearth of information on the benefits of bariatric surgery in people with or without diabetes on obstructive sleep apnoea, despite the resulting radical near-normalization of weight and metabolic abnormalities.

Alternative therapies

There are almost as many alternative therapies for blood pressure as there are for blood sugar levels and, as with blood glucose, unfortunately almost no well-conducted and adequately-powered trials; systematic reviews and meta-analyses under these circumstances are bound to yield dispiriting outcomes. Yet there are hints that some agents – perhaps many – may be of real value, and similar to the DASH form of multi-nutritional input, may be especially powerful in judicious combination. None can be firmly recommended and there are insufficient safety data for the nutraceutical and herbal remedies. Even therapies that would now be considered more mainstream, for example acupuncture, are not effective in hypertension. **Box 11.3** lists a selection of approaches. Cocoa flavanols have the best evidence-base and in meta-analysis systolic pressure falls by about 3 mm Hg, with greater effects in younger and hypertensive patients (Jumar and Schmeider, 2016). The difficulties are that the intake of active compounds is highly variable, as cocoa preparations are not standardized, and also if consumed as chocolate there will probably be a significant caloric load (100 g chocolate = 500 kcal), especially if high-sugar, low-cocoa 'milk' chocolate is the object of the 'chocaholic's' attention. Notably, cocoa has no adverse effects on lipid profiles and may improve insulin resistance.

> **Box 11.3** Some potential complementary and alternative therapies for hypertension.
>
> *Herbal*
> - Hawthorn.
> - Traditional Chinese herbal medicine formulas.
>
> *Nutriceuticals*
> - Flaxseed, folate, soy protein, fish oils, olive oil.
> - Vitamins/antioxidants/mineral supplements (especially potassium, calcium and vitamin D, possibly vitamin C).
> - Flavonoids: tea (perhaps a slightly larger effect with green rather than black tea), cocoa, wine, grapes.
> - High fibre.
>
> *Meditation-based interventions*
> - Yoga.
> - Qi Gong.
> - Zen Buddhist.
>
> *Biofeedback*
> - Respiratory exercises, isometric handgrip.
>
> *Source*: Woolf and Bisognano, 2011. Reproduced with permission of John Wiley & Sons.

Many neutraceuticals have reasonable controlled trials to support their use; they nearly all have a small individual effect on systolic blood pressure (e.g. −2 mm Hg), but they can be effectively combined in a portfolio, much like the possible dietary approaches to LDL reduction. Several interesting non-nutrient nutraceuticals, especially lycopene (tomatoes), co-enzyme Q10, aged garlic extract and probiotics also have supporting data. Resveratrol (derived from grapes) is a potentially powerful compound. For obvious reasons there is great interest in cocoa, which has multiple beneficial *in vitro* effects on endothelial function. A very large trial of isolated cocoa extract placebo-controlled began in 2016 (Borghi and Cicero, 2017).

> **Practice point**
>
> Instituting a portfolio of evidence-based non-pharmacological interventions is likely to be of value in managing hypertension.

DIAGNOSING HYPERTENSION: WHAT IS THE BEST MEASUREMENT TO USE?

Office/clinic, ambulatory blood pressure monitoring (ABPM) or home blood pressure monitoring (HBPM)?

Not everyone with diabetes (especially those with Type 1) is inevitably hypertensive. Making a precise diagnosis is critical but most guidelines are surprisingly slight on the practical details, especially when it comes to the use of newer and better office and out of office measurements. Evidence and opinion is moving away from routine office measurements using standard auscultatory techniques. These measurements are on average 9/6 mm Hg higher than in the research setting using the same equipment, resulting in

Table 11.1 Current criteria for the diagnosis of hypertension using different measurement methods (ESH/ESC Guidelines: Mancia *et al.*, 2013).

Category	Systolic BB (mm Hg)		Diastolic BP (mm Hg)
Office BP	≥140		≥90
Ambulatory BP			
Daytime (or awake)	≥135		≥85
Nighttime (or asleep)	≥120	and/or	≥70
24-hour	≥130		≥80
Home BP	≥135		≥85

significant overdiagnosis of hypertension when used in isolation. By contrast, automated oscillometric equipment, now widely available, gives results comparable to research-quality measurements. The devices are as reliable as auscultation methods in patients with atrial fibrillation (Cloutier *et al.*, 2015).

Where possible, elevated office measurements should be followed up by an out of office assessment, preferably with ambulatory blood pressure monitoring (ABPM) though probably more practical in most circumstances home blood pressure monitoring (HBPM). With this information the second physician visit – ideally within one month – should be sufficient to confirm the diagnosis or otherwise. Even when office measurements are apparently high (e.g. 140–179/90–109 mm Hg) an out of office assessment is recommended in order to exclude white coat hypertension. There is no agreed protocol for home measurements in diagnosis, but a study in UK general practice found that hypertension could be ruled out in most people by using the average of the first five consecutive days of self-monitored blood pressure (Nunan *et al.*, 2015). Current diagnostic criteria are shown in **Table 11.1**.

> **Practice point**
>
> In diagnosing hypertension, always suggest home blood pressure monitoring to confirm (or refute) the clinic results.

White coat and masked hypertension

White coat hypertension is the term for *untreated* individuals where office BP measurements are ≥140/90 mm Hg, while out-of-office measurements are normal. A better descriptive term would be 'isolated clinic hypertension'. It is important to consider this diagnosis early on and the recommended sequence of office measurements followed by confirmation with out of office measurements will usually help, though this idealized sequence is not usually followed in clinical practice, thus leading to a general underappreciation of white coat hypertension. It is more common in diabetes, as is the so-called 'white coat effect' – the same disparity in office compared with out of office measurements in people with *treated* hypertension. The current general view is that white coat hypertension is associated with increased cardiovascular risk and although there are no major longitudinal studies of white coat hypertension in diabetic compared with non-diabetic subjects, it is likely that diabetes carries additional adverse long-term consequences; there may also be higher risks of retinopathy and nephropathy (Kramer *et al.*, 2008).

Irrespective of the cardiovascular risks, there is sound longitudinal evidence that both white coat hypertension and masked hypertension (normal office values, elevated

Box 11.4 Factors associated with white coat hypertension and masked hypertension.

White coat hypertension:
• Age, female gender, non-smoking.
• Increased risk of sustained hypertension.

Masked hypertension:
• Younger age, smoking, alcohol consumption, family history of hypertension.
• Physical activity, exercise-induced hypertension.
• Asymptomatic organ damage.
• Increased risk of diabetes.
• Increased risk of sustained hypertension.
• Anxiety and job stress.
• Obesity, chronic kidney disease.
• Office BP measurements in the high-normal range.

out-of-office measurements) carry a four- to 10-fold increased risk of progressing from normotension to sustained hypertension over 12 years (Sivén *et al.*, 2015). Masked uncontrolled hypertension is common in all treated patients but slightly more so in people with diabetes (prevalence 35% compared with 30% of non-diabetic people). There is a particular burden of poorly-controlled nocturnal hypertension in these patients. It is a high-risk condition that is difficult to diagnose, and overlaps strongly with resistant hypertension (see later) (Banegas *et al.*, 2014). Factors associated with white coat hypertension and masked hypertension are shown in **Box 11.4**.

ANTIHYPERTENSIVE MEDICATION

The higher the baseline blood pressure the greater the fall with a single medication, but the majority of patients require two or more medications for adequate control. In the ACCORD study, an average of 3.4 drugs were needed to achieve the intensive outcome of mean systolic pressure 119 mm Hg and 2.6 drugs in the standard group (mean systolic pressure 134 mm Hg), but a high proportion needed four or five drugs – approximately 16% in the standard group and approximately 40% in the intensive group (ACCORD Study Group, 2010) (**Figure 11.4**). As with glycaemia, achieving ultimate degree of control requires even greater numbers of medications, with higher risks of non-adherence and side effects. Meticulous medicines management is needed.

The stepped therapy approach (initial monotherapy with dose titration) is nearly always still used, but combination therapy with drugs from two drug classes is much more effective. The European Society of Hypertension and European Society of Cardiology joint recommendation is to use combination therapy in high-risk people and those with high baseline blood pressure. Fixed-dose drug combinations of two or three agents have been around a long time, and preparations containing multiple different doses of each component are increasingly available, but in spite of evidence for better adherence they are rarely prescribed and physicians still have an irrational aversion to suggesting them, even though most are available in generic forms.

Nocturnal dosing may be helpful in people with poor control (Rossen *et al.*, 2014). Nocturnal blood pressure predicts cardiovascular events better than daytime values, and a crossover study in Type 2 patients with nocturnal hypertension (mean night-time

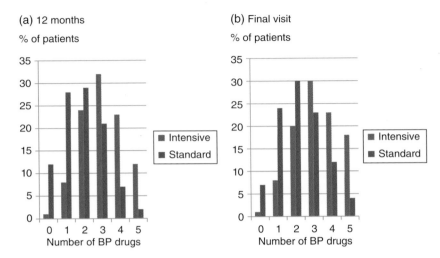

Figure 11.4 Numbers of antihypertensive medications needed (a) at 12 months and (b) at trial end in the ACCORD study (ACCORD Study Group, 2010). Nearly 40% of routinely treated patients required three or more drugs.

systolic >120 mm Hg) reduced mean nocturnal systolic values by 8 mm Hg and 24-h values by 3 mm Hg. Plasma C-reactive protein levels fell and urinary sodium excretion increased.

Practice point

Nocturnal dosing rather than morning dosing can improve control, especially in patients with high nocturnal BP (mean SBP >120 mm Hg)

Dose responses

Most antihypertensive drugs are now old or very old. There are few detailed dose-response studies in large patient groups, and where they have been published they often use diastolic blood pressure as the outcome measure, much less emphasized these days. For example, among the ACE inhibitors, lisinopril and perindopril may be the only agents with a meaningful dose-response relationship. The angiotensin receptor blockers have a small dose range – often only two steps, and the differences between the two doses in practice may not be clinically meaningful (though proteinuria shows a much stronger dose-response relationship, and proteinuric patients always require the higher doses; see **Chapter 4**). However, it is worthwhile remembering that absolute blood pressure reduction with any single agent is not as great as we imagine (though it should be obvious given the polypharmacy needed in all treat-to-target trials – see the example of the ACCORD study). For example, irbesartan, for which there is good dose-response data, reduces blood pressure by approximately 10/6 mm Hg at the full daily 300 mg dose, and approximately 8/5 mm Hg at 150 mg daily – and that was from a high mean baseline average ~150/100 (Reeves et al., 1998).

ANTIHYPERTENSIVE DRUGS

Not very long ago documents were full of protocols recommending specific sequences for the introduction of medication, for example 'ABCD' (angiotensin blocker/β-blocker/calcium channel blocker/diuretic), which rapidly changed to 'ACD' when β-blockers fell out of favour. There is now a sound pluralistic approach, similar to the one we are moving towards in blood glucose control. It recognizes that for a given BP reduction all classes of agents have the same benefits. Drug choices should then be based on the needs of particular groups of patients, and where there are specific contraindications.

Metabolic effects of thiazide diuretics and β-blockers

Since many patients will require three or more antihypertensive agents, it is difficult to avoid these important groups of drugs. There is no reason to do so, as their metabolic effects are minor and, much more importantly, there is no diminution of the beneficial cardiovascular effects when they are used. However, the myths are persistent and there is a trend to avoid them by using the triad of angiotensin blocking agent + calcium channel blocker + doxazosin. Doxazosin is safe and effective, and in the ASCOT study was an effective add-on agent; however, in the Antihypertensive and Lipid-Lowering Treatment to Prevent Heart Attack Trial (ALLHAT) the arm treated primarily with doxazosin was terminated early because of an increased risk of heart failure, and this was especially marked in people with diabetes, where there was a nearly twofold increased risk compared with the group treated with the diuretic chlortalidone (Barzilay et al., 2004). Doxazosin should therefore not be used in preference to a diuretic in diabetes. Patients with difficult hypertension must have a diuretic or they are more likely to develop resistant hypertension, and there is convincing evidence that combined diuretic treatment is invaluable in patients with resistant hypertension (see later).

Are the metabolic effects of these drugs meaningful for people with diabetes? Combined β-blocker and thiazide treatment raises fasting glucose by 0.1–0.3 mmol/l, triglycerides by 0.2–0.5 mmol/l and uric acid by about 20%, changes similar to the variability of the measurement. Beta-blockers have a greater adverse metabolic effect than thiazides, but these can be minimized or avoided using the newer vasodilator agents, for example carvedilol and nebivolol (see later).

There is no doubt that thiazides are associated with a substantially increased risk of developing diabetes (for example during ALLHAT new-onset diabetes occurred in 7.5% of patients treated with chlortalidone, compared with 5.6% in the amlodipine-treated group and 4.3% of those treated with lisinopril). Critically, however, the risk of mortality – cardiovascular, non-cardiovascular and all-cause – was lower in chlortalidone-treated subjects who developed diabetes during the trial than in those treated with amlodipine or lisinopril. (However, the same study also confirms that new-onset diabetes is associated with an approximately 50% increased risk of coronary heart disease compared with those who remain without diabetes; Barzilay et al., 2012.) Yet even in high cardiovascular risk people, chlortalidone emerged as the more valuable drug in reducing meaningful endpoints; so, for example, metabolic syndrome patients (in whom thiazides might be resisted as first line treatment in subjects with 'prediabetes') had fewer cardiovascular events – including heart failure – when treated with chlortalidone, and in black patients with the metabolic syndrome, the risk of stroke was reduced by 35–40% compared with the other agents (Wright *et al.*, 2008). Old habits, however convincing the evidence (and the evidence here is highly convincing), persistently decline repeated invitations to die.

> **Practice point**
>
> Thiazide- and thiazide-like diuretics should be used freely in people with diabetes. Their metabolic effects are minor yet event and mortality reduction is possibly greater than with other classes of drugs.

ANGIOTENSIN BLOCKING AGENTS (ACE INHIBITORS, TABLE 11.2 AND ANGIOTENSIN RECEPTOR BLOCKERS, TABLE 11.3)

These are groups of drugs which rival the statins in their importance in the management of cardiovascular disease – and without much of the statins' unfortunate lot of partisan opinion. The first ACE inhibitor, captopril, was introduced in 1981 and the first angiotensin receptor blocker, losartan, in 1995. Given this venerable age, we are still not as practised in their use as we should be. Traditionally, it is believed that patients with 'low renin' hypertension, especially the elderly and black people, do not respond as well to ACE inhibitors as to other antihypertensives. There is some support for this from ALLHAT, where systolic blood pressure in black subjects was on average 4 mm Hg lower in those treated with chlortalidone compared with lisinopril; more importantly, this translated into a higher risk of stroke with the ACE inhibitor. By contrast, in the important treat-to-target AASK study (Wright *et al.*, 2002), African-Americans with established hypertensive renal disease (eGFR 20-65 ml/min) treated with ramipril had a lower rate of hard renal end points than those taking either metoprolol or amlodipine, though by design achieved blood pressure was the same in all groups. Lack of responsiveness in huge trials cannot be used to justify not using them in individuals, though, especially as most patients will require multiple medications.

Table 11.2 ACE inhibitor agents in widespread use.

	Usual starting dose (mg)	Maximum dose (mg)	Comments
Enalapril	5	40	Serviceable, and used in many clinical trials, but out of fashion
Lisinopril	10	40	A first choice ACE inhibitor, with a documented dose-response relationship in hypertension
Perindopril	4	8	Perindopril arginine is available, starting dose 5 mg increasing to 10 mg daily. Perindopril may also have a valuable dose-response relationship
Ramipril	1.25–2.5	10	Higher doses have been used in RCTs
Trandolapril	0.5	4	

Table 11.3 Angiotensin receptor blocking agents in current use. All are taken once-daily. Where there are two starting doses, use the lower one initially in the elderly >75 years or volume depleted.

	Starting dose (mg)	Maximum dose (mg)
Candesartan	4, 8	32
Eprosartan	300, 600	800
Irbesartan	75, 150	300
Losartan	25, 50	100
Olmesartan	10	20–40
Telmisartan	20	40–80
Valsartan	40, 80	320

Practice point

Black patients may have a weaker blood pressure response to ACE inhibitor treatment than to other agents, but if they are treated to target (which may require additional medication) renal outcomes may be better.

ACE inhibitor or angiotensin receptor blocker?

One drug from either of these classes is a key component of any antihypertensive regimen. Within living memory there have been titanic efforts to demonstrate the superiority of angiotensin receptor blockers to the older ACE inhibitor drugs – to no avail. The ONTARGET study (ONTARGET Investigators, 2008) randomized patients at high cardiovascular risk to an ACE inhibitor (ramipril 10 mg daily), an angiotensin receptor blocker (telmisartan 80 mg daily) or a combination of the two. Although achieved blood pressure was slightly lower in the group treated with telmisartan, there was no difference in major cardiovascular outcomes, nor in intermediate objective measures such as left ventricular mass and volume. Telmisartan carried a slightly higher risk of hypotension (this has been noted in other studies of angiotensin receptor blockers), but ramipril was not as well tolerated (cough and angio-oedema). Importantly, the study was the first large-scale RCT to uncover significant harm as a result of combining ACE inhibitor with angiotensin receptor blocker treatment (see later). Now that drugs of both groups are out of patent protection it is most unlikely there will be further randomized trials that will help us prioritize one group over the other, though a huge meta-analysis confirmed the superiority of ACE inhibitor drugs that reduced all-cause mortality compared with angiotensin receptor blockers (van Vark et al., 2012). In the individual, however, quotidian considerations, such as the importance of using maximum recommended doses, efforts to maintain medication adherence and continued careful follow-up are likely to be more important in determining outcomes than very small blood pressure differences uncovered only in huge analyses, and in many cases these will move practitioners to recommending angiotensin receptor blockers.

Practice point

Where possible start angiotensin blockade treatment with an ACE inhibitor. They may have outcome benefits over angiotensin receptor blockers in hypertension.

Discontinuing and starting angiotensin blocking agents in advanced kidney disease

With such a long and distinguished record of significantly delaying hard renal endpoints, it is disappointing that there is still little information on whether there is a degree of renal impairment beyond which ACE inhibitor or angiotensin receptor blocker treatment is either no longer valuable or even counterproductive or, more important, what the effects are of withdrawing treatment in patients with advanced chronic kidney disease (CKD). There is a general reluctance to stop treatment even in the presence of continually sliding renal function, but persistence may be misplaced. In an observational report of elderly patients with CKD stage G4/5 (mean eGFR 22 ml/min) and heavy proteinuria, of whom nearly 50% had diabetic kidney disease, in the two years after discontinuing angiotensin blockade eGFR increased or remained stable in about 90%. In around one-third of patients eGFR increased by 50% or more and 20–25% changed CKD category. Blood pressure increased slightly but there was no change in proteinuria (Ahmed *et al.*, 2010). Plausible explanations for this phenomenon include reversing the adverse effects of angiotensin blockers on diffuse atherosclerotic disease and intrarenal hypoperfusion in structurally abnormal kidneys. This is an increasingly common clinical scenario and the results of an important trial (STOP-ACEi) will be available around 2019 (Bhandari *et al.*, 2016). A cautious trial of reduction and withdrawal of an angiotensin blocking agent is worthwhile, so long as patients are meticulously monitored. Heart failure would be a contraindication.

Practice point

If renal function continues to fall in patients taking angiotensin blockade in CKD 4–5, there is a case for temporarily withdrawing medication and observing closely for any recovery in renal function.

The converse situation – starting angiotensin blockade in people with established CKD – has a more sound basis, at least in patients with baseline serum creatinine levels in the range 150–280 µmol/l. In practice, this is much less of a problem than discontinuing angiotensin blocking agents because the majority of patients have been taking long-term medication. In non-diabetic nephropathies studied over five years in the REIN trial, ramipril reduced the number of patients entering end-stage renal disease by 30% from a baseline mean creatinine clearance 30 ml/min and serum creatinine 275 µmol/l (Ruggenenti *et al.*, 2001). Young Chinese people with non-diabetic renal disease and advanced renal impairment (mean baseline serum creatinine 350 µmol/l, eGFR 37 ml/min) treated with benazepril had a 40% reduction in renal end points at three years, although this study has been contested, and included patients clinically far removed from usual diabetes patients with renal disease (Hou *et al.*, 2006). In diabetes, patients treated with angiotensin receptor blockers in the RENAAL and IDNT studies, where baseline serum creatinine was 150–170 µmol/l (see **Chapter 4**), had clear benefit in reducing hard renal endpoints.

Adverse effects

Dry cough and angio-oedema

Dry cough is the commonest side-effect of ACE inhibitor treatment and is reported in 10–35% of patients. In an analysis of three large clinical trials of perindopril, it led to the withdrawal of about 4% of patients (Brugts *et al.*, 2014). Around 5–30% of patients, therefore, may experience cough without it causing them to discontinue treatment. It is a specific and unusual side effect and patients may not recognize it as such. Inform patients about the possibility of cough before starting treatment and enquire during the early treatment period. Combining results from this study and a UK primary care database study, cough is more common in:

- women
- people 65 or older
- those taking statins or calcium channel blockers
- people with a history of allergy, and those using anti-asthmatic and antihistamine drugs or taking systemic glucocorticoids

but not in smokers or Asian patients.

Angio-oedema with ACE inhibitor treatment is uncommon, but is the commonest identifiable cause of angio-oedema in the emergency care setting. Since it is probably mediated through the same mechanism as cough, that is, increased bradykinin production, emergency treatment with adrenaline does not help and may harm (Curtis *et al.*, 2016). Although the angio-oedema rate with angiotensin receptor blockers is only about one-third that with ACE inhibitors, about 7% of people with previous ACE inhibitor-associated angioedema develop it with an angiotensin receptor blockers. Because of the potential hazard, documented angio-oedema is a contraindication to both these classes.

Practice point

Angiotensin receptor blockers do not cause dry cough, but they can cause angio-oedema. Do not trial one in someone who has had angio-oedema with an ACE inhibitor.

Changes in renal function and hyperkalaemia

Renal function

Serum creatinine frequently increases after starting an ACE inhibitor, usually within the first four weeks of treatment. It then stabilizes within two months and returns to baseline if medication is discontinued. Vasodilatation of the efferent glomerular vessels, reducing intraglomerular pressure and lowering GFR, is the usual explanation. The average rise in serum creatinine in hypertensive people is approximately 30% but in heart failure a combination of reduced cardiac output, vasodilatation and diuretics can cause a rise of between 75 and 200%. The prognostic benefit of ACE inhibitor treatment, especially in heart failure, is not decreased by these changes in eGFR, which can return to baseline after long-term drug treatment.

In a large study in predominantly non-diabetic hypertensive patients from the early 2000s in which the average rise in serum creatinine was, as expected, 26%, ACE inhibitor discontinuation rates rose with increasing baseline serum creatinine (e.g. 5% in those with serum creatinine <130 µmol/l, 7% with creatinine 130–175 µmol/l and 12% with creatinine >175 µmol/l). Treatment was discontinued in the majority of patients even though the rise in creatinine within three months of starting was less than the usual criteria for stopping treatment (i.e. >30% or >0.5 mg/dl [44 µmol/l]). Cough may be a factor in discontinuation but this would not account for the higher cessation rates with increasing serum creatinine. Factors linked to discontinuation included coprescription of non-steroidal anti-inflammatory drugs, diuretics and β-blockers, but persistence with treatment was more frequent in males and people with heart failure and (surprisingly) baseline systolic blood pressure <100 mm Hg (Jackevicius *et al.*, 2014). This situation is probably unchanged in contemporary practice and in people with diabetes these discontinuation rates are likely to be magnified by concerns over hyperkalaemia.

Practice point

Expect up to a 30% rise in serum creatinine within three months of starting an ACE inhibitor. This is not associated with a worse clinical outcome.

Hyperkalaemia, hyporeninemic hyopoaldosteronism and type IV renal tubular acidosis

Hyperkalaemia, defined as either plasma potassium >5.5 or 6.0 mmol/l, is a real problem in diabetes even in the absence of complications (Sousa *et al.*, 2016). The pathophysiology is complex, the resulting hyperkalaemia common and very troublesome in therapy, and specific treatments few. Contributors include hyperosmolarity, insulin deficiency or resistance, and raised glucagon levels, but there are other factors that come into play once complications develop, especially renal disease, but also autonomic neuropathy; the problem is then further exacerbated by drugs, predominantly angiotensin blockers, but also potassium-sparing diuretics, non-steroidals, calcineurin inhibitors and β-blockers, and a potentially wide variety of alternative and complementary medications. These result in decreased renin synthesis or action, leading to decreased aldosterone secretion, hyporeninaemic hypoaldosteronism and chronic hyperkalaemia. Hyporeninaemic hyperaldosteronism is largely synonymous with type IV renal tubular acidosis.

In most patients with normal renal function, mild hyperkalaemia goes unnoticed until angiotensin blockade treatment starts. In the VA NEPHRON-D trial of dual angiotensin blockade in Type 2 patients with established diabetic renal disease (see **Chapter 4**), significant hyperkalaemia (serum potassium 5.5–6.0 mmol/l) developed in only 4.4% of patients treated with lisinopril 10–40 mg daily, and although patients with baseline serum potassium >5.0 mmo/l were excluded, they were at high risk (male, mean age 64 years, mean eGFR 54 ml/min, and with heavy proteinuria) (Fried *et al.*, 2013). Other studies have identified powerful risk factors for the development of hyperkalaemia: eGFR <45 ml/min and baseline serum potassium >4.5 mmol/l off angiotensin blockade (Lazich and Bakris, 2014). Statistically, angiotensin receptor blocker treatment may cause less hyperkalaemia than ACE inhibitors but in practice in the individual patient there is likely not to be a significant difference.

About one-third of diabetes patients newly-starting angiotensin blockade treatment do not have potassium monitoring; this is a very frequent reason for patients being sent to and admitted to hospital, sometimes recurrently. The general recommendation is for monitoring within a week of starting treatment or increasing the dose; this is sound but arduous for primary care teams and patients alike.

Practice point

Hyperkalaemia is likely if baseline eGFR <45 ml/min and serum potassium >4.5 mmol/l. Check potassium within a week of starting therapy.

There is much guidance on how to manage hyperkalaemia in the common situation of a patient with high-normal baseline serum potassium, depressed eGFR and heavy proteinuria starting on angiotensin blockade treatment, but in practice once culprit drugs have been excluded there is very little to do to ameliorate the problem (Palmer, 2004). Diuretics are uniformly recommended (thiazide, or loop diuretic when eGFR <30 ml/min) but there are no trial data on their efficacy in reducing serum potassium or permitting meaningful angiotensin blockade treatment in this situation. Starting very low-dose medication is recommended but patients often cannot be prescribed even minute doses because of the rapid onset of severe hyperkalaemia and even if they can, token angiotensin blockade will probably have no impact on renal disease or other meaningful outcomes. Rigorous control of blood pressure with other drugs that may have some antiproteinuric effect (non-dihydropyridine calcium channel blockers or β-blockers – though not in combination), optimum glycaemic control and LDL lowering become even more important in this situation.

Pregnancy

Both classes of angiotensin blocking drugs are harmful to the foetus in the second and third trimesters. It is not certain whether exposure in the first trimester is responsible for an increased rate of congenital malformations or whether any increased risk is due to factors associated with the need to take angiotensin blockade (hypertension, other medication, obesity or diabetes itself). Type 1 patients planning pregnancy will probably have been advised to discontinue these drugs and antihypertensives known to be safe during pregnancy substituted in their place. There is probably little harm in discontinuing them as soon as pregnancy has been confirmed; this is a common situation in women with known Type 2 diabetes, where much larger numbers of people will be hypertensive. Diabetic renal disease does not usually progress during pregnancy as long as there is normal renal function, and meticulous control of blood pressure is the most important clinical challenge.

Practice point

Angiotensin blocking agents during the 2nd and 3rd trimesters of pregnancy are toxic to the fetus, but probably not during the 1st. If not already discontinued, do so immediately pregnancy is confirmed.

Dual angiotensin blockade – combination ACE inhibitor and angiotensin receptor blocking treatment

Combination treatment became popular in the early 2000s after small studies reported additional reductions in intermediate measures, especially urinary albumin levels in patients with diabetic renal disease. Clinicians were further encouraged by the results of the COOPERATE trial (2003), which seemed to show a reduction in hard renal endpoints in non-diabetic renal disease, though the data were subsequently shown to have been falsified. There was also some hint of benefit from the complex CHARM series of studies in heart failure. There were, however, no data in patients with uncomplicated hypertension, but many patients with resistant or not-so-resistant hypertension ended up taking this combination. The rather sorry saga up to 2010 is reported by Messerli et al. (2010).

The ONTARGET study recruited patients at high cardiovascular risk, but not primarily hypertensive. Treatment was with ramipril or telmisartan or a combination of the two. Attained blood pressure was slightly lower in the telmisartan group but there was no difference in cardiovascular outcomes between the three groups. Combination therapy was associated with an increased risk of adverse effects (hypotension, syncope, and approximately 3% absolute increased risk of physician-defined renal dysfunction leading to discontinuation of the drug) and a trend towards more patients needing dialysis for acute kidney injury (ONTARGET Investigators, 2008).

In Type 2 patients with renal or cardiovascular disease, or both, dual therapy with the direct renin inhibitor aliskiren and an angiotensin receptor blocker in the ALTITUDE trial showed no reduction in cardiorenal end points (though blood pressure and albumin-creatinine ratio decreased to a greater extent in the dual-therapy group). Significant hyperkalaemia (serum potassium ≥6.0 mmol/l) occurred in 11% of the dual-therapy group compared with 7% in the single-therapy group, and hypotension was more common. There was a trend towards physician-defined renal dysfunction resulting in medication being stopped but no reports of dialysis being required (Parving et al., 2012). There were minor improvements in progression of albuminuria in Type 2 patients in ALTITUDE, but no differences in composite renal endpoints.

The results of the VA NEPHRON-D study (see **Chapter 4**) should finally have relegated dual angiotensin blockade to the annals of heroic negative studies in diabetes and thereby to therapeutic oblivion. But this – see later for the strangely analogous situation with renal denervation – has not quite happened. Regret at the unfulfilled promise of a therapy that has been studied for a long time is understandable, but pleas for further trials and for more studies that may allow selection of groups of patients to benefit from this treatment are misplaced, although sustained by general promissory claims of the pharmacogenomics industry. Messerli's statement in 2010 was clear then and now even more so: '…given the adverse effects and lack of consistent survival benefits, the use of dual renin angiotensin system blockade should be avoided unless ironclad data emerge to the contrary' (Messerli et al., 2010).

Practice point

Dual angiotensin blockade is of no advantage, may do harm and should not be used. Take active measures to find patients who are still taking combination treatment and ensure that only one agent is continued.

CALCIUM CHANNEL BLOCKERS

Dihydropyridine drugs (e.g. amlodipine, nifedipine)

Calcium channel blockers are the best 'broad-spectrum' antihypertensives. They are even older than ACE inhibitors; the prototype, nifedipine, was introduced in the 1970s, amlodipine, now the most widely prescribed, in the early 1990s. The dihydropyridines lower blood pressure as efficiently as any other group of drugs and have a rapid action that makes them valuable in hypertensive emergencies – but, as in the IDNT trial, where amlodipine was trialled against irbesartan, it neither reduced proteinuria nor delayed the onset of significant renal endpoints. However, amlodipine is particularly effective in reducing stroke risk in diabetes and, importantly, in renal disease there is no difference in cardiovascular events with amlodipine compared with any other antihypertensive drugs (Jeffers et al., 2015). In monotherapy there may be a slight increase in the risk of heart failure but this clearly does not have an impact on mortality outcomes. They are metabolically neutral and seem to be of particular benefit in high cardiovascular risk patients (see later). Nifedipine, the prototype agent, has largely been eradicated from therapeutic consciousness, partly because of confusion over the many preparations available.

> **Practice point**
>
> Amlodipine is as effective as angiotensin blocking drugs in reducing cardiovascular endpoints in diabetes, with or without impaired renal function.

The non-dihydropyridine drugs (diltiazem and verapamil)
The non-dihydropyridine calcium channel blockers diltiazem and verapamil are of the same vintage as the dihydropyridines. They are as effective in blood pressure reduction but much less widely used, especially verapamil, which has significant negative inotropic effects; cardiologists favour them for their antiarrhythmic properties when β-blockers are contraindicated. They seem to have some proteinuria-reducing activity, perhaps up to 20%, but there are very few studies and none of renal outcomes. Longer-acting formulations must be used for hypertension. Different formulations have different ranges of strengths and maximum recommended doses; the British National Formulary recommends they are prescribed by brand name.

Adverse effects
All calcium channel blockers can cause initial headache. Peripheral oedema is common. Amlodipine is often prescribed at the higher 10 mg dose and this frequently causes ankle swelling (12%, compared with 8% taking the 5 mg dose) (Ganz et al., 2005). Reduce the dose if it is troublesome to the patient, but in the ACCOMPLISH study (where even higher oedema rates were reported; see later) there were endpoint advantages of the higher dose, especially in Type 2 patients. There is an interaction with simvastatin and 20 mg is the highest dose recommended when coprescribed with calcium channel blockers. Gum hypertrophy is associated with all drugs, including amlodipine, and can be severe. This is important in people with diabetes who are already predisposed to gingival disease and periodontitis.

Combination treatment with a calcium channel blocker and ACE inhibitor – ASCOT-BPLA and ACCOMPLISH studies
There are huge numbers of clinical trials exploring combination therapy. In non-diabetic patients, the ASCOT-BPLA trial used a combination that was standard at the time the study was designed – a β-blocker and bendroflumethiazide – and compared it with amlodipine and perindopril (Dahlöf et al., 2005). Cardiovascular event rates and new-onset diabetes were lower in the amlodipine-perindopril group, but analysis of cardiovascular outcomes was hampered by its greater blood pressure lowering effects. Post hoc statistical matching hinted that clinical benefits were greater than would be expected on account of the differences in attained blood pressure, but this interpretation was considered too tenuous for recommending a change in treatment strategy.

However, a later trial – ACCOMPLISH – supported the provisional conclusions of ASCOT-BPLA and is particularly important because it recruited a high proportion of people with diabetes, and because attained blood pressure in both treatment arms were indistinguishable. By this time – some five years after ASCOT-BPLA (2010) – β-blockers had fallen out of favour as a mainstay of hypertension treatment. The most striking finding of the ACCOMPLISH study was that despite identical achieved blood pressure (132/73 mm Hg) in the groups taking a combination of the ACE inhibitor benazepril and amlodipine and those taking benazepril and hydrochlorothiazide there was a 2.2% difference in absolute risk reduction (20% relative risk reduction) in the primary cardiovascular outcomes favouring benazepril with amlodipine: the same difference was observed in diabetic and non-diabetic subjects. There were additional benefits in diabetes, for example reduction in the risk of an acute coronary event and revascularizations. In those judged to be at very high risk (previous cardiovascular or stroke events) absolute risk benefit was even greater at 3.7% (Weber *et al.*, 2010). Separation of outcomes in favour of benazepril-amlodipine occurred as early as 3–4 months. Since all patients were taking an ACE inhibitor, there was no difference between the treatment groups in the incidence of dry cough (21%), but with the amlodipine combination, 30% had peripheral oedema compared with 13% in the hydrochlorothiazide combination.

Practice point

The higher dose of amlodipine (10 mg daily) often causes ankle swelling, but in the ACCOMPLISH trial it had endpoint advantages when combined with an ACE inhibitor.

ACCOMPLISH contrasts with previous studies, including ALLHAT, in demonstrating a clear cardiovascular benefit of specific drugs beyond that of blood pressure lowering. It supports initial combination therapy in high-risk subjects, even if blood pressure does not reach the consensus level of the Seventh Report of the Joint National Committee on Prevention, Detection, Evaluation, and Treatment of High Blood Pressure (JNC 7) for starting a combination i.e. ≥20/10 mm Hg higher than treatment goals.

Further information on optimum progression of treatment may come with the results of a three-phase trial in the important PATHWAY series (there are some details on published studies later). This will randomize newly-diagnosed and known hypertensives previously on monotherapy to either monotherapy or combination therapy, then to open-label combination, and finally open-label combination with add-on therapy if blood pressure is still uncontrolled at >140/90 mm Hg (MacDonald *et al.*, 2015).

Practice point

Combination treatment with a calcium channel blocker and an ACE inhibitor is the preferred initial combination for reducing the risks of many vascular outcomes in high-risk patients.

THIAZIDES AND THIAZIDE-LIKE DIURETICS

Although the ALLHAT monotherapy trial reported after the turn of the millennium, it was designed in the 1990s when it was still not clear whether the thiazide diuretics, in use since the late 1950s, should be recommended as first line treatment. The comparator drug in the ALLHAT was the thiazide-like compound chlortalidone, widely used in many other clinical trials. The primary cardiovascular outcomes in ALLHAT were no different whether patients were treated with chlortalidone, lisinopril or amlodipine, but blood pressure control in this enormous trial was slightly better with chlortalidone than the other agents; this, in part, may have accounted for the reduced rate of stroke and heart failure with chlortalidone. A background concern may also have been the cost of the newer drugs compared with the diuretics whose patents had long expired. This is no longer significant in developed healthcare systems, as all antihypertensive drugs are now available in generic form.

Choice of thiazide diuretic

In people with diabetes unwarranted concerns about the adverse effects of diuretics still prevent these extremely valuable drugs being used (see previously). A broader difficulty is the lack of comparative clinical trials and even of studies of dose-responses for individual agents, resulting in heroic but indirect statistical attempts to compare the efficacy of different drugs. The clinician understandably remains perplexed by the lack of evidence, and worse by the capriciousness of the market. For example, hydrochlorothiazide is available in the United Kingdom only in the dose range 12.5–25 mg and in fixed-dose combinations, usually with angiotensin blocking drugs, but also with other diuretics. For example, the unjustly obsolete combination of hydrochlorothiazide with the potassium-sparing diuretic amiloride (e.g. hydrochlorothiazide 25 mg/amiloride 2.5 mg daily) was shown in the large INSIGHT study to have an identical effect on cardiovascular outcomes to modified-release once-daily nifedipine 30 mg daily (Brown *et al.*, 2000). However, when used alone, hydrochlorothiazide is probably more effective in the 25–50 mg dose range.

Chlortalidone, widely used in drug trials, is a very effective antihypertensive with a long action and emerged as a drug of choice in UK guidelines (NICE, 2011). In trials the minimum effective dose of chlortalidone is 12.5–25 mg daily (**Table 11**.4). In the United Kingdom it is a difficult drug to source and the last thing needed in a condition that depends on maximum adherence is uncertainty of supplies.

Bendroflumethiazide is much less widely used out of the United Kingdom, and there are few modern studies, but it has a flatter dose-response relationship than other agents.

Table 11.4 Thiazide and thiazide-like diuretics.

	Elimination half-life (h)	Usual dose range (mg)	Approximate dose for therapeutic equivalence (mg)	Comments
Bendroflumethiazide	9	2.5–5	2.5	The 2.5 mg dose is universally used
Hydrochlorothiazide	3–13	12.5–25	50	In the UK hydrochlorothiazide is not available as a single agent. It is widely combined as 12.5 or 25 mg options with other agents, especially angiotensin blockers. The 12.5 mg dose is subtherapeutic
Chlortalidone (chlorthalidone)	40–60	12.5–50	25	Potent and long acting (an occasional missed dose is probably secure) but not reliably available in the UK. Neither patients nor their doctors are experienced with it
Indapamide	14	2.5 (immediate release) 1.5 (modified release)	2.5/1.5	Minimal metabolic adverse effects. Widely-available, and in the UK currently the diuretic of choice for hypertension

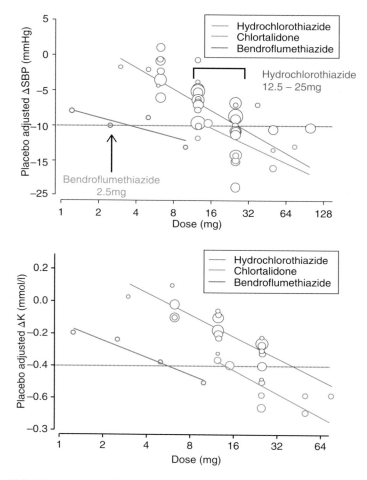

Figure 11.5 Dose-response relationships for thiazide diuretics. Upper panel: systolic blood pressure; lower panel: serum potassium. Bendroflumethiazide has a relatively flat dose-response relationship and at the usual dose of 2.5 mg daily is effective. Chlortalidone is more potent than hydrochlorothiazide at its usual dose of 12.5 or 25 mg daily. The hypokalaemic effect parallels the antihypertensive potency of these three agents. *Source*: Peterzan *et al.*, 2012. Reproduced with permission of Wolters Kluwer Health, Inc.

The 2.5 mg dose is widely prescribed (Peterzan *et al.*, 2012), though 1.25 mg was used in ASCOT-BPLA; 5 mg daily is slightly more effective, but little used. Dose-response relationships for these agents are shown in **Figure 11.5**.

Potassium-sparing diuretics

The aldosterone antagonist spironolactone has a particularly valuable role in patients with resistant hypertension (see later) but amiloride, previously widely used in combination with a thiazide, is valuable both in blood pressure reduction and because in combination at a dose of 10 mg it neutralizes the adverse effects of hydrochlorothiazide 25 mg daily on glucose and potassium levels, though it has not been studied in diabetes (Brown *et al.*, 2016). Eplerenone, a more recent aldosterone antagonist, is used in primary aldosteronism with bilateral adrenal disease and, as with spironolactone, there is some evidence it benefits proteinuria independently of its blood pressure lowering effects. Its main licensed indication is heart failure. There are no large-scale studies in diabetic hypertension. Hyperkalaemia, especially when used in combination with an angiotensin blocking agent, was highlighted early on as a concern and it was less effective than spironolactone in reducing diastolic blood pressure in a randomized study in patients with primary hyperaldosteronism. However, this same study confirmed that there was a much lower rate of male gynaecomastia (5% compared with 20% with spironolactone) and also of the less well-recognized side effect of breast pain in women (0% compared with 20%) (Parthasarathy *et al.*, 2011).

Indapamide

The thiazide-like drug indapamide is emerging as a valuable agent and is thought to be more potent than hydrochlorothiazide. By diuretic standards it is a relatively new drug, developed in the late 1970s, and has been used in several studies, though few that are comparative. In the HYVET study in the relatively healthy very elderly (mean age 83 years, only about 7% with diabetes), primary treatment of sustained systolic blood pressure >160 mm Hg with modified-release indapamide 1.5 mg daily, followed if necessary by low dose perindopril, 2–4 mg daily, had a profound effect in reducing stroke, all-cause death and heart failure (Beckett *et al.*, 2008). Modified-release indapamide is, moreover, glucose and lipid-neutral and carries a lower risk of hypokalaemia (<3.4 mmol/l) than the 2.5 mg immediate-release form, though it raises serum urate to the same extent as other diuretics.

Practice point

Chlortalidone is probably the most effective diuretic for hypertension but few clinicians have experience of it and it is not reliably available in the United Kingdom. Indapamide 2.5 mg daily (or modified-release 1.5 mg daily) is the best practical alternative.

Efficacy of thiazides in renal impairment

Thiazide and thiazide-like diuretics are widely thought to be ineffective once eGFR falls to <30 ml/min. Guidelines are strangely muted on this common therapeutic problem but expert opinion is that a thiazide should be replaced by a loop diuretic given twice daily – despite the poor adherence that inevitably results from the heavy diuresis – or perhaps supplementing the thiazide with a low-dose loop diuretic if there is oedema: both strategies will probably require specialist input (Elliott and Jurca, 2016). There is tentative evidence from a handful of small studies that adding hydrochlorothiazide or chlortalidone 25 mg daily to existing non-diuretic therapy in CKD G4/5 may have significant effects on blood pressure.

Practice point

Thiazides are ineffective below an eGFR of 30 ml/min.

Side effects: hyponatraemia and hypokalaemia

Thiazide-associated hyponatraemia is frequent and is the commonest identifiable cause of hyponatraemia requiring hospital admission. It is impossible to estimate accurately its incidence, because the two main contributors – extracellular volume depletion and syndrome of inappropriate ADH secretion (SIADH) – are common in people, especially the elderly, admitted to hospital (though there are many other possible pathogenic mechanisms operating). But in the SHEP trial of chlortalidone in the elderly, severe hyponatraemia (serum sodium <130 mmol/l) was common – 4% of patients compared with 1% of control patients. Given the high usage of thiazide diuretics, this represents a real clinical problem (Liamis *et al.*, 2016).

They key to preventing severe hyponatraemia with its associated neurological morbidity is meticulous biochemical monitoring. A valuable review (Barber *et al* 2015) established that severe hyponatraemia has a rapid onset after starting treatment (average three weeks, range between 8 and 30 days) and is usually associated with marked hypokalaemia (mean serum potassium 3.3 mmol/l), which may perpetuate the hyponatraemia. The vulnerable patient needs frequent biochemical monitoring in the first two months of treatment. The risk factors for severe hyponatraemia are well-established (**Box 11.5**). Of importance is definite but mild hyponatraemia before starting treatment, of a degree that may not be highlighted in routine biochemical reports, for example serum sodium approximately 135 mmol/l.

Most patients taking a thiazide will develop a lower serum potassium: in meta-analysis the mean fall is -0.2 mmol/l. The situation is the same as with sodium: be aware of the patients whose baseline serum potassium is borderline low, for example approximately 3.5 mmol/l, another result which might not be flagged up in automated biochemistry reports. The time course of hypokalaemia is not known, but its degree is dose-dependent (**Figure 11.5**).

Practice point

Serum potassium is likely to drop by about 0.2 mmol/l when starting a thiazide. Measure electrolytes frequently in patients with pre-existing borderline low serum potassium, and especially if there is ischaemic heart disease. Hyponatraemia is more frequent in patients with baseline low-normal serum sodium.

Box 11.5 Risk factors for thiazide-associated hyponatraemia in the elderly.

- Female.
- Type 2 diabetes (possible contribution from severe hyperglycaemia).
- Low-normal or unmeasured pretreatment sodium levels.
- Multiple comorbidities.
- Low body mass index (e.g. ~25).
- Co-administration of drugs affecting water homoeostasis, for example NSAIDs, SSRIs, benzodiazepines.
- Co-administration of amiloride or spironolactone.

Source: Adapted from Liamis *et al.*, 2016.

OTHER AGENTS

Beta-blockers

The heyday of β-blocker trials was between 1985 and 2005. There have been none since the ASCOT-BPLA 2005 trial, nor are there likely to be. Evidence for their use is now based mostly on meta-analysis of the 30 years of RCTs. They are widely viewed as ineffective – though their potency in lowering blood pressure is similar to that of other classes of agents – but there are recurrent hints from RCTs that outcomes for the same degree of blood pressure lowering may not be as good, for example stroke reduction in the over-60s. Their adverse metabolic effects and concern that they may not reduce central blood pressure as much as other agents have been frequently cited as reasons for the lack of uniformly beneficial outcomes, seen most dramatically in the diabetic substudy of LIFE (Lindholm *et al.*, 2002), where, for a similar degree of blood pressure reduction, losartan was much more effective in reducing cardiovascular outcomes in people with left ventricular hypertrophy.

Similar to the situation with diuretics, it is not clear what the optimum doses of the traditional β-blockers are, especially atenolol, previously used in high doses with a high associated rate of significant side effects. Currently they are used at only 25–50% of the maximum recommended doses, which fortunately are probably effective in cardioprotection. Even in clinical situations where they were particularly effective, for example angina, they have been supplanted by the calcium channel blockers and other agents. Traditional β-blockers have been replaced by the newer generation of metabolically neutral vasodilating dual α- and β-blockers (carvedilol and nebivolol), though they are not as effective in lowering blood pressure as traditional agents and there is no evidence for increased effect at doses higher than the recommended starting dose (e.g. 12.5 mg twice daily for carvedilol and the fixed single dose of 5 mg daily for nebivolol) (Wong *et al.*, 2015). The quality of evidence for blood pressure lowering is poor: these agents were introduced in the late 1980s and early 1990s without full-scale comparative Phase 3 RCTs, but with an emphasis on smaller physiological studies demonstrating their benign metabolic profile.

> **Practice point**
>
> The newer β-blockers, for example carvedilol and nebivolol, while metabolically neutral are less effective than traditional β-blockers in reducing blood pressure. Heart failure should remain their primary indication.

Alpha-blocking agents

The α-blockers have a long history, starting with the now obsolete prazosin. Immediate-release doxazosin was introduced in the mid-1980s, but inevitably studies compared it mostly with atenolol, then a first-line treatment. The modified-release form, now preferred, was introduced around the millennium. Investigation of its antihypertensive properties has been diluted somewhat by the energy devoted to other therapeutic areas, especially benign prostatic hypertrophy, and its metabolic profile. Only tentative conclusions about its current status can be gleaned from the two major comparative trials which used the modified-release form: ALLHAT and ASCOT-BPLA. The primary cardiovascular outcomes in the doxazosin arm of ALLHAT were similar to those using other drugs, though more add-on drugs were needed compared with the chlortalidone group. The increased risk of heart failure was robust in analysis, leading to the doxazosin arm being discontinued. In the ASCOT-BPLA trial modified-release open-label doxazosin 4–8 mg daily was added to the existing two trial agents if blood pressure was >140/90 mm Hg (or >130/80 in people with diabetes) (Chapman *et al.*, 2008). Mean fall after a year taking doxazosin was 11/7 mm Hg. There was no increase in heart failure, in contrast with ALLHAT, and this may be another example of an adverse effect exposed in a monotherapy trial being balanced by other agents when used in multiple therapies. In the PATHWAY-2 study in resistant hypertension (see later), doxazosin was less effective than spironolactone but was about as effective as bisoprolol. Modified-release doxazosin is therefore a moderately effective antihypertensive agent but should not be used in preference to a diuretic.

Practice point

The modified-release form of doxazosin should always be used in hypertension, starting at 4 mg daily. Side effects include dry mouth and erectile/ejaculatory dysfunction.

Other agents

A raft of other drugs have niche places in specialist areas of hypertension management, particularly in pregnancy where the once-popular dual α/β blocker labetalol is now confined, as is the poorly-tolerated methyldopa. Both require multiple daily dosing. The centrally-acting agent moxonidine was briefly popular but most people developed troublesome side effects. It should not be used. Hydralazine and minoxidil are frequently mentioned and almost never prescribed. However, the main therapeutic reason to avoid these drugs in general clinical practice is because patients requiring them nearly always have resistant or refractory hypertension, and there are now much clearer approaches to patients with this common and threatening problem – and they do not involve these drugs.

RESISTANT HYPERTENSION

Undoubtedly the favourite hypertension topic of the past few years, in part because of the meteoric appearance of renal denervation treatment in resistant hypertension, but also because many careful recent studies have reminded us how common the problem is. Most important, there is also a series of elegant old-fashioned physiological studies, now almost a thing of the past, that offer us sound guidance in the use of drugs that often cost pennies – and also an approach to clinical trials that is refreshingly different from that of the megatrials.

Background

Definitions vary slightly. The European Society of Hypertension (ESH) and JNC 7 define resistant hypertension as blood pressure ≥140/90 mm Hg in non-diabetic individuals, and ≥140/85 in diabetes (ESH) or >130/80 (JNC 7). Patients will be prescribed and adherent to agents from three antihypertensive classes including a diuretic and after exclusion of a secondary cause of hypertension. Unpacking the definition is complex; is it, as Brown frames the problem, a definitive subtype of hypertension, or an artefact of blood pressure measurement (white-coat, for example) or poor adherence to treatment (Brown, 2014)? Even the once clear-cut repertoire of secondary causes of hypertension is blurred by the emergence in several studies of a high prevalence of hyperaldosteronism that does not amount to Conn syndrome or even diffuse nodular hyperplasia of the adrenals but which outweighs by orders of magnitude the 'traditional' secondary causes, mostly associated with rare endocrine disorders. Further complexity has been added now that it is relatively easy to measure metabolites of antihypertensive agents in urine; for example, nearly one-quarter of patients referred for renal denervation had no detectable drugs in their urine. But regardless of its multiple causes it is common. In one large study it was found in 18% of diabetic patients, a prevalence about twice that of the non-diabetic population (Daugherty et al., 2012). Short-term cardiovascular morbidity and mortality is high.

> **Practice point**
>
> Resistant hypertension in diabetes is ≥140/85 mm Hg (ESH) or >130/80 (JNC 7) in people reliably taking three antihypertensives, including a diuretic.

Approach to the diagnosis of resistant hypertension

The diagnosis of resistant hypertension requires the same careful approach as that of newly-diagnosed hypertension: careful repeated BP measurements, as in making the diagnosis of hypertension, emphasizing home and ambulatory measurements to help exclude the white-coat effect. Once confirmed, consider the list of important reasons for poor blood pressure control not related to blood pressure itself (**Box 11.6**). The use of drugs that either antagonize antihypertensive agents (e.g. NSAIDs, which antagonize all drugs apart from calcium channel blockers) or themselves cause hypertension should be carefully explored. Few modern prescribed drugs will do this, but always remember to enquire sensitively about herbal supplements (e.g. ginseng) and anabolic steroids and cocaine. Remember the important contribution of excess alcohol and salt (see previously).

Secondary causes of hypertension

About 15% of hypertensive patients are usually stated to have a secondary (identifiable) underlying medical diagnosis and there is a standard list: primary renal disease, oral contraceptive use, obstructive sleep apnoea, cardiac rarities such as coarctation of the

> **Box 11.6** Causes of 'pseudo-resistant' hypertension.
>
> - Poor BP measuring technique.
> - White-coat effect.
> - Poor adherence:
>   - side effects
>   - complicated dosing regimen
>   - poor education and understanding
>   - memory, psychiatric problems.
> - Poor prescribing:
>   - inadequate doses (often of diuretic)
>   - inappropriate combinations
>   - inadequate use of appropriate combinations.
> - Physician inertia.
>
> *Source*: Adapted from Sarafidis and Bakris, 2008.

aorta – and endocrine disorders. In turn, these include Cushing's syndrome, phaeochromocytoma (which is as often associated with sustained hypertension as with the classical paroxysmal events) and primary hyperaldosteronism due to a Conn's adrenal adenoma. Fascinating but very rare syndromes associated with hypertension include defects in the family of 11β-hydroxysteroid dehydrogenase enzymes. In these conditions, presenting, as does Conn's syndrome, with hypokalaemia and hypertension (hence the term 'apparent mineralocorticoid excess'), it is not excess aldosterone, but excess cortisol which mediates elevated blood pressure, either through excessive activity (11βHSD1) or loss of glucocorticoid deactivation in the better-defined autosomal recessive 11βHSD2 deficiency. Intensive research is continuing to clarify the role of these important enzymes in more subtle manifestations of hypertension and the metabolic syndrome. In the clinical situation, it is less appropriate to consider the other items in the usual list of endocrine 'causes' of hypertension (e.g. acromegaly, hypo- and hyperthyroidism, hyperparathyroidism, vitamin D deficiency), which are associated with hypertension but almost never present with a primary query about blood pressure.

Investigations in people with resistant hypertension

The extensive list of investigations that patients endured in the past can now be shortened. We need not look for renal artery stenosis, as interventions are of no value. In the context of resistant hypertension diagnosing obstructive sleep apnoea is not helpful either, as hypertension does not meaningfully respond to treatment with continuous positive airway pressure. There should be increasing focus on diagnosing important endocrine causes (see Further reading):

- *Cushing's syndrome*: the best initial screening test is the overnight dexamethasone suppression test. A single dose of 1 mg dexamethasone orally is taken at 10:00 p.m. and a single serum cortisol taken the following day at 9:00 a.m. The normal response is complete suppression of cortisol (<50 nmol/l). Other tests used in different centres include two or three 24-hour urinary free cortisol measurements, two late-night salivary cortisol measurements, or first line in many endocrine centres, the low-dose dexamethasone suppression test.
- *Phaeochromocytoma*: triplicated 24-hour urinary free catecholamines, or simpler, where available, spot plasma metanephrines.
- *Primary hyperaldosteronism*: There is no agreement on who to screen but patients with resistant hypertension and those with either spontaneous or diuretic-induced hypokalaemia must be investigated. However, note that in most cases serum potassium is normal. The first step is to demonstrate true hyperaldosteronism with a random plasma aldosterone/renin ratio. Beta-blockers (which block renin release) should be stopped two weeks before testing and spironolactone six weeks before. Stable angiotensin blocking treatment can continue and calcium channel blockers and doxazosin are fine.

The protocol for testing will vary between centres, as will the reference ranges. The specimen should be taken into an EDTA container (purple top in the United Kingdom) and should be in the laboratory within 30 minutes. Do not transfer the sample on ice, which can increase pro-renin to renin conversion. Imperial College's endocrine department (UK) interprets aldosterone/renin ratios as follows:

>1700: Conn likely if renin <0.3 pmol/ml/h
850–1700: possible Conn, investigate further
<680 Conn unlikely

For diagnosis of Conn:

Plasma renin <0.3 pmol/ml/h (reference range 0.5–3.1)
Aldosterone usually >275 pmol/l (reference range 90–700), so may be normal or high

Thereafter, the recommended sequence is then an adrenal CT scan, adrenal vein sampling and laparoscopic adrenalectomy for a culprit adenoma. The field is moving rapidly and specialist endocrinology and radiology is always needed, but a properly measured aldosterone/renin ratio will move along the diagnosis more quickly in many centres.

The spectrum of hyperaldosteronism

It is becoming clear that the spectrum of hyperaldosteronism with an inappropriately low plasma renin but with no radiological evidence of adrenal adenoma or bilateral hyperplasia is broadening, and comprises approximately 10% of all hypertension, increasing to approximately 20–25% of patients with resistant hypertension, of whom only around one-half will have a unilateral adenoma (Brown, 2014). There is no reason to think that this prevalence is lower in people with diabetes, though there are no large studies. However, fewer than 50% of older people with aldosterone-producing adenomas are cured of hypertension and now that plasma aldosterone/renin measurements are relatively simple, younger people with difficult to control hypertension warrant a random measurement and an adrenal-protocol CT; laparoscopic adrenalectomy may well cure the condition without the need for long-term drug therapy. Type 1 diabetes does not preclude a coexisting secondary cause of hypertension and, given the growing importance of hypertension and premature vascular disease in this group, we should be especially vigilant.

Once endocrine tests are completed and negative and causes of pseudo-resistant hypertension excluded as far as possible, the key drug is spironolactone. In the PATHWAY-2 study in which 12% of participants had Type 2 diabetes, spironolactone at a dose of 25–50 mg daily was more effective than modified-release doxazosin 4–8 mg or bisoprolol 5–10 mg daily in reducing systolic blood pressure when added to standard triple therapy (angiotensin blocker, diuretic and calcium channel blocker) (Williams *et al.*, 2015) (**Figure 11.6**). The tolerability of spironolactone was impressive: discontinuations because of the typical side-effects of spironolactone – hyperkalaemia and gynaecomastia – were no more frequent than in the placebo-treated group. At baseline this group had a strictly normal mean potassium (4.1 mmol/l: patients were excluded if they had serum potassium outside the normal range on two occasions, i.e. usually >5.0 mmol/l). Serum potassium increased by a mean of 0.4 mmol/l in the spironolactone arm, and hyperkalaemia is likely to limit the use of this otherwise valuable drug in Type 2 diabetes (see previously). An important therapeutic pointer uncovered in this trial was that spironolactone shows a clear dose-response relationship in resistant hypertension, at least in the 25–50 mg dose range, whereas there was no evidence for such a relationship with either doxazosin or bisoprolol (see previously).

Practice point

In treatment-resistant hypertension, consider the careful use of spironolactone, which is more effective than doxazosin or bisoprolol. Hyperkalaemia is a limiting factor and requires frequent and regular laboratory monitoring.

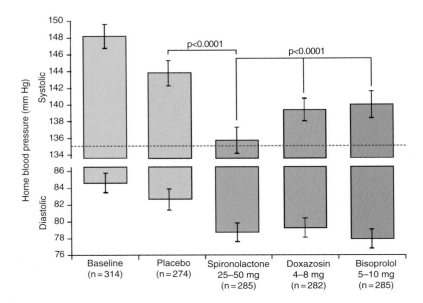

Figure 11.6 Blood pressure responses in the PATHWAY-2 study. Adding spironolactone was more impressive in treatment-resistant patients already taking recommended triple therapy than either doxazosin or bisoprolol, though all three agents had a detectable effect. *Source*: Williams *et al.*, 2015. Reproduced with permission of Elsevier.

Refractory hypertension

A more severe phenotype than resistant hypertension, refractory hypertension was defined in the REGARDS study as blood pressure ≥140/90 mm Hg while taking five or more classes of antihypertensive drugs (Calhoun *et al.*, 2014). This study oversampled black Americans and patients from the areas of the USA with very high stroke incidence (stroke buckle and belt). The overall prevalence of refractory hypertension was only 0.5%, but blacks had a threefold increased risk and people with diabetes a twofold increased risk. **Box 11.7** outlines the characteristics of these patients.

This group of patients is a major challenge, because in addition to possible diagnostic problems with drug side effects, poor adherence and white-coat hypertension, the prognosis is poor. But vigorous LDL reduction, reasonable glycaemic control and repeated education about salt, alcohol and weight reduction and increased activity will always be of substantial benefit if achieved. Specialist advice for medication review and refining diuretic therapy and introducing is important.

The meteoric rise and evidence-based fall of renal denervation

Invasive treatments for resistant hypertension, renal denervation and, more recently, baroreceptor stimulation were almost unheard of as recently as 2010. Renal denervation is a procedure based on sound physiology where radiofrequency energy applied to the renal artery wall is used to disrupt afferent and efferent sympathetic nerves. After the positive results of two preliminary trials, a bold, large, single-blinded trial – critically, using a sham control procedure – was published in 2014 (SYMPLICITY HTN-3). This

> **Box 11.7** Characteristics of USA patients with refractory hypertension (Calhoun *et al.*, 2014.)
>
> - Black ethnicity.
> - High BMI (33).
> - More social deprivation.
> - Impaired renal function (eGFR ≤60 in 35%).
> - Diabetes (two-thirds of patients).
> - Prior stroke or CHD.
> - Higher prevalence of depressive symptoms, but lower prevalence of heavy alcohol intake.
> - Low usage of drugs thought to be effective in resistant hypertensive states (chlortalidone 4%, amiloride 0%, mineralocorticoid receptor antagonist, 18%).
> - No differences in smoking status, medication adherence (90%) or DASH diet score.

was a study in a large group of patients with resistant hypertension, office systolic blood pressure ≥160 mm Hg and mean 24-hour ambulatory pressure ≥135 mm Hg. At six months there was no difference in achieved BP between the two groups (office systolic pressure fell by 12–14 mm Hg, ABPM by 5–7 mm Hg). Sham-treated patients could undergo denervation after six months if they fulfilled the original criteria; six months after their procedure they had a similar response to the original treated group. In those who did not have a procedure, office blood pressure reduction was very large at six months, probably reflecting increased adherence, but substantially attenuated at 12 months. Over 40% of the SYMPLICITY HTN-3 patients had Type 2 diabetes; results were identical to non-diabetic participants (Bakris *et al.*, 2015).

The apparent simplicity of the SYMPLICITY trial and its outcome is complicated by substantial questions of adherence (urine metabolites were not measured), white-coat effects, statistical matters such as regression to the mean, whether the procedures were technically complete, and the known difficulties of managing medication in people with complicated hypertension compared with the lure of a device-based 'cure'. Trials of renal denervation are still reporting and the debate on its value is as furious as ever, but the outlook for the procedure is not looking promising. For example, a randomized study of renal denervation compared with additional spironolactone in people with mean baseline systolic pressure 155–160 mm Hg found that both interventions had a similar effect (mean 24-hour reduction of 6–8 mm Hg systolic pressure); but in the admittedly less robust per-protocol analysis, spironolactone was significantly more effective (e.g. 15 mm compared with 6 mm reduction) (Rosa *et al.*, 2016).

A clear-cut answer on the effectiveness and indications for renal denervation may never emerge but in clinical practice it currently is not an option recognizing more optimistically that very few patients will have truly refractory hypertension using sophisticated combination drug therapy. There is a flurry of interest in carotid baroreceptor stimulation, which is a much older concept even than renal denervation, and being considered in other conditions such as heart failure.

References

ACCORD Study Group. Effects of intensive blood-pressure control in type 2 diabetes mellitus. *N Engl J Med* 2010;362:1575–85 [PMID: 20228401] PMC4123215.

Ahmed AK, Kamath NS, El Kossi M, El Nahas AM. The impact of stopping inhibitors of the renin-angiotensin system in patients with advanced chronic kidney disease. *Nephrol Dial Transplant* 2010;25:3977–82 [PMID: 19820248] Free full text.

Appel LJ, Moore TJ, Obarzanek E et al. A clinical trial of the effects of dietary patterns on blood pressure. DASH Collaborative Research Group. N Engl J Med 1997;336:1117–24 [PMID: 9099655] Free full text.

Bakris GL, Townsend RR, Flack JM et al. SYMPLICITY HTN-3 Investigators. 12-month blood pressure results of catheter-based renal artery denervation for resistant hypertension: the SYMPLICITY HTN-3 trial. J Am Coll Cardiol 2015;65:1314–21 [PMID: 25835443] Free full text.

Banegas JR, Ruilope LM, de la Sierra A et al. High prevalence of masked uncontrolled hypertension in people with treated hypertension. Eur Heart J 2014;35:3304–12 [PMID: 24497346] Free full text.

Barber J, McKeever TM, McDowell SE et al. A systematic review and met-analysis of thiazide-induced hyponatraemia: time to reconsider electrolyte monitoring regimens after thiazide initiation? Br J Clin Pharmacol 2015;79:566–77 [PMID: 25139696] PMC4386942.

Barzilay JI, Davis BR, Bettencourt J et al. ALLHAT Collaborative Research Group Cardiovascular outcomes using doxazosin vs. chlortalidone for the treatment of hypertension in older adults with and without glucose disorders: a report from the ALLHAT study. J Clin Hypertens (Greenwich) 2004;6:116–25 [PMID: 15010644] Free full text.

Barzilay JI, Davis BR, Pressel SL et al.; ALLHAT Collaborative Research Group. Long-term effects of incident diabetes mellitus on cardiovascular outcomes in people treated for hypertension: the ALLHAT Diabetes Extension Study. Circ Cardiovasc Qual Outcomes 2012;5:15–62 [PMID: 22396585] PMC3359874.

Beckett NS, Peters R, Fletcher AE et al. HYVED Study Group. Treatment of hypertension in patients 80 years of age or older. N Engl J Med 2008;358:1887–98 [PMID: 18378519] Free full text.

Bhandari S, Ives N, Brettell EA et al. Multicentre randomized controlled trial of angiotensin-converting enzyme inhibitor/angiotensin receptor blocker withdrawal in advanced renal disease: the STOP-ACEi trial. Nephrol Dial Transplant 2016;31:255–61 [PMID: 26429974] PMC4725389.

Blomster JI, Zoungas S, Chalmers J et al. The relationship between alcohol consumption and vascular complications and mortality in individuals with type 2 diabetes. Diabetes Care 2014;37:1353–9 [PMID: 24578358].

Borghi C, Cicero AF. Nutraceuticals with a clinically detectable blood pressure-lowering effect: a review of available randomized clinical trials and their meta-analyses. Br J Clin Pharmacol 2017; 83:163–71 [PMID: 26852373].

Brown MJ. Ins and outs of aldosterone-producing adenomas of the adrenal: from channelopathy to common curable causes of hypertension. Hypertension 2014;63:24–26 [PMID: 24082060] Free full text.

Brown MJ, Palmer CR, Castaigne A et al. Morbidity and mortality in patients randomised to double-blind treatment with a long-acting calcium-channel blocker or diuretic in the International Nifedipine GITS study: Intervention as a Goal in Hypertension Treatment (INSIGHT). Lancet 2000; 356;366–72 [PMID: 10972368].

Brown MJ, Williams B, Morant SV et al. British Hypertension Society's Prevention and Treatment of Hypertension with Algorithm-based Therapy (PATHWAY) Studies Group. Effect of amiloride, or amiloride plus hydrochlorothiazide, versus hydrochlorothiazide on glucose tolerance and blood pressure (PATHWAY-3): a parallel-group, double-blind randomised phase 4 trial. Lancet Diabetes Endocrinol 2016;4:136–47 [PMID: 26489809] PMC4728199.

Brugts JJ, Arima H, Remme W et al. The incidence and clinical predictors of ACE inhibitor induced dry cough by perindopril in 27,492 patients with vascular disease. Int J Cardiol 2014;176:718–23 [PMID: 25189490].

Calhoun DA, Booth JN 3rd, Oparil S et al. Refractory hypertension: determination of prevalence, risk factors, and comorbidities in a large, population-based cohort. Hypertension 2014;63:451–8 [PMID: 24324035] PMC4141646.

Chapman N, Chang CL, Dahlöf B et al. ASCOT Investigators. Effect of doxazosin gastrointestinal therapeutic system as third-line antihypertensive therapy on blood pressure and lipid in the Anglo-Scandinavian Cardiac Outcomes Trial. Circulation 2008;118:42–8 [PMID: 18559700] Free full text.

Cloutier L, Daskalopoulou SS, Padwal RS et al. A new algorithm for the diagnosis of hypertension in Canada. Can J Cardiol 2015;31:620–30 [PMID: 25828374] Free full text.

Curtis RM, Felder S, Borici-Mazi R, Ball I. ACE-I angioedema: accurate clinical diagnosis may prevent epinephrine-induced harm. *West J Emerg Med* 2016;17:283–9 [PMID: 27330660] PMC4899059.

Dahlöf B, Sever PS, Poulter NR *et al*. ASCOT Investigators. Prevention of cardiovascular events with an antihypertensive regimen of amlodipine adding perindopril as required versus atenolol adding bendroflumethiazide as required, in the Anglo-Scandinavian Cardiac Outcomes Trial-Blood Pressure Lowering Arm (ASCOT-BPLA): a multicentre randomised controlled trial. *Lancet* 2005;366:895–906 [PMID: 16154016].

Daugherty SL, Powers JD, Magid DJ *et al*. Incidence and prognosis of resistant hypertension in hypertensive patients. *Circulation* 2012;125:1635–42 [PMID: 22379110] PMC3343635.

Elliott WJ, Jurca S. Loop diuretics are most appropriate for hypertension treatment in chronic kidney disease. *J Am Soc Hypertens* 2016;10:285–7 [PMID: 26993218].

Espeland MA, Probstfield J, Hire D *et al*. Look AHEAD Research Group; ACCORD Study Group. Systolic blood pressure control among individuals with type 2 diabetes: a comparative effectiveness analysis of three interventions. *Am J Hypertens* 2015;28:995–1009 [PMID: 25666468] PMC4506323.

Estruch R, Sacanella E De la Sierra *et al*. Effects of alcohol withdrawal on 24 hour ambulatory blood pressure among alcohol-dependent patients. *Alcohol Clin Exp Res* 2003;27:2002–8 [PMID: 14691389].

Fleg JL, Evans GW, Margolis KL *et al*. Orthostatic hypotension in the ACCORD (Action to Control Cardiovascular Risk in Diabetes) blood pressure trial: prevalence, incidence, and prognostic significance. *Hypertension* 2016;68:888–95 [PMID: 27504006] PMC5016241.

Fried LF, Emanuele N, Zhang JH *et al*.; VA NEPHRON-D Investigators. Combined angiotensin inhibition for the treatment of diabetic nephropathy. *N Engl J Med* 2013;369:1892–903 [PMID: 24206457] Free full text.

Ganz M, Mokabberi R, Sica DA. Comparison of blood pressure control with amlodipine and controlled-release isradipine: an open-label, drug substitution study. *J Clin Hypertens (Greenwich)* 2005;7(Suppl 1):27–31 [PMID: 15858400] Free full text.

Hata J, Arima H, Rothwell PM *et al*. ADVANCE Collaborative Group. Effects of visit-to-visit variability in systolic blood pressure on macrovascular and microvascular complications in patients with type 2 diabetes mellitus: the ADVANCE trial. *Circulation* 2013;128:1325–34 [PMID: 23926207] Free full text.

Hedegaard U, Kjeldsen LJ, Pottegård *et al*. Improving medication adherence in patients with hypertension: a randomized trial. *Am J Med* 2015;128:1351–61 [PMID: 26302142].

Holman RR, Paul SK, Bethel MA *et al*. Long-term follow-up after tight control of blood pressure in type 2 diabetes. *N Engl J Med* 2008;359:1565–76 [PMID: 18784091] Free full text.

Hou FF, Zhang X, Zhang GH *et al*. Efficacy and safety of benazepril for advanced chronic renal insufficiency. *N Engl J Med* 2006;354:131–40 [PMID: 16407508] Free full text.

Jackevicius CA, Wong J, Aroustamian I *et al*. Rates and predictors of ACE inhibitor discontinuation subsequent to elevated serum creatinine: a retrospective cohort study. *BMJ Open* 2014;4:e005181 [PMID: 25232564] PMC4139635.

Jamerson K, Weber MA, Bakris GL *et al*. ACCOMPLISH Trial Investigators. Benazepril plus amlodipine or hydrochlorothiazide for hypertension in high-risk patients. *N Engl J Med* 2008;359:2416–27 [PMID: 19052124] Free full text.

Jeffers BW, Robbins J, Bhambri R, Wajsbrot D. A systematic review on the efficacy of amlodipine in the treatment of patients with hypertension with concomitant diabetes mellitus and/or renal dysfunction, when compared with other classes of antihypertensive agents. *Am J Ther* 2015;22: 322–41 [PMID: 25738570].

Jumar A, Schmeider RE. Cocoa flavanol cardiovascular effects beyond blood pressure reduction. *J Clin Hypertens (Greenwich)* 2016;18:352–8 [PMID: 26514936] Free full text.

Kim S, Shin DW, Yun JM *et al*. Medication adherence and the risk of cardiovascular mortality and hospitalization among patients with newly prescribed antihypertensive medications. *Hypertension* 2016;67:506–12 [PMID: 26865198].

Kivimäki M, Batty GD, Hamer M *et al*. Influence of retirement on nonadherence to medication for hypertension and diabetes. *CMAJ* 2013;185:E784–90 [PMID: 24082018] PMC3832579.

Kjeldsen SE, Berge E, Bangalore S et al. No evidence for a J-shaped curve in treated hypertensive patients with increased cardiovascular risk: the VALUE trial. *Blood Press* 2016;25:83–92 [PMID: 26511535].

Kramer CK, Leitão CB, Canani LH, Ross JL. Impact of white-coat hypertension on microvascular complications in type 2 diabetes. *Diabetes Care* 2008;31:2233–7 [PMID: 18768675] PMC2584170.

Krousel-Wood M, Joyce C, Holt E et al. Predictors of decline in medication adherence: results from the cohort study of medication adherence among older adults. *Hypertension* 2011;58:804–10 [PMID: 21968751] PMC3220657.

Ku E, McCulloch CE, Mauer M et al. Association between blood pressure and adverse renal events in type 1 diabetes. *Diabetes Care* 2016;39:2218–24 [PMID: 27872156] PMC5127223.

Lazich I, Bakris GL. Prediction and management of hyperkalemia across the spectrum of chronic kidney disease. *Semin Nephrol* 2014;34:333–9 [PMID: 25016403].

Levy D. Macrovascular complications, hypertension, and lipids. in Levy D: *Type 1 diabetes*, 2nd edn (Oxford Diabetes Library), Oxford, Oxford University Press, 2016, pp. 145–66.

Liamis G, Filippatos TD, Elisaf MS. Thiazide-associated hyponatremia in the elderly: what the clinician needs to know. *J Geriatr Cardiol* 2016;13:164–82 [PMID: 27168745] PMC4854958.

Lindholm LH, Ibsen H, Dahlöf B et al. LIFE Study Group. Cardiovascular morbidity and mortality in patients with diabetes in the Losartan Intervention For Endpoint reduction in hypertension study (LIFE): a randomised trial against atenolol. *Lancet* 2002;359:1004–10 [PMID: 11937179].

MacDonald TM, Williams P, Caulfield M et al. Monotherapy versus dual therapy therapy for the initial treatment of hypertension (PATHWAY-1): a randomised double-blind controlled trial. *BMJ Open* 2015;5:e007645 [PMID: 26253566] PMC4539389.

Mancia G, Fagard R, Narkiewicz K et al. Task Force Members. 2013 ESH/ESC Guidelines for the management of arterial hypertension: the Task Force for the management of the European Society of Hypertension (ESH) and of the European Society of Cardiology (ESC). *J Hypertens* 2013;31:1281–357 [PMID: 23817082].

Mancia G, Kjeldsen SE, Zappe DH et al. Cardiovascular outcomes at different on-treatment blood pressures in the hypertensive patients of the VALUE trial. *Eur Heart J* 2016;37:955–64 [PMID: 26590384].

Martinez-Garcia MA, Capote F, Campos-Rodriguez F et al. Spanish Sleep Network. Effect of CPAP on blood pressure in patients with obstructive sleep apnea and resistant hypertension: the HIPARCO randomized clinical trial. *JAMA* 2013;310:2407–15 [PMID: 24327037].

Menne J, Ritz E, Ruilope LM et al. The Randomized Olmesartan and Diabetes Microalbuminuria Prevention (ROADMAP) observational follow-up study: benefits of RAS blockade with olmesartan treatment are sustained after study discontinuation. *J Am Heart Assoc* 2014;3:e000810 [PMID: 24772521] PMC4187490.

Merino J, Guasch-Ferré M, Martinez-González MA et al. Is complying with the recommendations of sodium intake beneficial for health in individuals at high cardiovascular risk? Findings from the PREDIMED study. *Am J Clin Nutr* 2015;101:440–8. [PMID: 25733627] Free full text.

Messerli FH, Staessen JA, Zannad F. Of fads, fashion, surrogate endpoints and dual RAS blockade. *Eur Heart J* 2010;31:2205–8 [PMID: 20685681] Free full text.

Molmen-Hansen HE, Stolen T, Tjonna AE et al. Aerobic interval training reduces blood pressure and improves myocardial function in hypertensive patients. *Eur J Prev Cardiol* 2012;19:151–60 [PMID: 21450580].

Mori TA, Burke V, Zilkens RR et al. The effects of alcohol on ambulatory blood pressure and other cardiovascular risk factors in type 2 diabetes: a randomized intervention. *J Hypertens* 2016;34:421–8 [PMID: 26734954].

NICE. Hypertension in adults: diagnosis and management. Clinical guideline [CG127] Published: August 2011.

Nilsson PM, Kjeldsen SE. Blood pressure goals in type 2 diabetes – assessing the evidence. *Lancet Diabetes Endocrinol* 2017;5:319–21 [PMID: 28169174].

Nilsson PM, Cederholm J, Zethelius BR et al. Trends in blood pressure control in patients with type 2 diabetes: data from the Swedish National Diabetes Register (NDR). *Blood Press* 2011;20:348–54 [PMID: 21675827].

Nunan D, Thompson M, Heneghan CJ et al. Accuracy of self-monitored blood pressure for diagnosing hypertension in primary care. J Hypertens 2015;33:755–62 [PMID: 25915880].

ONTARGET Investigators; Yusuf S, Teo KK, Pogue J et al. Telmisartan, ramipril, or both in patients at high risk for vascular events. N Engl J Med 2008;358:1547–59 [PMID: 18378520] Free full text.

Palmer BF. Managing hyperkalemia caused by inhibitors of the renin-angiotensin-aldosterone system. N Engl J Med 2004;351:585–92 [PMID: 15295051].

Parikh A, Lipsitz SR, Natarajan S. Association between a DASH-like diet and mortality in adults with hypertension: findings from a population-based follow-up study. Am J Hyertens 2009;22:409–16 [PMID: 19197247].

Parthasarathy HK, Ménard J, White J et al. A double-blind, randomized study comparing the antihypertensive effect of eplerenone and spironolactone in patients with hypertension and evidence of primary aldosteronism. J Hypertens 2011;29:980–90 [PMID: 21451421].

Parving HH, Brenner BM, McMurray JJ et al. ALTITUDE Investigators. Cardiorenal end points in a trial of aliskiren for type 2 diabetes. N Engl J Med 2012;367:2204–13 [PMID: 23121378] Free full text.

Patel A; ADVANCE Collaborative Group, MacMahon S et al. Effects of a fixed combination or perindopril and indapamide on macrovascular and microvascular outcomes in patients with type 2 diabetes mellitus (the ADVANCE trial): a randomised controlled trial. Lancet 2007;370:829–40 [PMID: 17765963].

Peterzan MA, Hardy R, Chaturvedi N, Hughes AD. Meta-analysis of dose-response relationships for hydrochlorothiazide, chlorthalidone, and bendroflumethiazide on blood pressure, serum potassium, and urate. Hypertension 2012;59:1104–9 [PMID: 22547443] PMC4930655.

Reeves RA, Lin CS, Kassler-Taub K, Pouleur H. Dose-related efficacy of irbesartan for hypertension: an integrated analysis. Hypertension 1998;31:1311–6 [PMID: 9622147] Free full text.

Rönnback M, Fagerud J, Forsblom C et al. Finnish Diabetic Nephropathy (FinnDiane) Study Group. Altered age-related blood pressure pattern in type 1 diabetes. Circulation 2008;110:1076–82 [PMID: 15326070] Free full text.

Rosa J, Widimský P, Waldauf P et al. Role of adding spironolactone and renal denervation in true resistant hypertension: one-year outcomes of randomized PRAGUE-15 study. Hypertension 2016; 67:397–403 [PMID: 26693818] Free full text.

Rossen NB, Knudsen ST, Fleischer J et al. Targeting nocturnal hypertension in type 2 diabetes mellitus. Hypertension 2014;64:1080–7 [PMID: 25259747] Free full text.

Ruggenenti P, Perna A, Remuzzi G; Gruppo Italiano di Studi Epidemiologici in Nefrologia. ACE inhibitors to prevent end-stage renal disease: when to start and why possibly never to stop: a post hoc analysis of the REIN trial results. Ramipril Efficacy in Nephropathy. J Am Soc Nephrol 2001;12:2832–7 [PMID: 11729254].

Sarafidis PA, Bakris GL. Resistant hypertension an overview of evaluation and treatment. J Am Coll Cardiol 2008;52:1749–57 [PMID: 19022154] Free full text.

Sivén S, Niiranen T, Kantola I, Jula A. 1B:03: White-coat and masked hypertension as risk factors for progression to sustained hypertension: the Finn-Home Study. J Hypertens 2015;33(Suppl 1):e5–6 [PMID: 26102839].

Slagman MC, Waanders F, Hemmelder MH et al. Holland Nephrology Study Group. Moderate dietary sodium restriction added to angiotensin converting enzyme inhibition compared with dual blockade in lowering proteinuria and blood pressure: randomised controlled trial. BMJ 2011;343:d4366 [PMID: 21791491] PMC3143706.

Soliman EZ, Byington RP, Bigger JT et al. Effect of intensive blood pressure lowering on left ventricular hypertrophy in patients with diabetes mellitus: Action to Control Cardiovascular Risk in Diabetes blood pressure trial. Hypertension 2015;66:1123–9 [PMID 26459421] PMC4644090.

Sousa AG, Cabral JV, El-Feghaly WB et al. Hyporeninemic hypoaldosteronism and diabetes mellitus: pathophysiology assumptions, clinical aspects and implications for management. World J Diabetes 2016;7:101–11 [PMID: 26981183] PMC4781902.

Suh DC, Kim CM, Choi IS et al. Trends in blood pressure control and treatment among type 2 diabetes with comorbid hypertension in the United States: 1988–2004. J Hypertens 2009;27:1908–16 [PMID: 19491704].

van Vark LC, Bertrand M, Akkerhuis KM *et al*. Angiotensin-converting enzyme inhibitors reduce mortality in hypertension: a meta-analysis of randomized clinical trials of renin-aldosterone system inhibitors involving 158,998 patients. *Eur Heart J* 2012;33:2088–97 [PMID: 22511654] PMC3418510.

Walraven I, Mast MR, Hoekstra T *et al*. Real-world evidence of suboptimal blood pressure control in patients with type 2 diabetes. *J Hypertens* 2015;33:2091–8 [PMID: 26237580].

Weber MA, Bakris GL, Jamerson K *et al*. ACCOMPLISH Investigators. Cardiovascular events during different hypertension therapies in patients with diabetes. *J Am Coll Cardiol* 2010;56:77–85 [PMID: 20620720] Free full text.

Weber MA, Bloch M, Bakris GL *et al*. Cardiovascular outcomes according to systolic blood pressures in patients with and without diabetes: an ACCOMPLISH substudy. *J Clin Hypertens (Greenwich)* 2016;18:299–307 [PMID: 27060568] Free full text.

Williams B, MacDonald TM, Morant S *et al*. British Hypertension Society's PATHWAY Studies Group. Spironolactone versus placebo, bisoprolol, and doxazosin to determine the optimal treatment for drug-resistant hypertension (PATHWAY-2): a randomised, double-blind, crossover trial. *Lancet* 2015;386:2059–68 [PMID: 26414968] PMC4655321.

Wong GW, Laugerotte A, Wright JM. Blood pressure lowering efficacy of dual alpha and beta blockers for primary hypertension. *Cochrane Database Syst Rev* 2015;26:CD07449 [PMID: 26306578].

Woolf KJ, Bisognano JD. Nondrug interventions for treatment of hypertension. *J Clin Hypertens (Greenwich)* 2011;13:829–35 [PMID: 22051428] Free full text.

Wright JT Jr, Bakris G, Greene T *et al*. African American Study of Kidney Disease and Hypertension Study Group. Effect of blood pressure lowering and antihypertensive drug class on progression of hypertensive kidney disease: results from the AASK trial. *JAMA* 2002;288:2421–31 [PMID: 12435255].

Wright JT Jr, Harris-Haywood S, Pressel S *et al*. Clinical outcomes by race in hypertensive patients with and without the metabolic syndrome: Antihypertensive and Lipid-Lowering Treatment to Prevent Heart Attack Trial (ALLHAT). *Arch Intern Med* 2008;168:207–17 [PMID: 1822737] PMC2805022.

Yudkin JS, Richter B, Gale EA. Intensified glucose lowering in type 2 diabetes: tie for a reappraisal. *Diabetologia* 2010;53:2079–85 [PMID: 20688748].

Zoungas S, Chalmers J, Neal B *et al*. ADVANCE-ON Collaborative Group. Follow-up of blood-pressure lowering and glucose control in type 2 diabetes. *N Engl J Med* 2014;371:1392–406 [PMID: 2534206] Free full text.

Further reading

British Hypertension Society approved HBPM devices: http://www.bhsoc.org/index.php?cID=246 (last accessed 27 August 2017).

DASH diet: https://www.nhlbi.nih.gov/health/health-topics/topics/dash (last accessed 27 August 2017).

Endocrine test protocols

Imperial Centre for Endocrinology, Imperial College Healthcare NHS Trust, London: http://imperialendo.co.uk (Freely-available comprehensive and authoritative manual of endocrine tests, updated annually.) Link provided courtesy of Professor Karim Meeran.

12 Lipids

Key points

- Type 1 patients often have good lipid profiles: offer treatment to younger people only after carefully considering and discussing cardiovascular risk
- LDL lowering is the simplest and most cost-effective strategy for reducing cardiovascular events in Type 2 diabetes
- In patients with known cardiovascular disease, LDL reduction of ≥50% *and* achievement of a low LDL level (e.g. <1.7–1.8 mmol/l) can usually be achieved with a potent statin at a moderate or high dose (e.g. atorvastatin 40–80 mg daily or rosuvastatin 20–40 mg daily)
- If there is no overt vascular disease, moderate-intensity statin treatment is recommended (e.g. atorvastatin 10–20 mg daily, simvastatin 20–40 mg daily)
- Ezetimibe is effective in reducing cardiovascular outcomes, though it is less potent than a starting dose of a statin
- Fibrates and omega-3 fatty acids are reserved for patients with severe hypertriglyceridemia; niacin is obsolete
- Plant stanols/sterols taken regularly at 2 g daily as a spread or drink are useful adjunctive therapy
- The PSCK9 inhibitors (alirocumab and evolocumab) are very powerful LDL-lowering agents and potentially valuable

INTRODUCTION

Together with blood pressure control, management of lipids is of critical importance in Type 2 diabetes, though there is much less evidence in Type 1. The literature is full of major trials reporting clear outcomes but there is no sign that controversy is settling, despite the strong evidence over the past five years that lipid-modifying agents other than statins and ezetimibe carry little benefit (fibrates) or none (niacin, fish oils) in reducing cardiovascular events. The introduction of the PCSK9 inhibitors is of major academic and potentially clinical significance. Astonishingly, controversy over the benefits and risks of statin treatment is as vigorous as ever, and this translates into continuing concern among patients about taking these agents.

On the guideline front, in 2014 the American College of Cardiology and American Heart Association jointly proposed that numerical targets for LDL should be replaced by a therapeutic aim, that is either moderate or intensive lipid lowering based on the potency of the statin. The rationale was that comparative trials have used different statins, contrasting with targeting specific numerical targets, as for example in the glycaemia and blood pressure trials. This may be academically sound for populations but

Practical Diabetes Care, Fourth Edition. David Levy.
© 2018 John Wiley & Sons Ltd. Published 2018 by John Wiley & Sons Ltd.

individual patients do not always have an average or greater than average response to statins and there is good evidence that for LDL, though not for blood pressure and HbA_{1c}, lower may be better for event reduction. The unintended consequence of this intellectually sound approach was to confuse further the practicalities of lipid-lowering treatment, especially in high-risk individuals.

LIPIDS IN TYPE 1 DIABETES

Very poor glycaemic control and the linked insulin deficiency is associated with higher LDL-cholesterol (LDL-C) and triglyceride levels (to the point of risking acute pancreatitis), and depressed HDL-cholesterol. However, when patients are in fair and stable glycaemic control, and as long as there is no diabetic kidney disease, lipid profiles are no more atherogenic, and in some respects less so, than in non-diabetic individuals. Why the risk of macrovascular disease remains so high in Type 1 diabetes is not fully explained (see **Chapter 6**) and clearly not related to evidently poor conventional lipid profiles. However, abnormal LDL subfractions may be in part responsible, even in the presence of often very high total HDL.

Lipid profile in Type 1 diabetes

Lipid profiles in Type 1 patients are widely quoted to be indistinguishable from (or numerically better than) non-diabetic controls. This was the case in the DCCT cohort (mid-1980s), and in the more recent SEARCH study (Maahs et al., 2013) in under-20s (mid-2000s):

Total cholesterol, mmol/l	4.2
Triglycerides, mmol/l	0.6
HDL-cholesterol, mmol/l	1.4
LDL-cholesterol, mmol/l	2.5

Not all surveys paint such a flattering picture. In Norway one-third of young people had LDL levels above the maximum level previously recommended by the American Diabetes Association (2.6 mmol/l) and in 10–16 year olds in the United Kingdom, Canada and Australia all lipid measures were worse than in non-diabetic controls. In addition mean BMI was higher (22 vs 21) and systolic blood pressure meaningfully higher (117 vs 110 mm Hg) (Maftei et al., 2014).

Type 1 diabetes is characterized by high HDL-cholesterol levels, which are strikingly elevated in long-term survivors (Keenan et al., 2007) and can reach extremely high levels (e.g. >2.0 mmol/l). While overall there is a broad inverse relationship between HDL levels and cardiovascular events, both low (<1.2 mmol/l) and high (>2.1 mmol/l), levels in women were associated with higher event risks in the Pittsburgh Study, perhaps explaining some of the elevated cardiovascular risk in Type 1 females (**Figure 12.1**) (Costacou et al., 2011). There are many biochemical mechanisms potentially contributing to dysfunctional HDL-cholesterol, some of which, for example reduced protection of LDL from oxidation, suppression of nitric oxide activity and systemic and vascular inflammation, occur in vitro in diabetes, especially if it is poorly controlled. Many other minor abnormalities of the Type 1 lipid profile have been described even in well-controlled patients in DCCT, for example an adverse profile of HDL particle size and increased concentration of total atherogenic apolipoprotein (apo)B particles. Long-term these multiple minor abnormalities may cumulatively increase cardiovascular risk, even when the routine laboratory lipid profile looks creditable.

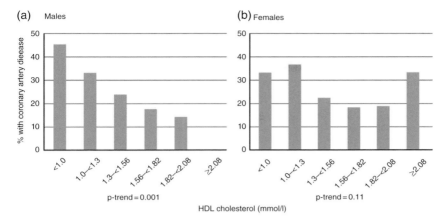

Figure 12.1 Strikingly different HDL distributions in (a) males and (b) females in the Pittsburgh epidemiological study of Type 1 diabetes. The straight-line relationship in men showing the familiar inverse relationship between HDL levels and incidence of coronary artery disease contrasts with the flat relationship in women, emphasizing the loss of coronary protection at high – supposedly 'good' – LDL levels. *Source*: Costacou *et al.*, 2011.

Practice point

HDL-cholesterol levels in Type 1 diabetes are often extremely high. In women very high levels may be associated with increased vascular risk, suggesting they have dysfunctional HDL.

Lipid effects of improving glycaemic control

In the SEARCH study, moving from very poor to rather better glycaemic control (e.g. HbA_{1c} from 10 to 8%, 86 to 64) resulted in an improved lipid profile (for example, mean LDL fell by about 0.2 mmol/l, triglycerides by about 9%); clearly the impact of even this substantial degree of improvement in glycaemia is much smaller than statin treatment, but statins would hardly be used in this group in any case, and the likely beneficial effect on vascular events is an additional reason to maintain optimum glycaemia (Maahs *et al.*, 2013). There is a balance to be struck: lipid profiles deteriorated in the intensively-treated DCCT group (mean HbA_{1c} 7.0%, 53), possibly because of weight gain and development of several insulin-resistance factors, but more important is the observation, also from DCCT, that all cardiovascular risk factors deteriorate with increasing HbA_{1c} (Writing Group for the DCCT/EDIC Research Group, 2016).

Practice point

Improving glycaemic control in Type 1 patients with high HbA_{1c} levels significantly improves LDL and triglyceride levels.

Assessment of risk

Standard risk calculators, for example Framingham, are of little value because few diabetic individuals and no Type 1 patients were included. The huge prospective database used for the UK QRISK system is unreliable in ethnic minorities, but it does include substantial numbers of Type 1 patients, and currently is probably the best for routine use (though others are in development). It is updated every year. Remarkably, however, several long-term studies in Type 1 patients, including EURODIAB and FinnDiane, did not identify LDL level as a significant risk factor for cardiovascular disease in Type 1 diabetes (Hero *et al.*, 2016). The total/HDL-cholesterol ratio is a more robust indicator, and this is the measure preferred in many risk equations, including QRISK2.

Practice point

Although no cardiovascular risk equation is wholly reliable in Type 1 diabetes, the UK QRISK, updated every year, is currently the best and is also very easy to use.

Many consensus documents conclude that risk is high in patients over 40; this is a reasonable judgement, given that, on average, patients will have had about 30 years of Type 1 diabetes at that age and will therefore probably be at higher risk. NICE (2015) proposes recommending a statin (atorvastatin 20 mg daily) for the following 'primary prevention' categories:

- age >40 years *or*
- diabetes duration 10 years *or*
- other vascular risk factors
- nephropathy is also included, but these patients are already firmly in the secondary prevention category.

Because of the consistent link between established microvascular complications and macrovascular disease, all patients with established retinopathy, persistent microalbuminuria or neuropathy should also have long-term statin treatment, but many of these patients are still young and improved glycaemia is always the primary strategy. A risk assessment is valuable for discussion with the under-40s, as it is important to take account of other, conventional, risk factors, for example hypertension, smoking and family history of premature vascular disease.

Practice point

Macrovascular events are increased in Type 1 with even relatively minor microvascular complications: consider statins in people with, for example, established background retinopathy (never forget improved glycaemia).

Statins

Statin treatment confers the same cardiovascular benefit in Type 1 and 2 and non-diabetic subjects (approximately 4% absolute and 22% relative risk reduction (see later)).

Ezetimibe

Lipid profiles in Type 1 patients may be less responsive to statins, on account of their increased tendency to absorb dietary cholesterol. Although this is commonly quoted, there is little evidence to support it. A small study found that ezetimibe lowered LDL more effectively than simvastatin in Type 1 patients (approximately 30% vs approximately 20% reduction) (Ciriacks *et al.*, 2015). The recently-established place of ezetimibe in secondary prevention is, therefore, particularly applicable to Type 1 patients (see later).

Aspirin
Further details can be found in **Chapter 6**.

TYPE 2 DIABETES

Contemporary studies, for example the Heart Protection Study (HPS), found that lipid profiles in Type 2 patients are broadly similar to those without diabetes (for example HDL levels were identical (mean 1.1 mmol/l), LDL lower by 0.2 mmol/l), in contrast to older studies and the widespread belief they are adverse. This finding is possibly due to greater awareness of lipids in diagnosed patients (Collins *et al.*, 2003). However, all studies show that at any level of LDL people with diabetes have a higher cardiovascular risk, though the absolute risk has very likely decreased over time. Individuals with multiple insulin resistance characteristics (e.g. ethnic minority subjects) have lower HDL levels and higher triglycerides, which increase vascular risk. Multiple other lipid abnormalities, not seen in the traditional lipid profile, further increase risk, much as in Type 1 diabetes (see previously), for example:

- Increased apoB, reflecting increased total numbers of atherogenic particles, even though LDL level may be normal.
- Increased small, dense, atherogenic LDL particles that are more prone to oxidation and glycation.
- Possibly increased lipoprotein(a).
- Subtly altered HDL subfractions (HDL_2 is the most powerful anti-atherogenic fraction and is reduced in diabetes; the antioxidant activity of the small dense HDL_3 fraction is also reduced).
- Increased non-HDL cholesterol (easily calculated from the standard lipid profile).

THE EFFECT OF CO-EXISTING CONDITIONS AND MEDICATION ON LIPID PROFILES IN TYPE 2 DIABETES

Newly-diagnosed or poorly-controlled diabetes
As in Type 1 diabetes, poor control, either at or after diagnosis, can be associated with deranged lipid profiles. The resulting severe hypertriglyceridaemia is a major clinical risk for acute pancreatitis; the combination of a hyperglycaemic emergency and acute pancreatitis can be life-threatening. **Figure 12.2** shows the complex interaction between diabetes and hypertriglyceridaemia. In clinical practice, routine biochemical tests at the onset of Type 2 diabetes often show markedly elevated total cholesterol and triglyceride levels with very low HD-cholesterol. It is the triglycerides that increase the pancreatitis risk. Statins do not help.

Practice point

Where available, look carefully at cumulative biochemical reports in newly-diagnosed Type 2 patients. Severely elevated triglycerides (>10 mmol/l) are a risk for acute pancreatitis. Oral lipid-lowering treatment, statin or fibrate, will not reduce this risk while there is uncontrolled diabetes.

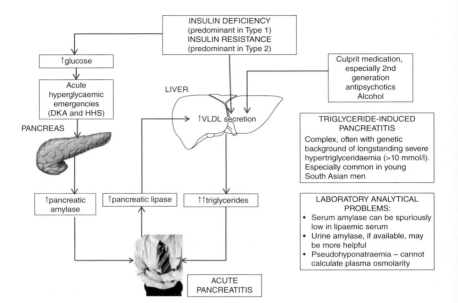

Figure 12.2 Acute pancreatitis and elevated triglycerides. A common and dangerous combination; the very high triglycerides make laboratory diagnosis and management especially complicated. *Source*: Levy, 2016.

Primary hyperlipidaemias

Familial hypercholesterolaemia (FH)

These conditions are more likely to be uncovered in people with diabetes, though they are not associated with it. Suspect FH in adults (aged 20 or older) if LDL-C ≥4.9 mmol/l (190 mg/dl) or if LDL-C is nowhere near target when the patient is reliably taking a reasonable statin dose. Even homozygous FH – rare, occurring in about 1 in 300 000 people – has a heterogeneous phenotype, so clinical features, family history, severity of atherosclerotic cardiovascular disease and response to treatment need to be taken into account. By contrast, heterozygous FH is common and occurs in about 1 in 200 of a northern European population. It is worthwhile making a formal diagnosis (genetic testing is not mandatory) because of the multiple existing risk factors in people with diabetes and the need for rigorous control of LDL (Santos *et al.*, 2016).

Familial combined hyperlipidaemia

Familial combined hyperlipidaemia is another common hyperlipidaemia and is found in 0.5–2.0% of the population. Its features overlap that of the metabolic syndrome and Type 2 diabetes. Despite its name, it is polygenic and modified by countless non-genetic factors. It is clinically the most frequent genetic hyperlipidaemia in patients with atherosclerotic cardiovascular disease and is clearly associated with premature cardiovascular disease: it is overrepresented – around 10% prevalence – in younger survivors of myocardial infarction (under 60 years). Diagnostic criteria are understandably vague but include LDL >4.1 mmol/l (>160 mg/dl), with or without triglycerides >2.3 mmol/l

Box 12.1 Secondary causes of hypertriglyceridaemia.

- obesity
- metabolic syndrome
- diet: high calorie, high fat or high glycaemic index
- increased alcohol consumption (perhaps as little as 3 units/day in males, 2 in females)
- diabetes (mainly Type 2)
- hypothyroidism
- renal disease (proteinuria, uraemia, or glomerulonephritis)
- pregnancy (particularly in the third trimester)
- paraproteinaemia
- systemic lupus erythematosus
- Drugs including corticosteroids, oral oestrogen, tamoxifen, thiazides, non-cardioselective β-blockers. In practice significant hypertriglyceridaemia with these agents is almost never seen. Also: cyclophosphamide, asparaginase, protease inhibitors, and second-generation antipsychotic drugs (e.g. clozapine and olanzapine).

Source: Hegele *et al.*, 2014. Reproduced with permission of Elsevier.

(200 mg/dl), and at least one other affected family member. Distinction from the metabolic syndrome is difficult but lifestyle factors are less apparent and inflammatory markers (high sensitivity C-reactive protein, fibrinogen) more abnormal. Apo B100 is consistently high (>125 mg/dl), but this is a specialized and non-standardized measurement. Carotid ultrasound for intima-media thickness and atherosclerotic plaque can be valuable in diagnosing subclinical atherosclerosis.

Severe hypertriglyceridaemia

Hypertriglyceridaemia is an independent risk factor for atherosclerotic cardiovascular disease, though the role of the triglyceride-rich lipoproteins is unclear, and the association is much less strong than for LDL-cholesterol levels. Postprandial hypertriglyceridaemia is strongly associated with vascular events and premature death, and non-fasting triglyceride measurements may be a valuable indicator of vascular exposure to extended peaks of triglycerides, which, in turn, may be a powerful cardiovascular risk factor.

There are several definitions. A scheme slightly modified from that proposed by European associations defines normal triglycerides as <2.0 mmol/l, mild-to-moderate hypertriglyceridaemia as 2–10, and severe >10.0 (885 mg/dl); the last group is likely to have a monogenic cause but cardiovascular risk is similar in all patients with a given level of hypertriglyceridaemia, so genetic testing is of no clinical value. Secondary causes of hypertriglyceridaemia are shown in **Box 12.1**.

Treatment

The potent statins atorvastatin and rosuvastatin remain the primary drug treatment in mild or moderate hypertriglyceridaemia, as no other drugs, even those with predominant effects on triglycerides, have been shown to reduce cardiovascular events (see later). However, their effect is modest: rosuvastatin 10 mg daily and atorvastatin 20 mg daily reduce triglycerides by only about 20% (Clearfield *et al.*, 2006). Fibrates and omega-3 fatty acids are slightly more effective and reduce triglycerides by about 40% and 30% respectively, depending on baseline values; they are recommended for reducing the risk of pancreatitis in patients with severe hypertriglyceridaemia (Hegele *et al.*, 2014). They should not be used in lesser degrees of hypertriglyceridaemia, as omega-3 fatty acids (at least taken as supplements) do not reduce cardiovascular events, and there is currently scant evidence for the value of fibrates either (see later).

Lifestyle is key to management in people with moderately elevated triglycerides. Modest reductions in weight and carbohydrate intake and severely limiting alcohol, together with moderately increased activity levels, are much more effective than drug treatment, and may help the non-alcoholic fatty liver disease associated with excessive hepatic VLDL secretion (see **Chapter 9**).

Practice point

The primary management of hypertriglyceridaemia up to about 10 mmol/l is weight loss and carbohydrate and alcohol reduction. Drug treatment does not reduce the increased risk of cardiovascular events associated with elevated triglycerides.

Hypothyroidism

Overt hypothyroidism (TSH ≥10 mU/l) reduces hepatic LDL clearance and profound hypothyroidism can be associated with very high cholesterol levels, but in subclinical hypothyroidism, thyroxine treatment will reduce LDL levels by only about 0.4 mmol/l (Tanis et al., 1996). This small change will rarely alter a decision to recommend statin treatment. Although there is little formal evidence, in patients with a poor response to statins, check thyroid function; there is a hint that statin-related muscle side effects are more common in hypothyroidism.

Renal disease

The lipid profile deteriorates as proteinuria progresses and lipid abnormalities can be particularly striking in patients with severely elevated albuminuria or the nephrotic syndrome. The high triglycerides and low HDL are probably caused by decreased Apo A1 synthesis. Patients with impaired renal function tend to have lower total and LDL-cholesterol levels than those with normal renal function. Cardiovascular disease risk markedly increases with decreasing eGFR and increasing levels of proteinuria (see **Chapter 4**), yet there are relatively few trials of statin treatment in this important group of patients (see later). A careful meta-analysis of patient-level data confirmed that dialysis patients do not benefit from statin treatment. In patients with non-dialysis levels of eGFR, and allowing for the lower LDL of patients with impaired renal function, statins are less effective in reducing cardiovascular events (Cholesterol Treatment Trialists' Collaboration, 2016).

Practice point

Patients on dialysis do not benefit from statin treatment, so there is no point in trying to intensify treatment. As eGFR falls, so do LDL levels.

LDL TARGETS IN TYPE 2 DIABETES?

Numerical targets for LDL lowering are accepted by most clinicians – and are being acted on. However, guidance by the American College of Cardiology and American Heart Association was published in 2013 refuting this approach on sound methodological grounds. It pointed out that LDL targets in widespread use (e.g. 1.7–1.8 mmol/l in high risk patients) were derived from *achieved* LDL levels in trials using specific drugs and specific doses (example: atorvastatin 10 mg daily in the 'primary' prevention CARDS trial: see later). No drug trials have been treat-to-target, as in glycaemia and BP studies (in practice mostly because there is only a handful of drugs that effectively reduce LDL, compared with the multiple effective agents use in managing glycaemia and blood pressure). The parsimonious conclusion was that treatment should be specified by [drug + dose of drug], the choice of which should be determined by the potency of the drug effect according to the level of individual patient risks used in trials, not the LDL level achieved.

This guidance required a major mental frame-shift and was widely 'discussed'. In 2015, the National Lipid Association issued its guidance, orientating clinicians back to more familiar ground and re-establishing the importance of numerical targets according to risk levels. There are now sound reasons for using either approach but clinicians are unlikely to change their practice to an unfamiliar system.

Justifying the use of numerical LDL targets

The justification for the approach is intuitively powerful and has consistently stood up to randomized control trial (RCT) evidence, in contrast to concerns about using the same approach in blood pressure and glycaemia management. The widely-reproduced linear regression (**Figure 12.3**) (Opie, 2015), regularly updated with the results of new trials, shows a striking linear relationship between achieved LDL values and incidence of coronary events. Achieved low LDL levels are therefore associated with reduced risk of events; this is common to both primary and secondary prevention (though the slope is both lower and shallower for the primary prevention relationship). Lowering LDL by a given amount reduces events to the same extent, regardless of the method used to reduce it (statins, diet, bile acid sequestrants, ileal bypass and ezetimibe) (Silverman *et al.*, 2016).

In secondary prevention in diabetes the slope is similar to that for non-diabetic people but is displaced upwards, reflecting the consistently higher risk of people with diabetes at every achieved LDL level. The linear relationship shows no signs of inflection at extremes of high or low LDL.

Practice point

While very low levels of glycaemia and systolic blood pressure are not inevitably accompanied by lower vascular risks, very low LDL levels are consistently associated with lower event rates.

Evidence from individual RCTs

'Primary' prevention: CARDS

The CARDS study (Colhoun *et al.*, 2004) found that maintaining LDL around 2.0 mmol/l (80 mg/dl) with low-dose atorvastatin (20 mg daily) reduced events in Type 2 patients without previous cardiovascular disease. (Whether this is primary or secondary prevention, given the high prevalence of asymptomatic or undetected cardiovascular disease in Type 2 diabetes, is moot, but the study population had no overt disease.) Atorvastatin works quickly: the risk of coronary events fell within six months and from 12 months until the end of the trial showed a consistent 37% relative risk reduction (Colhoun *et al.*, 2005). While there is no current explanation for this rapid onset of effect, the achieved LDL level of 2.0 mmol/l also happens to be the threshold where small interventional studies using

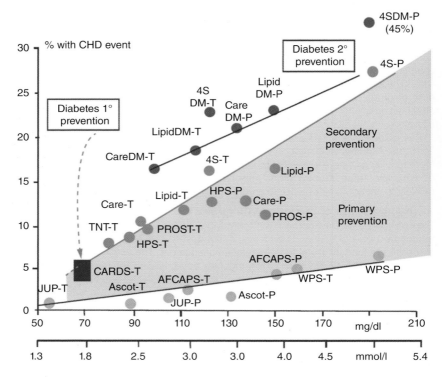

Figure 12.3 The striking and consistent linear relationships between achieved LDL values and incidence of coronary events. The relationship holds for non-diabetic subjects in both primary and secondary prevention (though the slope of the line is much less marked for primary prevention) and for secondary prevention in Type 2 diabetes. The excess events in diabetes at a given LDL is notable (Opie, 2015).

quantitative coronary angiography showed a high likelihood of at least stabilization of coronary and carotid atheroma, though none of these studies has been large enough to demonstrate a relationship between atheroma reduction and event reduction.

PROVE-IT TIMI 22

The PROVE-IT TIMI 22 trial (Cannon et al., 2004) compared the lower potency statin pravastatin 40 mg daily with high-dose atorvastatin 80 mg daily in patients who had had an acute coronary syndrome. It strikingly confirmed that events were significantly lower in the atorvastatin treated patients who had an achieved mean LDL of 1.7–1.8 mmol/l (66–70 mg/dl). Although this was not strictly a treat-to-target study, it is important because two different drugs were used, resulting in two stable and widely different LDL values.

Post hoc analysis of the same trial found that increased benefit in this high-risk group could be extended to patients who had achieved ultra-low LDL levels (<1.04 mmol/l, and 1.04–1.55 mmol/l, 40–60 mg/dl), many of whom were older males with diabetes. A substudy of the one-third of PROVE-IT patients with diabetes confirmed again that the rate of acute events was higher than in non-diabetic subjects (21% vs 14% in those who were intensively treated) but the risk reduction, approximately 25%, was similar in both groups (Ahmed *et al.*, 2006). This and other postcoronary syndrome studies led to European guidelines in 2012 urging an LDL target of <1.8 mg/dl in high-risk patients.

Effect on recurrent events

PROVE-IT TIMI 22 also confirmed a reduction in the total future burden of ischaemic events with the high-intensity regimen, not just a reduction in the next event (Murphy *et al.*, 2009). These events are a substantial burden, amounting to twice the number of initial events; not surprisingly, people with diabetes have an increased rate of multiple events, around one-third, compared with one-quarter of non-diabetic subjects. Several other studies have reinforced this point in post-ACS patients, for example the Treating to New Targets (TNT) study (LaRosa *et al.*, 2010) which used high-dose atorvastatin 80 mg day, and more recently the IMPROVE-IT study using simvastatin-ezetimibe where the main events contributing to the reduced total burden over the 6 year follow-up were non-fatal myocardial infarction and stroke (Murphy *et al.*, 2016).

Practice point

Intensive lipid-lowering reduces the cumulative risk of multiple future events, not just the next event, after an acute coronary syndrome. This is another reason to encourage continuing adherence.

Guidelines

USA guidance in 2004 (National Cholesterol Education Program Adult Treatment Panel III) considered Type 2 diabetes a coronary equivalent (though it probably no longer is; see previously) and, therefore, recommended a target LDL of 2.0 mmol/l or lower for all patients, with a desirable target of <1.7–1.8 mmol/l in people with established vascular disease. This simple and memorable set of rules was modified in the 2013 ACC/AHA guidelines (Stone *et al.*, 2014) because: 'the expert panel was unable to find RCT evidence to support titrating cholesterol-lowering drug therapy to achieve target LDL-C … as recommended by ATP III'. Treatment targets were replaced by the broad statin strategies used in clinic trials, classified as low-, moderate- and high-intensity treatment (**Table 12.1**): these remain valuable in initial assessment of patients and also when discussing the difficult topic of starting statin treatment. The established and proposed guidelines are shown in **Table 12.2**.

Table 12.1 Statin treatment classified by intensity (ACC/AHA guideline; modified from Stone *et al.*, 2014). Drugs either not licensed used in the United Kingdom (e.g. lovastatin) or little used in practice (e.g. fluvastatin) are omitted.

High intensity Average LDL reduction ≥50%	Moderate intensity Average LDL reduction 30–50%	Low intensity Average LDL reduction <30%
Atorvastatin 40–80 mg Rosuvastatin 20–40 mg	Atorvastatin 10–20 mg Rosuvastatin 5–10 mg Simvastatin 20–40 mg Pravastatin 40 (80) mg	Simvastatin 10 mg Pravastatin 10–20 mg

Table 12.2 Recommendations for statin treatment in Type 2 diabetes.

	NCEP ATP III and pre-2013	ACC/AHA 2013
Patients without overt vascular disease ('primary' prevention)	LDL target <2.0 mmol/l	Moderate-intensity statin
Overt vascular disease (secondary prevention)	LDL target <1.7–1.8 mmol/l	High-intensity statin (aim to reduce LDL 50% or more)

Secondary prevention

Similar to that for people without diabetes: high-intensity statin therapy with the aim of reducing LDL by 50% or more. This is congruent with the older guideline: most high-risk patients need this degree of LDL lowering to achieve a value of 1.8 mmol/l. Pragmatically NICE suggests using atorvastatin 20 mg daily for this purpose; it reduced LDL by a mean of approximately 45% in the valuable dose-response STELLAR study (Jones et al., 2003).

'Primary' prevention (people without overt vascular disease)

- Moderate-intensity statin (derived from CARDS).
- If 10 year vascular risk is 7.5% or greater using the Pooled Cohort Equations (http://my.americanheart.org/cvriskcalculator) consider high-intensity statin treatment.

Importantly, risks derived from the Pooled Cohort Equations and the Framingham Score are different: neither is familiar in clinical practice in the United Kingdom. Fortunately, diabetes is recognized in all guidelines as an important cardiovascular risk factor and most over-75s are taking either moderate- or high-intensity statin treatment (Tran et al., 2016). A critical clinical point is that individual responsiveness to statins varies, and there will be substantial proportions of patients who will not show the expected LDL reductions specified in the ACC/AHA document (**Table 12.1**). This will involve dose titration in many patients and perhaps a change in the potency of the statin, both of which comprise elements of a treat-to-target approach.

Adherence is probably a more important matter in overall success of treatment and while coronary artery disease is nearly always treated with a statin, the proportion of treated patients with non-coronary atherosclerotic disease (which includes peripheral arterial disease, abdominal aortic aneurysm and symptomatic carotid artery disease) in one study was only 75% compared with 100% in coronary disease (Thapa et al., 2015). Achieved LDL levels were also lower in the coronary group (2.1 compared with 2.4 mmol/l); not all vascular disease seems to be considered of equal importance in the eyes of the managing physician.

> **Practice point**
>
> Aim for LDL <2.0 mmol/l in all people with Type 2 diabetes, and <1.7–1.8 mmol/l if there is established vascular disease. In the very highest-risk patients (e.g. post-CABG) targets can be set lower without a significant risk of increased harm, as long as monitoring is diligent and there is frequent review for any emerging side effects.

STATIN TREATMENT

Statins are the most widely-prescribed drugs, among the most beneficial pharmaceutical products ever and among the safest too. As different agents have moved out of patent, furious financial arguments have receded (generic versions of rosuvastatin were introduced in the USA in 2016) to be replaced by seemingly never-ending conflicting data on side effects in real life and the still unclear role of statins in primary prevention, especially in very low risk individuals. This latter consideration is relevant in diabetes only in some Type 1 patients (see previously).

The arguments about adverse effects of the statins fall into several categories:

- muscle-related side effects
- low-grade, but chronic non-muscle-related effects that are very important to individuals expected to take lifelong treatment
- disease-related concerns, especially diabetes and cancer.

The continuing debate is not enlightened by the fact that the full spectrum of non-severe side effects is not captured in most clinical trials of statins, which also routinely exclude the elderly, the group most likely to be prescribed statins and to have comorbidities and polypharmacy that further increase the risk of side effects. There are multiple scoring systems and classifications for statin intolerance and more are proposed now that the PCSK9 inhibitors (see later) are being trialled in, among other groups, statin-intolerant patients, but they are still focused on muscle-related side effects. New drug interactions continue to emerge.

The impact of statin-related media stories

After such a long period in clinical use – nearly 30 years – it is unfortunate that we still do not have greater clarity on the range of side effects of statins or of groups who may be at risk of them. This uncertainty continues to fuel contradictory media stories in many countries that lurch between proposing universal statin use and exaggerated stories about serious side effects. In an enlightening study from Denmark, negative news stories translated into about 10% of statin users discontinuing treatment, and positive stories a similarly decreased risk of discontinuing them. Soberingly, early discontinuation was associated with a one-fifth to one-quarter increase in risk of myocardial infarction or cardiovascular death (Nielsen and Nordestgaard, 2016).

> **Practice point**
>
> Patients who discontinue statin treatment in response to negative media stories run a substantially increased risk of heart attack and cardiovascular death.

Muscle-related side effects

In population studies, the incidence of significant side-effects, usually musculoskeletal, appears to be around 5–10% compared with, for example the very low rate of 0.5% observed in the Heart Protection Study (Saxon and Eckel, 2016). The highest licensed dose of simvastatin, 80 mg daily, used in a few trials, is associated with an increased risk of muscle side-effects and should not be used. The nomenclature of muscle side effects is complex, but worth recalling:

- *Myalgia*: muscle discomfort resulting in pain, soreness, cramp, spasm or aches without elevation in serum creatine kinase (CK) values.
- *Myopathy*: muscle weakness with or without CK elevation.
- *Myositis*: muscle inflammation with elevated CK.
- *Myonecrosis*: muscle injury graded according to the degree of CK elevation. The most severe form, rhabdomyolysis, results in myoglobinuria or acute kidney injury and occurred in a very small proportion, 0.006%, of a large retrospective cohort.

Muscle strength and function have not been fully investigated but atorvastatin, at least, results in an increase in CK levels even in asymptomatic individuals, suggesting some degree of muscle injury. Electrophysiological evidence of peripheral neuropathy can often be detected but it is only very rarely symptomatic.

Although a convoluted statin clinical myalgia index score is available (Rosenson *et al.*, 2014), it will never be used in routine clinical practice, but it does highlight important clinical features:

- symptoms in bilateral hip flexors/thighs
- onset within four weeks of starting treatment
- improvement within two weeks of statin withdrawal
- similar symptoms returning within four weeks of re-challenge.

The race is on to identify a biomarker predicting muscle damage. The scenario is familiar: claims are high, current clinical utility very low. Nothing can alleviate the symptoms. Supplements of co-enzyme CoQ10 are popular but of no value. The requirement for routine liver function testing was dropped long ago, as hepatotoxicity is very rare and idiosyncratic. Statins are safe in patients with stable chronic liver disease.

Does statin intolerance increase cardiovascular risk through either poor adherence or suboptimal LDL control? Serban *et al.* (2017) used prescribing definitions of statin intolerance (e.g. down-titration, switching from statin to ezetimibe monotherapy, or changing to three or more types of statin within a year). If one of these definitions was recorded in the year after a myocardial infarction, the risk of coronary events and recurrent myocardial infarction in the following two years increased by 50% in diabetic and non-diabetic patients. Maintaining target LDL levels using the best-tolerated low-dose statin with ezetimibe and stringent lifestyle is clearly important in these very high-risk patients, but novel agents without muscle side effects are needed too.

Non-muscle side effects

In clinical practice, non-muscle side effects are common and not adequately quantified in clinical trials. There is concern about acute or subacute cognitive impairment, which may occur but has not been systematically studied (there is however no evidence that statins increase the risk of dementia or Alzheimer's disease) (Bitzur, 2016). Patients often mention joint pains; if troublesome they should be managed as muscle symptoms by temporarily stopping the medication, followed by a re-challenge if possible.

Disease-related concerns: cancer and new-onset diabetes

Cancer incidence has been studied in detail in many statin studies. The results are uniformly reassuring. There are some hints from retrospective and subgroup analyses that some specific tumours (for example, prostate cancer) may be less common in patients on long-term statin treatment.

There are clear data that statin treatment increases the risk of developing diabetes. For example, in the JUPITER study, which used rosuvastatin, this amounted to a 0.6% absolute increased risk (2.4% in the placebo-treated group, 3.0% in the rosuvastatin group). In meta-analyses, the increased relative risk is around 12%. There is statistically significant but clinically irrelevant weight gain (around 0.25 kg) and in Type 2 patients studied in CARDS there was also a statistically significant but similarly small absolute increase in HbA_{1c} (0.14%) over the first year of treatment, but no change thereafter. It did not attenuate the beneficial effect of atorvastatin on cardiovascular outcomes (Livingstone *et al.*, 2016).

> **Practice point**
>
> In extensive studies, statins do not increase cancer risk and may be associated with a slight decrease in certain tumours. The tiny increase in blood glucose in people with diabetes is not detectable on routine testing and does not reduce their cardiovascular benefit.

DRUG INTERACTIONS

Drug–drug interactions significantly increase the risk of statin side effects, usually through enhancing blood levels of statins. In general, atorvastatin and simvastatin have a higher risk of side effects than pravastatin and rosuvastatin because they are metabolised by CYP3A4. Commonly-prescribed drugs that inhibit CYP3A4 increase the circulating levels of simvastatin and atorvastatin. A few drugs that notably induce CYP3A4 (e.g. phenytoin) reduce the availability of these two statins. All calcium-channel blockers increase the risk of side effects. HIV specialists are well aware of the interactions between antiretroviral drugs and statins: pravastatin carries the lowest risk (**Table 12.3**).

> **Practice point**
>
> There are more drug–drug interactions with simvastatin and atorvastatin (metabolized by CYP3A4) than with pravastatin and rosuvastatin.

Table 12.3 Clinically significant drug interactions with statins.

Statin and CYP substrate	Drugs likely to cause severe interactions: do not use	Drugs likely to cause major interactions: use with caution	Other drugs to use with increased awareness
Simvastatin (CYP3A4)	Clarithromycin Erythromycin Red yeast rice	Amiodarone, dronedarone Amlodipine, nidefipine Diltiazem, verapamil Fibrates Ranolazine Ticagrelor	Dexamethasone Digoxin Esomeprazole Omeprazole Phenytoin Rifampicin
Atorvastatin (CYP3A4)	Red yeast rice	Clarithromycin Digoxin Diltiazem, verapamil Erythromycin Fibrates	Amiodarone Antacids Esomeprazole, lansoprazole, omeprazole Phenytoin Quinine Ranolazine Rifampicin Warfarin
Rosuvastatin (CYP2C9: minor interaction)	Red yeast rice	Antacids Clarithromycin	Colchicine Warfarin
Pravastatin (largely eliminated by other routes)	Red yeast rice	Bile acid resins Clarithromycin Erythromycin	Orlistat

Single drinks of grapefruit juice increase the bioavailability of simvastatin and atorvastatin but do not interact with pravastatin or rosuvastatin. A more significant acute interaction is between clarithromycin/erythromycin and simvastatin/atorvastatin; this will be widely over-looked in the absence of automated interaction alerts and therefore particularly likely to occur in hospitalized patients. Amiodarone is less widely used now but the lowest doses of atorvastatin and simvastatin are advised. Anticoagulant monitoring should be more frequent when starting or dose escalating any of the statins, apart from pravastatin.

Enquiring about over-the-counter, herbal and other complementary medicines is always important but is especially so with statins. For example, red yeast rice is widely available as a health food supplement in Europe (though patent claims exclude it from the USA) and it is widely reported to be very effective in reducing LDL levels. This is hardly surprising, since an early statin – lovastatin – was derived from the active LDL-lowering agent in red yeast rice – monacolin K. St John's Wort is well known to increase statin levels. Where there is a suspicion of side effects associated with drug interaction in patients taking simvastatin or atorvastatin, a trial of pravastatin or rosuvastatin is worth-while. Changing from simvastatin to atorvastatin is usually attempted but for sound reasons patients are likely to get the same side effects – and they are then often labelled as 'statin intolerant'. Although pravastatin is not much used these days, having been designated a weak statin, at its maximum dose, 40 mg daily, it reduces LDL by about 30%, so using the target LDL approach of <2.0 mmol/l, it may be of value if baseline LDL is about 3.0 mmol/l. Although higher doses have not been included in RCTs, pravastatin is licensed up to 80 mg daily in the USA. Patients who have had side effects with one or more statins are understandably reluctant to try other agents. Use the lowest doses in these trials. Alternate-day atorvastatin and rosuvastatin is effective, though not formally licensed, and may be of value in some patients with side effects; it is also a useful strat-egy in patients who have had poor experiences with other statins (Elis and Lishner, 2012).

Practice point

Specifically enquire about the over-the-counter food supplement red yeast rice. An early statin (lovastatin) was derived from it and side effects are likely to be enhanced if taken together with a statin.

Statins in people of South-East Asian origin

As cardiovascular disease increases in South-East Asia, statins are more widely used. The licensed maximum doses of all statins are lower than in countries with predominantly white populations. Serum statin levels are higher in Asians than in Caucasians, though where efficacy and side effects have been studied there seem to be no differences. There is a widespread clinical impression that South-East Asian patients are more sensitive to both the therapeutic and adverse effects of statins and it is wise to start with low doses. (Potential ethnic differences in responses to statins are another compelling reason not to treat according to statin 'potencies', which were established in clinical trials of predomi-nantly white people.)

Practice point

People from South-East Asia may be more sensitive to the effects and side effects of statins. Start with low doses.

INTENSIVE LDL LOWERING IN SEVERELY HYPERTENSIVE PATIENTS

Even when practitioners have reached the practical limits of improving glycaemic control in individual patients, managing blood pressure and LDL are very effective. Furthermore, even in patients with poorly controlled blood pressure, LDL lowering is still of major importance. This important general point was highlighted in an elegant analysis of treatment-resistant hypertension in the Treating to New Targets (TNT) study, which compared low- and high-dose atorvastatin (80 mg and 10 mg daily, respectively) in a general population of people with coronary artery disease. Although diuretic use was low and most patients therefore did not conform to the conventional definition of resistant hypertension, they undoubtedly had severe hypertension (e.g. systolic blood pressure $\geq$140 mm Hg with three agents). Coronary deaths were reduced by 45% in the high-dose patients (mean LDL 2.0 mmol/l) compared with the low dose, and all-cause mortality was reduced by a nearly-significant 30%, highlighting the importance of intensive LDL lowering in all high-risk patients. Stroke rates, however, more sensitive to blood pressure than LDL lowering, were not reduced by the high-intensity regimen (Bangalore et al., 2014).

Practice point

Intensive LDL lowering is important in all high-risk patients, including those with resistant hypertension – but do not give up continuing to manage the hypertension either, as stroke risk remains high.

AGE

While there are no formal trials of statins in people older than 75, CARDS (atorvastatin 10 mg daily) included 1100 Type 2 patients 65–75 years old at randomization, and therefore 70–80 years old at trial end after four years follow-up. Relative risk reduction for a first major cardiovascular event was identical in younger and older patients (37%) with a correspondingly higher absolute risk reduction (4% vs 2.7%) and no differences in the safety profile (Neil et al., 2006). Age itself is not a contraindication to statin treatment but there are more competing considerations than in younger populations (for example, frailty and sarcopenia). Formal studies in less highly-selected patients would be invaluable.

Practice point

Older people are not more prone to statin side effects and absolute benefits are greater. It is important to consider potential impact of side effects on mobility, but that mandates more careful discussion and follow up, not reluctance to prescribe.

STATINS AND NON-ALCOHOLIC FATTY LIVER DISEASE (SEE CHAPTER 13)

STATINS AND DIABETIC RETINOPATHY

There are strong epidemiological links between micro- and macrovascular complications in Type 1 and 2 diabetes. In addition, abnormal lipid measurements (usually elevated triglycerides and low HDL levels) have frequently been linked with worse microvascular outcomes, especially in Type 1 diabetes, though any association with LDL levels is at most weak. It is therefore no surprise that a great deal of data analysis has been done to find whether statins, so dramatically successful in reducing macrovascular events, might also benefit microvascular outcomes. There are no RCTs directly exploring this question and they will not happen now.

In Type 1 diabetes, a 30-year follow-up of the important Wisconsin retinopathy study found that there was a weak inverse relationship between HDL-cholesterol levels and prevalence of proliferative retinopathy, but no relationship with other lipid values. Importantly, statins did not reduce the incidence of proliferative retinopathy or macular oedema (Klein *et al.*, 2015). This is another reason not to promote wider statin use in otherwise uncomplicated Type 1 diabetes.

The data in Type 2 is not much more persuasive. There is tentative evidence that people who take statins before the onset of Type 2 diabetes are at slightly lower risk of subsequently developing neuropathy and retinopathy (and gangrene of the foot), but not nephropathy (Nielsen and Nordestgaard, 2014). Once Type 2 has developed, many patients will be long-term users of statins in any case, so the interest in whether statin treatment benefits microvascular outcomes is probably of more academic than practical relevance (there is no evidence that they increase the risk, despite their slight adverse impact on glucose levels). Occasional reports of exudative and plaque maculopathy regressing after intensive lipid therapy will remain occasional reports. There is more interest in microvascular complications being helped by the fibric acid drugs (see later).

Practice point

Microvascular complications of Type 1 diabetes are not helped by statins. There may be some benefit in Type 2 diabetes, especially if started before the onset of diabetes, but the majority of patients will already be taking statins for their dramatic macrovascular effects.

OTHER LIPID-MODIFYING DRUGS

The past five years have seen an extraordinary collapse in the evidence base for the use of lipid-modifying agents that were previously widely used and advocated as adjunctive treatment, especially in patients with an additional need for correction of the diabetic dyslipidaemia of modestly elevated triglycerides and depressed HDL. The most spectacular victim of trial-based evidence was niacin and its modified release and combination preparations, which are no longer available in Europe. Fibrates are still available, as are omega-3 fish oils, but with a more tenuous base for their use. To balance these failures, right at the end of ezetimibe's patent life, unequivocal evidence for its benefit in reducing cardiovascular endpoints emerged with the IMPROVE-IT study (Murphy *et al.*, 2016) and the parenteral PCSK9 inhibitors are emerging as possible treatments.

Fibrates

Fibric acid drugs (predominantly fenofibrate and bezafibrate) were previously widely used combined with statins in patients with insulin-resistant dyslipidaemia (low HDL-cholesterol, elevated triglycerides); the combination was seen as a more complete solution to the overall lipid abnormalities in Type 2 diabetes. Fibrates are pleiotropic PPAR-α agonist drugs acting on nuclear receptors, with beneficial effects on multiple detailed lipid and non-lipid characteristics. For example, they increase LDL particle size (large particles are anti-atherogenic in epidemiological studies), reduce pro-thrombotic factors, including fibrinogen, and promote flow-mediated vasodilatation (McKeague and Keating, 2011). Interest in fibrates was stimulated by the VA-HIT study of 1999 in which gemfibrozil treatment resulted in 4% absolute reduction in cardiovascular events. The study population was secondary prevention non-diabetic male patients with isolated low HDL-cholesterol levels (mean 0.8 mmol/l) but otherwise undramatic lipid profiles (Rubins et al., 1999).

The promise shown by their biochemical and in vitro effects was largely unfulfilled in two major cardiovascular outcome trials. In the FIELD study, which used fenofibrate monotherapy, coronary events were unchanged, though total cardiovascular events, including revascularization, were reduced (Keech et al., 2005). Pulmonary embolus and pancreatitis were more common with fenofibrate, events that in more recent cardiovascular outcomes trials would have been explored in greater detail.

In the ACCORD lipid study, patients at high cardiovascular risk were randomised to statin or statin plus fenofibrate treatment. As in the FIELD study, patients had undistinguished lipid profiles including a humdrum HDL-cholesterol level (mean total cholesterol 4.5 mmol/l, HDL 1.0 mmol/l and triglycerides 1.8 mmol/l). While vascular outcomes were overall unchanged in both the ACCORD and FIELD studies, some prespecified outcomes were reduced, for example below-knee amputations and the need for laser treatment for retinopathy in the FIELD study. In the ACCORD study – similar to findings in smaller previous studies – there was an additional 10–13% reduction in cardiovascular and coronary end points in the group with the most insulin-resistant lipid profiles (e.g. HDL <0.75 mmol/l and triglycerides >3.2 mmol/l) (ACCORD Study Group, 2010). This is consistent with the VA-HIT study result.

Practice point

Fibric acid–statin combinations do not improve cardiovascular outcomes. Mild retinopathy might benefit but standard multimodal intervention à la Steno-2 is probably more valuable overall.

Recurrent suggestions based mostly on the FIELD results to use fenofibrate in patients with specified degrees of retinopathy or specific lipid profiles have clinically fallen on deaf ears. Like their PPAR partners, the γ-receptor activating glitazones, they remain potentially valuable drugs in search of better-defined patient groups, and it is frustrating that the ACCORD and FIELD studies did not pursue the VA-HIT's striking finding of reduced events in people with isolated low HDL-cholesterol levels (mean HDL in the FIELD study was 1.1 mmol/l); but the search for clinical benefit in drugs with 'pleiotropic' effects was at it its most elaborate in the 2000s.

The most notable fibrate adverse effect is a reversible rise of up to 20% in serum creatinine, due to increased creatinine synthesis; at any eGFR <60 ml/min fenofibrate doses must be reduced. As with statins, non-specific side effects occur and need to be taken seriously, but the risk of muscle side effects is much lower and they were not more common in the combined statin–fibrate group in the ACCORD study. Gemfibrozil is available but not used in the United Kingdom and cannot be used in combination with a statin.

Discontinuing fibric acid drugs

Clinicians are unlikely to routinely start fibrates treatment, except in cases of marked hypertriglyceridaemia, but patients may well still be taking them. Should they be continued? Triglyceride-induced pancreatitis would be a definite indication for continuing but in the more common situation, where they were initially prescribed for a mild diabetic dyslipidaemia (usually with a statin), carefully monitored withdrawal is worthwhile, because of their minimal effect on the routine lipid profile. Statin treatment may need modifying.

> **Practice point**
>
> Consider carefully monitored withdrawal of fibrate treatment in patients where it was started for its potential cardiovascular protection effects. Intensifying statin treatment is of greater value.

Ezetimibe: finally a result

Ezetimibe inhibits intestinal cholesterol absorption but its dominant effect is not so much on reducing absorption of dietary cholesterol (which is small, 200–300 mg daily) but on the much larger pool of cholesterol contained in bile. While in large trials ezetimibe has detectable but minor effects on Apo B levels and triglycerides, which fall slightly, and on HDL, which increases, its dominant effect is on LDL, which it reduces by a fixed amount – around 15–20% — and the IMPROVE-IT trial results (ezetimibe + simvastatin) lie directly on the regression line in **Figure 12.3**. It acts synergistically with statins, and its effect is independent of baseline LDL levels; this is particularly important when considering up-titration of statins, where a doubling of the dose beyond the standard starting dose will cause a further LDL fall of only about 6% (**Figure 12.4**).

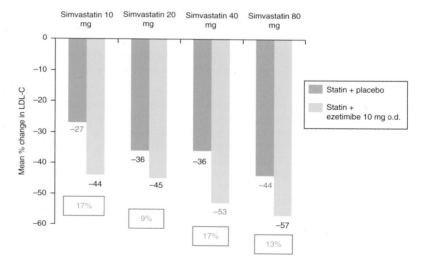

Figure 12.4 Practical pharmacology of ezetimibe. This dose-response study of ezetimibe, 10 mg daily added to simvastatin in doses of 10, 20, 40 and 80 mg daily, illuminates several practical points in LDL management: (i) the major impact of a statin is achieved at or near its starting dose; here 10 mg simvastatin reduced LDL on average by 27%. (ii) Statin dose effects are log-linear. Doubling the dose on average further reduces LDL by approximately 6%. (iii) The fixed effect of ezetimibe 10 mg daily is to further decrease LDL by between 9 and 17%, the equivalent effect of up to three dosage steps of a statin. (iv) In combination, maximum-dose simvastatin (80 mg is no longer recommended) and ezetimibe reduced LDL by nearly 60%. *Source:* Davidson *et al.*, 2002.

After several trials in non-ischaemic cardiac conditions where, not surprisingly, no benefit was seen, the huge (>18 000 patients) post-coronary syndrome IMPROVE-IT study found that ezetimibe in addition to simvastatin reduced vascular events by exactly the extent predicted from its LDL-reducing effect (approximately 0.4 mmol/l, from 1.8 to 1.4 mmol/l), amounting to about 7% risk reduction, but with a 2% absolute risk reduction in these high-risk patients. Ischaemic stroke was also reduced, haemorrhagic stroke very slightly increased. No major side effects were reported (Cannon et al., 2015). It does not increase the risk of cancer, a fear raised and dismissed several years ago. Subgroup results for patients with diabetes in IMPROVE-IT have not been reported but presumably are the same as in the whole study group, as in all the statin trials. The current indications for ezetimibe in clinical practice are therefore:

- As add-on to high-dose or maximum-tolerated dose statin where target LDL has not been reached; it may be of particular value in Type 1 patients who have a particularly good response to ezetimibe.
- As monotherapy where there is intolerance to any statin treatment.
- Chronic kidney disease. Ezetimibe is effective and safe in all degrees of renal impairment, including predialysis and dialysis patients.

Ezetimibe was licensed in 2000 and it is a pity that it was 15 years before the definitive RCT was published with reassurance about adverse effects, concerns which persisted for many years. Its patent expiry is imminent.

Niacin (nicotinic acid, vitamin B3)

Niacin had a long history of use in lipid disorders, with a broad profile that, like fibrates, reduced triglycerides and increased HDL. Early studies showed some benefit in postcoronary bypass patients. It briefly thrived, at the expense of ezetimibe (though the lipid actions of the two were hardly comparable), when extended-release niacin was shown to induce regression of carotid intima-media thickening while ezetimibe seemed to promote it (Villines et al., 2010). Its grudging uptake was limited by persistent cutaneous flushing and concerns about adverse effects, in particular raising blood glucose levels occasionally to a clinically significant degree in people with diabetes.

Its definitive and unexpected demise arrived with two studies, AIM-HIGH (2011) and HPS2-THRIVE (2014), both of which used an extended-release form of niacin coformulated with the largely untested laropiprant, a prostaglandin inhibitor that reduced the worst effects of flushing. Neither study showed a significant reduction in cardiovascular events and there was a significant excess of a variety of side effects. New-onset diabetes increased by 30% and in HPS2-THRIVE there was an alarming increase in hyperglycaemia-related hospitalization. Niacin preparations are no longer available in Europe. The usual pleas for further studies in subgroups will likely fall on deaf ears. As with other previously promising drugs which have fallen by the evidence-based wayside, niacin is still advocated by some, mostly on the grounds of positive mechanistic studies conducted within the large clinical trials, and by others interested in meta-analysis rather than the outcomes of definitive and substantial clinical trials.

Bile acid sequestrants

The first-generation bile acid sequestrants were poorly tolerated and fell out of use in lipid management when the statins were introduced. A second-generation agent, colesevelam, was introduced in 2000 and was found consistently to reduce HbA_{1c} in Type 2 diabetes by 0.3–1.1%, though its blood glucose lowering mechanism is not understood. It is licensed in the USA for blood glucose lowering. LDL falls by a further 10–16%

when added to a statin. Despite gastrointestinal side effects typical of this group, discontinuation rates in clinical trials are reported to be low. However, it has to be given in large and divided doses, and is prohibitively expensive.

Omega-3 (n-3) fatty acids

In their pharmaceutical form, omega-3 fatty acids have suffered the same fate as fibrates. They retain their value in people with hypertriglyceridaemia (see previously) where they reduce hepatic VLDL synthesis and increase hepatic β-oxidation and peripheral VLDL clearance, although they must be taken in large doses for meaningful reductions in triglycerides, for example 8 g daily for about 40% reduction. At much lower doses – 1 g daily – sudden death was reduced in the well-remembered GISSI-Prevenzione trial (1999), and hospitalization for heart failure in GISSI-HF (2008). The large Alpha Omega Trial (Kromhout et al., 2010) treated older secondary prevention patients (60–80 years) with low dose n-3 fatty acids or the plant-derived alpha-linoleic acid. There were no consistently beneficial effects on cardiovascular outcomes, except in people with diabetes in a post hoc analysis.

Pharmaceutically-refined products were previously but are no longer licensed in the United Kingdom for event prophylaxis after myocardial infarction. The heart failure indication was not pursued. The small benefits observed in these earlier studies have been obliterated by a series of factorial studies that, as well as a pharmaceutical product, included omega-3 fatty acids, though usually in the small 1 g daily dose used in GISSI-Prevenzione. The huge ORIGIN study (ORIGIN Trial Investigators, 2012) treated more than 12 000 dysglycemic subjects at high cardiovascular risk with 1 g daily of pharmaceutical-grade omega-3 fatty acids for up to six years with no reduction in events (insulin glargine, in the same factorial study, was also neutral for cardiovascular event outcomes; see **Chapter 10**). These results contrast strongly with the striking and consistent epidemiological evidence that oily fish intake is strongly associated with reduced cardiovascular events, even though a 2–3 ounce (56–84 g) portion of fish contains only about 1 g omega-3 fatty acids.

Practice point

Omega-3 fatty acids are almost certainly better consumed as food (e.g. regularly eating oily fish) rather than as food supplements, which have no meaningful cardiovascular benefits.

Phytosterols/phytostanols

Plant sterols, hydrogenated to stanols, reduce cholesterol absorption. This effect seems to be independent of the cholesterol absorption-inhibiting effect of ezetimibe and is additive to the effect of statins. They are recommended as part of the non-pharmaceutical approach to LDL-lowering treatment. They are certainly effective up to a daily dose of 2 g, possibly 3 g daily; when taken regularly, mean LDL falls by approximately 12% (Ras et al., 2014) – a meaningful effect, similar to a fourfold increase in a statin dose. Because they are fat-soluble they are incorporated into dairy products such as margarine (daily requirement 1½ tablespoons – possibly unpalatable) or more conveniently as a small yoghurt drink each containing about 2g per portion. The products are expensive and there are no studies of real-life adherence, and certainly none of cardiovascular outcomes, but they are potentially valuable, especially in people where statin treatment is not practicable, for example the young, women of childbearing age and Type 1 patients, and in patients requiring portfolio medication for severe hypercholesterolaemia. Advise patients to be aware of the carbohydrate content of the products, though several readily-available drinks have <40 kcal per serving.

Practice point

2 g plant sterols/stanols taken daily as a spread (margarine) or yoghurt drink daily can meaning-fully reduce LDL by about 12%. Ensure a low-sugar product is chosen.

PCSK9 inhibitors (alirocumab, evolocumab)

The most recently introduced LDL-lowering agents, with a completely novel mode of action. A tsunami of clinical trials is presently investigating them. They have elicited considerable excitement among lipidologists; their place in standard lipid management in the clinic will take longer to establish and in many patients careful combination therapy using a potent statin with ezetimibe may approach the LDL levels achievable with these undoubtedly powerful agents. We must also remain aware of the cautionary lessons from the seemingly established drugs that have fallen by the wayside as a result of well-conducted large-scale clinical trials (see previously), and the even more salutary lessons learned from agents such as the CETP inhibitor torcetrapib, which despite its dramatic HDL-raising effect also, for unknown 'off-target' reasons, increased the risk of adverse cardiovascular outcomes.

PCSKP9 (plasma proprotein convertase subtilisin/kexin type 9) is synthesized in the liver and binds to LDL receptors. Recycling of the LDL receptors to the cell surface is reduced, LDL clearance is reduced and plasma LDL levels increase. Inhibiting PCSK9 prevents LDL receptor degradation in the lysosomes and preserves receptor recycling, thereby increasing LDL receptor activity on hepatocytes. This is the same end result as statin treatment, but through a different mechanism. Two human monoclonal antibodies to PCSK9, alirocumab and evolocumab, were approved in 2015 for hypercholesterolaemia (e.g. heterozygous familial hypercholesterolaemia, very high cardiovascular risk patients, and those not at target because of statin intolerance). As they are monoclonal antibodies they are given subcutaneously by injection, either two-weekly (alirocumab 75 mg or 150 mg) or monthly (evolocumab 420 mg, but also 140 mg every two weeks). There have been no studies conducted with the ideal of placebo injections.

Like the potent statins, in addition to substantial LDL-lowering effects they have a modest impact on other lipids, for example up to 25% triglyceride lowering and 8% HDL elevation. A high proportion of patients reach LDL levels <1.4 mmol/l. The results for evolocumab are the same in Type 2 as non-diabetic people, and are not affected by insulin use or any other baseline characteristics (Sattar et al., 2016). These drugs were in clinical trials around the time the ACC/AHA guidelines were proposed and the trial results place greater emphasis on their LDL-lowering potency than achieved LDL values. In addition, because statin-intolerant patients were often included, baseline LDL values are often higher than in other trials (e.g. about 3 mmol/l). The field is muddied by the multiple definitions of statin intolerance; a unified definition is needed even more urgently with the advent of these drugs.

Injection-site reactions, myalgia, neurocognitive disorders, mostly related to memory, and ophthalmological side effects are documented, but the full range of adverse effects may take a while to emerge. Analysis of adverse effects in the first small tranche of patients treated in clinical trials does not highlight any specific major adverse effects, but reassurance will come only with the scale of trials now mandated for cardiovascular outcomes in diabetes (Jones *et al.*, 2016). The results of two massive placebo-controlled trials indicate some benefit on cardiovascular outcomes. The three-year FOURIER study using evolocumab (140 mg every two weeks or 420 mg monthly) reduced events including ischaemic stroke to the expected extent in patients with established cardiovascular disease and other associated risk factors, for example diabetes. However, inclusion required baseline LDL ≥1.8 mmol/l. Actual mean baseline LDL was 2.3 mmol/l, so lipid-lowering treatment was not optimum at the start of the trial. Achieved mean LDL was 0.8 mmol/l and, although there were no signals of specific side effects, this was a relatively short study (Sabatine *et al.*, 2017). The critical comparative study between a PCSK9 inhibitor and highly active treatment with a high-potency statin, ezetimibe and optimum diet is awaited, but probably for a long time. Another PCSK9 inhibitor, bococizumab was withdrawn from clinical trials because of a high level of antidrug antibody formation, attenuation of its LDL-lowering effect with time and injection-site reactions. In the prematurely-terminated cardiovascular outcome studies, there was no cardiovascular benefit in lower-risk patients, but a 20% risk reduction in a higher-risk group with baseline LDL ≥2.6 mmol/l studied for 12 months. Overall, early outcome trials of these agents are modestly encouraging but there is no shortage of articles proclaiming a new dawn in lipid-lowering treatment.

Practice point

The injected PCSK9 inhibitors evolocumab and alirocumab are promising in patients with advanced atherosclerotic disease, severe statin intolerance and some familial hypercholesterolaemias. Safety is not established in long-term trials.

References

ACCORD Study Group; Ginsberg HN, Elam MG, Lovato LC *et al.* Effects of combination lipid therapy in type 2 diabetes mellitus. *N Engl J Med* 2010;362:1563–74 [PMID: 20228404] PMC2879499.

Ahmed S, Cannon CP, Murphy SA, Braunwald E. Acute coronary syndromes and diabetes: is intensive lipid lowering beneficial? Results of the PROVE IT-TIMI-22 Trial. *Eur Heart J* 2006;27:2323–9 [PMID: 16954134] Free full text.

Bangalore S, Fayyad R, Laskey R *et al.* Treating to New Targets steering committee and investigators. Lipid lowering in patients with treatment-resistant hypertension: an analysis from the Treating to New Targets (TNT) trial. *Eur Heart J* 2014;35:1801–8 [PMID: 23990605] Free full text.

Bitzur R. Remembering statins: do statins have adverse cognitive effects? *Diabetes Care* 2016;39 Suppl 2:S253–9 [PMID: 27440840].

Cannon CP, Braunwald E, McCabe CH *et al.* Intensive versus moderate lipid lowering with statins after acute coronary syndromes. *N Engl J Med* 2004;350:1495–504 [PMID: 15007110] Free full text.

Cannon CP, Blazing MA, Giugliano RP; IMPROVE-IT investigators. Ezetimibe added to statin therapy after acute coronary syndromes. *N Engl J Med* 2015; 2387–97 [PMID: 26039521] Free full text.

Cholesterol Treatment Trialists' (CTT) Collaboration. Impact of renal function on the effects of LDL cholesterol lowering with statin-based regimens: a meta-analysis of individual participant data from 28 randomised trials. *Lancet Diabetes Endocrinol* 2016;4:829–39 [PMID: 27477773] Free full text.

Ciriacks K, Coly G, Krishnaswami S *et al.* Effects of simvastatin and ezetimibe in lowering low-density lipoprotein cholesterol in subjects with type 1 and type 2 diabetes mellitus. *Metab Syndr Relat Disord* 2015;13:84–90 [PMID: 25490061].

Clearfield MB, Amerena J, Bassand JP *et al*. Comparison of the efficacy and safety of rosuvastatin 10 mg and atorvastatin 20 mg in high-risk patients with hypercholesterolemia – Prospective study to evaluate the Use of Low doses of the Statins Atorvastatin and Rosuvastatin (PULSAR). *Trials* 2006;7:35 [PMID: 17184550] PMC1770361.

Colhoun HM, Betteridge DJ, Durrington PN *et al*.; CARDS Investigators. Primary prevention of cardiovascular disease with atorvastatin in type 2 diabetes in the Collaborative Atorvastatin Diabetes Study (CARDS): multicentre randomised placebo-controlled trial. *Lancet* 2004;364:685–96 [PMID: 15325833].

Colhoun HM, Betteridge DJ, Durrington PN *et al*. CARDS Investigators. Rapid emergence of effect of atorvastatin on cardiovascular outcomes in the Collaborative Atorvastatin Diabetes Study (CARDS). *Diabetologia* 2005;48:2482–5 [PMID: 16284747].

Collins R, Armitage J, Parish S *et al*. Heart Protection Study Collaborative Group. MRC/BHF Heart Protection Study of cholesterol-lowering with simvastatin in 5963 people with diabetes: a randomised placebo-controlled trial. *Lancet* 2003;361;2005–16 [PMID: 12814710].

Costacou T, Evans RW, Orchard TJ. High-density lipoprotein cholesterol in diabetes: is higher always better? *J Clin Lipidol* 2011;5:387–94 [PMID: 21981840] PMC3190122.

Davidson MH, McGarry T, Bettis R *et al*. Ezetimibe coadministration with simvastatin in patients with primary hypercholesterolaemia. *J Am Coll Cardiol* 2002;40:2125–34 [PMID: 12505224] Free full text.

Elis A, Lishner M. Non-every day statin administration – a literature review. *Eur J Intern Med* 2012;23:474–8 [PMID: 22726380].

Hegele RA, Ginsberg HN, Chapman MJ *et al*. European Atherosclerosis Society Consensus Panel. The polygenic nature of hypertriglyceridaemia: implications for definition, diagnosis, and management. *Lancet Diabetes Endocrinol* 2014;2:655–66 [PMID: 24731657] PMC4201123.

Hero C, Svensson AM, Gidlund P *et al*. LDL cholesterol is not a good marker of cardiovascular risk in Type 1 diabetes. *Diabet Med* 2016;33:316–23 [PMID: 26498834].

Jones PH, Davidson MH, Stein EA *et al*. STELLAR Study Group. Comparison of the efficacy and safety of rosuvastatin versus atorvastatin, simvastatin, and pravastatin across doses (STELLAR Trial). *Am J Cardiol* 2003;92:152–60 [PMID: 12860216].

Jones PH, Bays HE, Chaudhari U *et al*. Safety of alirocumab (a PCSK9 monoclonal antibody) from 14 randomized trials. *Am J Cardiol* 2016;118:1805–11 [PMID: 27729106] Free full text.

Keech A, Simes RJ, Barter P *et al*. FIELD study investigators. Effects of long-term fenofibrate therapy on cardiovascular events in 9795 people with type 2 diabetes mellitus (the FIELD study): randomised controlled trial. *Lancet* 2005;366:1849–61 [PMID: 16310551].

Keenan HA, Costacou T, Sun HK *et al*. Clinical factors associated with resistance to microvascular complications in diabetic patients of extreme disease duration: the 50-year medalist study. *Diabetes Care* 2007;30:1995–7 [PMID: 17507696].

Klein BE, Myers CE, Howard KP, Klein R. Serum lipids and proliferative diabetic retinopathy and macular edema in persons with long-term type 1 diabetes mellitus: the Wisconsin Epidemiologic Study of Diabetic Retinopathy. *JAMA Ophthalmol* 2015:133:503–10 [PMID: 25502808] PMC4433425.

Kromhout D, Giltay EJ, Geleijnse JM; Alpha Omega Trial Group. n-3 fatty acids and cardiovascular events after myocardial infarction. *N Engl J Med* 2010;363:2015–26 [PMID: 20929341] Free full text.

LaRosa JC, Deedwania PC, Shepherd J *et al*. TNT Investigators. Comparison of 80 versus 10 mg of atorvastatin on occurrence of cardiovascular events after the first event (from the Treating to New Targets [TNT] Trial). *Am J Cardiol* 2010;105;283–7 [PMID: 20102935].

Levy D. Acute pancreatitis, in *Levy D: The Hands-on Guide to Diabetes Care in Hospital*. Chichester: John Wiley & Sons Ltd, 2015, pp. 62–65

Livingstone SJ, Looker HC, Akbar T *et al*. Effect of atorvastatin on glycaemia progression in patients with diabetes: an analysis from the Collaborative Atorvastatin in Diabetes Trial (CARDS). *Diabetologia* 2016;59:299–306 [PMID: 26577796] PMC4705133.

Maahs BM, Dabelea D, D'Agostino RB *et al*. SEARCH for Diabetes in Youth Study. Glucose control predicts 2-year change in lipid profile in youth with type 1 diabetes. *J Pediatr* 2013;162:102–7. [PMID: 22795314] PMC3807690.

Maftei O, Pea AS, Sullivan T; AdDIT Study Group. Early atherosclerosis relates to urinary albumin excretion and cardiovascular risk factors in adolescents with type 1 diabetes: Adolescent type 1 Diabetes cardio-renal Intervention Trial (AdDIT). *Diabetes Care* 2014;37:3069–75 [PMID: 25071076].

McKeague K, Keating GM. Fenofibrate: a review of its use in dyslipidaemia. *Drugs* 2011;71:1917–46 [PMID: 21942979].

Murphy SA, Cannon SP, Wiviott SD *et al*. Reduction in recurrent cardiovascular events with intensive lipid-lowering statin therapy after acute coronary syndromes from the PROVE-IT TIMI 22 (Pravastatin or Atorvastatin Evaluation and Infection Therapy-Thrombolysis in Myocardial Infarction 22) Trial. *J Am Coll Cardiol* 2009;54:2358–62 [PMID: 2008293] Free full text.

Murphy SA, Cannon SP, Blazing MA *et al*. Reduction in total cardiovascular events with ezetimibe/ simvastatin post-acute coronary syndrome: the IMPROVE-IT Trial. *J A Coll Cardiol* 2016;67:353–61 [PMID: 26821621].

Neil HA, DeMicco DA, Luo D *et al*. CARDS Study Investigators. Analysis of efficacy and safety in patients aged 65–75 years at randomization: Collaborative Atorvastatin Diabetes Study (CARDS) *Diabetes Care* 2006;29:2378–84 [PMID: 17065671].

NICE. *Type 1 diabetes in adults: diagnosis and management*. NICE guidance [NG17] 2015. www. nice.org.uk/guidance/ng17 (last accessed 1 September 2017).

Nielsen SF, Nordestgaard BG. Statin use before diabetes diagnosis and risk of microvascular disease: a nationwide nested matched study. *Lancet Diabetes Endocrinol* 2014;2:894–900 [PMID: 25217178].

Nielsen SF, Nordestgaard BG. Negative statin-related news stories decrease statin persistence and increase myocardial infarction and cardiovascular mortality: a nationwide prospective cohort study. *Eur Heart J* 2016;37:908–16 [PMID: 26643266].

Opie LH. A proposal to incorporate trial data into a hybrid American College of Cardiology/American Heart Association algorithm for the allocation of statin therapy in primary prevention. *J Am Coll Cardiol* 2015;66:1412–3 [PMID: 26383733].

ORIGIN Trial Investigators; Bosch J, Gerstein HC, Dagenais DR *et al*. n-3 fatty acids and cardiovascular outcomes in patients with dysglycemia. *N Engl J Med* 2012;367:309–18 [PMID: 22686415] Free full text.

Ras RT, Geleijnse JM, Trautwein EA. LDL-cholesterol-lowering effect of plant sterols and stanols across different dose ranges: a meta-analysis of randomised controlled studies. *Br J Nutr* 2014;112:214–9 [PMID: 24780090] PMC4071994.

Rosenson RS, Baker SK, Jacobson TA *et al*. The National Lipid Association's Muscle Safety Expert Panel. An assessment by the Statin Muscle Safety Task Force: 2014 update. *J Clin Lipidol* 2014;8(3 Suppl):S58–71 [PMID: 24793443].

Rubins HB, Robins SJ, Collins D *et al*. Gemfibrozil for the secondary prevention of coronary heart disease in men with low levels of high-density lipoprotein cholesterol. Veterans Affairs High-Density Lipoprotein cholesterol Intervention Trial study group. *N Engl J Med* 1999;341:410–8 [PMID 10438259] Free full text.

Sabatine MS, Giugliano RP, Keech AC *et al*. FOURIER Steering Committee and Investigators. Evolocumab and clinical outcomes in patients with cardiovascular disease. *N Engl J Med* 2017;376:1713–22 [PMID: 28304224].

Santos RD, Gidding SS, Hegele RA *et al*. International Atherosclerosis Society Severe Familial Hypercholesterolemia Panel. Defining severe familial hypercholesterolaemia and the implications for clinical management: a consensus statement from the International Atherosclerosis Society Severe Familial Hypercholesterolemia Panel. *Lancet Diabetes Endocrinol* 2016;4:850–61 [PMID: 27246162].

Sattar N, Preiss D, Robinson JG *et al*. Lipid-lowering efficacy of the PCSK9 inhibitor evolocumab (AMG 145) in patients with type 2 diabetes: a meta-analysis of individual patient data. *Lancet Diabetes Endocrinol* 2016;4:403–10 [PMID: 26868195].

Saxon DR, Eckel RH. Statin intolerance: a literature review and management strategies. *Prog Cardiovasc Dis* 2016;59:153–64 [PMID: 27497504].

Serban MC, Colantonio LD, Manthripragada AD *et al*. Statin intolerance and risk of coronary heart events and all-cause mortality following myocardial infarction. *J Am Coll Cardiol* 2017;69: 1386–95 [PMID: 28302290].

Silverman MG, Ference BA, Im K et al. Association between lowering LDL-C and cardiovascular risk reduction among different therapeutic interventions: a systematic review and meta-analysis. JAMA 2016;316:1289–97 [PMID: 27673306].

Stone NJ, Robinson JG, Lichtenstein AH et al. American College of Cardiology/American Heart Association Task Force on Practice Guidelines. 2013 ACC/AHA guideline on the treatment of blood cholesterol to reduce atherosclerotic cardiovascular risk in adults: a report of the American College of Cardiology/American Heart Association Task Force on Practice Guidelines. Circulation 2014;129(25 Suppl 2):S1–45. [PMID: 24222016] Free full text.

Tanis BC, Westendorp GJ, Smelt HM. Effect of thyroid substitution on hypercholesterolaemia in patients with subclinical hypothyroidism: a reanalysis of intervention studies. Clin Endocrinol (Oxf) 1996;44:643–9 [PMID: 8759176].

Thapa R, Sharma S, Jeevanantham V et al. Disparities in lipid control and statin drug use among diabetics with noncoronary atherosclerotic vascular disease vs those with coronary artery disease. J Clin Lipidol 2015;9:241–6 [PMID: 25911081].

Tran JN, Kao TC, Caglar T et al. Impact of the 2013 cholesterol guideline on patterns of lipid-lowering treatment in patients with atherosclerotic cardiovascular disease or diabetes after 1 year. J Manag Care Spec Pharm 2016;22:901–8 [PMID: 27459652] Free full text.

Villines TC, Stanek EJ, Devine PJ et al. The ARBITER 6-HALTS Trial (Arterial Biology for the Investigation of the Treatment Effects of Reducing Cholesterol 6-HDL and LDL Treatment Strategies in Atherosclerosis): final results and the impact of medication adherence, dose, and treatment duration. J Am Coll Cardiol 2010;55:2271–6 [PMID: 20399059] Free full text.

Writing Group for the DCCT/EDIC Research Group. Coprogression of cardiovascular risk factors in type 1 diabetes during 30 years of follow-up in the DCCT/EDIC study. Diabetes Care 2016;39: 1621–30 [PMID: 27436274] PMC5001148.

Guidelines

Stone NJ, Robinson JG, Lichtenstein AH et al. American College of Cardiology/American Heart Association Task Force on Practice Guidelines. 2013 ACC/AHA guideline on the treatment of blood cholesterol to reduce atherosclerotic cardiovascular risk in adults: a report of the American College of Cardiology/American Heart Association Task Force on Practice Guidelines. Circulation 2014;129(25 Suppl 2):S1–45. [PMID: 24222016] Free full text.

NICE. Type 1 diabetes in adults: diagnosis and management. NICE guidance [NG17] 2015. www.nice.org.uk/guidance/ng17 (last accessed 1 September 2017).

13 Clinical aspects of the metabolic syndrome

Key points

- Focus on clinical aspects of the metabolic syndrome, rather than the definitional cut points of glucose, blood pressure and waist circumference
- The key treatment for non-alcoholic fatty liver disease is caloric restriction and weight loss. No drugs are of proven value
- Treatment of obstructive sleep apnoea with continuous positive airway pressure (CPAP) should be targeted at symptoms and quality of life. To date there are no metabolic or cardiovascular benefits
- Enquire about clinical gout. Episodes may have occurred many years ago
- Polycystic ovarian syndrome is common in both Type 1 and 2 diabetes, but the phenotype is different

INTRODUCTION

The terms insulin resistance and the metabolic syndrome are still used interchangeably. This is because insulin resistance (the inability of insulin to exert its normal actions at concentrations found in normal subjects) is enormously complex and difficult to measure, while the phenotypic manifestations of insulin resistance – the metabolic syndrome – are simpler to define. Short cuts have been devised to measure insulin resistance in the clinical setting but even these are not routinely available. Even the simplest, homoeostatic model assessment (HOMA), calculated from a single fasting measurement of glucose and insulin, is rarely used in practice. This difficulty led to countless attempts to use even simpler clinical manifestations of insulin resistance (fasting glucose, blood pressure, routine lipid measurements and anthropometric measurements) to define the metabolic syndrome. These attempts ended up as largely fruitless arguments between epidemiologists about minute differences in cut points of, for example, waist measurement and fasting glucose levels. This phase peaked around 2009–10 with an attempt to 'harmonize' the various definitions that were then in use (Simmons et al., 2010). Since then a more pragmatic approach has been used; important clinical syndromes thought to have insulin resistance as their fundamental defect are being investigated in much more detail with a view to helping the very large numbers of patients with clinically significant conditions.

Practice point

Because it is so difficult to measure insulin resistance, it is best to discuss its clinical correlate – metabolic syndrome – and its specific components.

Practical Diabetes Care, Fourth Edition. David Levy.
© 2018 John Wiley & Sons Ltd. Published 2018 by John Wiley & Sons Ltd.

The concept of insulin resistance is old and predates by decades the laboratory measurement of insulin levels. Harold Himsworth (1905–1993) was the first to investigate insulin sensitivity and resistance in the modern era in important papers published in the 1930s. He was an endocrinologist and his later work focused on the pituitary hormones, not insulin, mediating insulin resistance. Progress was mostly halted by World War II. Gerald Reaven (b. 1928) resurrected the notion of insulin resistance in his famous 1988 Banting lecture, where he initiated the crucial process of defining the links between a nexus of laboratory abnormalities associated with insulin resistance and clinical abnormalities (Reaven, 1988). He was unaware of Himsworth's work until recently but has graciously acknowledged its importance.

DEFINITIONS

The agreed components of the metabolic syndrome – though these are largely for epidemiological and research purposes – are central obesity together with two or more other factors. In 2010 the World Health Organization firmly concluded that further attempts to define it would be of limited help. The broad cluster of factors is, however, still valuable in alerting clinicians to people who should be observed for the clinically important syndromes associated with it. These numbers are the definitional cut-points issued in 2014 by the International Diabetes Federation:

- *Central obesity*. There is a great deal of debate how this can be measured simply. Obesity is assumed if BMI >30. In European males, waist >94 cm, females >80 cm are proposed, and >90 cm for males of other ethnicities.
- *Hypertension* (e.g. ≥130/≥85) or treated hypertension.
- *Raised fasting glucose* ≥5.6 mmol/l (100 mg/dl), but below the threshold for the diagnosis of diabetes (i.e. <7.1 mmol/l).
- *Dyslipidaemia*: elevated triglycerides (e.g. >1.7 mmol/l) or low HDL (e.g. <1.0 mmol/l in males, <1.3 mmol/l in females).

Practice point

Definitions of the metabolic syndrome require (i) central obesity, (ii) hypertension, (iii) glucose level between normality and diabetes and (iv) low HDL/elevated triglycerides.

Much analytical energy was devoted to trying to show how different combinations of these factors might be more or less strongly linked to cardiovascular outcomes. None were conclusively shown to be more strongly predictive of meaningful vascular outcomes than standard risk factors (diabetes, hypertension, smoking, LDL and obesity). Focusing on cardiovascular outcomes was always too limited, given the multiple different organs where insulin resistance can be measured or inferred.

In addition, the core measurements are not always present, and in truth they just happened to be elements of the data set that was collected in epidemiological studies. Striking exceptions may not be all that uncommon, for example the lean phenotype of the polycystic ovarian syndrome; and while dyslipidaemia is a clear manifestation of insulin resistance (for example the failure of insulin to suppress free fatty acid metabolism, leading to elevated VLDL production and hypertriglyceridaemia), non-alcoholic fatty liver disease (more a manifestation of the inflammatory aspects of insulin resistance, which are omitted from the epidemiologically-derived definition above) has much more serious clinical consequences. Inevitably the more unusual – but still common – clinical manifestations of insulin resistance are the most difficult situations to manage and nested within them is a spectrum of clinical severity that is still not understood, has not yielded to multifactorial analysis and is likely to remain relatively resistant to the efforts of the new biomarker movement – though it must be said not through lack of trying.

THE SCOPE OF INSULIN RESISTANCE

Although the clinical consequences of insulin resistance are most vividly seen in the three tissues where insulin has its major effects (muscle, adipose tissue and liver), insulin acts at a wide variety of other tissues and organs, and new aspects of insulin resistance continue to be described. Even in organs traditionally thought not to require insulin-mediated glucose uptake, for example the brain, there are certain anatomical areas where the importance of insulin action is increasingly recognized. The hippocampus is one such region; insulin resistance here may be significant in Alzheimer's disease (Rani *et al.*, 2016).

In general clinical practice it is important to recognize the variety of clinical syndromes that are considered to be associated with insulin resistance (**Figure 13.1**), or at least to acknowledge that items in this and the many other lists may be more or less strongly linked. 'Association' is a critical qualifier here: ascribing a single causality to these

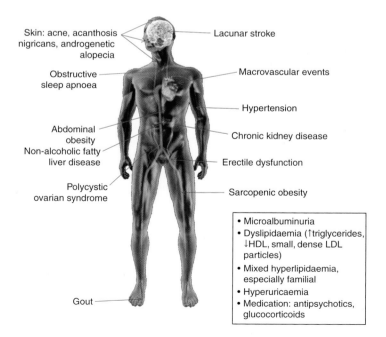

Figure 13.1 Clinical associations of insulin resistance.

evidently different conditions is very difficult to establish and attempts to do so are often the subject of prevailing fashion, for example sympathetic overactivity or changes in the intestinal microbiome.

NON-ALCOHOLIC FATTY LIVER DISEASE (NAFLD)

Up to three-quarters of Type 2 patients have some form of fatty liver (broadly defined as >5–10% histological fat in people who drink <20 g alcohol daily) and NAFLD is justifiably raising concern as a public health problem. It is increasing as a common form of chronic liver disease; in the USA, NAFLD-associated cirrhosis or hepatocellular carcinoma is the second most common reason for liver transplantation. It is detectable in 25–30% of non-diabetic people. Important associations in Type 2 diabetes have been established (Hazelhurst et al., 2016), for example:

- Increased (approximately twofold) risk of cardiovascular events.
- Increased risk of chronic kidney disease (CKD) and retinopathy.
- Type 2 diabetes co-existing with biopsy-proven NAFLD increases the risk of progression to fibrosis.
- Type 2 diabetes may further worsen the prognosis of hepatocellular carcinoma.

Practice point

About 75% of Type 2 patients have NAFLD.

NAFLD is no more common in Type 1 diabetes than it is in non-diabetic individuals matched for obesity. However, it probably does exist in patients in very poor control on account of the dyslipidaemia, which is broadly similar to that of poorly-controlled Type 2 diabetes (**Chapter 12**). Mauriac syndrome, comprising growth failure, Cushingoid appearance and hepatomegaly, was common in children in the early years of insulin treatment and is still sporadically reported in patients with chronically very poor control. Fatty change is seen on liver biopsy. Short of Mauriac syndrome glycogen hepatopathy is described, also in poorly-controlled children. Given the low overall frequency of liver disease in younger people with Type 1 diabetes, the differential diagnosis needs pursuing; remember the rare association between Type 1 diabetes and autoimmune liver disease.

Pathogenesis and diagnosis

Although the general view is that NAFLD has a 'multihit' pathogenesis, the major underlying problem is excessive hepatic triglyceride accumulation, which correlates with hepatic VLDL production, and which is not adequately suppressed by insulin. There are several sources of the triglycerides; dietary and de novo lipogenesis from conversion of carbohydrates to lipid (up to 25% of liver triglycerides in NAFLD); fructose, which in its various forms constitutes a substantial proportion of the western diet, is considered particularly potent at promoting intrahepatic triglyceride accumulation. Hepatic fat results in increased insulin requirements, with the potential exacerbating effect of stoking up weight further. Other pathogenic processes include oxidative stress.

Formal diagnostic criteria are fraught with definitional minutiae. Standard liver function tests can be normal even when there is quite advanced hepatic fibrosis, promoting the use of various panels of tests with better discriminatory power. Where transaminases are abnormal, alanine transaminase (ALT) levels are usually greater than aspartate transaminase (AST); the converse suggests fibrosis or cirrhosis. Liver fat is 'bright' on ultrasound and radiographers and radiologists can readily detect it, but it is difficult to discriminate simple fat accumulation (steatosis) from the more advanced inflammatory state of steatohepatitis. FibroScan techniques, which rely on the tissue properties of the homogeneous liver tissue to transmit and reflect ultrasonographic waves in different ways according to the level of hepatic fibrosis, are not yet routinely used; biopsy is considered the 'gold standard' but rarely used outside the research arena.

Management

Weight loss

There are no specific drug treatments but even short-term caloric restriction can have dramatic effects on hepatic steatosis and the associated metabolic abnormalities. For example, a low-fat diet of 1200 kcal/day for seven weeks resulted in about 10% reduction in body weight in very insulin-resistant Type 2 patients, and fasting glucose fell from 8.8 to 6.4 mmol/l. Hepatic and muscle fat both decreased and hepatic insulin sensitivity improved. It may not be as difficult for patients in the real world to achieve these outcomes as they believe: mean weight in this study fell from 86 to 78 kg, BMI from 30.0 to 27.5, so they were still overweight (Petersen et al., 2005). High-intensity physical training (e.g. 30–40 min a week for 12 weeks) has been shown to reduce hepatic fat independently of weight loss (see **Chapter 9**). However, given the dietary contribution to fat overload, dietary restriction is probably overall the most important non-pharmacological treatment; histological measures of hepatic steatosis decrease in proportion to the degree of weight loss.

Practice point

NAFLD responds to about 10% body weight loss.

Can bariatric surgery improve hepatic structure? In a very large study patients with a mean BMI of 48 underwent either Roux-en-Y bypass or gastric banding. In sequential liver biopsies over five years after surgery NAFLD improved more after bypass than banding; much of the effect was explained by the differences in weight loss (Caiazzo et al., 2014). Bariatric surgery is safe in people even with advanced fibrosis and although small studies show improvement in the histology of non-alcoholic steatohepatitis, and hint that hepatic fibrosis may improve, there are no definitive studies in more advanced stages of NAFLD (Nostedt et al., 2016). Hopefully these will be performed soon.

Medication

Much literature is devoted to possible beneficial effects of antidiabetic agents on fatty liver disease (Corrado et al., 2014). Though the use of glitazones is now minuscule, and the evidence weak that they meaningfully improved hepatic structure, they are still widely discussed as possible therapies in NAFLD. Metformin is now considered safe in patients even with advanced liver disease and, while it does not improve liver histology in patients with lesser degrees of NAFLD, it may be of value in more advanced disease. Other antihyperglycaemic agents in current use have not been shown to help NAFLD, though insulin paradoxically may, certainly in comparison with the liver-neutral GLP-1-RA agents (Corrado et al., 2014). Optimistic animal studies of SGLT2 inhibitors support the liver-friendliness of these agents in promoting weight loss (fat mass, not just via osmotic effects and glycosuria) and hint at possible metabolic switching from glucose to lipids, but history should warn us against extrapolation to humans without definitive RCTs (Hazelhurst *et al.*, 2016).

The literature is full of small trials of various combinations of alternative therapies and vitamins in the treatment of NAFLD. High-dose vitamin E (800 units daily) taken for two years improved histological measures of non-alcoholic steatohepatatis (NASH), the advanced inflammatory and fibrotic state of NAFLD, at the expense of increasing insulin resistance and plasma triglycerides. The substantive trial is unlikely ever to be performed (in the same study, pioglitazone showed no benefit in NAFLD) (Sanyal *et al.*, 2010).

Statins, safe in liver disease, probably reduce the heightened cardiovascular risk in NAFLD patients, as they do in other higher-risk individuals. There is tentative evidence in a small group of patients that histological appearances improve (Kargiotis *et al.*, 2015), as opposed to normalizing the liver function tests, a false reassurance widely observed with the glitazones and omega-3 fatty acids.

Practice point

Although no drugs improve the progression of NAFLD, all patients are at high cardiovascular risk, and need intensive statin treatment, which may help liver histology.

OBSTRUCTIVE SLEEP APNOEA (OSA)

In obstructive sleep apnoea there are repeated upper airway occlusions during sleep that result in intermittent hypoxia and a fragmented sleep pattern, associated with daytime somnolence. It is common: 10–17% of men and 3–9% of women have a moderate or severe form. The sleep disturbances lead to a series of physiological and biochemical abnormalities, possibly unified by sympathoadrenal activation, which in turn increase the risk of the metabolic syndrome and Type 2 diabetes. Using simple indices, such as the number of apnoeic and hypopnoeic episodes per hour (apnoea-hypopnoea index) longitudinal studies confirm that moderate-to-severe OSA is an independent risk factor for developing Type 2 diabetes (Pamidi *et al.*, 2010).

Practice point

Simple clinical indicators of OSA (witnessed apnoea, heavy snoring, daytime somnolence) should prompt a focus on metabolic abnormalities that may not have been identified.

Obesity is the dominant common risk factor for both Type 2 diabetes and OSA, but other conditions associated with the metabolic syndrome conditions may play a part, for example, the chronic intermittent hypoxia of OSA has been linked to increased structural abnormalities in the fatty liver. Hypertension and OSA share the common aetiological factor of sympathetic nervous system activation and resistant hypertension is commonly associated with OSA (see **Chapter 11**). Other cardiovascular associations with OSA are variably documented, including stroke, myocardial infarction and heart failure. Increased left ventricular mass and hypertrophy are also associated with OSA, independent of obesity and hypertension, and possibly also left ventricular function and heart failure. There are hints that OSA may promote atrial fibrillation independent of the degree of obesity and also that untreated OSA reduces the efficiency of treatments for atrial fibrillation including medication, cardioversion and ablation (Goudis and Ketikoglou, 2017).

Treatment of OSA and its effect on Type 2 diabetes

Overnight continuous positive airway pressure (CPAP) treatment is widely used in treatment. Its main objectives are to improve sleep quality for the patient and their partner, and to relieve daytime somnolence. Conducting properly randomized studies is difficult and there is evidence that a substantial effect of CPAP on somnolence when used at recommended levels is placebo-associated, or related to patient expectation.

Practice point

Successful CPAP treatment probably has no meaningful impact on glycaemic control.

Although studies are small-scale, CPAP treatment does not improve overall glycaemic control. Although a large-scale trial might demonstrate some benefit, glycaemia is better and more easily treated with conventional methods. The hoped-for improvement in measures of insulin sensitivity could not be demonstrated in a well-conducted sham-control randomized controlled trial (RCT) lasting 12 weeks; there were no reductions in visceral abdominal or liver fat either (Hoyos *et al.*, 2012). Hypertension has been a more hopeful candidate but trials have been small and results equivocal; in a large six-month RCT (Muxfeldt *et al.*, 2015) in resistant hypertension, there was a small reduction in night-time BP, but no overall changes. OSA, independent of the degree of obesity and hypertension, is associated with increased left ventricular mass and hypertrophy, and possibly also with left ventricular systolic and diastolic function. A cross-sectional study within the Look AHEAD study found a strong relationship between measured apnoea-hypopnoea index and self-reported stroke but not with other cardiovascular events (Rice *et al.*, 2012), and although weight loss in the same study led to improvement in sleep apnoea, increased fitness itself did not.

Practice point

Sleep apnoea improves after losing weight but not with increasing fitness.

Does CPAP treatment reduce cardiovascular risk?

No, according to the results of the large and definitive SAVE study (McEvoy *et al.*, 2016). In a group of patients with established coronary or cerebrovascular disease followed up for four years, CPAP did not reduce the risk of recurrent events, either in the whole group or the approximately 30% of patients in the trial who had diabetes (blood pressure did not improve either). However, quality of life meaningfully improved: snoring and daytime sleepiness decreased, and CPAP improved mood and health-related quality of life, as well as tending to reduce accidents causing injury, though not road traffic accidents. Adherence to treatment was about the same as in other studies (average 3.3 hours each night during the trial) and claims that a more positive effect on cardiovascular events might be seen with better adherence is another example of special pleading for even more model trial participants.

It seems that successful treatment of OSA with CPAP can lead to real symptomatic improvement but does not have meaningful benefits on biomedical outcomes.

Practice point

Do not use CPAP in diabetic patients with OSA expecting that glycaemia or blood pressure will improve, or that the risk of cardiovascular events will fall. However treatment improves symptoms and several measures of quality of life. Equipment is relatively inexpensive but continuing specialist follow-up is needed.

'Lifestyle' treatment of OSA

As obesity is central to OSA, weight reduction is important in its management. In the sleep substudy of the Look AHEAD study, weight loss improved OSA, and in spite of the 50% weight regain between years 1 and 4 of the study, the improvement in OSA persisted. Other short-term studies of weight loss have shown the same degree of improvement. Statistically, weight loss did not explain the improvement in all patients – some randomized to the intensive lifestyle arm of the Look AHEAD study showed an improvement in OSA without significant weight loss, so other interventions not easily quantified may contribute (Kuna et al., 2013). Sadly, there are no robust studies of the effect of bariatric surgery on OSA.

GOUT

Gout was previously considered the province of the rheumatologists; fortunately, like rheumatoid, the destructive arthropathies common in the past are now very rare. Gout – or at least hyperuricaemia – is now a focus of metabolic physicians. The literature and speculation on elevated serum urate as a cardiorenal risk factor hugely outweighs the fortunately relatively simple management of clinical gout. Epidemiologically both Type 1 and – surprisingly – Type 2 diabetes are associated with a lower risk of gout, but there is a strong association between the metabolic syndrome, however defined, and gout (Roddy and Choi, 2014). Nephrologists are also interested in the role of hyperuricaemia in chronic kidney disease generally, and although probably not as widespread as in the past, urate stone disease is still common. Fructose intake, increasing recently through high consumption of sugar-sweetened drinks, especially by young people, is associated with increased insulin resistance, and some of this may be mediated through uric acid; in the Nurses' Health Study, women with high fructose intake had an increased risk of articular gout. Increased alcohol intake is also associated with increased gout risk: beer is a particular culprit, followed by spirits, but not moderate wine intake (Choi et al., 2004). The association with drinking port will, with luck, remain embedded in the history, culture and folk memory of medicine, unenlightened by evidence-based medicine.

The relationship between hyperuricaemia and the metabolic syndrome and thereby cardiovascular disease has been established in many epidemiological studies but the mechanism of the link is less clear, and the critical therapeutic question – whether or not treatment of asymptomatic hyperuricaemia reduces cardiovascular risk – is still open. Serum uric acid level is strongly associated with the development of CKD (though not of proteinuria) in Type 2 patients (De Cosmo et al., 2015). Speculative documents of the 'hype or hope' variety vastly outweigh the almost non-existent trial data. Even the metabolic effects of insulin and hyperinsulinaemia are unclear, except for old data showing that both in normal and insulin-resistant states, insulin reduces renal clearance of uric acid (and of sodium).

An isolated attack of gout many years ago, characteristically in the great toe (podagra) is common in middle-aged people with the metabolic syndrome, but specific enquiry is needed. Like their physicians, patients may not make the connection between a remote and perhaps isolated episode of pain in the big toe and a cluster of cardiovascular risk factors. Nevertheless, any history of gout should alert the physician to other components of the metabolic syndrome.

Management

Until the discovery of allopurinol (the first ever enzyme inhibitor drug) in 1956, weight loss and dietary manipulation were the only therapies available. In total more has probably been written on the dietary management of gout than of obesity. Because gout is strongly associated with obesity, achieving normal BMI is recommended. There is now a lot of epidemiological data on specific foods associated with gout and hyperuricaemia but almost nothing on the effects of exclusion of the same foods, so a portfolio approach is suggested (**Figure 13.2**). As with all interventions, careful monitoring is needed and a combination of dietary and pharmacological treatments will generally be required. All thiazide and loop diuretics markedly increase serum urate (see **Chapter 11**).

Recurrent attacks warrant prophylactic treatment, with either allopurinol or febuxostat, which at its higher dose of 80 mg daily is more effective in lowering serum urate than allopurinol 300 mg daily at any level of renal function; both agents are equally well

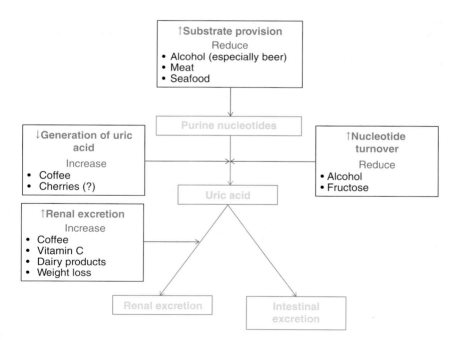

Figure 13.2 Dietary strategies in managing hyperuricaemia and gout. *Source:* Chaichian *et al.*, 2014. Reproduced with permission of Elsevier.

tolerated and safe in people with diabetes (Becker *et al.*, 2013). While allopurinol is a very safe drug, its use is associated with a variety of hypersensitivity reactions, including DRESS (Drug Rash with Eosinophilia and Systemic Symptoms), which can be fatal, especially in South-East Asian patients. Start treatment at a low dose, for example 100 mg daily, and titrate against serum urate levels. There are high hopes for, but no evidence yet, of cardiovascular events being reduced with prophylactic treatment in people with elevated serum urate but no clinical gout and in CKD. Where there are recurrent episodes of articular gout, ask for a rheumatology review.

> **Practice point**
>
> Ask people with metabolic syndrome about episodes of gout affecting the great toe even in the remote past.

ECTOPIC FAT ACCUMULATION IN ORGANS OTHER THAN THE LIVER

Adipose tissue itself may not be deleterious; its metabolic impact may depend more on its site (e.g. lower body adipose tissue, dominant in females, may be protective compared with upper body adiposity; fat accumulation in muscle and liver may be more deleterious than accumulation elsewhere). New syndromes of fat accumulation in and around other organs, mostly related to overnutrition, continue to be described and the proximity of these fat stores to critical organs may be particularly harmful. Areas of current interest include:

- *Heart*. Both intramyocardial and epicardial fat appear to be important in different ways. Excess intramyocardial lipid probably has both structural and functional effects, increasing the risk of fibrosis and altering the metabolic pathways of the myocardium. For example in insulin resistance the already small proportion of myocardial energy generated from glucose (around 25%) falls further, promoting fatty acid metabolism. This spectrum of abnormalities has led to speculation about a specific metabolic cardiomyopathy (Mandavia *et al.*, 2012). The amount of fat surrounding the atria may be important in determining the risk, and persistence and severity, of atrial fibrillation. Epicardial fat is anatomically very close to the coronary arteries and its volume is associated with several cardiovascular risk factors, including diabetes. It is thought of as a paracrine and endocrine promotor of coronary calcification though increased production of inflammatory cytokines.
- *Pancreas*. Pancreatic fat and its postulated centrality in Type 2 diabetes made the headlines in 2011, when a mechanistic study of a 600 kcal diet for eight weeks reversed the major abnormalities of Type 2 diabetes in patients with less than four years known duration of diabetes: dynamic insulin responses improved towards normal and hepatic glucose output was more fully suppressed by insulin, all well-known from earlier studies (see **Chapter 4**). MRI-measured fat in the liver and pancreas fell (Lim *et al.*, 2011). The excess intrapancreatic triglyceride and its decrease with weight loss is specific to Type 2 diabetes, as it did not occur in matched non-diabetic subjects undergoing bariatric surgery with the same degree of weight loss (Steven *et al.*, 2016).
- *Kidney*. The kidney is a metabolically highly active organ, regulated by insulin. In addition to the increasing interest in the specific glomerulopathy associated with

obesity (see **Chapter 4**), ectopic lipid accumulation in the kidney may also be associated with adverse functional and structural effects on renal cells, especially the mesangial cells, podocytes and proximal tubular cells (de Vries *et al.*, 2014).

POLYCYSTIC OVARIAN SYNDROME (PCOS)

While PCOS is not part of any definition of the metabolic syndrome, it is universally considered a manifestation of insulin resistance. Its aetiology remains obscure, hence it is described in terms of phenotype (oligomenorhea, hirsutism and biochemical hyperandrogenism, with clinically broad definitions: **Box 13.1**). It is common in Type 1 diabetes, probably because of peripheral hyperinsulinaemia, and can be detected in up to 50% of young Type 1 women in their 20s (compared with 5–10% in people without diabetes). In Type 1 diabetes, PCOS is unlikely to be associated with obesity, hypertension or dyslipidaemia. They are therefore similar to the frequently-encountered lean phenotype of PCOS seen in non-diabetic women. In premenopausal women with Type 2 diabetes, PCOS is bound to be common but estimates of prevalence are unreliable. Regardless, clinicians should always be aware of the condition. The long sought-after link between PCOS and increased risk of cardiovascular disease remains elusive but, as in all aspects of the metabolic syndrome, its presence should prompt the practitioner to consider other associated cardiovascular risk factors, especially hypertension and cigarette smoking, Insulin-resistant dyslipidaemia (low HDL, elevated triglycerides) is common but would not warrant treatment in young women. It is not yet known whether women with 'double diabetes' (Type 1 plus metabolic syndrome, usually associated with obesity) have phenotypically more severe PCOS. Always bear in mind the most extreme manifestations of insulin resistance/PCOS, including infertility and the very unpleasant cutaneous hidradenitis suppurativa. Other skin conditions associated with insulin resistance include acanthosis nigricans (thickening and darkening of skin folds, especially the neck, axillae, antecubital fossa and groin), acne and hirsutism (classically associated with PCOS but not part of its definition), and androgenetic alopecia.

Practice point

Be aware of simple clinical features that may point to insulin resistance, including oligo-amenorrhoea in PCOS, and skin problems including acne, acanthosis nigricans and hirsutism.

METABOLICALLY HEALTHY OVERWEIGHT ('FIT FAT')

The protective effect of current physical activity on cardiovascular and all-cause mortality is now well established in obese people without diabetes. The effect is the same whether over the previous 10 years obesity developed, remitted or remained unchanged (Dankel *et al.*, 2016). About 9% of obese younger people in the USA population have high

Box 13.1 Rotterdam criteria for diagnosis of PCOS (2003). All are contentious.

- Oligo-anovulation (cycle length >35 days or fewer than eight episodes of menses in a year).
- Hyperandrogenism (biochemical definition not agreed).
- Polycystic ovarian morphology on ultrasound (≥12 follicles 2–9 mm in diameter in each ovary or increased ovarian volume, >10 cm³). Elevated serum anti-Müllerian hormone assay is emerging as a more reliable measure of follicular count.

cardiovascular fitness, though this is a small proportion compared with 17% of the overweight population, and 30% of normal weight people. It is not known how this relationship is changed by the presence of Type 2 diabetes. The related 'obesity paradox' describes improved outcomes, including survival in mildly, but not severely obese people. It has turned out to be one of the knottiest statistical problems in medicine, a common explanation being 'collider stratification bias', unmeasured confounding induced by selection bias. In the general population the paradox is reasonably well established for diverse conditions such as heart failure, critical illness and CKD, as well as postoperative complications and cancer surgery (Chang et al., 2016). Practically, it seems preferable to urge normalization of weight in all people with the aim of reducing Type 2 diabetes in the first place, then doing the same in people with uncomplicated diabetes in the hope of improving important endpoints, rather than statistical hair-splitting over optimum weight once a severe complication like heart failure has developed.

References

Becker MA, MacDonald PA, Hunt BJ, Jackson RL. Diabetes and gout: efficacy and safety of febux-ostat and allopurinol. *Diabetes Obes Metab* 2013;15:1049–55 [PMID: 23683134] PMC3902994.

Caiazzo R, Lassailly G, Leteurte E et al. Roux-en-Y gastric bypass versus adjustable gastric banding to reduce nonlcoholic fatty liver disease: a 5-year controlled longitudinal study. *Ann Surg* 2014;260:893–8 [PMID: 25379859].

Chaichian Y, Chohan S1, Becker MA. Long-term management of gout: nonpharmacologic and pharmacological therapies. *Rheum Dis Clin North Am* 2014;40:357–74 [PMID: 24703352].

Chang HW, Li YH, Hsieh CH et al. Association of body mass index with all-cause mortality in patients with diabetes: a systemic review and meta-analysis. *Cardiovasc Diagn Ther* 2016;6:109–19 [PMID: 2754100] PMC4805755.

Choi HK, Atkinson K, Karlson EW et al. Alcohol intake and risk of incident gout in men: a prospective study. *Lancet* 2004;363:1277–81 [PMID: 15094272].

Corrado RL, Torres DM, Harrison SA. Review of treatment options for non-alcoholic fatty liver disease. *Med Clin North Am* 2014;98:55–72 [PMID: 24266914].

Dankel SJ, Loenneke JP. Loprinzi PD. Does the fat-but-fit paradigm hold true for all-cause mortality when considering the duration of overweight/obesity? Analyzing the WATCH (Weight, Activity and Time Contributes to Health) paradigm. *Prev Med* 2016;83:37–40 [PMID: 26687100].

De Cosmo S, Viazzi F, Pacilli A et al. AMD-Annals Study Group. Serum uric acid and risk of CKD in type 2 diabetes. *Clin J Am Soc Nephrol* 2015;10:1921–9 [PMID: 26342044] PMC4633786.

Goudis CA, Ketikoglou DG. Obstructive sleep and atrial fibrillation: pathophysiological mechanisms and therapeutic implications. *Int J Cardiol* 2017; 230:293–300 [PMID: 28040290].

Hazelhurst JM, Woods C, Marjot T et al. Non-alcoholic fatty liver disease and diabetes. *Metabolism* 2016 656:1096–108 [PMID: 26856933] PMC4943559.

Hoyos CM, Killick R, Yee BJ et al. Cardiometabolic changes after continuous positive airway pressure for obstructive sleep apnoea: a randomised sham-controlled study. *Thorax* 2012;67:1081–9 [PMID: 22561530].

Kargiotis K, Athyros VG, Giouleme O et al. Resolution of non-alcoholic steatohepatitis by rosuvastatin monotherapy in patients with metabolic syndrome. *World J Gastroenterol* 2015;21:7860–8 [PMID: 26167086] PMC4491973.

Kuna ST, Reboussin DM, Borraidaile KE et al. Sleep AHEAD Research Group of the Look AHEAD Research Group. Long-term effect of weight loss on obstructive sleep apnea severity in obese patients with type 2 diabetes. *Sleep* 2013;36:641–649A [PMID: 23633746] PMC3624818.

Lim EL, Hollingsworth KG, Arbisala BS et al. Reversal of type 2 diabetes: normalisation of beta cell function in association with decreased pancreas and liver triacylglycerol. *Diabetologia* 2011;54:2506–14 [PMID: 21656330] PMC3168743.

Mandavia CH, Pulakat L, DeMarco V, Sowers JR. Over-nutrition and metabolic cardiomyopathy. *Metabolism* 2012;61:1205–10 [PMID: 22465089] PMC3393834.

McEvoy RD, Antic NA, Heeley E *et al*. SAVE Investigators and Coordinators. CPAP for prevention of cardiovascular events in obstructive seep apnea. *N Engl J Med* 2016;375:919–31 [PMID; 27571048] Free full text.

Muxfeldt ES, Margallo V, Costa LM *et al*. Effects of continuous positive airway pressure treatment on clinic and ambulatory blood pressures in patients with obstructive sleep apnea and resistant hypertension: a randomized controlled trial. *Hypertension* 2015;65:736–42 [PMID: 25601933].

Nostedt JJ, Switzer NJ, Gill RS *et al*. The effect of bariatric surgery on the spectrum of fatty liver disease. *Can J Gastroenterol Hepatol* 2016;2059245 [PMID: 27777925] PMC5061986.

Pamidi S, Aronsohn RS, Tasali E. Obstructive sleep apnea: role in the risk ad severity of diabetes. *Best Pract Res Clin Endocrinol Metab* 2010;24:703–15 [PMID: 21112020] PMC2994098.

Petersen KF, Dufour, Befroy D *et al*. Reversal of nonalcoholic hepatic steatois, hepatic insulin resistance, and hyperglycemia by moderate weight reduction in patients with type 2 diabetes. *Diabetes* 2005;54:603–8 [PMID: 15734833] PMC2995496.

Rani V, Deshmukh R Jaswal P *et al*. Alzheimer's disease: is this a brain specific diabetic condition? *Physiol Behav* 2016;164(Pt A):259–67 [PMID: 27235734].

Reaven GM. Banting lecture 1988. Role of insulin resistance in human disease. *Diabetes* 1988;37:1595–607 [PMID: 3056758].

Rice TB, Foster GD, Sanders MH *et al*. Sleep AHEAD Research Group. The relationship between obstructive sleep apnea and self-reported stroke or coronary heart disease in overweight and obese adults with type 2 diabetes mellitus. *Sleep* 2012;35:1293–8 [PMID: 22942508] PMC3413807.

Roddy E, Choi HK. Epidemiology of gout. *Rheum Dis Clin North Am* 2014;40:155–75 [PMID: 24703341] PMC4119792.

Sanyal AJ, Chalasani N, Kowdley KV *et al*. NASH CRN Research Group. Pioglitazone, vitamin E, or placebo for non-alcoholic steatohepatitis. *N Engl J Med* 2010;362:1675–85 [PMID: 20427778] PMC2928471.

Simmons RK, Alberti KG, Gale EA *et al*. The metabolic syndrome: useful concept or clinical tool? Report of a WHO Expert Consultation. *Diabetologia* 2010;53:600–5 [PMID: 20012011].

Steven S, Hollingsworth KG, Smith PK *et al*. Weight loss decreases excess pancreatic triacylglycerol specifically in type 2 diabetes. *Diabetes Care* 2016;39:158–65 [PMID: 26628414].

de Vries AP, Ruggenenti P, Ruan XZ *et al*. ERA-EDTA Working Group Diabesity. *Lancet Diabetes Endocrinol* 2014;2:417–26 [PMID: 24795255].

Consensus document

IDF Consensus worldwide definition of the metabolic syndrome (2014) https://www.idf.org/e-library/consensus-statements/60-idfconsensus-worldwide-definitionof-the-metabolic-syndrome (last accessed 12 October 2017).

14 Youth and emerging adulthood; old age

Key points

Youth and emerging adulthood

- Persistent HbA$_{1c}$ >90% (75) is a very high risk level for microvascular complications in both Type 1 and 2 diabetes
- In Type 1 diabetes glycaemic control has probably slowly but steadily improved over the past 20 years, but significant regional and national differences persist
- Exercise improves diabetes control; spending more time watching screens does not
- Young Type 2 patients can develop significant microvascular complications years in advance of Type 1
- All healthcare professionals should take time to discuss contraception and prepregnancy counselling

Old age

- The numbers of Type 1 patients living into healthy old age without significant complications are rapidly increasing
- An older person taking insulin may have Type 1 diabetes and must never be without insulin or insulin supplies
- Frailty is strongly associated with Type 2 diabetes and is a powerful predictor of death and disability
- There is little clinical trial evidence on the use of newer agents in Type 2 in elderly patients
- Hypoglycaemia is an ever-present risk, especially in people taking sulfonylureas and insulin. Low HbA$_{1c}$ values, for example <7.0% (53), even without hypoglycaemia, may impair everyday abilities. Do everything possible to minimize insulin usage in people living with dementia

YOUTH AND EMERGING ADULTHOOD

There are no agreed definitions of the age ranges of these groups and, in practice, organizational definitions are more widely used than social or physiological ones. Traditionally, people with diabetes have been supervised by their paediatric teams until they are around 16, when they transition to an 'adolescent' or 'young adult clinic', where they will usually see a paediatrician and an adult physician with an interest in young people's diabetes, together with a team of variable composition, including nurses with a specialist interest in young people and a clinical psychologist. Some teams include administrative staff, such as a navigator to help young people negotiate their way around an often complex medical system. Thereafter, further transition to the adult clinic occurs once they reach their early 20s. These limits are not always helpful in clinical practice but for the purposes of this chapter diabetes will be discussed in those aged 16 and above.

Practical Diabetes Care, Fourth Edition. David Levy.
© 2018 John Wiley & Sons Ltd. Published 2018 by John Wiley & Sons Ltd.

The wide disparity in organizational arrangements for assisting young people through these transitions directly reflects equal uncertainty about how to do it well.

The upper age limit that defines adulthood is also contentious. It is gradually increasing as full psychosocial maturity is lengthening in urban Western societies. It should not be an arbitrary number established by authoritarian figures. In Denmark, nearly one-half of the general population aged between 25 and 29 did not consider themselves to be fully adult. Characteristics that young people themselves would consider to be adult included personal responsibility, and independence in making decisions, including financial ones (Arnett and Padilla-Walker, 2015).

The group is still dominated by young people with Type 1 diabetes. Monogenic and other forms of diabetes (see **Chapter 2**) comprise a small but relatively fixed proportion of cases, but Type 2 diabetes is highly variable between countries. It is becoming very important in the USA, but despite increased concern over the past two decades about a possible 'epidemic', it has not yet emerged as a significant problem in the United Kingdom and Europe. In the comprehensive SEARCH study of young people (USA) the prevalence of both Type 1 and Type 2 diabetes has increased markedly over the decade 2001–2009, and in all major ethnic groups (non-Hispanic Whites, Hispanic, African-American).

Type 1 diabetes: glycaemic control

By the mid-teens, the average Type 1 patient will be coming to the end of their first decade of diabetes. The concern highlighted by the Diabetes Control and Complications Trial (DCCT) and amply supported by evidence over not far off three decades is that poor glycaemic control during this period will imprint a harmful legacy for the development of microvascular and macrovascular complications, and possibly for excess mortality too (see **Chapter 7**). More positively, most studies are now highlighting significantly improved overall glycaemic control over the past 10–15 years. Several studies (for example those from Denmark, Germany/Austria and Slovenia) have documented a mean fall in HbA_{1c} of about 1% towards the low 8% region (approximately 64 mmol/mol) in the first decade of the millennium, but these are not always population studies and selection bias is a concern (Levy, 2016).

There are, however, three concerns concealed within this positive trend.

Trends in glycaemia during adolescence and young adulthood

All studies show that glycaemic control in Type 1 diabetes consistently deteriorates from around age 10 to the late teens. At this point HbA_{1c} tends to plateau, but it does not return to around 8% until the late 20s (see **Figure 7.2**). Even in the large and important T1D registry study in the USA, which has a significant overrepresentation of upper socioeconomic class young people and a high proportion using insulin pumps, peak HbA_{1c} is currently still around 9% (73) and remains at this level for around five years (15–19) (Clements et al., 2016).

Disparities in control between countries

In international studies, there are striking differences in glycaemia between countries (**Figure 14.1**). For example, in all age groups of younger people (under 15, those between 15 and 25, and older than 25 years), the UK mean HbA_{1c} is about 1% higher than Germany, which has the lowest values in Europe. Even within the countries of the United Kingdom, there are significant differences, Scotland having the highest mean HbA_{1c} values, England slightly lower. These differences will, if they persist, result in higher rates of microvascular complications, and probably of macrovascular complications later in life (McKnight et al., 2015).

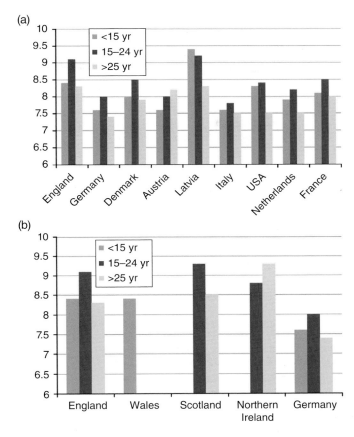

Figure 14.1 HbA$_{1c}$ in European countries and USA (2010–2013) in young Type 1 patients. (a) Data from regional or national registries. Latvia and England have the highest HbA$_{1c}$ values. (b) UK countries compared with Germany, which had the lowest values in this study. *Source*: McKnight *et al.*, 2015. Reproduced with permission of John Wiley & Sons.

Glycaemic tracking

There is increasing evidence that HbA$_{1c}$ levels tend to track consistently over time, and this period may be long. For example, a large study in Germany and Austria documented tracking over 15 years in one-third to one-half of a young population between the ages of 7 and 22 (Hofer *et al.*, 2014). More detailed analysis identified two groups: one continued in reasonable control (HbA$_{1c}$ ~8%, 64) with only a slight upward trend; however, 10–30% started with poor control (HbA$_{1c}$ ~9%, 75) that then markedly worsened (up to ~11%, 97). This group had less paternal monitoring and input, less functional autonomy and lower levels of self-control. The importance for practitioners is that while overall glycaemia tends to settle by the mid-20s, in a substantial group it fails to do so. These patients would benefit from more intensive input and astute authors have proposed that there is a valuable window of opportunity during adolescence; once out of this period when personal independence is complete it may be even more difficult to make positive changes. However, the extended and extending reach of young adulthood with more young people remaining much longer in the parental home may also extend the opportunity for valuable intervention in at least a reasonably stable domestic environment – a possible benefit in an otherwise rather gloomy scenario for some Type 1 patient and their guardians.

Practice point

Up to one-third of young people with Type 1 diabetes continue to have poor glycaemic control beyond their mid-20s. They need especially intensive input.

Type 2 diabetes

Type 2 diabetes was first recognized in young people in the USA during the early 1980s but it was not formally reported in the United Kingdom until 2002. In the USA, most patients are from ethnic minority groups, with especially high rates in American Indians and Native Alaskans, while in Europe both white and ethnic minority patients are described. The numbers managed in clinics are still very small. In an international study, only 1.3% of under-20s had Type 2 diabetes, lower than the proportion with either monogenic diabetes or cystic fibrosis-related diabetes (Pacaud et al., 2016). Type 2 diabetes is diagnosed later than Type 1 (usually in the 10–19 year age group) at a time when young people are becoming less dependent on parents and where peer influences on diet are becoming more important. As in adults, treatment with atypical antipsychotics increases the risk of Type 2 diabetes two- to threefold. Many drop out of clinic supervision, so there is little reliable information on glycaemic control in these underserved and threatened patients. In the USA SEARCH study, insulin-treated Type 2 patients had similar glycaemic control compared with their Type 1 counterparts (HbA$_{1c}$ 9.1%, 76) and it was only slightly better in those using insulin with oral hypoglycaemics (HbA$_{1c}$ 8.6%, 70) (Badaru et al., 2014).

Management

Young people with Type 2 diabetes have the cluster of insulin resistance characteristics that in adults often warrants multiple medication, so a key aim is to minimize drug treatment and the associated problems of adherence and side effects. Lifestyle interventions (increased activity, daily caloric deficit) in obese youth both with and without diabetes have given variable results, mostly quite disappointing, at least from the point of view of glycaemic outcomes (Huang et al., 2016) (see the TODAY study, next section) but the more intensive the input the better the outcome, and reports of highly structured programmes are encouraging – though costly in time and money. As in adults, dietary restriction, not exercise, is the mainstay of weight reduction, whereas activity (documented to be low in young Type 2 subjects compared with both Type 1 and non-diabetic individuals) more benefits cardiometabolic measures.

Medication

The TODAY study is the only medication trial in young Type 2 subjects, aged 10–17 years (TODAY Study Group, 2012). Although a combination of metformin and rosiglitazone was marginally more effective than metformin alone or metformin plus lifestyle intervention in preventing deterioration in control, there were no meaningful differences between the three interventions. Metformin remains the mainstay of pharmacological treatment but there is no agreement at what stage it should be started (in practice, most young people present symptomatically and in very poor glycaemic control, so immediate metformin, possibly with insulin in the acute stage, would be appropriate). Regardless, the failure rate in TODAY, defined as HbA_{1c} persistently $\geq 8.0\%$ (64) or the need for permanent addition of insulin, was around 50% at four years and was highest in African-Americans, followed by Hispanics and non-Hispanic whites, and there was a hint that metformin was less effective in black subjects. Patients unable to achieve non-diabetic HbA_{1c} values of 6.3% (45) or less on metformin were much more likely to lose glycaemic control by four years and warrant especially careful supervision (Zeitler et al., 2015).

Practice point

Metformin, widely used in young peope with Type 2 diabetes, has a failure rate around 12% per year. The failure rate is highest in African-Americans and in those not achieving HbA_{1c} <6.3% (45) on metformin.

By custom, metformin is widely used off-licence in young people (as it is in pregnancy). Sulfonylureas, again used in pregnancy, are probably safe. Insulin is naturally licensed but may be of limited help in obese people. There are no data on incretin-related drugs and in these patients who may be ketosis-prone, SGLT2 inhibitors should not be used until there is convincing evidence that they are safe (see **Chapter 10**).

Complications in young people

The picture is still dominated by emerging microvascular complications but in both Type 1 and Type 2 diabetes powerful risk factors are already present for premature macrovascular disease. The few reports of outcomes in Type 2 make consistently depressing reading. Because of the inevitably long prodrome, associated insulin-resistance characteristics and poor overall control, not only are all complications more prevalent than in age-matched Type 1 subjects, major microvascular outcomes (dialysis, blindness or amputation) begin to occur within 10 years of diagnosis (Dart et al., 2014; see later). The SEARCH study systematically compared the complications in young people with Type 1 and 2 diagnosed under 20 years of age. Microvascular complications (retinopathy, neuropathy and diabetic kidney disease) were all 2.0–2.5 times more likely in the Type 2 subjects but after full statistical adjustment markers of early arterial disease (hypertension and arterial stiffness) were just as common in Type 1 patients. These are early years in the comparative follow-up of young people, but it is clear that both diabetes types remain at high risk (Dabelea et al., 2017).

Practice point

Monitor young Type 2 people very carefully for emerging vascular complications. Microvascular complications seem to be especially prevalent in Type 2.

Microvascular complications

Retinopathy

The reduction in risk of progression of retinopathy with tight control (HbA_{1c} 7%, 53) was the same in the adolescent cohort of the DCCT (~60%) as in the adults. Adolescent females are at greater risk of retinopathy than males and develop it about 1.5 years earlier, presumably on account of worse glycaemic control. Although annual retinal screening is recommended from 12 years of age, retinopathy of greater severity than transient minor background changes is fortunately uncommon, but its frequency is inevitably related to overall long-term control. For example, in the USA SEARCH cohort of Type 1 patients under 20, which includes 20% ethnic minorities, 17% had some degree of retinopathy. However, Type 2 patients had a threefold increased prevalence of retinopathy – mean HbA_{1c} was very poor (9.4%, 79) compared with 8.6% (70) in those without retinopathy (Mayer-Davis et al., 2012).

Practice point

Stress the importance of regular retinal screening, especially in people with about 10 years of Type 1 diabetes in persistent poor control, for example HbA_{1c} ≥9.0% (75), and Type 2 patients.

Diabetic renal disease – albuminuria and nephropathy

Nephropathy behaves much as retinopathy in this age group, though microalbuminuria (mildly elevated albuminuria) is much more common than retinopathy. Overt diabetic renal disease (**Chapter 4**) is most unusual, but in a poorly-controlled population of UK Type 1 patients, mean age 19, duration 10 years, 3% had proteinuria (Amin et al., 2008). This fortunately small group may run the same course of diabetic renal disease that was seen in previous eras, with a high risk of end-stage renal disease after a further 10 years. Once again, young people with Type 2 diabetes fare worse than those with Type 1: in the SEARCH cohort, 9.2% of Type 1 patients, but 22% of Type 2, had microalbuminuria. At the start of the four-year interventional TODAY study, 6.3% had microalbuminuria, rising to 16% over the course of four years.

Like retinopathy, microalbuminuria is powerfully related to glycaemia, with a hint from several studies that HbA_{1c} persistently above about 9% (75) carries a greatly increased risk (Daniels et al., 2013) (**Figure 14.2**). However, it is now clear that microalbuminuria does not inevitably progress to proteinuria and nephropathy, and spontaneous regression in this group that almost never needs treatment for hypertension occurs in approximately 50%, with only around 10% progressing. NICE recommends screening using annual urinary ACR screening from the age of 12; the American Diabetes Association proposes screening from 10 years of age or 5 years duration.

Practice point

Do not treat microalbuminuria in this age group with angiotensin blocking agents unless there is clear evidence of progression on multiple repeated tests of ACR or definite hypertension. Smoking is probably a risk factor for microalbuminuria.

Macrovascular risk factors

Indicators of structural arterial changes (carotid intima-media thickness [CIMT], arterial stiffness)

The precise measurement by ultrasound of the combined thickness of the intima and media of the common carotid artery is considered a structural correlate of vascular risk (though it probably does not add to the predictive power of conventional risk factor assessment). Increased intima-media thickness can be detected shortly after Type 1 is

% of patients

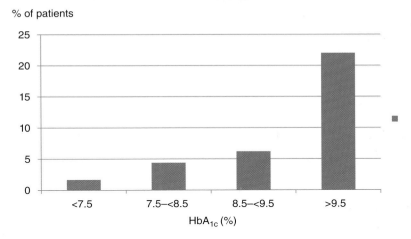

Figure 14.2 Microalbuminuria in 18–20 year olds in the T1D Exchange Network. *Source*: Data from Daniels *et al*., 2013. This and other studies indicate that the risks of microvascular complications rise rapidly at HbA$_{1c}$ values persistently higher than 9.0% (75).

diagnosed, but at this stage is most unlikely to indicate established arterial disease. However, by adolescence increased intima-media thickness is frequent and may be established. It also occurs in the aorta, where it may be an earlier and more reliable marker of abnormal arterial structure. In both carotid and aorta intima-media thickness is linked to traditional cardiovascular risk factors as well as glycaemic control (Harrington *et al*., 2010). Measures of arterial stiffness (most simply pulse pressure, or alternatively carotid-femoral pulse wave velocity) are of increasing interest and are also abnormal at an early age in Type 1 diabetes. Not surprisingly, in the SEARCH study arterial stiffness was greater and distensibility lower in the Type 2 subjects than Type 1.

Hypertension
Although important and reasonably frequently measured, blood pressure measurements in young people should be interpreted using percentile charts or significant hypertension is likely to be overlooked (National High Blood Pressure Education Program Working Group, 2004). Subtle but important changes in blood pressure occur between pre-puberty and young adulthood in Type 1 diabetes: for example, centile-related hypertension increases from 4% in prepuberty to 14% postpuberty. Up to age 17, blood pressure persistently ≥120/80 mm Hg is always abnormal – though it is the benchmark for strictly normal blood pressure in adults with or without diabetes. During adolescence systolic pressure rises more steeply than in the non-diabetic population and there is a premature fall in diastolic pressure, leading to increased widening of pulse pressure. In a large international survey of 10–16-year-old subjects with Type 1 diabetes of only six years duration, casual blood pressure was significantly higher than in age-matched controls (113/62 mm Hg vs 110/58) (Bradley *et al*., 2016). About three-quarters of the Type 2 patients in the SEARCH study were hypertensive. In the newly-diagnosed subjects in the TODAY study, only 12% were hypertensive, but during the trial about 5% developed hypertension each year, predicting SEARCH-like prevalences after a decade.

> **Practice point**
>
> Use percentiles to interpret blood pressure measurements in young people. Up to age 17, blood pressure ≥120/80 mm Hg is meaningfully elevated and requires careful monitoring and follow-up.

Lipids

In most historical studies, lipid profiles in Type 1 patients were overall better than those of non-diabetic subjects. In a more recent survey in 10–16 year olds from the United Kingdom, Canada and Australia, while mean HDL cholesterol was higher than in controls (typical for Type 1), total cholesterol was also higher (4.5 vs 4.0 mmol/l), and probably as a result of a higher body mass index, mean triglycerides were also higher (1.1 vs 0.8 mmol/l). The resulting higher LDL cholesterol (2.4 vs 2.2 mmol/l) may contribute from an early age to premature macrovascular events (Maftei et al., 2014). Not surprisingly, in Type 2 patients in the SEARCH study, dyslipidaemia (low HDL with elevated triglycerides) was found in nearly two-thirds.

Smoking

Type 1 patients are as likely to smoke as non-diabetic people. For example, 20% of all late-teenagers, controls and Type 1 subjects alike, were smokers in a 2014 report from the USA SEARCH study (Shah et al., 2014) – identical to the average prevalence of smoking in the EU28 countries (OECD/EU, 2016). Young people are perfectly aware of the hazards. Hardly surprisingly, other adverse cardiovascular risk factors (diastolic BP, lipids) cluster in the smokers, who also have worse glycaemic control (Hofer et al., 2009).

> **Practice point**
>
> We have made little impact on smoking in Type 1 patients compared with the general population. About 15–20% of Type 1 and non-diabetic people in their late teens are smokers. This is a shocking educational deficit.

Exercise

The effect of exercise on even short-term glucose control is not known. The risk of hypoglycaemia increases during aerobic exercise, followed by a sharp rebound in glucose levels about 2–3 hours after the end of exercise. Thereafter, between 7–11 hours and up to 30 hours after exercise there is an increased risk of further hypoglycaemia, especially in adolescents and in people exercising in the morning; afternoon exercise is probably better from this point of view. The general advice is to reduce prior fast-acting insulin by at least 25%, and to supplement with 15–30 g fast-acting carbohydrate every 30 minutes. The reduction should be 70–80% before prolonged exercise, for example, long-distance running. Pump patients are advised to reduce the basal rate by at least 50% but it is probably safer to suspend basal insulin completely (McAuley et al., 2016).

More Type 1 patients are doing endurance events such as marathon runs and long-distance cycling. Even with generous carbohydrate supplementation hypoglycaemia during and after the event can occur. Increasing availability of personal continuous glucose monitoring will help individuals monitor their response and take preventive action, and superb control can be achieved (**Figure 14.3**).

In a study of Germans between 3 and 18 years old, regular physical activity was associated with an HbA$_{1c}$ approximately 0.3% lower in all age groups and with lower diastolic BP.

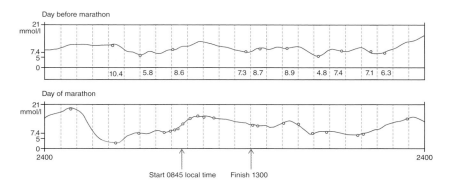

Figure 14.3 Continuous glucose tracing during an endurance event (Paris Marathon, 2015) in a 47-year old Type 1 patient in very good control (HbA$_{1c}$ 6.1–7.1%, 43–54). Record from FreeStyle Libre personal glucose system (Abbott). She was mildly hypoglycaemic the morning before the run, but glucose levels were stable throughout the marathon. Post-exercise hyperglycaemia is less marked in physically active Type 1 pump patients compared with those using multiple-dose insulin.

The effect is not consistent between studies and HbA$_{1c}$ differences of greater than 1% have been described. The lipid profile was better in exercising older teenagers (15–18 years old) but nearly 50% of the patients were inactive (Herbst *et al.*, 2007). Not surprisingly, young Type 2 patients exercise less than their Type 1 counterparts (Lobelo *et al.*, 2010).

Screen watching time

There is concern that increased screen time might be causally related to worse glycaemia and obesity in Type 1 diabetes. Back in 2008–9, a daily average of three hours screen time was to a certain extent balanced by five hours exercise a week in Type 1 German adolescents. Type 1 youngsters indulge in the same screen time as their non-diabetic peers but total sedentary time is high (mean 10 hours a day) and, in the SEARCH study in 2010, 50–70% of participants were using electronic media for more than two hours a day (Lobelo *et al.*, 2010). For a given screen consumption there may be greater adverse cardiovascular risk effects in diabetes and although glycaemia deteriorated in all SEARCH study subjects followed for five years, the rise was moderated if the time watching TV decreased rather than increased. Increased screen time was associated with increases in LDL and triglyceride levels (Li *et al.*, 2015).

There are probably important recent changes, such as a major increase in screen time recently in boys, but not girls. Any impact will be difficult to dissociate from general trends in obesity, rapid changes in technology calculated to keep young people glued ever-longer to their screens, and in some countries from counterbalancing improvements in glycaemia.

Practice point

Young Type 1 patients do the same amount of exercise and view screens for as long as non-diabetic people but, with increasing screen viewing time, HbA$_{1c}$ deteriorates more in both Type 1 and 2

Exercise and microvascular complications

Several cross-sectional studies have found a link between exercise and a lower risk of microvascular complications, but the long-term FinnDiane study found that higher levels of leisure-time physical activity carried a lower risk of developing microalbuminuria and of progressing nephropathy, allowing for the likely lower exercise tolerance of microalbuminuric patients (Wadén *et al.*, 2015).

Psychosocial functioning

In Type 1 diabetes, caregivers report higher levels of stress than the young people themselves. Also unexpectedly, Type 1 patients have less anxiety and depression than their non-diabetic peers (Kristensen *et al.*, 2014). This is not to say (see below) that some people with Type 1 diabetes do not have major self-management problems, especially during adolescence and young adulthood, but it is not a period of inevitable maladjustment. Mild depression occurred in 14% and moderate-to-severe depression in around 9% of young Type 1 people in the SEARCH study, but these rates were the same in non-diabetic controls. Young women who reported acute diabetes problems (for example diabetic ketoacidosis, emergency department attendance, hypoglycaemia) were more likely to be depressed. Little is known about these important matters in Type 2 diabetes, other than an occasional intriguing and not always intuitively obvious finding, for example that young males were more depressed than their Type 1 counterparts (Lawrence *et al.*, 2006).

Practice point

Depressed mood is common in young people with diabetes, but no more so than in the non-diabetic population. Type 2 males, and Type 1 females with acute diabetes problems are more likely to be depressed

---

Quality of life (QoL) has been extensively studied, with only a few unexpected results. After the first year of pump treatment, QoL is consistently better than in patients using multiple daily injections (Birkebaek *et al.*, 2014). There are no associations with simple measures of 'glycaemia' and even long-term studies may not help further illuminate this contentious question. Not surprisingly, health-related QoL is better in young Type 1 than Type 2 people; regardless of the type of diabetes, girls have lower QoL than boys. QoL decreases during adolescence in girls, and increases in boys.

Family structure and dynamics

Family structure is relatively easy to quantify. The factors consistently associated with worse glycaemic control in young people include:

- single-parent households compared with two-parent environments;
- living with biological parents is associated with better glycaemic control than any other family arrangement;
- in the USA, glycaemic control is consistently worst in African-Americans, followed by Hispanics, then white people. There are no comparable data for UK ethnic minorities.

Low income and single parenthood often covary with ethnicity, so causality is difficult to establish. In an important prospective study starting at diagnosis, African-Americans had worse control than young white people, even shortly after diagnosis; glycaemia deteriorated in both groups thereafter, but more rapidly in African-Americans, with a difference of 1.2% HbA$_{1c}$ emerging after two years (Frey *et al.*, 2007). Counterintuitively, income itself is not a significant effect. Single parenthood is the most powerful predictor of poor glycaemia.

> **Practice point**
>
> Single parenthood is strongly associated with poor glycaemia. Young people and guardians in single-parent households need intensive supervision and support.

Negative family dynamics account for about one-third of the variance in metabolic control – more important than adherence. General and diabetes-specific disagreements are important, the latter especially focused around blood glucose monitoring. Poor parental, especially maternal, psychological well-being, is thought to be important. However, fathers are important in diabetes, especially in the over-14s. They should be encouraged to participate in their offspring's diabetes management.

Eating disorders

Classical anorexia is fortunately rare in Type 1 diabetes; however, when it occurs the prognosis is grim, with a reported 12-year mortality of over one-third. Bulimia or binge eating disorder is common, in perhaps up to 30% of a British cohort aged 11–19. A 'disordered eating' syndrome is also prevalent (Pinhas-Hamiel *et al.*, 2015) (**Box 14.1**). Success with all forms of management is poor (though counterintuitively insulin pump treatment may help) and four out of five patients with disordered eating drop out of therapy.

Insulin omission

A widespread, unrecognized problem in Type 1 diabetes. The aim is to lose weight or prevent weight gain. Restricting insulin carries a poor outlook, with a threefold increased mortality in women. There is a close link with disordered eating: in a nationwide survey from Norway, one in three adolescent females occasionally omitted insulin entirely after overeating (Wisting *et al.*, 2013). More extreme practices are rarely reported to clinical teams; Bryden *et al.* (1999) described women taking insulin only twice a week, and some omitted it entirely for up to two weeks over prolonged periods during adolescence and early adulthood. Clinicians are therefore justified in starting a discussion of this important topic by stating that insulin omission is very common.

> **Box 14.1** Features of disordered eating in Type 1 diabetes (adapted from Pinhas-Hamiel *et al.*, 2015).
>
> - Much more prevalent in females (e.g. 25% vs 10% in males).
> - Prevalence increases rapidly throughout adolescence (e.g. 8% in 11–13 year old, 40% in 17–19 year olds)
> - Poor glycaemic control.
> - Recurrent DKA.
> - Missed medical appointments.
> - Declining to be weighed.
> - Tendency to vegetarianism.
> - Preoccupation with the caloric value of food.
> - Depression, decreased self-worth and poor body image.
>
> Features less commonly seen in diabetic subjects, compared with non-diabetic subjects, include skipping meals, fasting, vomiting and laxative or diuretic use

Table 14.1 Maternal and foetal risks in diabetes.

Maternal risks	Risks for foetus
Miscarriage	Miscarriage
Pre-eclampsia	Malformations (especially cardiac and neural tube)
Caesarean section	Stillbirth
Prematurity	Prematurity
	Macrosomia
Risks of diabetes	
Progression of microvascular complications	***Risks for baby***
Hypoglycaemia	Shoulder dystocia
Associated medication (especially Type 2)	Neonatal hypoglycaemia
	Future risk of developing diabetes and insulin-resistance characteristics

Source: Courtesy of Dr Nicoletta Dozio.

Prepregnancy counselling

A matter of the utmost importance for all diabetes practitioners, and for all forms of diabetes. Pregnancy and contraception are often difficult topics to tackle in clinics, but the health and wellbeing of mother and child are at risk if they are avoided (**Table 14.1**).

Type 1 diabetes

About one-third of pregnancies in Type 1 subjects in the United Kingdom are unplanned, about one-half in the USA. Glycaemia thereafter improves rapidly but HbA_{1c} levels still run consistently about 0.5% higher (Cyganek *et al.*, 2010). Prepregnancy counselling (including ready access to contraception and family planning services) need improving, recognizing that unwanted pregnancies occur most commonly in the age group with the worst glycaemic control. However, even where there are intensive programmes for prepregnancy care, only 30–40% access them and the benefits were seen in Type 2 but not Type 1 patients (Murphy *et al.*, 2010). Spontaneous pregnancy losses occur in nearly 20% of pregnancies and malformation rates are 2–4 times higher than in the background population. Stillbirths and neonatal deaths, though fortunately infrequent, are minimum at a periconception HbA_{1c} of approximately 6.7% (50) and increase consistently with higher values. Since glycaemic control during pregnancy is the most important factor predicting outcome, stringent control is needed. In both the United Kingdom and USA, HbA_{1c} <6.5% (48) is recommended if it can be achieved without hypoglycaemia (**Figure 14.4**). Glycaemic control during pregnancy is associated with incrementally better control using insulin pumps, sensor-augmented pumps and closed-loop insulin delivery (Stewart *et al.*, 2016) but trials are too small to demonstrate meaningful improvements in pregnancy outcomes using this burden of technology.

Practice points:

- One-third of Type 1 pregnancies are unplanned.
- Repeated education and access to family planning services are important. Target HbA_{1c} during pregnancy is <6.5% (48) if it can be achieved without hypoglycaemia.
- Emphasize the importance of prepregnancy folic acid, 5 mg daily.

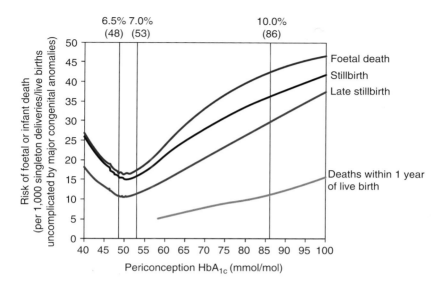

Figure 14.4 Glycaemic control around the time of conception and subsequent risks of foetal or infant death in Type 1 and Type 2 diabetes combined. Two specific targets for preconception HbA_{1c} are shown: the NICE recommendation in the UK is <48 (6.5%); <53 (7.0%) that of the American Diabetes Association. 86 mmol/mol (10%) or above is the level at which NICE recommends avoiding pregnancy because of unacceptably high risks for all four outcomes. *Source*: Tennant *et al.*, 2014. Reproduced with permission of Springer.

Type 2 diabetes

An increasing area of interest and of concern, highlighted in several earlier studies and confirmed in the TODAY study. Because of potential rosiglitazone treatment in this randomized study, a requirement in consent was for contraception, yet only 5% of the patients who became pregnant during the study, at an average age of 18, were actually using contraception (Klingensmith *et al.*, 2016). The reported outcomes are sobering: 10% were electively terminated and nearly 25% resulted in pregnancy loss. There were two stillbirths, and of the live-born infants 15% were preterm and 20% had a major congenital abnormality. Contributors to this very high abnormality rate (the comparable UK figure is around 5%) include marked obesity (median BMI 35), a smoking history in about one-half, low reported income and educational status. Interestingly, however, the median HbA_{1c} nearest to the onset of pregnancy was no different to the group without congenital abnormalities, (7.0–7.5%, 53–58, falling to around 6% (42) at the end of pregnancy). Glycaemia in some patients was very poor and there were not sufficient numbers of patients to clarify the role of glycaemia.

This study presents particularly poor outcomes. Probably more representative is a large study of native and non-native Dutch women with Type 2 diabetes who were much older (average age 32), less obese (mean BMI 30–32), with a short duration diabetes (median 1–2 years) and in good control throughout pregnancy (median HbA_{1c} values 5.5–6.9%,

37–52). Outcomes were still poor, highlighting the intrinsic risks of Type 2 diabetes in pregnancy: perinatal mortality was 4.8%, and congenital malformations occurred in 6%. However, there were no differences in outcomes between the native and non-native Dutch populations. Access to good local health provision is a critically important factor in equalizing these outcomes (Groen *et al.*, 2013).

Practice point

Women with pre-existing Type 2 diabetes have poor outcomes, though any differences due to ethnicity can be mitigated by ensuring access to high-quality pregnancy services.

Gestational diabetes

The burden of gestational diabetes worldwide is huge. The International Federation of Gynecology and Obstetrics (FIGO) estimates that it complicates 1 in 6 pregnancies in the developing world, which accounts for nearly 90% of total births (Hod *et al.*, 2015). Diagnosis is usually made between weeks 24 and 28 of pregnancy, so treatment must be prompt and effective. Criteria include fasting glucose levels of 5.1–6.9 mmol/l and a two-hour blood glucose level on a glucose tolerance test of 8.5–11.0 mmol/l. Blood glucose targets are fasting glucose <5.3 mmol/l, one-hour postprandial <7.8 mmol/l, and two-hour postprandial <6.7 mmol/l. Most women will achieve these with nutritional medical therapy alone, but metformin and insulin are fully safe. Glibenclamide is also widely considered to be safe for the foetus but it is no longer used in treatment out of pregnancy because of the risks of hypoglycaemia.

OLD AGE

People with Type 1 diabetes are now living much longer and, in many cases, in good health; the same is likely to be the case in Type 2 diabetes. Although there is much information about pathophysiology and epidemiology, there is almost no evidence base for practice in old people. Upper age limits for recruitment for clinical trials continue to rise but the numbers recruited to Type 1 studies are small and, in any case, they are mostly trials comparing insulin preparations, unhelpful when it comes to thinking about broader management strategies, though possibly of value in addressing concerns about some aspects of hypoglycaemia. Even in Type 2 diabetes there is very little to help guide management in the elderly or – increasingly – the very elderly. (Interestingly, because many of the Type 2 cardiovascular outcome studies recruit postacute coronary syndrome patients, mean age is still only in the early 60s, so that very few people in their late 70s or beyond are recruited.) We are left with the unsatisfactory prospect of proposing individualized treatments based on trials in people 10–20 years younger than the much more fragile elderly population increasingly seen in the community and hospital practice. Heavy-handed management with overmedication is a common problem in people who always require a more subtle approach, especially to drug interactions and side effects.

Type 1 diabetes

The happy trend to greater longevity with Type 1 diabetes – often with few or no microvascular complications – is reflected in the rapidly increasing number of celebratory medals awarded by *Diabetes UK* and the *American Diabetes Association* to individuals with long-duration Type 1 diabetes. In the United Kingdom, a 50-year medal (named after Sir John Nabarro) was once a rarity but many people, now mostly in their late 70s and 80s, are being awarded the UK 70-year medal (the McLeod medal), and the 75- and 80-year medals in the USA. The clinical corollary is that there is a substantial number (if a low proportion) of old people with insulin-treated diabetes who are genuinely insulin requiring and ketosis prone.

Practice point

Never assume that an older person using insulin has Type 2 diabetes. Some will have long-standing Type 1 diabetes. Continuity of insulin treatment is critical and they must always have adequate supplies.

In general, HbA_{1c} tends to drift down gradually from early middle age onwards. In the T1D Exchange cohort of USA Type 1 patients over 65, with a mean duration of 29 years, mean HbA_{1c} was 7.4% (57). HbA_{1c} was low (<7.0%, 53) in more than one-third, with the expected high rates of severe hypoglycaemia (1 in 6 subjects in the past year) but correspondingly low diabetic ketoacidosis rates (**Figure 14.5**). HbA_{1c} was identical (7.5%, 58) in a more representative survey from Germany and Austria with an even longer duration (32 years) in which only 20% in this age group used pumps, compared with 60% in the US study. There were significant differences between the groups. For example macroalbuminuria was more prevalent in the European population, albeit in an overall narrow range between 3 and 6%, and stroke and myocardial infarction were more prevalent – 6–10% compared with 2–7%. Medication use was higher in the USA (statins in 70% vs 40%, antihypertensives in 85% vs 60% and aspirin in 80% vs 21%). The groups are obviously not directly comparable (the major difference being the greater age of the European population) but the differences in medication are very striking, and

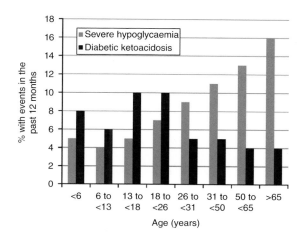

Figure 14.5 Rates of severe hypoglycaemia and diabetic ketoacidosis across the age range surveyed in the T1D Registry. The consistent rise in hypoglycaemia and fall in ketoacidosis from the 3rd decade onwards is very striking. The over-65s are particularly prone to severe hypoglycaemia, yet this group has the 'best' mean HbA_{1c}. About 1 in 6 over-65s will have a severe hypoglycaemic episode every year. *Source*: Data from Beck *et al.*, 2012.

given the similar HbA$_{1c}$ levels – though the long-term trajectories are not known – perhaps evidence-based resistance to using standard prophylactic medication in younger people continues with less justification into older age.

Practice point

Frequently review the need for aspirin, antihypertensive and lipid-lowering treatment in older Type 1 patients based on individual risk factors and risk calculations, for example QRISK in the United Kingdom.

Practice point

Type 1 patients in their 60s and beyond with long-standing diabetes tend to have low HbA$_{1c}$ values (e.g. 7.5%, 58) and are at increased risk of severe hypoglycaemia but at lower risk of diabetic ketoacidosis.

Clinically important features of Type 1 diabetes in older people (though there is almost no evidence for the real-life impact of these factors):

- They often require low or very low doses of insulin (0.5–0.7 U/kg in the DPV and T1D Exchange groups); dosage changes of even one unit may represent major proportional shifts and dose titration needs the gentlest of touches.
- They may have lower numerical skills than younger people. The calculation burden of carbohydrate-counting programs such as DAFNE may be taxing for them.
- Visual disability, not always apparent, for example in people with the diffuse but disabling consequences of extensive retinal laser treatment. Equipment with large or high-contrast scales is available.
- Advanced neuropathy or cheiroarthropathy affecting dexterity and the ability to give insulin injections, especially in multiple dose regimens.
- Increased risk of falls, fractures and other injuries: contributing factors include vitamin D deficiency, neuropathy and low bone mineral density related to low BMI.
- Autonomic neuropathy and postural hypotension.
- Higher risk of early cognitive impairment which may not be otherwise apparent (e.g. remembering precise insulin doses and how to dial them up in pen devices).
- Life environment. Some have lost their life partners who may have been major players in managing the patient's diabetes and often did so with astonishing intuitive skill that may not be apparent to other carers and healthcare professionals.
- Patients with very long-standing Type 1 diabetes are usually highly resilient and take pride in their self-management skills. Needs assessments must be done with care and sensitivity.

'Brittle' diabetes in the elderly

As in the much younger patients, 'brittle' diabetes is defined as glycaemic instability that disrupts life and results in long hospital admissions. Despite the same term, it is clinically quite different from brittle diabetes in the young, where it is usually dominated by recurrent diabetic ketoacidosis. In the elderly, approximately equal numbers of patients have predominant ketoacidosis and hypoglycaemia, or a mixed picture. Psychological problems, a major feature in the young, are rarely seen in the elderly and it is usually not associated with memory problems. It is commoner in women, but this may be a survivor effect – the mean age in a UK-wide survey in 2001 was 74 (Benbow et al., 2001). It is fortunately uncommon but management is difficult and patients require much thought and support especially in relation to their home circumstances.

Features of very long-standing Type 1 diabetes (duration greater than 50 years)

People surviving more than 50 years of Type 1 diabetes have been described in separate cohorts in the United Kingdom (the Golden Years Cohort; Bain et al., 2003) and the USA (the Joslin 50-year Medalist Study; Sun et al., 2011). The two groups, mean age 70 and mean duration 57 years when they were studied, are strikingly similar, and share much in common with the DPV and T1D cohorts mentioned earlier:

- insulin sensitive, requiring low doses of insulin (~0.5 U/kg/day)
- normal BMI (~25)
- high HDL (mean 1.8 mmol/l)
- males and females equally represented.

Microvascular complications

In the USA group, only 5% had proteinuria (similar to the T1D cohort), confirming the poor outlook in patients with nephropathy. Only 50% had proliferative retinopathy and more than one-third never had retinopathy more severe than mild non-proliferative disease, suggesting that many of these patients tracked with excellent glycaemic control over many decades. Forty percent had no evidence of neuropathy and 50% did not have cardiovascular disease. These are intriguing findings, with no obvious explanation, but processing of advanced glycation end-products (AGEs), only weakly linked to HbA_{1c}, may be important in predicting long-term complications (Sun et al., 2011). They also have well-preserved levels of endothelial and circulating progenitor cells compared with age-matched non-diabetic subjects, which were higher than younger patients and age-matched Type 2 patients. The proposal is that these high numbers may be protective against the inevitable metabolic disturbances of even well-controlled long-term Type 1 diabetes (Hernandez et al., 2014).

The DPV and T1D cohorts had 20 fewer years of diabetes than these extreme long survivors, yet they are similar. Once patients have reached 30 years of diabetes with no significant complications, they may be set fair for at least a further 20 years.

Practice point

Although people with very long-standing well-controlled Type 1 diabetes are at low risk of significant complications, be vigilant.

Type 2 diabetes

Vascular complications of Type 2 diabetes develop slowly. The cohort of trials in the 2000s in patients with longer-standing diabetes – around 10 years since diagnosis – provided no support for the reduction in microvascular complications with even ultratight glycaemic control, and while there is no evidence that glycaemia is any *less* important in the elderly, the focus of most reviews, which is glycaemia (and secondarily the risk of hypoglycaemia), is unjustified when lipids and hypertension both contribute so much more than glycaemia to cardiovascular disease at this stage of life. Because clinical trials focus on lower targets for glycaemia, the problem is framed in a biased way, questioning whether tight glycaemic control is harmful to the elderly rather than whether there is a reasonable level of glycaemia below which, over a given remaining life expectancy, evolution of complications is unlikely. Individualization is critical and a framework proposed by Sinclair *et al.* (2015) must be modified by factors such as:

- total or active life expectancy
- risk of complications
- competing risks
- need for carer or social support
- hypoglycaemia and risks of adverse drug reactions.

This proposes a range of HbA_{1c} for independent people and the frail or those with mild disability between 7 and 8% (53–64), and under 8.5% (69) where there is moderate or severe disability or cognitive impairment.

> **Practice point**
>
> Glycaemic control in older groups should lie between 7 and 8.5% (53–69) depending on the individual's degree of independence, level of frailty and disability.

One properly highlighted area is the substantial population of people with diabetes in care homes, where severe hyperglycaemia is probably common and a symptomatic burden. Since hyperglycaemic symptoms, especially urinary, infective and cognitive, are often difficult to isolate in people with impaired cognition, exercise judgement in considering reasonable individualized targets. Society recommendations are particularly unhelpful here and documents often focus on clinically important areas, such as falls, sarcopenia and frailty, which are associated with poor glycaemia, but are not meaningfully reversed by good glycaemia.

In this age group cardiovascular risk reduction is even more important compared with glycaemia than in younger subjects. Management of statin treatment, using the same targets as in younger people and blood pressure (e.g. <140/90 mm Hg) are important. Patients without cardiovascular disease may still be taking aspirin treatment started years ago in the era when all patients with diabetes were assumed to benefit. Aspirin may need to be discontinued.

Over-tight control in Type 2 patients

The problem of overtight control has been at least quantified in older Type 1 patients (see earlier) but there is little data in Type 2. As in younger patients, very low HbA_{1c} measurements should not be accepted uncritically as a prompt for mutual congratulation, though in the world of payment-by-results they often are. Beyond about 65 years of age, appetite and body weight progressively fall; impairment of cognition and mobility may further reduce individuals' access to food. A falling HbA_{1c}, especially into or below the non-diabetic range (<6.5%, 48) is particularly hazardous in patients taking insulin and sulfonylureas. Doses should be progressively and gradually reduced assisted by increased frequency of home blood glucose and HbA_{1c} monitoring, though this is difficult and time consuming. Nevertheless, it is an important but rarely-described form of clinical inertia that is difficult enough to counter in younger free-living individuals, much less the frail elderly person, especially those in care homes. Acute hypoglycaemia is a real problem. About 20% of diabetes-related admissions in the over-80s are hypoglycaemia-related. Once admitted, then inappropriate doses of insulin and sulfonylureas are often identified, but this cohort represents only the tip of the iceberg of people with more subtle, chronic hypoglycaemia in the community, which may be especially difficult to detect. Although the autoimmune conditions associated with new-onset hypoglycaemia (especially Addison's and coeliac) are much less likely in Type 2 compared with Type 1 diabetes, many normal-weight Type 2 patients will have autoimmune forms of diabetes.

The much-quoted and debated ACCORD study (**Chapter 10**) was unable to find a clear relationship between severe hypoglycaemia, low HbA_{1c} levels and the excess of all-cause death that caused premature termination of the glycaemic part of the trial. However, it reminds us that although low HbA_{1c} values are clinically a risk factor for severe hypoglycaemia, high values are frequently accompanied by hypoglycaemia, though usually in insulin- and not sulfonylurea-treated patients.

The lack of systematic evidence should not blind us to obvious clinical risks. Data are likely to emerge. For example, a large cross-sectional study of people with diabetes in Italian nursing homes found that glycaemia was already very tight (mean HbA_{1c} 7.0%, 53) in people who were barely overweight (mean BMI 25.5). Importantly, impairments of activities of daily living progressively worsened with decreasing tertiles of HbA_{1c} (8.4%, 68; 6.9%, 52; 5.8%, 40), especially in patients taking sulfonylureas and repaglinide. Glycaemia, and not hypoglycaemic events, was associated with impaired activities (Abbatecola *et al.*, 2015).

Frailty

Frailty is a concept growing in importance and becoming of major clinical significance in diabetes. As in many other chronic disease areas, frailty is now recognized as an important factor determining morbidity and mortality independent of the underlying disease entity. For example, in diabetes classical comorbidities, hypertension and cardiovascular complications account for only 15–40% of the excess risk of frailty, but the links are so strong that diabetes is considered a model of frailty (Sinclair *et al.*, 2015). It is complex and comprises features of several domains, but is broadly a state of physiological sensitivity that easily results in disequilibrium and consequent vulnerability, especially in the over-75s. Factors associated with frailty in diabetes include:

- bone fragility (see **Chapter 5**)
- sarcopenia (in turn strongly linked to disability)
- increased muscle fat (insulin resistance)
- mood disturbance and depression (see **Chapter 15**)
- cognitive impairment
- falls (linked to polypharmacy, cerebrovascular disease, hypoglycaemia, orthostatic hypotension and visual impairment).

The severity of baseline frailty in Type 2 patients in their mid-70s is a significant predictor of increased risk of death and incident disability over the next 6–7 years (Castro-Rodríguez *et al.*, 2016).

Practice point

Frailty in Type 2 patients over the age of 75 is more important in determining mortality and disability than standard macrovascular characteristics.

Individual antihyperglycaemic agents (Chapter 10)

Although not formally reported, some older people may make quite radical changes to their diet when diagnosed, so desisting from the automatic prescription reflex is particularly important in this situation.

- *Metformin*. Still a mainstay in most patients; adjust dose according to renal function. Remember the occasional anorexia-like syndrome in some elderly people who have been taking metformin for a long time, characterized by falling weight and severely impaired appetite, without the overt and usually acute bowel and upper gastrointestinal symptoms encountered in younger people.
- *Sulfonylureas (SUs)*. Widely condemned and avoided, but used carefully and with due regard for hypoglycaemia and low HbA$_{1c}$, especially if prescribed in maximum or near-maximum doses, they can still be valuable. However clinicians are properly cautious about a de novo start of a sulfonylurea in an elderly newly-diagnosed Type 2 patient (normally in addition to metformin). Many would observe the effect of a DPP-4 inhibitor first.
- *DPP-4 inhibitors*. Overall weak agents, but free of hypoglcyaemia risk, and once daily with an established record of low side effects. Valuable in this age group, especially those that can be used in varying degrees of renal impairment.
- *GLP-1-receptor agonists*. Their potential for weight loss may be of value in the obese elderly person, but not to be used in the normal weight and thin patient. Use with caution in patients with long-standing diabetes, where they may uncover subclinical gastroparesis.
- *SGLT2 inhibitors*. Should not be used until further information is available. They are powerful glucose-reducing agents but may exacerbate urinary frequency and possibly incontinence, and are contraindicated in the large number of patients already taking diuretics.
- *Insulin*. Vigorously promoted, especially for patients with long-standing diabetes and supposedly 'exhausted' β-cells, but it can be a real challenge to initiate and continue successfully and with minimum risk, especially in the care-home environment where staff cannot administer insulin in variable dosages according to meal size. There is almost no evidence on which to base practice, particularly in the very old, and in those where the aims are for reasonable glycaemia, and minimizing the number of injections and hypoglycaemia risk. In the German/Austrian registry reporting in 2016, Type 2 patients with comorbid dementia had a 40% increased risk of severe hypoglycaemia and a twofold increased risk of hypoglycaemic coma compared with oral hypoglycaemic-treated patients, though overall glycaemia was no different (HbA$_{1c}$ 7.7%, 61). Perversely, dementia patients were more likely to be insulin-treated (Prinz *et al.*, 2016).

Practice point

Repeatedly assess whether or not Type 2 patients with dementia really need insulin treatment. They are at high risk of severe hypoglycaemia and hypoglycaemic coma, with little or no benefit for overall glycaemia compared with non-insulin agents.

Adding basal analogue insulin to an existing non-insulin regime would be standard practice in younger people; it was successful in the short-term in a group of older people, too (Papa *et al.*, 2008), without increasing the risk of hypoglycaemia. However, this does not address critical problems in the elderly requiring insulin:

- Ensuring injections are given reliably and technically appropriately if self-administered.
- Supervision of injections in supported environments.
- Timing of injections if the patient is relying on community nursing staff.

- Erratic meal patterns, omitting food through volition, forgetfulness or cognitive impairment.
- Visual impairment and musculoskeletal problems that may impair efficient or safe injections.

Practical matters in insulin treatment in the elderly

Make a full assessment of the practicalities of insulin administration and set realistic targets for blood glucose and HbA$_{1c}$ before proposing insulin treatment. The hazards of insulin and the potential lack of benefit should be the primary considerations, not the often unpredictable and unquantifiable benefits. However, there are continual improvements in insulin types and delivery devices that may be of practical benefit in the individual patient. Specialist teams must be involved right from the start. Examples of products that may be of value include:

- *Easier-to-inject devices*, for example FlexTouch, low injection force, minimal extension disposable pens (NovoNordisk) available with long-acting analogues detemir and degludec; Innolet.
- *Biphasic mixtures*, analogue (e.g. Humalog Mix 25 and 50, NovoMix 30, Ryzodeg (degludec 70%/aspart 30%)) or human (e.g. Humulin M3). All, apart from Ryzodeg, are cloudy and need mixing before injection.
- *High-strength analogues*, for patients needing large doses of basal insulin, in order to avoid multiple injections of the same insulin (e.g. U200 degludec (Tresiba), U300 glargine (Toujeo)).
- Fixed-dose GLP-1/long-acting analogue mixture, for example Xultophy (degludec/liraglutide), in obese patients.

References

Abbatecola AM, Bo M, Armellini F et al. Tighter glycemic control is associated with ADL physical dependency losses in older adults using sulfonylureas or miglitinides: results from the DIMORA study. Metabolism 2015;64:1500–6 [PMID: 26318196].

Amin R, Widmer B, Prevost AT et al. Risk of microalbuminuria and progression to macroalbuminuria in a cohort with childhood onset type 1 diabetes: prospective observational study. BMJ 2008;336:697–701 [PMID: 18349042] PMC2276285.

Arnett JJ, Padilla-Walker LM. Brief report: Danish emerging adults' conceptions of adulthood. J Adolesc 2015;38:39–44 [PMID: 25460678].

Badaru A, Klingensmith GJ, Dabelea D et al. Correlates of treatment patterns among youth with type 2 diabetes. Diabetes Care 2014;37:64–72 [PMID: 24026554] PMC3867996b.

Bain SC, Gill GV, Dyer PH et al. Characteristics of Type 1 diabetes of over 50 years duration (the Golden Years Cohort). Diabet Med 2003;20:808–11 [PMID: 14510860].

Beck RW, Tamborlane WV, Bergenstal RM et al. T1D Exchange Clinic Network. The T1D Exchange clinic registry. J Clin Endocrinol Metab 2012;97:4383–9 [PMID: 22996145].

Benbow SJ, Walsh A, Gill GV. Brittle diabetes in the elderly. J R Soc Med 200;94:578–80 [PMID: 11691895] PMC1282243.

Birkebaek NH, Kristensen LJ, Mose AH, Thastum M. Danish Society for Diabetes in Childhood and Adolescence. Quality of life in Danish children and adolescents with type 1 diabetes treated with continuous subcutaneous insulin infusion or multiple daily injections. Diabetes Res Clin Pract 2014;106:474–80 [PMID: 25451903].

Bradley TK, Slorach C, Mahmug FH et al. Early changes in cardiovascular structure and function in adolescents with type 1 diabetes. Cardiovasc Diabetol 2016;15:31 [PMID: 26879273] PMC4754808.

Bryden KS, Neil A, Mayou RA, Peveler RC et al. Eating habits, body weight, and insulin misuse. A longitudinal study of teenagers and young adults with type 1 diabetes. *Diabetes Care* 1999;22:1956–60 [PMID: 10587825] Free full text.

Castro-Rodríguez M, Carnicero JA, Garcia-Garcia FJ et al. Frailty as a major factor in the increased risk of death and disability in older people with diabetes. *J Am Med Dir Assoc* 2016;17:949–55 [PMID: 27600194].

Clements MA, Foster NC, Maahs DM et al. T1D Exchange Clinic Network. Hemoglobin A1c (HbA1c) changes over time among adolescent and young adult participants in the T1D exchange clinic registry. *Pediatr Diabetes* 2016;17:327–36 [PMID: 26153338].

Cyganek K, Hebda-Szydlo A, Katra B et al. Glycaemic control and selected pregnancy outcomes in type 1 diabetes women on continuous subcutaneous insulin infusion and multiple daily injections: the significance of pregnancy planning. *Diabetes Technol Ther* 2010;12:41–7 [PMID: 20082584].

Dabelea D, Stafford JM, Mayer-Davis EJ et al. SEARCH for Diabetes in Youth Research Group. Association of type 1 diabetes vs type 2 diabetes diagnosed during childhood and adolescence with complications during teenage years and young adulthood. *JAMA* 2017;317:825–35 [PMID: 28245334].

Daniels M, DuBose SN, Maahs DM et al. T1D Exchange Clinic Network. Factors associated with microalbuminuria in 7,549 children and adolescents with type 1 diabetes in the T1D Exchange clinic registry. *Diabetes Care* 2013;36:2639–45 [PMID: 23610082] PMC3747908.

Dart AB, Martens PJ, Rigatto C et al. Earlier onset of complications in youth with type 2 diabetes. *Diabetes Care* 2014;37:436–43 [PMID: 24130346].

Frey MA, Templin T, Ellis D et al. Predicting metabolic control in the first 5 yr after diagnosis for youths with type 1 diabetes: the role of ethnicity and family structure. *Pediatr Diabetes* 2007;8:220–7 [PMID: 17659064].

Groen B, Links TP, van den Berg PP et al. Similar adverse pregnancy outcome in native and non-native dutch women with pregestational type 2 diabetes: a multicentre retrospective study. *ISRN Obstet Gynecol* 2013;2013:361435 [PMID: 24294525] PMC3833010.

Harrington J, Peña AS, Gent R et al. Aortic intima media thickness is an early marker of atherosclerosis in children with type 1 diabetes mellitus. *J Pediatr* 2010;156:237–41 [PMID: 19853860].

Herbst A, Kordonouri O, Schwab KO et al. DPV Initiative of the German Working Group for Pediatric Diabetology Germany. Impact of physical activity on cardiovascular risk factors in children with type 1 diabetes: a multicentre study of 23,251 patients. *Diabetes Care* 2007;30:2098–100 [PMID: 17468347].

Hernandez SL, Gon JH, Chen L et al. Characterization of circulating and endothelial progenitor cells in patients with extreme-duration type 1 diabetes. *Diabetes Care* 2014;37:2193–201 [PMID: 24780357] PMC4113171.

Hod M, Kapur A, Sacks DA et al.The International Federation of Gynecology and Obstetrics (FIGO) Initiative on gestational diabetes mellitus: a pragmatic guide for diagnosis, management, and care. *Int J Gynaecol Obstet* 2015;131(Suppl 3):S173–211 [PMID: 26433807] Free full text.

Hofer SE, Rosenbauer J, Grulich-Henn J et al. DPV-Wiss. Study Group. Smoking and metabolic control in adolescents with type 1 diabetes. *J Pediatr* 2009;154:20–3 [PMID: 18804216].

Hofer SE, Raile K, Fröhlich-Reiterer E et al.; German Competence Network for Diabetes Mellitus. Tracking of metabolic control from childhood to young adulthood in type 1 diabetes. *J Pediatr* 2014;165:956–61 [PMID: 25151197].

Huang TT, Ferris E, Tripathi D. An integrative analysis of the effect of lifestyle and pharmacological interventions on glucose metabolism in the prevention and treatment of youth-onset type 2 diabetes. *Curr Diab Rep* 2016;16:78 [PMID: 27380713].

Klingensmith GJ, Pyle L, Nadeau KJ. TODAY Study Group. Pregnancy outcomes in youth with type 2 diabetes: the TODAY study experience. *Diabetes Care* 2016; 39: 122–9 [PMID: 26628417] PMC 4686849.

Kristensen LJ, Brikbaek NH, Mose AH et al. Symptoms of emotional, behavioural, and social difficulties in the Danish population of children and adolescents with type 1 diabetes – results of a national survey. *PLoS One* 2014;19:e97543 [PMID: 24842772] PMC4026318.

Lawrence JM, Standiford DA, Loots B et al. SEARCH for Diabetes in Youth Study. Prevalence and correlates of depressed mood among youth with diabetes: the SEARCH for Diabetes in Youth study. Pediatrics 2006;117:1348–58 [PMID: 16585333].

Levy D. Adolescence and emerging adulthood, in Levy D: Type 1 Diabetes (Oxford Diabetes Library). Oxford: Oxford University Press, 2016, pp. 167–187.

Li C, Beech B, Crume T et al. Longitudinal association between television watching and computer use and risk markers in diabetes in the SEARCH for Diabetes in Youth Study. Pediatr Diabetes 2015;16:382–91 [PMID: 25041407] PMC4291304.

Lobelo F, Liese AD, Liu J et al. Physical activity and electronic media use in the SEARCH for diabetes in youth case-control study. Pediatrics 2010;125:e1364–71 [PMID: 20457683].

Maftei O, Peña AS, Sullivan T et al. AdDIT Study Group. Early atherosclerosis relates to urinary albumin excretion and cardiovascular risk factors in adolescents with type 1 diabetes: Adolescent type 1 Diabetes cardio-renal Intervention Trial (AdDIT) Diabetes Care 2014;37:3069–75 [PMID: 25071076].

Mayer-Davis EJ, Davis C, Saadine J et al. SEARCH for Diabetes in Youth Study Group. Diabetic retinopathy in the SEARCH for Diabetes in Youth Cohort: a pilot study. Diabet Med 2012;29:1148–52 [PMID: 22269205] PMC4495729.

McAuley SA Horsburgh JC, Ward GM et al. Insulin pump basal adjustment for exercise in type 1 diabetes: a randomised crossover study. Diabetologia 2016;59:1636–44 [PMID: 27168135].

McKnight JA, Wild SH, Lamb MJ et al. Glycaemic control of Type 1 diabetes in clinical practice early in the 21st century: an international comparison. Diabet Med 2015;32:1036–50 [PMID: 25510978].

Murphy HR, Roland JM, Skinner TC et al. Effectiveness of a regional prepregnancy care program in women with type 1 and type 2 diabetes: benefits beyond glycemic control. Diabetes Care 2010;33:2514–20 [PMID: 21115765] PMC2992180.

National High Blood Pressure Education Working Group on high blood pressure in children and adolescents. The fourth report on the diagnosis, evaluation, and treatment of high blood pressure in children and adolescents. Pediatrics 2004;114(2 Suppl 4th report):555–76 [PMID: 15286277].

OECD/EU (2016), Health at a Glance: Europe 2016 – State of Health in the EU Cycle. OECD Publishing, Paris. 10.1787/9789264265592-en (last accessed 31 August 2017).

Pacaud D, Schwandt A, de Beaufort C et al. SWEET Study Group. A description of clinician reported diagnosis of type 2 diabetes and other non-type 1 diabetes included in a large international multicentered pediatric diabetes registry (SWEET). Pediatr Diabetes 2016;17(Suppl 23):24–31 [PMID: 27748026].

Papa G, Fedele V, Chiavetta A et al. Therapeutic options for elderly diabetic subjects: open label, randomized clinical trial of insulin glargine added to oral antidiabetic drugs versus increased dosage of oral antidiabetic drugs. Acta Diabetol 2008;45:53–9 [PMID 18180864].

Pinhas-Hamiel O, Hamiel U, Levy-Shraga Y. Eating disorders in adolescents with type 1 diabetes: Challenges in diagnosis and treatment. World J Diabetes 2015;6:517–26 [PMID: 25897361] [PMC4398907].

Prinz N, Stingl J, Dapp A et al. DPV Initiative. High rate of hypoglycaemia in 6770 type 2 patients with comorbid dementia: a multicentre cohort study on 215,932 patients from the German/Austrian diabetes registry. Diabetes Res Clin Pract 2016;112:73–81 [PMID: 26563590].

Shah AS, Dabelea D, Talton JW et al. Smoking and arterial stiffness in youth with type 1 diabetes: the SEARCH Cardiovascular Disease Study. J Pediatr 2014;165:110–6 [PMID: 24681182] PMC4074551.

Sinclair A, Dunning T, Rodriguez-Mañas L. Diabetes in older people: new insights and remaining challenges. Lancet Diabetes Endocrinol 2015;3:275–85 [PMID: 25466523].

Stewart ZA, Wilinska ME, Hartnell S et al. Closed-loop insulin delivery during pregnancy in women with type 1 diabetes. N Engl J Med 2016;375:644–54 [PMID: 27532830] Free full text.

Sun JK, Keenan HA, Cavallerano JD et al. Protection from retinopathy and other complications in patients with type 1 diabetes of extreme duration: the Joslin 50-year medalist study. Diabetes Care 2011;34:968–74 [PMID: 21447665] PMC3064059.

Tennant PW, Glinianaia SV, Bilous RW et al. Pre-existing diabetes, maternal glycaemic haemoglobin, and the risks of fetal and infant death: a population-based study. Diabetologia 2014;57:285–92 [PMID: 24292565].

TODAY Study Group; Zeitler P, Hirst K, Pyle L et al. A clinical trial to maintain glycemic control in youth with type 2 diabetes. N Engl J Med 2012;366:2247–56 [PMID: 22540912] PMC3478667.

Wadén J, Tikkanen HK, Forsblom C et al. FinnDiane Study Group. Leisure-time physical activity and development and progression of diabetic nephropathy in type 1 diabetes: the FinnDiane Study. Diabetologia 2015;58:929–36 [PMID: 25634228].

Wisting L, Frøisland DH, Skrivarhaug T et al. Disturbed eating behaviour and omission of insulin in adolescents receiving intensified insulin treatment: a nationwide population-based study. Diabetes Care 2013;36:3382–7 [PMID: 23963896] PMC 3816868.

Zeitler P, Hirst K, Copeland KC et al. TODAY Study Group. HbA1c after a short period of monotherapy with metformin identifies durable glycemic control among adolescents with type 2 diabetes. Diabetes Care 2015;38:2285–92 [PMID: 26537182] PMC4657618.

Further reading

Extended early adulthood/stay at home kids

http://www.telegraph.co.uk/women/mother-tongue/8474569/Stay-at-home-kids-a-worldwide-phenomenon.html (last accessed 31 August 2017).

Reference values for blood pressure in young people

National High Blood Pressure Education Working Group on high blood pressure in children and adolescents. The fourth report on the diagnosis, evaluation, and treatment of high blood pressure in children and adolescents. Pediatrics 2004;114(2 Suppl 4th report):555–76 [PMID: 15286277].

Youth-onset Type 2 diabetes

Nadeau KJ, Anderson BJ, Berg EG et al. Youth-onset Type 2 diabetes consensus report: current status challenges, and priorities. Diabetes Care 2016;39:1635–42 [PMID: 27486237].

Levy D. Adolescence and emerging adulthood, in Levy D: Type 1 Diabetes (Oxford Diabetes Library), Oxford: Oxford University Press, 2016, pp. 167–188.

15 Psychological aspects of diabetes

> **Key points**
>
> *Type 1 diabetes*
>
> - Quality of life in childhood diabetes is not impaired, though that of parents can be
> - Single parenthood is the most important risk factor for poor glycaemic control in children
> - Family dysfunction is common and family-based interventions consistently beneficial
> - Depression is not as prevalent as previously thought and has often been confused with diabetes-related distress (which is very common)
> - When depression occurs, it is more severe and lasts longer than in non-diabetic subjects; it is much more common in females
> - Psychological interventions for depression are more effective than antidepressant drugs
> - Severe hypoglycaemia (e.g. with seizure) in young children with Type 1 diabetes is a risk factor for impairment of selective aspects of IQ and possibly lower educational achievement
>
> *Type 2 diabetes*
>
> - The causal links between Type 2 diabetes and depression operate in both directions
> - Screening for depression is of no value in itself
> - Frequent medical interventions improve both diabetes and depressive symptoms in Type 2 patients. Psychological interventions seem not to benefit medical aspects of diabetes, but they improve depression more effectively than antidepressants
> - There is a significant excess mortality risk in depressed people with foot ulceration

INTRODUCTION

The psychological aspects of a long-term, often lifelong condition such as diabetes have been explored for a long time. Much of the literature still focuses on cross-sectional studies using an array of psychological tests, some generic, others specific for diabetes, and the associations uncovered are often predictable and unsurprising. However, therapies for psychological problems, especially depression, which is highly prevalent in both Type 1 and 2 diabetes, are still not well established and the number of prospective studies, either controlled trials or longitudinal cohort studies, is still small in comparison with the acknowledged scale of the problem. However, long-established prospective cohort studies, especially in Type 1 diabetes, are now delivering valuable information. Clinicians are now much more aware of the psychological problems of diabetes, though health systems deliver any evidence-based therapies variably and in general rather inefficiently, and earnest exhortations markedly outweigh clinical activity. Because the life-stories of people with Type 1 and Type 2 diabetes are quite different, especially when considering

Practical Diabetes Care, Fourth Edition. David Levy.
© 2018 John Wiley & Sons Ltd. Published 2018 by John Wiley & Sons Ltd.

family functioning, a particular problem in Type 1 diabetes, it is worthwhile discussing them separately.

TYPE 1 DIABETES

The features of psychological and psychosocial stress in Type 1 patients are mostly subtle and are not reliably captured by the profusion of questionnaires that have been developed. Because of the young age of many Type 1 patients, psychological functioning is strongly influenced by sociodemographic factors, which are directly related to barriers to good health.

Psychological problems around the time of diagnosis

There is increasing interest in familial and personal factors that may precipitate the onset of Type 1 diabetes in childhood. Life stresses seem not to be associated but hospitalization or serious illness are, and this sequence is frequently encountered in clinical practice. In a large Swedish study (Nygren *et al.*, 2015) serious life events experienced by the child or parents, including a death and serious illness, carried a threefold increased risk of developing Type 1 diabetes and a new family structure, for example divorce, was also associated, though more weakly. Other factors identified include unemployment, parental dispute and the trauma of war.

Practice point

Major life events can precipitate the clinical onset of Type 1 diabetes in children. These include a family illness or death and parents divorcing.

The onset of Type 1 diabetes in young people is a major crisis for them, their parents, siblings and peers. Neurocognitive functioning, especially psychomotor speed, is markedly impaired within the first few days of diagnosis but is not caused solely by the severity of the metabolic state at diagnosis, as it persists for at least a year and is correlated with glycaemic control (Schwartz *et al.*, 2014). This is an important reason for heightened awareness and early interception of Type 1 diabetes. Adjustment problems immediately after diagnosis are common and, if present, can become chronic. Post-traumatic stress disorder can be detected six weeks after diagnosis in about one in five mothers and fathers; adjustment disorders in mothers largely resolve by the end of the first year.

Because of the high rate of psychological disorders in children and their families, psychological intervention is often advocated, but in most situations is not delivered, as resources are limited, and because so much of the focus over this period is the biotechnical aspects of establishing blood glucose control.

Childhood

Surprisingly little is known. Early-onset diabetes is associated with poorer working memory and a higher risk of learning problems. There is conflicting evidence on the impact of diabetes on school performance. In a large study from Australia, pupils with Type 1 diabetes lost 3% of school days but overall test outcomes were the same as their non-diabetic peers. However, there were significant relationships between glycaemic control, test scores and poorer attendance; for example, a 2% worse attendance record for each 1% increase in HbA_{1c}, though severe hypoglycaemia and diabetic ketoacidosis had no impact (Cooper et al., 2016).

Parents believe their child's quality of life (QoL) is lower than that of their non-diabetic peers but this view is not shared by the children themselves, who have a quality of life similar to their non-diabetic peers. Boys self-rate their quality of life higher than girls, as do children from higher socioeconomic backgrounds. Higher numbers of daily injections and lower frequency of home blood glucose monitoring are associated with worse quality of life, as well as higher total daily insulin doses and – linked – body mass index. Psychological interventions are sparse in pre-adolescents but coping skills training, focusing on the day-to-day problems of stress management and conflict resolution, resulted in improved life satisfaction more than group education, which focuses more on diabetes management (Ambrosino et al., 2008). Both approaches improved psychosocial adaptation.

Adolescence and emerging adulthood

Teenage angst is by no means universal in Type 1 diabetes. A large study of young Danish people aged 8–17 found depression and anxiety was more prevalent in non-diabetic children compared with Type 1 peers. There was also no evidence of a higher prevalence of severe symptoms. As in younger children, caregivers reported a higher level of psychological stress than the patients themselves (Kristensen et al., 2014). Studies do not agree on the relationship between quality of life and glycaemia in this age group. In the diabetes control and complications trial (DCCT), the highly-pressured intensively-treated group experienced a lower quality of life than the conventionally-treated group, but in the real-life Hvidøre study better glycaemia was associated with higher quality of life. However, this did not apply in significant groups, for example, girls, ethnic minorities and single-parent families. Long-term insulin pump treatment is associated with better quality of life than multiple dose insulin, but any difference takes a year to emerge after starting treatment (see **Chapter 7**).

FAMILY STRUCTURE

Cross-sectional studies consistently agree on the following:

- Glycaemia in young people is worse when they are in single-parent households compared with living with two parents.
- Best glycaemic control occurs when children are living with their biological parents.
- In the USA, African-Americans have worse glycaemic control than Hispanics. White children have the lowest HbA_{1c} values.

Interestingly, low income itself is not associated with worse control and the general view is that single parenthood is the single most powerful predictor of poor diabetes outcome. There are strong ethnic differences: for example, from shortly after diagnosis until five years later African-Americans have higher HbA_{1c} levels than white people.

Practice point

Single parenthood is a very powerful predictor of poor diabetes control in in Type 1 children. Single-parent children merit intensive multidisciplinary care.

FAMILY FUNCTIONING

About one-third of the variance in metabolic control can be attributed to family functioning, while adherence accounts for only about 10%. Good family dynamics (a well-engaged family working positively with the young person, cohesion and good organization) are consistently associated with successful management. Negative aspects of family dynamics are just as unsurprising:

- Conflict over matters specifically related to diabetes, especially disagreement over responsibility for blood glucose monitoring.
- Transition from less parental to more individual responsibility, often pushed too fast by parents.
- General disagreements.
- Poor parental (especially maternal) psychological well-being.
- Obsessionality in either the young person or parents. Creditable glycaemia may come at the cost of low mood and anxiety.

Family-based interventions have repeatedly been shown to improve self-testing and glycaemia outcomes, and reduce hospitalizations. A potentially modifiable specific factor is eating home-prepared meals with the family.

EATING DISORDERS

These are discussed in **Chapter 14**.

DEPRESSION

Depression in Type 1 diabetes has not been as extensively studied as it has in Type 2 diabetes. There is a widespread belief that it is more common in Type 1 patients than in the general population. This may be the case during the first five years after diagnosis, where general practitioners in the United Kingdom recorded twice the rate both of diagnosis of depression and prescription of antidepressants in comparison with the general population (Morgan et al., 2014). Other evidence on depression in Type 1 diabetes once out of these early years is more reassuring. In the USA T1D Exchange Registry, the rate of major depressive symptoms was approximately 5–11% (Trief et al., 2014), no different from the general population, and this was replicated in a study from California, which also showed that one of the standard questionnaires (PHQ-8) yielded high false-positive rates compared with a structured interview. The false-positivity was due to failure of the questionnaire to differentiate between depression and diabetes-related distress, which at 40% was high (Fisher et al., 2016).

When clinical depression does occur, in comparison with the non-diabetic population episodes last longer and the relapse rate is high – half of the episodes occur within six years of the initial problem. Ninety percent of depressive episodes occur in females. Diagnosis is difficult and three-quarters of initial episodes were untreated, though one-half of relapses were treated, presumably because of heightened general awareness. Maternal depression is associated with a threefold increased risk of depression in the young person and with higher health resource use (visits to the emergency department and hospitalization), emphasizing the particular relationship between the psychological well-being of mothers and their offspring with diabetes (Jaser, 2010). In adults newly diagnosed with Type 1 diabetes, worsening depressive symptoms were associated with higher HbA$_{1c}$ (8.2 vs 7.2%, 66 vs 55) at the end of five years – and with reduced quality of life and increased diabetes-related distress (Kampling *et al.*, 2017).

> **Practice point**
> Depressive symptoms are probably no more common in young people with Type 1 diabetes than the general population. However, episodes of depression are severe and last longer. Poor maternal psychological health is a strong risk factor for depression in their children with diabetes.

Treatment

Antidepressants are widely prescribed (for example in a German study, half of the under-25s diagnosed with depression were treated with drugs, nearly one-third with a selective serotonin reuptake inhibitor (SSRI)) (Plener *et al.*, 2015) but there is little evidence that they are more beneficial than placebo. Psychological interventions are better studied and the results more encouraging. The primary aim of most studies is – correctly – improved self-management. Changes in glycaemic control are often quoted but interventions are usually short-term and any reported improvements must be interpreted cautiously.

Potentially useful techniques include peer-based group therapies (emphasizing problem solving, support, and coping strategies), family-based therapies and mindfulness-based cognitive therapy. Motivational interviewing is promising because it can be used in the routine clinic setting and emphasizes a neutral, rather than a traditional, educational style, reducing the risk of confrontation and circular arguments (see Powell *et al.*, 2014 for a practical case history).

Depression in later life and diabetes complications

Little-studied, but the factors associated with depression in later life are the same in Type 1 and Type 2 diabetes. Insulin omission persists in older people, with a prevalence of 5–10%, depending on the definition; it is strongly associated with depression, non-white ethnicity, lower household income, educational and exercise levels, and vascular complications (Trief *et al.*, 2014). In the FinnDiane study, middle-aged women using antidepressants had a high (20%) 10-year mortality mostly from or with microvascular complications, whereas mortality in women not taking antidepressants was more associated with macrovascular complications.

Although subjects in the DCCT were not representative, a long-term quality of life follow-up found that in EDIC year 17 (when the average age was 51 and diabetes duration nearly 30 years) prior intensive treatment had no overall effect on diabetes quality of life domains of satisfaction, impact, diabetes worry and social/vocational worry) (Jacobson *et al.*, 2013). However, females were more likely to have a clinically meaningful decrement in quality of life score than males. The following individual factors were also associated with lower quality of life:

- severe hypoglycaemia
- advanced microvascular complications
- higher HbA$_{1c}$, blood pressure and BMI
- symptoms: chest pain, decreased vision, paraesthesiae, urinary incontinence and erectile dysfunction, especially marked when several of these were present
- self-reported anxiety and treated depression.

Depression is associated with a substantially increased risk of established complications. In a mixed population of Type 1 and 2 patients with a first episode of foot ulceration, associated depression was associated with a threefold increased mortality over 18 months; this increase persisted up to five years (Winkley *et al.*, 2012).

There are only tiny numbers of interventional studies in depression at this stage of diabetes but small-group cognitive behavioural training, individual mindfulness-based cognitive therapy and cognitive behavioural training improved depressive symptoms, anxiety, well-being and diabetes-related distress, compared with a waiting-list control group of Type 1 and 2 patients (Tovote *et al.*, 2014).

> **Practice point**
>
> Increased mortality persists for up to five years in patients with co-existing depression and diabetic foot ulceration.

TYPE 2 DIABETES

Much of the literature concerns the important problem of depression and the linked distress. There is a long-unfulfilled promise of more data from longitudinal and interventional studies. The co-existence of diabetes and depression is acknowledged as a significant health problem, largely because the two conditions contribute more than additively to perception of decreased health state, with an additional deleterious contribution from the impact of economic hardship. However, it should not need emphasizing that many psychological factors, not just depression, operate widely at all stages of Type 2 diabetes (**Figure 15.1**).

Depression is equally common in Type 1 and Type 2 diabetes, with an overall reported prevalence of 10–20% (though depression in Type 1 diabetes may be overdiagnosed: see previously). It is uncommon at diagnosis, but becomes more common with increasing intensity of diabetes treatment. For example, at baseline in the Look AHEAD study, with

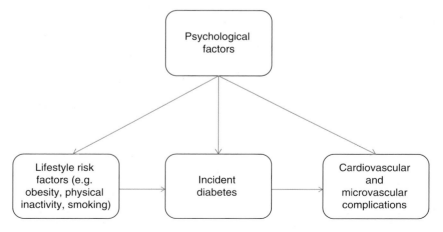

Figure 15.1 Simplified conceptual diagram of the impact of psychological factors throughout the lifetime of people with Type 2 diabetes.

a mean diabetes duration of seven years, 16% were taking antidepressant medication. Over their lifetime, depressed Type 2 patients experience about two episodes of depression, totalling nearly two years, though in patients with multiple relapses, subsequent episodes become progressively shorter (de Groot et al., 2016). The cumulative disablement process – contributory factors including increased treatment demands, functional limitation and loss of social roles – increases the risk of depression and, in addition to its obvious personal cost, depression in diabetes is costly to the health economy, incurring a 4.5-fold increased expenditure. Distress, the emotional response to unpleasant stress factors, is linked, but not always strongly, to depression; the two partly overlap but have common non-diabetes-related determinants (Snoek et al., 2015). Likewise, there are inconsistent links between depression and diabetes-distress and glycaemic control.

Diabetes and depression – cause or association?

A huge research effort has investigated the link between diabetes and depression, the principal question focusing on the direction of causality. The conclusion is that the link is bidirectional: Type 2 diabetes is associated with an increased risk of depression and conversely depression increases the risk of Type 2 diabetes. There is increasing speculation that the two have common biological origins, possibly reaching back to foetal development, including cytokine-mediated inflammatory responses caused by overactivity of innate immunity, and possibly abnormalities of the stress pathway mediated through the hypothalamo-pituitary-adrenal axis. Other candidate endocrine abnormalities may be relevant. For example, men in the metformin arm of the Diabetes Prevention Program experienced better mood if they generated a higher level of testosterone during the trial, though metformin itself had no effect on testosterone levels. Though this more likely represents play of chance in a highly-analysed cohort, it continues to focus on the neuroendocrine abnormalities that may contribute to the high morbidity of depression in Type 2 diabetes (Kim et al., 2016).

Psychological explanations abound, most obviously that the psychological burden of a chronic disorder leads to a higher risk of depression (the prevalence of depression is greater in people with diagnosed Type 2 diabetes than those with impaired glucose tolerance or undiagnosed diabetes). Alternatively, the two conditions may share similar psychosocial roots, for example reduced activity levels, socioeconomic deprivation and childhood adversity; work stress in adults carries a higher risk of both Type 2 diabetes and depression (Moulton et al., 2015).

Practice point

Type 2 diabetes increases the risk of depression, and vice versa. Stress responses – including to the work environment – increase the risk of both.

Finally, and less intuitively, depression (with or without its associated treatments) may predispose to Type 2 diabetes. There is some evidence for this from the Diabetes Prevention Program, where the diagnosis of diabetes was very precisely defined. Raised depression scores at entry to the study were not associated with the progression of impaired glucose tolerance to diabetes, but in the intensive lifestyle and placebo metformin groups, baseline antidepressant use and continuous antidepressant use during the study were associated with a two- to 3.5-fold increased risk of diabetes independent of other factors (Rubin et al., 2010). Type 2 diabetes could, therefore, be an adverse effect of antidepressant treatment, which is prevented by metformin taken in the third arm of the study. Supporting their adverse metabolic effects, antidepressant use during the Diabetes Prevention Program predicted a higher risk of weight regain. A more mundane explanation is that more severe depression, indicated by antidepressant usage, is associated with the risk of developing diabetes, as has been suggested in one meta-analysis. Regardless of which of these explanations turns out to be correct, the message for the clinician is that depression and Type 2 diabetes are very closely related. The diagnosis of Type 2 diabetes is not surprisingly much less traumatic than that of Type 1 diabetes; there is short-lived anxiety, followed by a transient rise in antidepressant use in the following year. But the consequences of depression in longer-term diabetes are much more significant.

Practice point

Antidepressants in people with prediabetes may increase the rate of progression to diabetes and also lower the likelihood of maintaining weight loss after intensive lifestyle input.

Associations with depression in Type 2 diabetes

Depression of all degrees of severity is equally prevalent among all ethnic groups in USA studies. Of all the self-care behaviours studied (adherence to diet and medication, and glucose monitoring, for example) the one most consistently associated with depression is missed medical appointments. This was also seen in the otherwise high-retention Look AHEAD study, which also found that depression scores and antidepressant use were independently associated with:

- hypertension and use of hypertensive medication
- current smoking
- obesity
- lower peak exercise activity.

The management corollary of these unspectacular findings is evident: identification of clusters of these factors should alert practitioners to the possibility of depression. In patients with established neuropathy, neurological disability predicts increased depressive symptoms, which, in turn, is most strongly associated with the symptom of unsteadiness, an important factor limiting a spectrum of activities. The important causal link between depression, foot ulceration and premature death is worth reiterating; even in the absence of specific comorbidities, men with symptomatic depression and diabetes had a 3.5-fold increased risk of death over 18 years' follow-up, and there was an independent though less powerful association with anxiety (Naicker et al., 2017).

There are considerable practical barriers to identifying depression, especially in those who are most likely to suffer it, namely those with a higher burden of chronic complications. Time-limited consultations are more likely to be taken up with biomedical priorities and targets, and the busy-ness surrounding the complexities of managing these makes it a real challenge to diagnose, especially in those who are most likely to benefit from treatment.

Screening for depression

Screening for depression is frequently recommended and occasionally mandated as a performance target, but it is much more important than this. Rising above the heated question of whether the Beck Depression Inventory, the Center for Epidemiologic Studies

Depression Scale, the Hospital Anxiety and Depression Scale, or the Patient Health Questionnaire is preferable, is the more important matter of the value of screening for depression in the first place. (This complexity is magnified by the distinct but related distress, which has its own screening tests, for example PAID (Problem Areas in Diabetes) and the WHO-5 Well-Being Index.) Everyone agrees that isolated screening, without associated follow-up and management planning is of no value, though in RCTs it leads to greater, but presumably non-systematic, use of mental health-care services, though no improvement in symptoms (Petrak *et al.*, 2015). Collaborative care, however, does improve outcomes of depression (see later).

Practice point

Depression is prevalent in Type 2 diabetes but routine screening for it is of no demonstrable value.

Interventions in depression in Type 2 diabetes

A key question is whether the aims of treatment are primarily medical or psychological. An ideal intervention would improve symptoms of depression and simultaneously diabetes outcomes, but it is evident that the latter is barely captured by detecting a fall in HbA_{1c}, and the treatment timescales are quite different – a matter of weeks or a few months for a severe depressive episode, years perhaps decades for meaningful changes in diabetes outcomes. The hope – that improvement in mood will permit improved diabetes-related self-care – has no evidence base yet. Regardless of treatment modality (antidepressants, mental health provider, alternative healers) patients report a uniform high degree of satisfaction (60–80%).

Intervention modalities include:

- intensive lifestyle interventions (e.g. Look AHEAD)
- collaborative-care interventions
- psychological (e.g. problem solving techniques, counselling, cognitive behavioural therapy)
- pharmacological (e.g. antidepressants, SSRIs).

Intensive lifestyle interventions

The Look AHEAD trial of intensive versus routine lifestyle input into patients with Type 2 diabetes did not achieve its primary outcome of reducing cardiovascular events. However, depression was carefully and prospectively studied, and concluded, as in most studies in Type 1 patients, that intensive management does not worsen quality of life and improves significant aspects. For example, intensive lifestyle intervention reduced the risk of developing mild or more severe depression by about 15%. Those with mild or worse depression at baseline benefited more with intensive lifestyle input at one year but not thereafter, though all patients, intensively or conventionally treated, remained in the non-depressed range, and this probably reflects the natural history of depression to improve over the short- to medium-term. While the physical component score of the Short Form 36 quality of life questionnaire worsened throughout the study, it did so less in the intensively treated group, and physical function (measured walking speed, grip and thigh muscle strength) was improved up to eight years. The mental component score did not change (Look AHEAD Research Group, 2014).

Collaborative-care interventions

Complex care arrangements, popular in the USA, involve collaboration between primary and secondary care in patients with linked comorbidities, for example diabetes and coronary heart disease. The framework for the benefits of this approach is well known. The Pathways study (Katon *et al.*, 2004) randomized depressed diabetic patients to usual care or specific intervention with enhanced education and antidepressants. Routine and intensive input were equally effective in patients with fewer complications but patients with one or more macrovascular complications did especially well with the intensive input. A more recent randomized study in patients with depression, and poorly controlled diabetes, coronary heart disease, or both, was reported in 2010 (Katon *et al.*, 2010). Intervention over a year was every two or three weeks in primary care, and delivered by trained practice nurses implementing guideline-based treatment protocols. Both biomedical outcomes and depression scores improved in the intervention group:

- HbA$_{1c}$ by 0.6%
- LDL by 0.2 mmol/l
- systolic BP by 5 mm Hg
- depression score
- improved QoL, greater satisfaction with care.

More adjustments were made to medication, including antidepressants, though adherence to both diet and exercise plans did not differ between the groups. Interestingly, there was no specific psychological intervention other than the medical management by study nurses, emphasizing, as in Look AHEAD, the importance of intensive intervention in the management of patients with depression and multiple morbidity. A similar study using the collaborative TEAMcare approach came to the same broad conclusions, but although initiation and adjustment rates of diabetes-related medication were much higher in the intensive group, medication adherence rates did not change (Lin *et al.*, 2012). There is potential and aspiration for this kind of care in many health systems but it cannot be done without increased resources.

Psychological

Purely psychological treatments have not been studied as rigorously. Many different interventions have been reported and meta-analysis to determine effects is thereby largely thwarted. Most individual studies have shown a moderate benefit on depressive symptoms, but not on glycaemic control, up to and beyond six months after the end of treatment.

Cognitive behavioural therapy, mindfulness-based therapy, psychosocial and psychoeducational approaches all seem to have some benefit on depression severity (Petrak *et al.*, 2015). In a large controlled trial in Type 1 and 2 patients, internet-based guided self-help was highly effective in reducing depressive symptoms, well-being and emotional stress, but there were no changes in glycaemic control or self-management skills (Ebert *et al.*, 2017).

Pharmacological

Symptoms consistently improve in reported placebo-controlled studies, which have mostly used paroxetine or alprazolam, but small numbers have been reported using sertraline, fluoxetine and nortriptyline. In the small number of studies using active comparisons, no meaningful differences between agents have emerged, but no trials reported long-term follow-up after treatment stopped.

Practice point

Antidepressant medication in Type 2 diabetes is not obviously superior to non-medical treatments when used alone. It may be valuable in people with established complications.

The important Diabetes and Depression (DAD) Study (Petrak *et al.*, 2015) compared a year of cognitive behavioural therapy (bibliotherapy) and continuing sertraline treatment in the nearly 50% of Type 1 and 2 patients who had responded significantly to three months of treatment. The year-long treatment phase improved depression scores with either intervention but outcomes were better with sertraline. There was no improvement in the baseline poor control (mean HbA_{1c} 9.3%, 78) in either group. Early antidepressant treatment for depressive symptoms, preferably accompanied by some modification of the collaborative-care system for glycaemic and other medical measures, seems to be the best combination in depressed poorly-controlled patients with diabetes complications, but implementing it in practice is quite another matter.

BRAIN FUNCTION AND IMPACT ON EDUCATION AND EMPLOYMENT IN TYPE 1 DIABETES

The effect of diabetes on brain function has been investigated in several long-term studies, in relation to exposure both to severe hypoglycaemia and chronic hyperglycaemia. Methodological problems, significant in Type 1 diabetes, become more so in Type 2, where multiple factors other than dysglycaemia are likely to have important effects on brain function.

Metabolic insults leading to impairment of brain function start at diagnosis. Impairment of some neuropsychological functions can occur in the short-term when Type 1 diabetes presents in childhood with diabetic ketoacidosis (see previously). There is concern that severe hypoglycaemia in childhood, followed by many years of marked hyperglycaemia, especially in adolescence and early adulthood, may have particularly deleterious effects on brain function, though there are no studies so far that have been able to take into account both these important factors (Cameron, 2015).

Severe hypoglycaemia in childhood is a risk factor for impaired neurocognition (e.g. example memory and learning deficits) but there is no consistent picture for functional outcomes. Brain glucose consumption peaks around five years of age, and it is not surprising that memory and learning function are impaired later on in those with early childhood onset of Type 1, especially in those diagnosed under the age of 2. It is not clear whether these result from recurrent acute hypoglycaemia-induced neuronal damage or impaired brain development. Mild cognitive impairments seem to result in worse academic primary and secondary school outcomes, resulting in lower rates of completing school education (Cameron, 2015).

Studies of neurocognitive outcomes over nearly two decades in the DCCT are broadly reassuring, though participants were adolescent or older at diagnosis, and not the very young children who seem to be at the highest risk. Beyond young adulthood, cognition may continue to decline more rapidly in Type 1 subjects as a result of the cumulative effects of chronic hyperglycaemia, hypertension and microvascular complications. This is another reason for careful vascular risk management in people with long-standing Type 1 diabetes and any indications of microvascular disease. The pathology may be a mixed picture, as it shares some cerebrospinal fluid markers with Alzheimer's disease (Moran *et al.*, 2015).

Education and employment in Type 1 diabetes

In addition to younger age at onset, hypoglycaemic seizures are associated with a more rapid fall in certain domains of IQ (for example verbal and full-scale, though not performance) and youngsters in these groups warrant – though probably do not receive – monitoring and educational support (Lin *et al.*, 2015). Verbal IQ remains lower in students in their early 20s. Management of Type 1 diabetes in schools and colleges at school and college is not always as good as it should be. Documents on good practice abound but individual management is the key, especially as family structure and dynamics are so important and continuing personal liaison between the patient, their specialist diabetes nurses and key school personnel is time consuming and often not optimal, especially for older students.

Shamefully little is known about the realities of having Type 1 diabetes in the modern workplace. Even non-severe hypoglycaemia can result in loss of working time but there have been no systematic studies of work time loss in Type 1. The burden of self-care at work is a real stress for many, particularly as a result of time pressures and unpredictable work schedules, and especially in the retail trades and public services that involve high levels of contact with the public. They also find less time to exercise, both during and outside work (Balfe *et al.*, 2014). In the United Kingdom, under the Equality Act (2010), it is illegal for an employer to discriminate against people with Type 1 diabetes (which for the purposes of the Act is considered a disability). Appeals under the Act may be disallowed if employees fail to disclose diabetes, but Type 1 people are reluctant to do this, and the first inkling of the diabetes may be an acute emergency at work. Despite large numbers of documents from national organizations, such as Diabetes UK and the American Diabetes Association, urging best practice in the work place and emphasizing education and negotiation, anecdotal reports of poor employment practice show no signs of decreasing.

References

Ambrosino JM, Fennie K, Whittemore R *et al.* Short-term effects of coping skills training in school age children with type 1 diabetes. *Pediatr Diabetes* 2008; 9:74–82 [PMID: 18540868] PMC2936820.

Balfe M, Brugha R, Smith D *et al.* Why do young adults with type 1 diabetes find it difficult to manage diabetes in the workplace? *Health Place* 2014;26:180–7 [PMID: 24480739].

Cameron FJ. The impact of diabetes on brain function in childhood and adolescence. *Pediatr Clin N Am* 2015;62:911–27 [PMID: 26210624].

Cooper MN, McNamara KA, de Klerk NH et al. School performance in children with type 1 diabetes: a contemporary population-based study. Pediatr Diabetes 2016;17:101–11 [PMID: 25423904].

Ebert DD, Nobis S, Lehr D et al. The 6-month effectiveness of internet-based guided self-help for depression in adults with Type 1 and 2 diabetes mellitus. Diabet Med 2017;34:99–107 [PMID: 27334444].

Fisher L, Hessler DM, Polonsky WH et al. Prevalence of depression in Type 1 diabetes and the problem of over-diagnosis. Diabetic Med 2016;33:1590–7 [PMID: 26433004].

de Groot M, Crick KA, Long M et al. Lifetime duration of depressive disorders in patients with T2D. Diabetes Care 2016;39:2174–81 [PMID: 27729427] PMC5127229.

Jacobson AM, Braffett BH, Cleary PA et al. DCCT/EDIC Research Group. The long-term effects of type 1 diabetes treatment and complications on health-related quality of life: a 23-year follow-up of the Diabetes Control and Complications/Epidemiology of Diabetes Interventions and Complications cohort. Diabetes Care 2013; 36:3131–8 [PMID: 23835693] PMC3781542.

Jaser SS. Psychological problems in adolescents with diabetes. Adolesc Med State Art Rev 2010;21:138–51 [PMID: 20568561] PMC3721971.

Kampling H, Petrak F, Farin E et al. Trajectories of depression in adults with newly diagnosed type 1 diabetes: results from the German Multicenter Diabetes Cohort Study. Diabetologia 2017;60:60–8 [PMID: 27787619].

Katon WJ, Von Korff M, Lin EH et al. The Pathways Study: a randomized trial of collaborative care in patients with diabetes and depression. Arch Gen Psychiatry 2004;61:1042–9 [PMID: 15466678].

Katon WJ, Lin EH, Von Korff M et al. Collaborative care for patients with depression and chronic illnesses. N Engl J Med 2010; 363:2611–20 [PMID: 21190455] PMC3312811.

Kim C, Barrett-Connor E, Aroda VR et al. Diabetes Prevention Program Research Group. Testosterone and depressive symptoms among men in the Diabetes Prevention Program. Psychoneuroendocrinology 2016;72:63–71 [PMID: 27371769] PMC5070975.

Kristensen LJ, Birkbaek NH, Mose AH et al. Symptoms of emotional, behavioural, and social difficulties in the Danish population of children and adolescents with type 1 diabetes – results of a national survey. PLoS One 19;e97543 [PMID: 24842772] PMC4026318.

Lin A, Northam EA, Werther GA, Cameron FJ. Risk factors for decline in IQ in youth with type 1 diabetes over the 12 years from diagnosis/illness onset. Diabetes Care 2015;38:236–42 [PMID: 25488913].

Lin EH, Von Korff, Ciechanowski P et al. Treatment adjustments and medication adherence for complex patients with diabetes, heart disease, and depression: a randomized controlled trial. Ann Fam Med 2012;10:6–14 [PMID: 22230825] PMC3262469.

Look AHEAD Research Group. Impact of intensive lifestyle intervention on depression and health-related quality of life in Type 2 diabetes: the Look AHEAD Trial. Diabetes Care 2014;37:1544–53 [PMID: 24855155] Free full text.

Moran C, Beare R, Phan TG et al. Alzheimer's Disease Neuroimaging Initiative (ADNI). Type 2 diabetes mellitus and biomarkers of neurodegeneration. Neurology 2015;85:1123–30 [PMID: 26333802].

Morgan E, Patterson CC, Cardwell CR. General practice-recorded depression and antidepressant use in young people with newly-diagnosed Type 1 diabetes: a cohort study using the Clinical Practice Research Datalink. Diabetic Med 2014;31:241–5 [PMID: 24111949].

Moulton CD, Pickup JC, Ismail K. The link between depression and diabetes: the search for shared mechanisms. Lancet Diabetes Endocrinol 2015;3:461–71 [PMID: 25995124].

Naicker K, Johnson JA, Skogen JC et al. Type 2 diabetes and comorbid symptoms of depression and anxiety: longitudinal associations with mortality risk. Diabetes Care 2017;40:352–8 [PMID: 28077458].

Nygren M, Carstensen J, Koch F et al. Experience of a serious life event increases the risk for childhood type 1 diabetes: the ABIS population-based prospective cohort study. Diabetologia 2015; 58:1188–97 [PMID: 25870022].

Petrak F, Herpertz S, Albus C et al. Cognitive behavioural therapy versus sertraline in patients with depression and poorly controlled diabetes: the Diabetes and Depression (DAD) Study: a randomized controlled multicentre trial. Diabetes Care 2015;38:767–75 [PMID: 25690005].

Plener PL, Molz E, Berger G *et al*. Depression, metabolic control, and antidepressant medication in young patients with type 1 diabetes. *Pediatr Diabetes* 2015;16:58–66 [PMID: 24636613].

Powell PW, Hilliard ME, Anderson BJ. Motivational interviewing to promote adherence behaviors in pediatric type 1 diabetes. *Curr Diab Rep* 2014;14:531 [PMID: 25142716] PMC4447119.

Rubin RR, Ma Y, Peyrot M *et al*. Diabetes Prevention Program Research Group. Antidepressant medicine use and risk of developing diabetes during the diabetes prevention program and diabetes prevention program outcomes study. *Diabetes Care* 2010;33:2549–51 [PMID: 20805256] PMC2992187.

Schwartz DD, Axelrad ME, Anderson BJ. Neurocognitive functioning in children and adolescents at the time of type 1 diabetes diagnosis: associations with glycemic control 1 year after diagnosis. *Diabetes Care* 2014;37:2476–82 [PMID: 24969580].

Snoek FJ, Bremmer MA, Hermanns N. Constructs of depression and distress in diabetes: time for an appraisal. *Lancet Diabetes Endocrinol* 2015;3:450–60 [PMID 25995123].

Tovote KA, Fleer J, Snippe E et al. Individual mindfulness-based cognitive therapy and cognitive behaviour therapy for treating depressive symptoms in patients with diabetes: results of a randomized controlled trial. *Diabetes Care* 2014; 37:2427–34 [PMID: 24898301].

Trief PM, Xing D, Foster NC *et al*. T1D Exchange Clinic Network. Depression in adults in the T1D Exchange Clinic Registry. *Diabetes Care* 2014; 37: 1563–72 [PMID: 24855157].

Winkley K, Sallis H, Kariyawasam D *et al*. Five-year follow-up of a cohort of people with their first diabetic foot ulcer: the persistent effect of depression on mortality. *Diabetologia* 2012;55:303–10 [PMID: 22057196].

Further reading

Moulton CD, Pickup JC, Ismail K. The link between depression and diabetes: the search for shared mechanisms. *Lancet Diabetes Endocrinol* 2015;3:461–71 [PMID: 25995124].

Petrak F, Baumeister H, Skinner TC *et al*. Depression and diabetes: treatment and health-care delivery. *Lancet Diabetes Endocrinol* 2015;3: 472–85 [PMID: 25995125].

Snoek FJ, Bremmer MA, Hermanns N. Constructs of depression and distress in diabetes: time for an appraisal. *Lancet Diabetes Endocrinol* 2015;3:450–60 [PMID 25995123].

Index

Note: Page number followed by "*b*" denotes text box, "*f*" denotes figure, and "*t*" denotes table

Index 453